Gary Null's

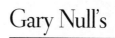

ULTIMATE
LIFETIME DIET

Also by Gary Null

Gary Null's Ultimate Anti-Aging Program

Get Healthy Now!

The Encyclopedia of Natural Healing

For Women Only

Gary Null's
ULTIMATE
LIFETIME
DIET

A REVOLUTIONARY ALL-NATURAL PROGRAM FOR
LOSING WEIGHT AND BUILDING A HEALTHY BODY

Gary Null, Ph.D.

BROADWAY BOOKS, NEW YORK

BROADWAY

BROADWAY BOOKS titles may be purchased for business or promotional use or for special sales. For information, please write to: Special Markets Department, Random House, Inc., 1540 Broadway, New York, NY 10036.

BROADWAY BOOKS and its logo, a letter B bisected on the diagonal, are trademarks of Broadway Books, a division of Random House, Inc.

Visit our Web site at www.broadwaybooks.com

Library of Congress Cataloging-in-Publication Data
Null, Gary.
    [Ultimate lifetime diet]
    Gary Null's Ultimate lifetime diet: a revolutionary all-natural program for
losing weight and building a healthy body / Gary Null—1st ed.
        p. cm.
    Includes index.
    1. Reducing diets.   2. Natural foods.   3. Weight loss.   I. Title.

RM222.2.N85 2000
613.2'5—dc21   99-048028
                                                                        CIP

FIRST EDITION

Designed by Carla Bolte

ISBN 0-7679-0473-7

00   01   02   03   04   10   9   8   7   6   5   4   3

Acknowledgments

With thanks to the people who have assisted with editing and research on this project, including Ann Campbell at Broadway Books; Lois Zinn; Vicki Riba Koestler; Andres Garcia; Debora Rasio, M.D.; Martin Feldman, M.D.; Katherine Cantrill; Rue Murray; Kimberly Coombs; Sloan Seal; Carol Schneider; and Diane Feeney.

A special thanks to Mitchell Waters, my agent at Curtis Brown, Ltd., for his invaluable help with this book.

Disclaimer

Readers are advised to consult with healthcare providers knowledgeable in alternative/complementary/preventive medicine to determine which vitamins, minerals, and food supplements would be beneficial for their particular health needs and the dosages that would be best for them. Also, if you are using any medications, you must consult with your physician and pharmacist to determine if any vitamin, mineral, phyto-chemical, herb, juice, or food may be counter indicated.

Contents

Introduction

One of the more underserved segments of our society is the over 90 million individuals who are constantly fighting the battle of the bulge. Our misconceptions and biases overflow when they concern people who are overweight. Over the years I've counseled thousands of people who are trying to lose weight and I've seen that, contrary to popular myth, overweight people are anything but lazy. They go to great lengths to try to get themselves trimmer, making every honest effort to follow the advice of diet books and weight-loss "experts." The fact that they usually don't succeed is due not to lack of will or work but rather to the quality of advice they're following.

Well, the advice here is going to be a little different from what you're used to. You probably purchased this book with the hope that this is the last diet you'll ever have to use. That's certainly my intention too. But at the outset, I would ask you to understand the difference between this book on weight control and all the other diet books out there—namely that this isn't really a diet book! There is no diet here, at least not in the sense of a traditional deprivation-oriented regimen. Instead, this is an altogether new way of helping you understand why it's not your fault you're fat and of getting you on the road to never being fat again. I'm confident that if you simply approach this with an open mind and a sense of determination, you'll soon be seeing positive results.

First, let's get an overview of the problem. More American adults are overweight than ever before—about 97 million. This constitutes over half the adult population, up from 43 percent in 1960. We spend about $33 billion a year in efforts to slim down, but obviously all that money isn't doing the trick. Many overweight people have been grappling with the problem for years and have been on just about every diet there is. They have gone on high-protein diets, on calorie-counting diets, and on fat-free diets. With each attempt there is a belief that "This time I'll succeed," but in the end they ultimately fail.

Nobody wants to be overweight, although sometimes our society implies they do. We blame people for being chronically lazy and suggest that it's their fault that they're fat. But I don't believe that they are necessarily to blame. There are so many factors that influence a person's level of fitness—and fatness—and if we're not aware of how these factors affect us, we can end up battling extra pounds for an entire lifetime and never understanding what's going on or why we are losing the battle. The physical factors include food sensitivities and allergic reactions, carbohydrate intolerance, and hormonal imbalances. Also, misunderstandings about what constitutes proper eating—for instance, isn't a fat-free diet ideal for a fat individual?—can perpetuate a weight problem. We'll be looking at all of these factors in this book as well as at how to overcome them.

But factors that go beyond the physical are even more important in determining whether you conquer your problems with your weight. What I'm referring to are some basic misconceptions that you may have. First, have you, like many Americans, bought into the idea that there's a magic-bullet solution to all physical problems? If so, not only will you probably not lose weight, but you may ultimately *gain* weight as you become disillusioned with each "miracle" weight-loss supplement or approach you try. We'll be discussing some of these illusory approaches here and why they fail.

Second, if you believe that losing weight involves feeling deprived and unhappy, you're not going to succeed. You'll sabotage yourself first, out of fear of feeling awful. The good news is that the truth is just the opposite—after a short period of adjustment, the healthy lifestyle you adopt in order to lose weight the right way will make you feel more energetic, fulfilled, and happy than you did previously. And to take this one step further, or perhaps one step deeper down into the heart of the matter: I don't believe you have a good shot at controlling your weight until you *are* happy.

That's why it's never just a person's weight that I'm concerned with. In fact, I never put anyone on a diet, even when guiding a health-study group of people from my radio audience who are desperately seeking to lose some girth in order to reduce the dangers of diabetes, heart disease, or other illnesses that are running parallel to their chronic overweight condition. Instead, my initial purpose is always to try to get a person to be happy. Now, why would I want a happy person instead of a slim one? Well, for one thing, it's because you can be slim and still be unhealthy. You can be a model on a runway doing cocaine or heroin and starving yourself to keep your figure. You could be of average weight but an angry and aggressive person, thus harming not only yourself but others. For another thing, it's rare to find people who are truly, genuinely happy and honoring their higher emotional and spiritual self who do anything that contributes to body toxicity and a resulting weight problem. In other words, happy people are less likely to intentionally harm their bodies. And I'll even go beyond that to say that you will not be as healthy until you're happy.

It was about ten years ago that I began to notice in my own day-to-day clinical experiences that most of the individuals I encountered were overweight. They were coming to me hoping that there would be some magic pill or herb that would melt away fat, painlessly and effortlessly. Or maybe it would be some miraculous supplement that could expand in the stomach and suppress the appetite mechanism. People were coming to me who had had part of their stomach stapled together, or part of their intestines resectioned, or had tried drastic liquid diets, all in a futile effort to shed those unnecessary pounds.

They didn't want to be overweight because they didn't like how they looked and they liked even less how they felt. They felt that people were making judgments about them, which people do. Even worse, they were making even more critical judgments about themselves.

So I would recommend what I still consider a very good diet, one that was primarily vegetarian, with all organic produce. And I would suggest appropriate supplements. People would walk out of the office with three or four pages of notes and a couple of books for reading and reference. But then I would see them six months later, and they would sheepishly say, "Well, I tried, but it just wasn't working." Sometimes they'd even gained weight. Clearly, the tools I had been using were inadequate for the job at hand.

Naturally I wondered, "What's wrong here?" At that point I decided to take a step back and examine the problem from a wider perspective—that of all of our modern-day physical ills. Looking at the war on cancer, I knew that what we needed was not more money, doctors, chemotherapy, or new technologies. Even with all of those things, we hadn't made a major change in the incidence or outcome for most adult types of cancer. The same was true for heart disease. What we needed was not more people taking beta-blockers and other medication or undergoing coronary bypass surgery or balloon angioplasty. At that time, 50 million people were dutifully fitting themselves into the accepted medical paradigm, and hypertension was going up instead of down. The incidence of people dying from heart disease was actually on the rise. Similarly, increasing numbers of people with arthritis were merely learning to live with their pain and taking nonsteroidal anti-inflammatory hormone drugs for their temporary effects. People with depression were taking mood alterers, like Valium, Thorazine, lithium, and later Prozac.

Then a few years ago we began to pathologize childhood. Just being a child meant that you were now at risk for a disease to which Ritalin would be the answer. Millions of children were classified as having attention deficit disorder, and many were ordered to take a prescription medication or forfeit going to school. It was largely genetic, the experts said. What I wondered, though, was how just one generation before, in the 1950s and 1960s when I was in school, we had had no attention deficit disorder and kids were able to function normally. How was this possible? Did we develop this genetic predisposition in one generation? The answer clearly was no.

It seemed that suddenly everyone had diseases resulting from a deficiency of some medication and that the blame was increasingly being put on inherent predispositions. Outside of cigarette smoke and alcohol, nothing *external* was ever blamed for anything. It was all in our genes. Whether you were overweight or depressed, suffering from cancer, arthritis, diabetes, or Crohn's disease, you could always say "It's in my genes." Then you were given a medicine that would supposedly correct the problem.

I looked at this trend toward medicalization and it made no sense to me, as other societies around the world were experiencing less of the conditions we were, and their citizens were living longer and healthier lives. So I went on a journey. From the mid-1980s to the early 1990s I spent a lot of time traveling the world and studying other cultures to see if there was something I could learn from what they were doing differently. What I found was that diet was not always the most important thing, and genes certainly were not. The key was in *lifestyle*.

Upon my return to the United States, I put a major effort into creating a new protocol for health using whatever tools would work. I took nearly 5,000 people over a two-year period, divided them into categories, and put each group on a different six-month program. The programs were not geared to disease conditions but to improving overall wellness.

There were five main groups. Group 1 experienced a change in diet. I gave people what, for all intents and purposes, would be considered a perfect diet, meaning that I excluded animal protein, including all dairy products. The only animal-derived food they could have would be six ounces of fish a day. Otherwise they had ample servings of grains, fruits, vegetables, and legumes and moderate amounts of nuts and seeds—all organic. Participants consumed about fifty grams of fiber daily. No processed sugars were allowed. They could have raw, unheated, unfiltered honey and crude molasses or rice syrup, but no other sweeteners. Also, they had to give up all processed foods, and everything had to be as close to its natural state as possible, with minimal heating, so that the food was rich in enzymes, antioxidants, and phytochemicals. And they had sea vegetables, such as sea palm, wakame, kombu, and nori—one serving per day. Men averaged 3,000 calories a day, and women, about 2,500. It was a dynamic diet, but—and this is the crucial factor—nothing else in their lives was changed. These people lost, on average, one to two pounds per week until they reached their ideal weight and stabilized.

They were very happy about the weight loss—while it lasted. The problem was that at the end of the six months, fewer than 5 percent of group members were able to sustain the diet. They gave such excuses as "It's too difficult." "Too many changes had to be made." "It was upsetting my social life." "I don't know how to make this food." "I feel deprived." But the diet did work, because those who did stick with it experienced significant health benefits and lost a considerable amount of weight.

A second group was put on an energetic exercise program—without a change in diet. This program was so vigorous that it enabled participants to run the New York City Marathon. They went from total novices to marathon-ready in just six months. It was a graduated program, with general exercise five days a week, up to an hour a day, plus exercises geared to specific body parts every other day for one hour. These were in the form of sit-ups and presses that affected every muscle in the body to create strength all over. This group talked about how much better they felt and how their overall sense of well-being had improved. Fewer than 10 percent were able to complete the six-month program, but the ones who did certainly lost a substantial amount of weight as their bodies became strengthened and toned. Even this 10 percent did not continue after the six months.

A third group was not given a special diet or exercise regime but was put on an ideal supplement and juicing protocol. I suggested vitamins, such as C, E, and B complex as well as oil of primrose, phosphatidylcholine, and coenzyme Q10, among other natural supplements. In addition to the supplement program, the participants drank a variety of fresh, organic juices, starting with one 10-ounce glass of juice a day for the first month and increasing intake by one glass per day each month, so that by month 6 they were drinking six glasses per day. Carrot juice was excluded because of its high sugar content, but any other combination of diluted vegetables with mineral water and aloe vera juice could be used. At first, they would drink only vegetable juice, but by the third month they could begin to add fruit juice, including grapefruit with lemon, orange, or lime, using the whole peel and skin. Added to the mix was nondairy acidophilus and raw flaxseed. Participants also did eat meals, although breakfast was generally a juice-only meal.

Again, everything in participants' lives stayed the same, except for the supplements and juices. If they did not already exercise, they weren't to start. They were given no dietary instructions except that they had to drink a total of one gallon of liquid per day, which included filtered or mineral water plus their juices. This group also lost weight and experienced other health improvements, although many were glad to get off the protocol—they hadn't been used to drinking a lot of juice, which can be an acquired taste.

Another group made no changes whatsoever in their exercise, diet, or supplementation, but they were to clean up their work and home environment. That meant that they were to go room by room and see what they could do to minimize the impact of that environment on their well-being. They had to get rid of carpets and get down to hardwood floors. They had to seal all cabinet insides with shellac to make sure that no particleboard—from which much modern cabinetry and furniture is made—would outgas, or emanate fumes. They had to clean their basements and garages of all toxic chemicals: lawn pesticides, paint cleaners and thinners, furniture-finishing products. And they had to install proper air and water filters in their house. Water filters would get rid of lead, cadmium, mercury, parasites, industrial solvents, viruses, and bacteria. And in the air at work and at home, they needed to get rid of animal danders, molds, fungi, and formaldehyde—anything that could cause the body's internal milieu to become imbalanced. This group had no weight changes, but they did experience improvement in some of their allergies and felt that breathing was easier.

The last group was to keep everything physical the same, except they were to answer a series of questions that were presented at monthly lectures. The questions had them examine their core values and attitudes, with an eye to destressing their lives and raising their self-esteem. Generally I would give them fifty questions: twenty per lecture and an additional thirty to take home with them. I also provided my own answers to these questions, explaining that these were not *the* answers, merely a springboard from which to formulate their own. Following are examples of these questions and the ways I had answered them:

Were you given negative messages as a child?

As a child, you probably believed whatever your parents told you. You accepted their messages, positive or negative, at face value. The question is, how have you dealt with the negative messages they conveyed to you? To sort through this issue, make a list of your parents' attitudes, noting whether they are positive or negative. Then go back and note which attitudes you have adopted as your own, both toward yourself and regarding your expectations about the world.

Until you evaluate these messages and discard the negative ones, they will remain a guiding force in your life. With your adult mind and adult ego strength, you have the ability to tolerate pain that you could not understand or handle as a child. You also have the opportunity to make important changes in yourself, provided you can find the courage to ask the hard questions about your past and present. When you stop blocking your awareness of your past hurts and current fears, you will gradually become energized, and your pain and fear will be less each time you make contact with them.

Do you have attitudes and behaviors that sabotage your health, happiness, and growth?

Some of your attitudes and behaviors can prevent you from doing things that are in your own best interest. If you are somewhat lazy, for example, you might like to sit around and watch television on Saturday mornings. Then, when a friend suggests going for a jog, power walk, or bicycle ride, you find it difficult to break your routine. You might get defensive and deny the benefits of exercising, and you might even overreact and make your friend feel bad for having suggested it. Since you work hard all week, you argue, you need Saturday mornings to do what you want to do. You feel upset that someone is infringing on your time and wants you to do something else.

That sort of thinking can undermine you. Why not look instead at the benefits that come from a change of pace? Ask yourself, is this something that will make me feel healthier, live longer, be happier, have more energy, and be a better person?

Do you avoid responsibilities for fear of failure?

Society measures success by what you have accomplished. You are deemed a failure if you attempt something new and fail. This concept is reinforced when others praise you for your successes and reprimand you for your failures. You do not receive credit for having tried; rather, you are considered inadequate for not having succeeded.

A fear of failure prevents many people from taking on new responsibilities that would allow them to grow. In reality, however, most successes are preceded by many failures. Go back in your life and assess your own failures. What did you learn from these experiences? Acknowledge yourself for having tried and for the lessons learned.

Are you looking to the right people for support?

You must share your dreams and goals with the people who offer positive support. Some people will always find a hole in your plans, yet you may return to these unsupportive people time and again for support. Since their advice will only discourage you, be more aware of whom you turn to for help. Watch your patterns and learn to interact with people who will be the most supportive and understanding of your needs and goals.

These are the types of questions that the fifth study group grappled with on their own and discussed as a group. They weren't told to make any physical changes whatsoever, and none of the other groups ever dealt with these issues.

The results of this experiment? At the end of the study, no group had retained more than a small fraction of its original members, except for the group that had focused on examining their life choices, value systems, and destressing. Most members of the other groups had dropped out. It was interesting to note that although the values-examining group had been given no dietary guidance, a number of its members had lost some weight and now reported feeling more energetic. Perhaps it was because while doing so much questioning about what went into their attitudes they were also learning to question what went in to their bodies.

What I learned from these groups is that trying to implement physical changes without taking into account what's going on in our inner lives rarely works. Sure, it did work in a few cases, but by and large the one-approach-only method was a failure. What I did after that initial study was combine the protocols for each of the individual study groups and put them into one single study, to see what the synergistic effect would be. Just as I'd suspected, the dropout rate plummeted, and people reported dramatic improvements in their health and vitality, with impressive weight loss in many of the participants for whom weight had been a problem. That's why now I use only the integrative approach when I organize health support groups and weight-loss seminars. Today the groups always combine diet—with an emphasis on detoxification—with exercise, supplements and juicing, an environmental clean sweep, and a thorough examination of life choices and values.

And that's also why now, when someone asks me, "Gary, what supplement should I take for my arthritis?" or "How do I lose weight real quick?" I no longer have an easy answer, as I might have had years ago. I'll say, "It's not about an arthritis supplement," or "It's not about a quick-fix diet." I tell him or her, "It's about the whole body. You've got to look at your whole body. And you've got to look at your mind."

Some people get frustrated by this kind of answer, and you can see their eyes kind of glaze over and disconnect. "Look at my *mind*?" you can almost hear them thinking. "Give me a break! Maybe I can go to my doctor and get a pill."

In today's society, we have been led to believe that being overweight is a medical problem, which therefore requires medical intervention. And it will probably be a superficial intervention, because we tend to want to change the symptoms of a problem without getting to the root of it. That we may have created the problem ourselves is not something we want to see; our idea is to resolve it simply by masking the symptoms. If you've got arthritis, get rid of the pain. If you've got a headache, get rid of the pain. If you're overweight, get rid of the fat. And we want the fastest, least taxing way of doing it: a quick fix. As for the side effects or consequences—well, we'll think about those later. Maybe they'll have come up with a quick-fix solution for the problems created by the original quick fix by then.

This book is designed to be a comprehensive, long-term fix to your weight problem. As a result, it is not a crash program but a slower, carefully managed one. What I have done here is taken everything that I have seen work for weight loss and explained it so that you can adapt it intelligently to your life. While implementing what's here will take time and effort, you won't have to count calories, you won't have to go on a fat-free anything, and you won't ever have to feel guilty about going off your weight-loss diet because you won't ever be on one. Rather, you'll be on a long-term body and mind cleanup and refueling program that will make you feel great.

Everything you'll be reading about has been put into practice by those multifaceted wellness-oriented support groups I now organize. In addition to substantial weight loss, members report high levels of success in ameliorating or even eliminating such conditions as arthritis, heart disease, diabetes, high cholesterol, depression, and chronic fatigue. In the process, these people also often find that their looks improve: Their skin becomes smoother, their eyes gain sparkle, and their hair thickens and reverts from gray to its original color.

In this book, we'll be looking at these people's success stories. We'll also, of course, be explaining exactly what they did in order to lose the weight and achieve other health benefits. We'll be looking at diet, particularly from a cleansing and detoxification point of view, because you don't want to be "throwing good stuff in on bad." We'll be looking at what, when, and how to eat, at what not to eat—and why. You may be surprised to find that some of your former "no-nos" have turned into "yes-yeses." Recipes are included, so you'll never be at a loss for how to turn all that healthful stuff in your refrigerator into actual meals. Supplements, exercise, and other aids to weight loss and health will be covered. Also, we'll be exploring the all-important area of your core beliefs and attitudes.

In addition, for those of you with Internet access, I'm going to be going online with people who have this book. I'm arranging for a two-hour session through my website to answer questions from people free of charge, as a public service. Or you may live near a city where I have a video conferencing health support group: New York, Washington D.C., Atlanta, Miami, or other cities up and coming. For more information on these high-tech extras, you can visit my website, www.GaryNull.com.

I wish you not just success in using this book but joy—in eating, drinking, moving, and living in exciting new ways.

—Gary Null

Part 1

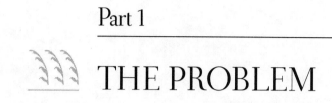

THE PROBLEM

Chapter 1

An Overview of
Overweight

Twenty years ago I was doing a lecture, one of my first for the Huxley Foundation. Afterward a couple came over to me to tell me the problems they had had with their son, who had been institutionalized his entire adult life. They showed me a picture of him. He was obese, weighing almost 300 pounds. He had been labeled a manic-depressive, incapable of functioning in society. When he went through periods of mania, he was deemed a danger to himself and others. When depressed, he would lie in his bed for days on end. They told me he had been to see over twenty psychiatrists but to no avail. They were desperate and asked if I had any advice for them.

I asked what their son's diet was like and was told that he ate institutional food plus almost $100 a week of what his parents gave him in confections, such as candies and potato chips. He was also a milk junkie, consuming large amounts of dairy products such as butter, cheese, and ice cream. I asked if their son had ever been through a detoxification program. They didn't know what detoxification was, so I outlined what a full-body cleansing program entailed and gave them suggestions for what they could do if they chose to put their son on this type of health-rebuilding program. I told them that the only sure-fire way to help their son lose weight and feel better both emotionally and physically was to remove the toxins from his diet and direct him toward healthier eating habits. They would start with a complete detoxification program and gradually remold his dietary lifestyle.

So they tried it. First they stopped bringing him sweets and restricted him to no junk food within the hospital setting. Believe it or not, in just three weeks, enough of an improvement had occurred that he could be moved from the institution to a therapeutic house. He had also lost fifteen pounds. While he was not able to go home at this point, he could now take charge of his own eating habits and create whatever diet protocols he wished. I guided them in mapping out a diet that included fresh vegetable juices each day, plenty of salads, grains, and legumes, and nutrients for rebalancing brain chemicals. Within one month of his arrival at the therapeutic house, the son no longer manifested any manic-depressive tendencies and was able to go home. Within a year and a half he was down to 165 pounds and was functioning normally.

This is an extreme example of someone who was a victim not only of an excessive weight condition but of an emotionally stunting chemical imbalance due to a junk-food diet. This man's poor dietary habits along with an allergic addiction to milk had seriously distorted both his brain chemistry and his behavior, not to mention his body shape. He had just never found a therapist who understood what was happening and made the connection between what was going on with his body and what was going on in his mind. Fortunately, with some nutritional guidance and a lot of determination on his part, this man was able to turn his life around.

I begin my book on weight control with this example not because I think that most people with weight problems have severe mental problems—that's obviously not the case. But I do want to stress my point that dietary and other lifestyle habits are closely connected not just with your shape and what your scale says but with how you think, feel, and act. All of these factors are intertwined to an extent that our society doesn't generally acknowledge. If you are overweight, you should understand at the outset that changing your eating habits for the better could change *all* of these factors for the better. You also should know that if you are overweight, you are far from alone. There are millions of people out there just like you, who share your feelings of frustration as well as your desire for a slimmer body and more fulfilling life.

THE STATISTICS

While obesity has been present since prehistoric times, as evidenced by early drawings, never before has the problem reached such epidemic proportions. Overweight conditions and obesity are rapidly increasing throughout the world, afflicting adults and children alike. In the United States, tens of millions of Americans are classified as either overweight or obese, with 20 percent of men and 25 percent of women falling into the obese category. These percentages have increased dramatically since the 1960s, with most of the gain seen in the 1990s. Ironically, despite the advent of diet centers on practically every corner and a national obsession with the rail-thin model look, the average American weighs eight pounds more than a decade ago.

All age groups are affected by this trend, and of particular concern is the frightening rise in childhood obesity. In a recent study of four- and five-year-old girls, for example, 10 percent were found to be overweight, which is almost double the amount found in 1971. Another investigation, this one focused on New York City grade-school children, found a third of the subjects to be overly fat. Adolescent incidence of this problem has gone up too; in fact, the number of overweight twelve- to seventeen-year-olds has more than doubled in recent years. These figures are particularly disturbing, as overweight children and adolescents tend to become overweight adults who run an increased risk of medical debilitation and premature death.

Socioeconomic factors seem to play a role, with women in less advantaged groups exhibiting obesity twice as often as women in higher socioeconomic brackets do. Black American women have a particularly high rate, at 40 percent. These differentials are probably due to a greater emphasis on being slim in more affluent groups as well as to differences in education, the availability of wholesome foods, and even housing. If you want to create wholesome meals you need good access to decent cooking and refrigeration facilities. If these facilities are less than adequate, people are more likely to rely on fast food and processed or junk items.

The most widely accepted standard for judging weight problems and obesity is the body mass index (BMI), a system that we will discuss in more detail in Chapter 6. Any adult with a BMI between 25 and 29.9 is classified as overweight, and measures beyond that signify obesity. The BMI is used to compare levels of obesity worldwide. Researchers have found that excessive weight is a global problem that is on the rise, particularly in urban populations.

Financially, the costs related to obesity are phenomenal. For the year 1990, the overall U.S. expenditure for obesity-related illness and lost productivity from missed work days was conservatively estimated at $68.8 billion. Moreover, the weight-loss industry, which includes everything from diet programs to surgical intervention and medications, costs the dieting population millions more. Were these methods successful, they might save money in the long run as obesity-related health disorders declined. The unfortunate reality is that after following these programs, most dieters regain their lost weight plus some extra, which then poses an even greater hazard to their health.

To what can we attribute this epidemic? While genetic and biological factors may explain why some individuals succumb to obesity, the overriding factor is the present-day environment where high-calorie, high-fat foods predominate, along with exertion-saving technological advances and the concomitant greater levels of inactivity. This raises questions about the standard approach to obesity today, which emphasizes medical intervention. If obesity and its related disorders are diseases of diet and lifestyle rather than infection, wouldn't it be more logical to take a holistic approach in their treatment? The modern hospital may be a technological marvel, but it is more suited to the treatment of acute conditions and trauma than to the correction of obesity, high cholesterol, or even heart disease, cancer, and other chronic diseases.

Unless drastic changes are made in our society that influence the overall behavior of communities, the problem of obesity is expected to escalate further, a fact that should be a cause for alarm. Let's take a more in-depth look at why we should be concerned.

LOST VITALITY

The costs of obesity go way beyond the financial, extending into many areas of health, and beginning with the way we feel and function every day. There's no getting around the fact that, on average, the more overweight you are, the less energy you're going to have to accomplish daily tasks and even enjoy daily pleasures. There's simply more of you to carry around.

Also, despite the quantity of food you consume, you may be malnourished. It may seem paradoxical, but being overweight and undernourished often go hand in hand. That's because the calorie-packed processed foods that overweight people tend to eat do not contain the full spectrum of nutrients. Also, sometimes a weight problem can be compounded by a system that does not properly absorb the nutrients that *are* in food. As the body becomes run down due to nutritional deficiencies, the first thing we might notice is that we are just not in top form. This condition is what Dr. Paul Bergner, author of *The Healing Power of Minerals*, calls "the blahs," which, he says, "are probably the American plague. People feel tired and sick, a first manifestation of mineral deficiency." Some of the results include depression, anxiety, irritability, immune problems, and fatigue. Dr. Jeffrey Bland, a research scientist at the Linus Pauling Institute in Washington state and the author of *The 20 Day Rejuvenation Diet Program*, has a name for this segment of the population—"the walking wounded." He asserts, "These people are not sick enough to be sick but not well enough to be well. These are the people who wake up tired in the morning, go to bed tired at night, have sore joints and muscles of unknown origin, and have digestive problems, headaches, and sensitivities to an environment that they used to be able to tolerate easily."

Most people in these circumstances believe there is nothing they can do but learn to live in a state of compromised vitality. What they fail to realize is that lost vitality is an early sign of deteriorating health, which, if left uncorrected, will pave the way for a variety of chronic conditions, including diabetes and cardiovascular disease. Nor do most conventional doctors understand the nutritional basis of "the blahs." They will either dismiss them as imaginary or treat the patient with an antidepressant drug.

In reality, lack of energy needs to be recognized and treated as a nutritional deficiency. Other important lifestyle choices also need to be taken into consideration, not the least of which is exercise, which we'll be discussing in Chapter 11.

LOST HEALTH

Being significantly overweight opens the door to a range of chronic health conditions that threaten quality of life, including cardiovascular disease and cancer—two major killers in the United States today. Too much fat is also related to hypoglycemia, noninsulin-dependent diabetes, high blood pressure, osteoarthritis, gastrointestinal disorders, peripheral vascular disease, and glandular dysfunction. Other risks to health include an increase in bad (LDL) cholesterol and a lowering of good (HDL) cholesterol; low back pain; gastrointestinal problems, especially gallbladder disease; and respiratory difficulties, including sleep apnea.

In addition, overweight conditions, especially obesity, have emotional ramifications. Being overweight is socially unacceptable, and society expresses disdain for overweight individuals, often viewing them as lazy and immoral. Children, in particular, have problems interacting with their peers and are more likely to suffer from alienation.

Obesity is clearly visible as a cosmetic issue, but its importance as a health issue has been largely ignored. Considering the many complications arising from obesity, addressing this problem is of utmost importance. In fact, the 1997 World Health Organization Consultation on Obesity concluded that obesity is one of the greatest health problems facing the world today, the impact of which may be equal to that of smoking.

Heart Disease

There is a well-established relationship between obesity and heart disease. Being overweight makes you prone to several risk factors for the illness: hypertension, dyslipidemia (raised cholesterol and triglyceride levels), high blood pressure, and glucose intolerance. Studies in the United States and throughout the world reveal that obesity, by itself, poses increased danger to the heart, and that the more overweight the individual, the quicker the onset of heart disease. Also, the way fat is distributed appears to make a difference, with fat around the abdomen being more dangerous than fat that's distributed evenly on the body.

Risks are further heightened when being overweight starts in childhood. Autopsies of obese children who died in car accidents show the early formation of arterial plaque. And studies reveal overweight youngsters to have high levels of LDL cholesterol and low levels of HDL cholesterol.

There is some evidence suggesting that certain types of foods are especially hazardous to the heart. Perhaps the worst heart offenders are foods containing free fats, for instance, margarine, mayonnaise, and fried foods. When we increase the amount of fats, principally animal fats—dairy, meat, chicken, pork, french fries—in the diet, we create unhealthy clumping in the red blood cells. The cells literally stick together. This can lead to a clot, which in turn can lead to a heart attack or stroke. Switching to a more wholesome diet, one that emphasizes whole grains, fruits, and vegetables, can reverse heart-related risks, as evidenced in the now-famous study by Dr. Dean Ornish.

Alcohol is falsely believed to help the heart, when, in actuality, it contributes to a fatty heart muscle. It also destroys protective antioxidants, folic acid, and B complex vitamins and contributes to various cancers and stroke. The compounds found in wine that protect the arteries from the damaging effects of LDL cholesterol actually can be obtained more healthfully through fruits and vegetables, particularly grapes and grape juice.

Eating poorly contributes to heart disease in yet another way. A deficiency of minerals, especially magnesium, is related to heart attacks. In fact, research has found many heart attack patients to have 30 percent less magnesium in their hearts than do normal controls. Without sufficient magnesium, the heart muscle and arteries become prone to spasm, which increases the likelihood of a heart attack.

Something we should remember is that heart disease is tied in to the functioning of other body systems. Western medicine tends to compartmentalize organ systems, as if one had nothing to do with the other, when their functioning is actually highly integrated. A good example of this is the liver's relationship to the heart. Devoted to a host of vital functions, including fat metabolism and toxin breakdown, the liver is one of our largest and hardest-working organs. When functioning properly, it keeps blood fats under control, thus helping to reduce cardiovascular disease. But when people are overweight, the liver becomes overburdened and stops functioning properly. Instead of burning fat and regulating fat metabolism, the liver begins to store fat. Often this is a precursor to fatty degeneration of the arteries and subsequent heart attacks and strokes.

Candida

Candida albicans, a yeastlike fungus, is a normal inhabitant of the intestinal tract that begins to wreak havoc if the healthy bacteria that normally keep it in check begin to die off. The problem usually begins with a series of antibiotics, which are overly prescribed. Antibiotics are designed to kill bacteria, which they do, but often they kill both harmful and good bacteria. With the good bacteria gone, the candida begin to proliferate. Once in charge, the candida upset the chemistry of the colon walls, causing local inflammation and the fermentation of sugars and carbohydrates. This leads to gas pain, diarrhea or constipation, and a spastic type of irritable colon. Candidiasis, or an overgrowth of candida, eventually can impair immunity and ultimately make toxins that poison the immune system. Thus a simple yeast infection can lead to an autoimmune condition, such as thyroiditis.

One symptom of candidiasis is a strong desire to eat carbohydrates for their sugar content and bread products for their yeast. These cravings are actually prompted by the candida themselves, which thrive on these substances. Unless corrected, the urges brought on by candida and their associated food allergies will most likely contribute to weight gain and make losing weight that much more difficult in the long run.

Diabetes

There is a strong link between obesity and type 2 (or adult-onset) diabetes. In one fourteen-year study of women between the ages of thirty and fifty-five, the risk was found to be forty times greater for obese women than for slimmer subjects (those with a BMI below 22). The link between obesity and type 2 diabetes is made stronger by certain factors, including obesity in childhood and adolescence, progressive weight gain from age eighteen, and intra-abdominal fat accumulation. Several studies emphasize the last factor as a particularly strong predictor.

One reason for the connection between obesity and diabetes is that overweight people tend to develop an intolerance to glucose where they require more and more insulin to break down sugar. At a certain point they become unable to produce enough insulin. As a result, they develop diabetes.

There is definitely a correlation between diabetes and a high-fat diet. This is evident in cultures that never experienced the condition until recent times, when their diet changed drastically to emphasize high-fat foods. The Pima Indians of southern Arizona, for example, knew nothing of diabetes at the beginning of the twentieth century. Their language didn't even have a word for it. Today these people get about 50 percent of their calories from fat, a 40 percent increase from 1900, and half of them are diabetic. Too much fat in the diet may cause fat to coat insulin, which then becomes less effective, or to clog insulin receptors on the cells themselves. Either way, the result is a situation in which sugar is prevented from moving out of the bloodstream and into the cell itself.

Early symptoms of diabetes to watch for include increased thirst, increased hunger, and increased urination. Sometimes there are no symptoms, though, and a routine physical exam reveals the problem. Many cases have been known to respond well to changes in diet, particularly when more fiber is added. Moreover, physical activity has been shown to help lower the risk.

Osteoarthritis

While it may not be life threatening, the crippling, painful disease of osteoarthritis dramatically impairs the quality of life. In the obese individual, osteoarthritis may develop due to too much weight being borne by the body's skeletal frame. Changes in metabolism brought on by an overweight condition also may promote arthritis. When we increase the weight-bearing load on the joints, the inner joint pressure on the synovial tissue is intensified, which can be harmful. In addition, allergens in the diet can cause inflammatory responses in the body's joints. One particular painful joint condition connected to excess weight is gout, an inflammation, stiffness, and swelling of the joints caused by the buildup of lactic acid and uric acid in the cells.

Cancer

There is a clear relationship between obesity and certain cancers, particularly those that are hormone-dependent (endometrial, ovarian, breast, cervical, and prostate) or gastrointestinal (colorectal, gallbladder, pancreatic, liver, and renal). When we increase the amount of animal proteins in the diet, we are also increasing the amount of animal hormones and estrogens. These can bind to receptor sites on the breast and increase the risk of cancer. Specific hormonal changes that result in increased abdominal fat are also thought to be linked to these higher risks. The more abdominal fat you have, the more you are susceptible to the harmful effects of the toxins, pesticides, and phenobiotics that accumulate in fatty tissue. This predisposes the body to acute toxemia, which can have mutagenic effects on cells that result in cancer.

Although science has not yet determined whether increased cancer risk is the effect of a high-fat diet or if it is obesity itself that is the important association, doctors with a background in nutrition say there is much people can do to lower their risk through eating. They warn against certain foods that tend to promote carcinogenic changes. These include the brown-drink group—coffee, cola, and chocolate—and foods that contain a lot of free fats, such as mayonnaise and margarine. The brown-drink group promotes carcinogenic changes by giving us increased amounts of sugar, fats, chemical preservatives, artificial flavors and sweeteners, and caffeine—one very unhealthy brew. Dairy products and red meat also have been implicated, due to their high percentage of animal fat.

The problem, however, may be due less to the animal fats themselves than to contaminants in them. When people are eating animal fat they are also ingesting a barrage of toxic chemicals. Because many of the poisons, such as pesticides and fertilizers, that get dumped into the environment are fat-soluble, they gradually collect in an animal's fat, making that creature, and later the person ingesting it, toxic. The poisons we ingest may not harm us all at once; rather, over time they inhibit enzymatic action, slowing all our systems. Thus the immune system becomes depressed and less able to ward off cancer and other diseases.

Gastrointestinal Disorders

Being overweight can lead to a host of disorders that affect the gastrointestinal organs, including the gallbladder, liver, and stomach. Studies have clearly demonstrated an association between obesity and gallbladder disease. In fact, the condition is seen three to four times more often in obese individuals than in people of normal weight. Other gastrointestinal complications of obesity are liver abnormalities. When we have more fat in the body than is necessary for normal metabolic activity, the organs become infiltrated with fat. This can be very disruptive to normal biological processes. It also strains the gallbladder to secret extra bile, which is necessary to break down the fat.

Another problem that overweight and obese individuals encounter is the hiatal hernia, a gradual sliding of the upper stomach above the diaphragm, where it doesn't belong. A hernia can manifest itself as a pulled muscle with ripped or torn tissue surrounding it, bulging into the abdominal cavity. If you have a hernia, any extra physical stress due to irritating medications, gas-producing foods, or nutrients that are difficult to digest (protein, fats, and carbohydrates) can cause a severe irritation. This problem can be difficult to diagnose, as the pain may come and go as well as mimic that of other medical conditions. The sensation may be similar to the pain of a peptic ulcer, or it might imitate angina, a heart-related pain that is found in a similar location, or heartburn. When there is uncertainty about what is going on a doctor will sometimes perform an endoscopy, a test that examines inside organs using a thin tube with a light and lens.

Excessive eating during meals is one factor connected to the hiatal hernia, as the volume of food can push the stomach outside its normal position in the abdominal cavity. Other irritants that can exacerbate this condition include medications that irritate the lower esophagus and stomach. The ones that tend to be especially bad are nonsteroidal anti-inflammatory drugs as well as tricyclic antidepressants, many asthma medications, and certain contraceptive medicines. Alcohol and caffeine also will act as irritants.

Stress

Stress is both a cause of weight gain and a result of it. It is common for people experiencing emotional strain to turn to food as a source of comfort. But making poor food choices and gaining weight throws the body's chemistry off, resulting in nutrient deficiencies that set off more emotional problems. People with low magnesium levels, for example, are more likely to experience anxiety, tension, and emotional upsets than those with normal magnesium levels. Compounding the problem is the fact that being overweight, in itself, can be stressful. The constant pressure to lose weight through dieting takes an emotional toll, especially since the result is usually failure.

Stress is also brought on by societal attitudes. Overweight people, most especially those who are obese, are stigmatized in most segments of American society and viewed as lazy, weak-willed, and even unintelligent. Others' disapproving attitudes have a negative effect on self-esteem, and this is especially true for adolescents.

Studies indicate that normal-weight individuals go further in life than obese people, who, on average, receive less education, are more frequently rejected from reputable schools, get hired less often, and earn less money at their jobs than do people of normal weight. It should be noted that even physicians show a more negative attitude toward obese patients, resulting in obese people seeking less counseling for both their weight problems and the emotional issues that result.

Hypertension

Much data supports the connection between obesity and hypertension, or high blood pressure. This silent disorder is nearly six times as likely to affect obese adults than it is to affect individuals of average weight. Obese children also commonly have this condition. The longer one is obese, the greater the risk of hypertension. On the positive side, weight loss is positively associated with a lowering of blood pressure.

The reason for the connection between an increased BMI and elevated blood pressure may be the fact that weight gain is connected to increased levels of circulating insulin. Excess insulin causes the kidneys to retain sodium, which, in turn, increases water retention, leading to more fluid in our veins—and thus higher blood pressure.

LOST LIFE

Studies on the impact of BMI on death rates conclude that there is a clear inverse relationship between how overweight people are and how long they live. Of course, no one can predict how long any particular individual, of whatever weight, will remain alive. But when you look at large groups, the negative effect of excess weight on longevity is unquestionable, due to the remarkable number of health- and life-threatening conditions that result. This relationship is seen most clearly in carefully designed studies that control for such factors as cigarette smoking. Overweight individuals often use cigarette smoking as a means to control their appetite, which can result in lung cancer and other medical conditions. Conversely, persons of an average weight, those whose BMI falls between 18 and 25, have the lowest mortality rates. The bottom line is that weight control isn't just a matter of how you look in the mirror—it could be a matter of life and death.

Ultimately, attempting to lose weight is not just about being able to look in the mirror with pride or fit into a size-6 dress—it's about avoiding the larger, far-reaching consequences of what obesity can do to our bodies, minds, and lives. I have outlined these consequences not to scare you but to give you a clear picture of what you stand to gain by following the program presented here. You can avoid and overcome these conditions, and you can improve the quality of your life. Now let's take a closer look at why we gain weight—and what we can do to remedy the problem.

Chapter 2

The Causes of Obesity

I grew up in the small town of Parkersburg, West Virginia. In that time and place, eating was an entirely different experience than it is for most Americans now. More often than not, people ate together as a family. Mothers insisted that their children eat three square meals a day. Breakfast usually consisted of eggs, orange juice, milk, toast, or hot cereal—oatmeal or Wheatena. But then there was also fruit. In my house, there was always a large bowl of fruit on the table or the counter. The milk we drank was unhomogenized and without extra hormones. Dinner was the meal during which the family shared the experiences of the day. It was an enjoyable time of coming together that people respected and appreciated. People respected and appreciated their food as well, perhaps because they had to expend more effort preparing it than is required today. Meals were much more leisurely, without the interruption of phone calls or television or people rushing off to the office or gym.

I don't remember seeing many grossly overweight people in my community. Of course everyone was naturally more active then. We walked to most destinations. In fact, on Sundays you'd find people purposely not taking their car places so they could walk downtown or to the local city park. There were no videos and no computers, and television viewing was relegated to a few hours a week. As I remember it, we kids were much more involved in socializing and doing active things than kids are today. We were outside a lot of the time, exercising and breathing fresh air while we had fun.

Sometimes I'd visit an older friend, a woman in her seventies, who tended a beautiful ornamental garden in her backyard. She'd make me fresh sassafras tea from her garden, and we'd drink it with honey as we sat on her back porch and she talked about life. That was the extent of "take-out food" back then! I treasure those memories and the feeling of calm that goes with them. Even if we weren't necessarily eating all the "right" foods, there was definitely a sense of rightness and order about our meals and our days.

Today things are different. We have lost that sense of order and rightness about food, and as a result, obesity is rampant. Most of my old childhood friends are overweight. People don't eat as a family; they eat on the run. What's more, they eat only what tastes good, without any thought to what may or may not be good for them. People drive everywhere, and even when they do exercise, they still drive to the gym or the track. And many people today, especially children, seem to just about live in front of televisions or computers or malls.

Recently I went back to my hometown, and after three days of visiting with a friend off and on, I realized that I never saw his kids. They were always out, always on the run, eating at fast-food places with their friends. Not once during my entire stay did my friend's family sit down together at the dining room table. I felt surprised and saddened that the lifestyle I had remembered so fondly had given way to these impersonal family interactions and eating habits. Unfortunately, as I know from my travels and from talking with others, what has happened in my town is typical of what's happening all over America: While the pace of our lives has become more frenetic, people actually are becoming less active physically. They're also becoming less home- and kitchen-centered and less thoughtful about what they eat. It all adds up, on average, to lower feelings of contentment—and higher numbers on the scale.

No two individuals are alike, and we all gain and lose weight for different reasons. In this chapter we'll take a more in-depth look at some of the leading contributors to excess weight. While not every scenario here will apply to you, it's important to identify the habits or health problems that seem most relevant to your situation, and I encourage you to use this chapter as a jumping-off point for honest self-reflection. Understanding how and why we gained weight in the first place is one of the keys to successful, long-term weight loss.

A CULTURE OF CONSUMPTION

While people have always loved to eat, the profound differences in the way we eat today contribute to the growing trend of obesity. Many of these differences are a result of the commercialism that has, to a large extent, taken control of our daily lives. We may not even notice it any more because it has become such a prominent part of our world, but we are constantly being encouraged by the media to buy things, whether it's a sleek, new Volkswagen Beetle or the latest laundry detergent. The barrage of these messages is unceasing, and the question of whether we actually need what we're consuming is irrelevant. So is whether the products we're consuming are good for us. This applies to every type of consumer product, including—and especially—food. "If someone's willing to eat it, someone's willing to make it" pretty much describes what's being sold as food today.

For most of the American population, a tremendous variety of foods are available almost anywhere and at any hour. Twenty-four-hour supermarkets, fast-food franchises, and vending machines make it easy to fill our stomachs any time we choose. Because of advertising and marketing strategies—after all, who can resist those mouth-watering M&M commercials, or the Burger King ads that wave a Whopper, fresh off the grill, under your nose?—we learn at a young age to make processed foods a part of our everyday diet. Even schools, beginning at the primary level, are setting bad examples by forming partnerships with cola companies and offering soda rather than juice. Junk-food meals and snacks accompanied by sugary beverages have largely replaced the traditional homemade meal, as evidenced by the skyrocketing sales of these products. In 1992 it was reported that fast-food sales in the United States alone totaled $78 billion and that every second of the day over 200 people were being served a hamburger.

HOW CALORIES COUNT

In Part II of this book we're going to look at how you can solve your weight problem, but we won't be dealing in calories. However, in order to understand the problems behind obesity, you should know that most processed and fast foods are calorie-dense simply because they're high in fat. Fat gives us nine calories per unit of weight, while carbohydrates and proteins supply us with only four. Thus the secret to losing weight is not to count calories but to count grams of fat and sugar. It seems easy enough to limit our high-fat food choices, but, to paraphrase a potato chip commercial, "It's hard to eat just one." Fat makes everything taste better, and the food industry exploits this fact with every new high-fat food product that it markets.

Sweetening processed foods also increases their addictive quality, enticing us to eat more refined carbohydrates than we should. Our cravings for simple sugars override our desire for natural fare; hence, we eat far fewer fresh fruits and vegetables than we need. The body is a complex organism that will send satisfaction signals to the central nervous system once it gets the nutrients it needs. If we eat too many natural sweets, our bodies have a built-in mechanism that will stop us, so, for instance, we won't find ourselves bingeing on raisins—we'll eat a reasonable quantity and then put them away. This won't occur, however, when we eat empty calories from refined sugars or fats. The body doesn't respond to nonnutritious foods with satisfaction, and in its quest for nutrients, the drive to eat heightens rather than disappears. That's why, while it's nearly impossible to eat too much fruit, we can easily devour a box of cookies or several candy bars.

The extra calories we get from eating excess fat are likely to be stored when we lead a sedentary lifestyle, as so many of us do in this automobile-replete society. The new inventions created to make our lives ever easier also result in our becoming ever more sedentary. We click a remote control, for example, instead of getting up to change channels. We shop over the Internet, without even leaving our homes. With such a dramatic increase in the fat calorie content of our diets and a marked decrease in the amount of physical activity in our lives, the pressing question shouldn't be "Why are so many people fat?" but rather "How does anyone manage to stay thin?"

EATING OFF SCHEDULE

Besides the easy availability of high-fat food and energy-saving devices, another factor in unwanted weight gain is eating at the wrong time. In an attempt to diet, people often skip breakfast, only to end up eating more at the end of the day. From a physiological point of view, the end of the day is the worst time to eat because our bodies are slowing down and burning fewer calories. Combine this physical response with the fact that typical evening foods, such as desserts, alcohol, chips, and other appetizers, tend to be more caloric than typical morning foods, such as cereal and juice, and you have a recipe for weight gain.

To ensure that you effectively metabolize calories and still get all the nutrients you need, always start the day with a good, hearty breakfast and finish with a light supper. This way you have plenty of energy to get you through the day, and your body won't have trouble burning all those calories as it becomes more sedentary in the evening.

Emotional Eating

Often we eat at the wrong time because we're not following physical cues but emotional ones. The body is a wise instrument that will tell us when and which foods we need to eat, but we are often out of touch with these natural signals. When we are babies, our bodies give us clear hunger and satiation signals that we receive without interference, but the older we grow, the more we stop using food strictly as a fuel and begin to attach extra significance to eating.

The "Oy! or Joy" Response. A lot of us turn to food unthinkingly when we're having a rough day and looking for a way to feel better. Powerful associations between food and love stem from our earliest memories of being held and fed at the same time by our mothers. As adults, when we don't feel loved we often turn to food, using it as a tranquilizer. The phrase we use to describe many of the foods we grew up with, "comfort food," says it all. Meatloaf, mashed potatoes, chocolate pudding, and pie are not just easy to swallow; they evoke images of a simpler, easier time in the protective environment of our family and first home. Indeed, "motherhood and apple pie" are almost synonymous in the American consciousness.

All of us go through difficult times. We lose a job, a loved one dies, a relationship ends. Overeating can be a way of dealing with these losses. Sometimes, deep-rooted traumas are the cause of overeating. For example, eating to excess and the resultant weight gain may be a subconscious strategy for protecting oneself against unwanted sexual interest, especially for those who were once victims of sexual abuse. Dr. Jane Hirshman, author of *Overcoming Overeating* and a founder of "antidiet" groups that help people recover from compulsive eating behaviors, suggests that we reach out for food because "we cannot sit with ourselves through the moment of difficulty. Many people don't really have eating problems—they have 'calming problems.' They use food to calm down." The problem, of course, is that food is not a healthy antidote for anxiety.

Although the negative feelings associated with emotionally triggered eating—depression, anxiety, boredom, loneliness, and anger—are probably familiar to us all, it seems that the use of food to suppress and cover up these feelings, especially feelings of anger, is most common among women. Throughout history, girls have been socialized into believing that negative emotions such as anger are unladylike. Even today, after years of "raised consciousness," there seems to be a double standard as to how much expressed dissatisfaction is acceptable from a man versus how much is acceptable from a woman. So rather than talk back to a spouse or speak up to a boss who gives an unjust reprimand, many women will go home and head to the kitchen cupboard for cookies.

Sometimes the situation is a little simpler, and food becomes a tool for procrastination. For instance, when we're alone, we might rummage in the kitchen and eat to put off tasks we really don't want to do. We might find ourselves saying "First I'm going to do something I enjoy," and often that enjoyment is eating.

Psychologist Judi Hollis, author of *Fat and Furious: Women and Food Obsession*, points out that we also turn to food to celebrate the happy things that happen in life, such as a promotion at work or joy in a relationship. Think about the social events that help us celebrate special occasions and bond with friends and family. At weddings, birthday parties, and holiday celebrations we feast on spectacular, rich edibles. Indeed, eating is central at all of these affairs, and if we dare to hold back, we risk the wrath of loved ones who, feeling offended, accuse us of not enjoying ourselves. "I've kept my weight off now for twenty-five years," Hollis says, "and I found out that people generally eat over the good stuff and that the happy times are often the most dangerous. When I'm having a good day is when I have to be the most careful about my food."

Facing your feelings, both sad and joyful, is the best way to overcome emotional eating. Working with a trained therapist may help, especially if you are confronting deep-rooted problems. However, there also are ways you can assist yourself. For some basic ideas to help you get started, see Chapter 14.

PHYSIOLOGICAL CRAVINGS

It should be noted that not all food cravings are emotionally related. Some are our body's way of telling us which nutrients we need. For instance, chocolate cravings are often a symptom of a magnesium deficiency. Our bodies use up a lot of magnesium when we're under stress, and as a result we can become magnesium deficient. Chocolate is a high-magnesium food, and hence we crave it. You may not actually want the sugar or the chocolate flavor at all but rather the minerals within the chocolate itself.

Cravings for sugar can sometimes indicate a blood sugar imbalance connected to an overgrowth of *Candida albicans*. Women often experience vaginal yeast infections, but yeast can overgrow throughout the body in both men and women. Many times this condition stems from a diet that contained a lot of drugs, sugar, or alcohol in the past. To conquer this common craving, it's best to see a healthcare practitioner who can run a test to see if an overgrowth of candida is present. Or follow an anticandida program, like the one described in Dr. William Crook's book, *The Yeast Connection*, and see if the sugar craving goes away. By eating as though you have a blood sugar imbalance, you may be able to overcome your desire for sugar. We will explore some of these physiological cravings in greater detail in the upcoming chapters.

Denatured Food and Nutrient Deficiencies

By altering the natural foods that have sustained us for thousands of years, we are harming ourselves more than we realize. Attractive packaging and titillating tastes should not deceive us into believing that we are eating anything of substance nutritionally. The food business places nutrition low on its list of priorities, and even attempts to fortify foods with vitamins are paltry compared to nature's offerings.

Dr. Donald Davis, a research associate at the University of Texas at Austin, notes that the whole foods that have sustained us for thousands of years have a complex metabolic machinery very similar to our own. When we eat plants, we ingest the amino acids, vitamins, minerals, trace minerals, fiber, and fatty acids that our cells need. Processing, though, destroys this natural synergy. For instance, when sugar is separated out from the sugar cane or beets, the nutritious elements of these plants are destroyed. Similarly, bran and germ, the most important parts of wheat and rice, are removed when white flour or white rice are made. When oils are extracted from beans and vegetables, their wholesome value is destroyed by heat, light, and the addition of heavy solvents. "If you think about that a minute," Davis states, "sugar, shortening, and white flour is the basic recipe for a cookie. The sad fact is that Americans, on average, get close to two-thirds of their calories every day from those three things. Basically, we're getting 1,500 calories a day from cookies and missing a tremendous number of vital nutrients."

Processed foods have long been endorsed by governments as an inexpensive way to feed large populations. Since the mid-1800s, when food manufacturing techniques were first introduced, the world's population has grown to depend more and more on these products. Davis surmises that the results of this trend will do more harm than good. "You could not convince any farmer to feed mostly cookies to his animals," says Davis. "The animals would undoubtedly become sick and die. The strange fact is that we can tolerate a great deal more ill health among humans than farmers could ever afford in their animals."

Another problem is that a lot of food eaten in the typical American diet is grown in nutrient-depleted soil, and as a result we lose the full spectrum of minerals so important for good health and metabolic balance. Food does not "grow" minerals. A food can get its minerals only by absorbing whatever is in the soil. Throughout the ages, plants have benefited from the natural process of decay that creates mineral-rich soil. Today, though, modern agricultural practices, such as monocrop farming, strip the soil, and thus our food, of some of their mineral content. Ways to counteract this are choosing organic produce when possible, because organic farmers practice environmentally conscious agriculture, and eating sea vegetables, which have been called "mineral concentrators" because of the way they absorb these elements from sea water. But most people don't do these things, and so most are not getting the minerals they should.

THE FAT-FREE FOOD TRAP

It's true that we should limit the fat in our diets, but several years ago a major campaign by food retailers convinced us that by eliminating fat completely, we could prevent ourselves from becoming fat. That's not the way it works, though. If it were, we wouldn't be seeing such a rise in obesity running parallel to the rising availability of fat-free foods. The truth is that the body needs a balanced diet, one that includes proteins, carbohydrates, and *good* fats. We require essential fatty acids in our diet to preserve good health, and when we totally eliminate fat from our diet, the imbalance sets off cravings that make us prone to binges. Afterward we feel mad at ourselves for losing control and hopeless as our lost weight returns. It's not really our fault, however, because we are only reacting to our body's need for fat—good fat, such as that found in foods such as salmon, walnuts, pumpkin seeds, flaxseeds, and uncooked flaxseed oil.

You should know that overrestriction of fat will adversely affect your looks, and it can even endanger your health. A fat-free diet will result in weak nails and lackluster hair and may lead to depression, kidney damage, and liver injury. Women who eliminate too much fat from their diet may stop menstruating. It's especially important to give overweight children enough good fatty acids. Young people need good fats to feed their rapidly growing brains and nervous systems and to have adequate energy to support their active lifestyles. Eating sufficient amounts of good fats may even help to prevent such childhood epidemics as attention deficit disorder, asthma, allergies, and earaches.

THE FOOD-MOOD CONNECTION

Foods can wreak havoc on our psychological health as well as our physical appearance, notes Dr. Elson Haas, director of the Preventive Medical Center in San Rafael, California, and author of *The Detox Diet*. Sugar is a particular culprit. "A number of my patients were on medicines for depression and other disorders," says Haas. "When I interviewed them about their diets, which their psychiatrists or doctors never did, it turned out that they were drinking a quart of colas every day. They were getting in the neighborhood of forty to fifty teaspoons of sugar daily."

Depressed people tend to love sugar because of the initial lift it provides. Sugar stimulates serotonin (an essential mood elevating hormone) levels, which, in turn, temporarily alleviates depression and makes a person feel good. But the initial charge disappears in a matter of minutes. The reason for this up-and-down pattern is that sugar, in any form, does not require digestion and passes directly into the bloodstream, where it raises the blood sugar level dramatically and overstimulates the pancreas to produce too much insulin. The excess of insulin then causes the sugar level to career down. The result is that twenty-five minutes after the initial consumption the blood sugar has dropped to very low levels and feelings of fatigue, irritability, and anxiety are generated. Feeling low again, the individual craves more sugar, and the cycle starts all over.

Numerous studies support the removal of sugar from the diet. Haas reports that when he helps his patients stop the sugar habit, they are able to reduce their medications and become more stable without psychoactive drugs. "This says a lot about how eating habits affect our health," Haas states. "When people don't feel well, they need to look at their lifestyle first and see if there are factors that are contributing."

The effect of diet on behavior is a growing field, notes Dr. Larry Christensen, psychologist and author of *Diet Behavior Relationships*, who agrees that sugar, along with caffeine, is a major contributor to depression, premenstrual syndrome (PMS), and other mood disorders. Women experience these sugar cravings more than men, and they are also the ones more likely to experience depression and other mood disorders. As Christensen points out, once depression sets in, people tend to adopt a more sedentary lifestyle, which of course then translates into weight gain. One of the key factors in overcoming the depression-nonactivity rut so common to overweight people is giving up sugar.

But if you're thinking of turning to artificial sweeteners to help your mood, think again. These chemicals also have been shown to contribute to feelings of sadness, fatigue, and depression. It is interesting to see how their popularity surge in recent years has run parallel to the rise in Prozac sales. To replace sugar, health food stores and even supermarkets offer more wholesome, natural alternatives. You can sweeten baked items with easy substitutes such as raw honey and rice syrup. Use these sparingly, however.

FOOD ALLERGIES

One of the most commonly overlooked causes of obesity is allergies to common foods. Often the allergy masks itself behind fairly benign symptoms while disrupting the body's digestion and metabolism and causing substantial weight gain. I'll give you an example.

A young, overweight girl was put on a diet that her pediatrician suggested was appropriate, yet her health went from bad to worse. In addition to being overweight, the child had constant ear infections and puffiness under the eyes, which her pediatrician said was congenital, normal, and nothing to worry about. Every morning she woke up completely congested. She also had problems with bedwetting and nightmares. And no matter how much activity and exercise she had, she continued to gain weight.

As the girl grew into her teen years, she tried every form of diet, but nothing seemed to work. She restricted her calories greatly, practically starving herself, but she always remained overweight. The situation was frustrating, to say the least.

The mother brought this girl to me when she was thirteen years old, and I asked the mother about what the girl had eaten. She said the child was very diligent. She didn't eat candy. She didn't eat sugar. What she did eat was the "good American diet," exactly the way the doctor had told her to. "The doctors told us that she just has more fat cells than most people. It's genetic," the mother said. "But I don't have the same problem, so how could it be genetic?"

I asked the mother to try an experiment. I told her to take her daughter off every single food that she was eating and put her on completely different foods. She had been eating white bread twice a day. I had her eat no bread or a spelt (whole grain, nongluten alternative to wheat) bread. She had been drinking soy milk, and I had her drink rice milk. She had been eating hamburger and steak; I had her eat fish. In fact, after two weeks there was virtually nothing in her diet that was similar to anything she had been eating before. No vitamins were used, just a simple elimination diet.

The first thing that happened was that the girl went through some excruciating headaches and nausea. But those symptoms went away after three days. Her face—which had been broken out with an ongoing case of acne, treated unsuccessfully with antibiotics—cleared up completely. The puffiness under her eyes went away totally. Her excess mucus stopped. She had been hyperagitated, but that problem was gone. And she lost seven pounds. Yet the number of calories she was consuming remained the same. Then, during the next two weeks, we put her back on the diet she had been on before, and all the old symptoms came back: acne, weight gain, puffiness under the eyes. When I again took her off that diet and put her on the new one, they went away again.

This was an instance in which a child had struggled her whole life, not only physically, but emotionally, because of all the abuse and innuendo about her so-called laziness, when she was actually suffering from allergies to the foods she had had since she was a baby.

Two years later I bumped into this girl on the street. She looked completely different. She was clearly in good shape, as you could see her muscle structure. Her skin was clear, and she had a healthy, youthful glow. She told me that she hadn't had a problem with her weight since, other than when she started indulging in a few of the old allergenic foods. Once she stopped, the problems disappeared.

Most mainstream doctors do not acknowledge the existence of this type of food allergy, which is not the classic, or "fixed," allergy with immediate and unmistakable symptoms, such as hives. This cyclic food allergy can have more subtle signs. What's important to know is that experts in the field *do* see a strong connection among food allergies, cravings, and the retention of fat and fluid. If you're beset by these problems, you owe it to yourself to investigate a possible allergy connection. Seek the help of a holistic physician versed in this area.

How Allergy Triggers Obesity

While you may be eating a restricted number of calories from good-quality foods, if you are allergic to any one of them—wheat, dairy, soy, or corn are common culprits—you may not lose weight. This is because allergens in your system lead to a slowing of metabolic and digestive processes, and as a result, your body's natural ability to regulate hunger becomes impaired. Normally, your body sends out a signal when it is hungry, but allergies may interfere with that mechanism, resulting in your eating when you are not really hungry.

Allergens also cause fluid retention, a condition known as edema. This is often the reason why your stomach feels bloated after a meal. When we eat a food to which we are allergic, our small blood vessels enlarge, and fluid from the blood plasma seeps into nearby tissues. These tissues begin to swell with the excess fluid and remain swollen until the allergen is removed from the body. But since many people eat the same allergy-producing foods over and over, the swelling never leaves for long. Edema caused by allergens in the diet may contribute to up to 4 percent of a person's total body weight.

The Coco Pulse Test

An easy way to determine what foods you are allergic to is to use the Coco pulse test. For two weeks, upon waking in the morning, sit quietly in bed and take your pulse for sixty seconds. Then take a small amount of a single item of food that you have ready at your bedside, put it under your tongue, and keep it there for one minute. Don't swallow it, and remain still because any movement will raise your pulse rate. Wait twenty minutes and take your pulse again while sitting still in bed. If your pulse has gone up more than five beats per minute you may be allergic to that food. At the end of two weeks, you will have been able to test almost all the common foods in your diet. Avoid those foods you seem to be allergic to for one week.

It is a good idea to test your drinking water as well, because fluoride is a common allergen. Actually, fluoride is a toxin that has been shown to affect the immune system. Switch to bottled water for one week and see how you feel. Also, remember to use bottled or filtered water in cooking so that fluoride does not end up in your meals.

At the end of the week, reintroduce those foods you've eliminated from your diet. Eat them totally separately, at least two hours removed from any other foods. For example, if you suspect that you are allergic to corn, eat some fresh corn separately and see what effect it has on your system. If you have properly cleansed your system of the toxins from a particular food to which you are allergic, your body will respond immediately by trying to eliminate them through the usual allergy symptoms such as excess mucus or watery eyes.

Carefully observe the signals from your body. In a short time you will be able to determine which foods you are allergic to, eliminate them, and begin to lose weight. Some people may lose up to fifteen pounds in one week simply by eliminating foods they are allergic to, even if their calorie consumption stays the same.

GENETICS

Have you ever wondered why some of your friends can eat all day long without ever gaining a pound while you seem to gain weight just thinking about food? The reason, in part, may be an inborn propensity to either hold on to fat or to burn it. In recent years a great deal of research has been performed on the role of genetic factors in overweight conditions and obesity. The hormone leptin, for instance, seems to be tied to a specific gene and affects satiety, or the feeling of fullness that signals us to stop eating. Some people seem to be resistant to the effects of leptin, and there may be a genetic link here as well. Much is yet to be learned in this complex field, but scientists have associated several genes with such proclivities as the likelihood of gaining weight over time, the propensity for abdominal fat, and appetite control.

This is not to suggest that you adopt a fatalistic approach to controlling your weight. In most instances genetic factors depend on an environment conducive to their expression. While overweight parents commonly have overweight children, this is not due solely to genetics but to the way these children have learned to live. If you place these same children in different surroundings where they can learn better eating and exercise habits, chances are they will slim down. Consider youngsters who spend summers at weight-loss camps, where they become significantly thinner, but who start putting on the pounds again over the winter, when they are in less health-promoting home environments. Consider also countries where entire populations remained slim for thousands of years until fast-food diets began to replace the traditional style of eating. Now obesity is rampant in places where none was ever seen before. Obviously, the genetic makeup of the people did not suddenly change; rather, the environmental factors did.

Genetic Taste Variations

One interesting area of research is the study of genetic taste variations and their possible implications for obesity. Awareness of differences in the ability to detect taste began in 1931, when Dupont scientist Arthur Fox was synthesizing a chemical called PTC. By accident, some of it blew into the air, creating a terribly bitter taste for another man who inhaled the substance but making no noticeable impression on Fox. Further investigation revealed that some people could not taste this substance while another group could and that there was a third group in the middle. The terms "nontasters," "supertasters," and "medium tasters" were used, respectively, to describe these groups, and it was learned that there was a genetic component that helped explain the variations.

So, how does this relate to weight loss? If supertasters have an unusually intense response to bitterness, they may tend to avoid healthful fruits and vegetables, foods that help keep people slim. Some researchers also theorize that supertasters may have a greater sensitivity to more pleasant-tasting sweets, salt, and fats, which makes them more likely to favor these foods. Others counter this contention, however, asserting that a liking for fat is universal. Dr. Adam Drewnowski, director of the nutritional sciences program at the University of Washington, holds this view, pointing out that "there's a very sensitive censure mechanism that turns you off to sugar, and it kicks in in an adult's life. For example, children like very, very sweet things; adults do not. Adults find sugar candy way too sweet. But this mechanism does not exist for fat. Things are never too rich or too creamy or too fatty; there's no limit. I suspect that this is because we were never really meant to eat fat. Fat was fairly rare in the food supply until 200 years ago when we had vegetable fats being turned out cheap by the industry. And as a result we do not have a natural physiological protection against eating too much of it."

Further research needs to be done on these issues. But even if we don't understand everything about how we accumulate extra weight, we do know how to control the tendency, which is the important thing.

Chapter 3

The Hormonal Connection

A hormone is a messenger of our body, whether it's adrenaline, catecholamines, DHEA, human growth hormone, or dozens of others secreted by the adrenal gland, the pituitary, the thyroid, or other glands. Hormones allow the body to function properly. When a hormonal system becomes imbalanced due to toxins in the environment—lead, cadmium, mercury, silver amalgam fillings in our teeth, fluoride or chlorine in our water, viruses, bacteria, or even electromagnetic stressors—a dysregulation can result. It can be subtle, with no obvious symptoms, but significant nevertheless because the person's metabolism changes, and his or her energy level generally does as well.

Metabolic changes can mean a state in which the body is not efficient in burning its fuel. The body stores more fat, the person is generally more fatigued, and then, because he or she is not as vitally energized as before, the individual begins to lose some of his or her earlier enthusiasm about everyday activities. In time, this can cause a depression that in itself can cause hormonal imbalances and the releasing of stress hormones.

After a number of years, the body adapts to a reduction in the central hormones and/or an imbalance in how they are used. Often careful examination and testing of a person's hormone systems can determine if that individual is out of balance. If that is the case, by going through a comprehensive detoxification program and then a hormonal rebalancing, the person is frequently able to lose weight without dieting, regain a sense of energy, and avoid the Yo-Yo syndrome (losing weight only to regain it). By contrast, placing people on high-protein diets or just giving them vitamins or having them count calories and skip meals does not correct the underlying imbalance.

Obviously, not everyone suffers from a hormone imbalance, but it is a good idea to rule out such conditions before embarking on your weight-loss program. Hormone problems are actually more common than you might think, and if your weight-control struggle is hormone-related, all the dieting and exercising won't automatically help you shed those extra pounds. Read the information presented here and if any of the symptoms sound familiar, make an appointment with an endocrinologist who can perform a simple hormone test to determine if you are producing adequate levels of melatonin, estrogen, thyroxin, and other critical hormones. If your tests come back normal, clearly your weight-control problem is not hormonally related. If they do identify an imbalance, the treatment you receive may improve both your weight and your overall health. Either way, the peace of mind you will derive is well worth the expense of having the tests done.

INSULIN RESISTANCE

While insulin's vital role in the prevention of diabetes is common knowledge, few people realize the relationship of this hormone to weight management. If you find that losing weight around the middle becomes increasingly difficult with age despite a wholesome diet rich in grains, fruits, and vegetables, you may be experiencing one of the effects of insulin resistance.

After eating, the body produces the hormone insulin to take food particles to the cells. Once at the cells, it enters through points on cell membranes called receptor sites. But for many people, there's a glitch in the process, and the insulin receptors become insensitive, failing to respond adequately. As a result, the insulin is forced to remain in the bloodstream, where it starts to build tissue, including fat tissue. Nutritionist Robert Crayhon from the Designs for Health Institute and author of *Robert Crayhon's Nutrition Made Simple* explains, "It reminds me of B. B. King's song 'The Thrill Is Gone.' The relationship is just not working. What happens then is a lot more insulin is hanging out in the bloodstream. This creates a lot of problems. One of them is too much adipose [fat] tissue, and we gain weight."

Along with weight gain, other symptoms begin to manifest. Levels of harmful triglycerides rise and protective HDL cholesterol drops. Other problems can include a rise in uric acid, gout, clogged arteries, and even polycystic ovary disease. Also, too much sugar in the blood eventually can lead to type 2, or adult-onset, diabetes. And some researchers are suggesting a possible link to cancer and heart disease. An overabundance of insulin also creates an imbalance of other hormones, such as the circulating thyroid hormone, and cortisol, produced by the adrenal glands. In the latter instance, the adrenal glands respond to a perceived fight-or-flight state of emergency when the blood sugar fails to drop. Too much cortisol means that you're not only storing fat, you're retaining water and becoming bloated. This complex problem is sometimes called metabolic syndrome, or syndrome X.

Several factors appear to precipitate insulin resistance. For most people, just gaining ten or fifteen pounds above what's normal throws the system off. This may explain why it's so difficult to lose those last few extra pounds. The condition also is related to a lack of trace minerals, such as chromium and zinc; too many refined carbohydrates; genetics, where there is a family history of diabetes; and a sedentary lifestyle.

Carbohydrates, especially simple sugars from refined foods and alcohol, raise blood glucose quickly. The body responds by producing greater amounts of insulin. When this happens, people are said to be carbohydrate intolerant. The relationship between carbohydrate intolerance and weight gain has led to a resurgence of the high-protein diet. Such a diet, which allows an unrestricted amount of meat, cheese, and eggs but eliminates bread, pasta, fruit, and sugary, starchy vegetables, is based on the premise that while carbohydrates destabilize blood sugar and should be avoided, protein stimulates ketosis, a process by which the body burns its own fat. Since fats slow down sugar's entry into the bloodstream, they are also permitted.

Lately Dr. Robert Atkins, the doctor who originally introduced this style of eating in his 1972 book, *Dr. Atkins' New Diet Revolution*, has been promoting the benefits of his plan in the updated 1992 version of this best-seller. Atkins calls his protocol safe and claims to have helped over 60,000 patients. Critics of the method, however, say that such a diet is unnatural and therefore impossible to maintain for any length of time. It also has been called unhealthful, resulting in constipation or diarrhea; fatigue; toxins, such as uric acid and ammonia (a damaging product of the breakdown of protein); bad breath; and body odor. In addition, too much meat is associated with higher incidences of cancer and heart disease. Furthermore, opponents of the plan point out that high-protein diets only give the illusion of working. Initial weight loss is rapid, as protein-induced toxins are flushed from the system. But this is not fat loss. Rather, tissues are dehydrating to get rid of ammonia.

Many doctors and nutritionists advocate a less extreme approach, citing success with higher amounts of complex carbohydrates. Research performed by Dr. Bernard Wolf and published in the October 1995 edition of the *Canadian Journal of Cardiology* seems to support this approach. In this study, slight alterations were made to the diets of twenty people with markers for insulin resistance. Specifically, individuals began eating in the ratio of 50 percent carbohydrates (instead of their usual 65 percent), 25 percent protein (instead of their usual 10 or 11 percent), and 25 percent fat (an unchanged amount). Both health and appearance improved.

New York City nutritionist Colette Heimowitz uses this moderate approach to overcoming insulin resistance with her patients and cuts back further only when necessary. She begins with what she calls a "change-in-lifestyle" plan in which people are taught to differentiate between complex and simple carbohydrates, guided toward appropriate food choices, and asked to record what they eat in a food diary. Often this alone is enough to make a dramatic difference in health and appearance. Heimowitz reports that at the beginning of treatment, laboratory tests commonly reveal high triglyceride and low HDL levels, which is the opposite of what should be found. But with a diet consisting of complex carbohydrates, sufficient protein, no sugar, and no chemicals, these levels often reverse. This reversal coincides with an improved appearance, where a thick waist and stomach paunch transform into a lean look.

Exercise and supplements help to control blood sugar levels. Some recommended supplements include:

- Pantothenic acid or pantetheine (500–1,000 milligrams [mg]) for adrenal support
- Chromium picolinate (200–800 micrograms [mcg]) for controlling blood sugar levels
- Vanadyl sulfate for hypoglycemia and hyperglycemia
- Lecithin and niacinamide for controlling blood lipid elevations
- L-carnitine (1,000–2,000 mg) on an empty stomach to aid thermogenesis (fat burning)
- Coenzyme Q10 (200 mg) to increase cellular energy

Additionally, the following nutrients may be added:

- Glutamine (2–4 grams [g])
- Choline (750–1,500 mg)
- Inositol (1,000–2,000 mg)
- Methionine (400–800 mg)
- Lipoic acid (100–400 mg)
- Linoleic acid (2–4 g)
- Taurine (1,000–2,000 mg)
- Vitamin C (2–8 g)
- Zinc (30–70 mg)
- For obese individuals with thyroid deficiencies, acetyl-L-tyrosine (500–1,000 mg)

Other good nutrients are vitamin B3 and the minerals magnesium and manganese. These help to control blood sugar levels and stabilize energy so that people don't have the ups and downs that produce cravings. Also important are fiber and selenium. In two to three months, the body starts to return to its normal weight.

Herbs can be used as well, although they should be taken on an interim basis, as their continual use diminishes effectiveness. One hundred million mg of Siberian ginseng, for example, can be helpful when taken for three weeks on and three weeks off. As Heimowitz notes, "The body is a symphony. Patients respond better when they have a broad spectrum of nutritional support." In addition, exercise should become part of the program, even if a person has to build up to it.

Commenting on why moderate changes to the protein/carbohydrate ratio work, nutritionist Crayhon states, "Protein helps support the endocrine system nicely, particularly the adrenal glands' ability to support blood sugar. And protein goes to the liver to participate in a process called gluconeogenesis, in which protein is turned into blood sugar slowly, keeping blood sugar levels stable so cravings decrease. Hypoglycemia is helped too. This is the kind of eating program that helps people lose weight, feel more energetic, have no cravings. And it's so easy."

Simple carbohydrates, found in refined foods such as alcohol, white flour, and white rice, wreak havoc on blood sugar and should be avoided by the carbohydrate-sensitive person at all cost. Because these foods lack fiber, the body quickly converts them to sugar, causing blood glucose levels to rise rapidly. As mentioned earlier, complex carbohydrates burn more slowly and, for the most part, are better tolerated. But you should note that certain complex carbohydrates have been found to increase blood sugar faster than others. The rate at which blood sugar levels rise after a specific food is eaten is called its glycemic index. The potato, in particular, is a high-glycemic-index food and should be consumed less frequently than beans, legumes, and brown rice, which are low-glycemic-index choices.

Sugar Substitutes

When reducing your sugar intake, focus on retraining yourself to want wholesome foods rather than turning to artificial sweeteners. The most popular of these today is Nutrasweet, a product containing aspartame and glutamate. These are excitatory amino acids (or excitotoxins) that can have negative effects on the central nervous system. While glutamate is a naturally occurring substance needed to help nerve cells transmit messages, ingesting extra amounts can result in an overstimulation of brain cells, which can alter brain chemistry. The popular seasoning monosodium glutamate, or MSG, also can cause this problem. It's easy enough to request no MSG at a Chinese restaurant but harder to eliminate it in grocery store purchases. Check your labels for such names as hydrolyzed vegetable protein, hydrolyzed protein, plant protein extract, texturized protein, yeast extract, or autolyzed yeast. These may be deceptive names for MSG.

Should dieters risk long-term artificial sweetener use? Apparently not, as research indicates no relationship to weight loss. In fact, despite the absence of calories, these chemicals can mess up metabolism so that you actually gain, instead of lose, weight.

Hypoglycemia

Having a "sweet tooth" or a habitual sugar craving is a good tip-off that something is wrong with your glucose metabolism. Another sign is that you get irritable, nervous, and shaky from eating just a little sugar. Even a small piece of fruit may be enough to trigger the symptoms.

Hypoglycemia, or low blood sugar, seems to occur episodically. One day you feel all right; then the next day it suddenly hits you. The first indication is a dramatic drop in energy. You may find that you are so exhausted you have to stop and rest because you just can't function. Usually this occurs in the late afternoon, when the body's natural drop in blood sugar is exacerbated by the hypoglycemic condition. Because you are feeling so low, you may overeat at this time and indulge particularly in sugar snacks. Gradually, as your glucose levels begin to rise, you feel better until the symptoms finally disappear.

Most physicians dismiss these symptoms as psychosomatic. However, if a hypoglycemic person does not receive treatment through changes in diet and lifestyle, eventually the condition can develop into weight gain and then diabetes. Fat distribution often takes on a pattern in which the circumference of the waist becomes greater than that of the hips. In the healthy adult, the circumference of the waist is less than hip circumference.

Warning: Beware the Coffee Break Trap. To counter feelings of fatigue from low circulating blood sugar levels, a common response is to reach for coffee and an empty-calorie sugary snack. But such an attempt at feeling better is ultimately fruitless, as the initial energy jolt you get from the caffeine and sugar quickly evaporates and your energy level plummets. People who take coffee and pastry breaks throughout the day typically find themselves in a vicious cycle of overstimulation and exhaustion. Plus too many simple carbohydrates lead to B-vitamin deficiencies and extra poundage.

THE HIDDEN PROBLEM OF HYPOTHYROIDISM

"Hypothyroidism is probably the most misunderstood illness," states Dr. Mark Leder, supervisor of nutritional services at New York's Natural Wellness Center. "It has so many ramifications on so many different systems of the body."

Indeed, every cell in the body needs thyroid hormone to function properly, and hypothyroidism, or low thyroid function, slows down all body processes, including metabolism. Since our metabolism controls the rate at which we burn calories, once metabolism becomes sluggish, people have trouble losing weight and are prone to gaining it easily. In addition to weight gain, symptoms of hypothyroidism can include fatigue, even chronic fatigue syndrome; cold hands and feet; cold intolerance; lethargy; weakness; dry, coarse skin; a puffy face or hands; loss of the outer third of the eyebrow; cramping; infertility; an absence of periods or, conversely, excessive menstrual bleeding; loss of appetite; thinning of hair; swelling of the neck or abdomen; constipation; arthritis; fibromyalgia; and allergies. When the brain is affected, the results might be depression, poor memory, an inability to concentrate, and slow speech. Long-standing hypothyroidism can be an underlying factor in diabetes, hyperlipidemia (elevated cholesterol), heart disease, stroke, and kidney failure. And because hypothyroidism depresses the immune system, it can cause chronic infections and set the stage for cancer later in life. Dr. Raphael Kellman, an internist and founder of the Center for Progressive Medicine in New York City, states, "Thyroid deficiency could be called the great masquerader because virtually every type of thing can go wrong."

The thyroid gland sets the body's temperature. When it is not functioning up to par, body temperature goes down, throwing off homeostasis, or the body's naturally balanced functioning. Dr. Alan Cohen, a leading nutritionist, elaborates: "The last time you had a fever, even if your temperature was just half a degree elevated, you felt ill, and you knew that something was wrong. Conversely, when your body temperature is always a little bit below normal, you may not feel as dramatically sick, but over time things begin to slow down and not function well."

Cohen goes on to explain that every cell has to be within a very narrow range of temperatures to function optimally. "We have enzymes that control every function that occurs in the body, and they are all temperature-sensitive. When your body temperature is low because of a low thyroid, then everything begins to slow down and every cell can begin to malfunction. You can have a constellation of symptoms and go from doctor to doctor without realizing the etiology."

To detect hypothyroidism, most doctors rely on two types of tests. Standard blood tests check levels of thyroid hormone—an iodine-containing compound released by the thyroid gland as thyroxine (T4) and a more powerful component, triiodothyronine (T3). A more sensitive test also looks at levels of thyroid stimulating hormone (TSH)—a substance released by the pituitary gland that regulates T4 and T3. Unfortunately, both measures pick up only severe deficiencies. Many people experience subclinical levels of hypothyroidism, which these tests do not detect.

In real life, this translates into too many people being told by their doctors that nothing is wrong when searching for answers to chronic problems. One unfortunate result is that Prozac and similar medications are prescribed for growing numbers of depressed patients when proper diagnosis and treatment of hypothyroidism may be all that is needed. Fatigue, common among women after pregnancy, is often due, at least partially, to an underactive thyroid, and it can be missed with the standard diagnostics. Pregnancy puts a great demand on the thyroid; after giving birth, many women experience fatigue, dry hair, thinning hair, and hair loss. Yet the common response by doctors is "You just had a baby. Get more rest." Further, hypothyroidism is a leading cause of infertility that frequently goes unrecognized.

"I classify people with hypothyroidism as the walking wounded," states Dr. Cohen. "They just do not feel well; they're tired; they can't concentrate; and they can't lose weight. They're able to function, but not at their optimal level of health. When they go to their doctor their blood tests are normal, and they're put on medication for depression. But that doesn't get to the underlying cause of the problem."

Causes

Mineral deficiencies are common underappreciated causes of hypothyroidism. While people tend to associate the condition with an iodine deficiency, due to the widespread use of iodized salt most Americans are not lacking in this mineral. Other nutrients, though, may be in short supply. Two of the primary minerals involved in thyroid metabolism are selenium and zinc. A deficiency in either of these can prevent proper conversion of T4 to T3.

Stress and excessive refined carbohydrate intake are also major contributors to the condition. Refined carbohydrates push blood sugar levels higher and affect cortisol delivery, and stress has an impact on cortisol delivery as well. When cortisol levels are too high, the thyroid can become overworked and exhausted.

Low-calorie diets can contribute to hypothyroidism as well, although they are not the most prevalent cause. Many individuals restrict their caloric intake to a dangerous degree. Eating too little or fasting excessively can lead to a slowing down of the metabolic rate and, thus, a decrease in the body's ability to burn fat and calories. Also important to consider are food allergies and a diet that includes too much caffeine.

Going beyond the issue of proper food intake, our digestive system itself has to be in proper working order for the thyroid gland to function correctly. Thyroid hormone remains inactive until it is broken apart by enzymes in the intestines. Factors that may cause a disruption in this process include repeated antibiotic therapy, a poor diet, and intestinal problems. If any of these cause a microflora imbalance, the result may be a decrease in the intestines' ability to reabsorb, or "reuptake," the active thyroid hormone.

Chemical and metal toxicity, from such sources as secondhand smoke or organic compounds, such as softeners found in plastics and food wrap, may result in a thyroid problem. Mercury from dental amalgam fillings and exposure to pesticides can be problematic for the thyroid as well. Even tap water, due to its fluoride and chlorine additives, may affect thyroid function negatively. In addition, any exposure to radiation can harm the thyroid gland.

The liver plays a large role in the healthy functioning of the thyroid gland. Dr. Leder asserts that the liver is probably the most "abused, overworked, and stressed organ at this time in history." The liver turns absorbed toxins into soluble substances that can then be eliminated from the body as waste. The same enzymes that break down many environmental toxins break down thyroid chemicals. If our livers are overworked because of an overexposure to poisons, these enzymes will speed up, and too much thyroid hormone is going to be moved out of the body.

Antidepressants constitute another type of toxin that can interfere with thyroid function. This type of drug intake is not a particularly common cause of thyroid dysfunction, but it can affect the gland's ability to work correctly and should be considered when investigating the problem.

Dr. Leder and others believe that these are the core factors of thyroid illness and that this country's medical establishment has, for too long, labeled hypothyroidism as idiopathic—that is, as a disease for which the cause is unknown. This categorization tends to let doctors off the hook in terms of looking at causes as well as at effective treatment, which encompasses detoxification, improving diet, and decreasing stress levels.

Diagnosis

Proper identification and treatment of hypothyroidism would resolve a number of health problems in a great many people. Diagnosis should begin with a basal temperature test using an oral thermometer. This is a simple way to determine whether a body is "running cold." Shake down the thermometer before going to bed for the night. Immediately on arising, place it under an armpit for about seven minutes. (Menstruating women need to do this after the first day of their blood flow.) The temperature should be above 97.8 degrees Fahrenheit. If it is lower, it may be an indication of hypothyroidism. But this is not always the case, as a low body temperature can be brought on by other factors, such as a low-grade chronic infection. And some people simply have a lower-than-average body temperature. Temperature-taking is thus a start, but not enough of a measure to determine whether hypothyroidism exists.

The gold standard for detecting hypothyroidism is the TRH stimulation test, an easy-to-administer test that is far more sensitive to thyroid hormone deficiencies than are standard measures. According to Dr. Kellman of the Center for Progressive Medicine, a significant percentage of people who test normally with the TSH test are found to be subclinically deficient in thyroid hormone when given the TRH test. "We've seen over and over again how this one simple test can change people's lives," Kellman states. "Other tests only show pathology. This one can show if the gland is not functioning as well as it should."

At the Natural Wellness Center, a person's environment is examined as well. To do this, an interview is conducted so that factors such as diet and stress levels can be considered when developing a plan for treatment. The patient is asked to fill out a seven-day "diet diary," which can turn a difficult case into one that is easily diagnosed. For example, eating too much of certain foods, such as broccoli, cauliflower, and cabbage, can contribute to hypothyroidism. Such foods are wonderfully healthful when eaten in moderation, but an overabundance can lead to problems in some people.

Treatment

Holistic protocols for restoring thyroid balance are multifaceted. They include:

Stress Management. Important for everyone, stress management is critical to the individual who exhibits symptoms of hypothyroidism. Physical exercise helps to reduce stress, which can, in turn, diminish symptoms of hypothyroidism when combined with high-quality multiple vitamins and minerals and a healthful well-balanced diet.

Detoxification. It is necessary to minimize the body's exposure to harmful substances that prevent the thyroid gland from producing thyroid hormone. Chlorinated tap water can limit iodine uptake and should be replaced with distilled or filtered or spring water. Fluoridated toothpaste should be eliminated as well. Many people with thyroid problems "miraculously" improve just by following a detoxification program.

Diet. Nutrients are key in resolving thyroid difficulties. Soy foods help T4 convert to its active and usable form, T3. Sea vegetables, such as kelp or dulse, are also beneficial because they are high in iodine, which is important for thyroid function.

Supplements. People with symptoms of a subclinical thyroid deficiency are often lacking in a number of important nutrients, including vitamins A, B2, B3, B6, C, and E as well as glutathione, L-tyrosine, selenium, iodine, copper, zinc, magnesium, and manganese. A nutritionist can assist you with an individual nutrient profile to see which nutrients are needed.

Addressing Psychological Issues. The workings of the body are profoundly affected by the mind. When we ignore psychological issues, they eventually express themselves as physical symptoms. Dr. Kellman, who lectures on mind/body medicine, has observed this connection with thyroid disease: "For many people it's a derailing of personal meaning in their lives that ends up as thyroid dysfunction. They've suspended their life goals, or what is meaningful to them, for some later time. And they continue with jobs they're not happy with or with lives that they're finding no personal meaning in." This dissatisfying life situation ends up being manifested as a thyroid problem.

In these instances, treating a person's physical symptoms is never enough. Rather, you must listen to what the body is trying to say and then do something about it. First, one must wake up to the problem and define it. "That, in itself, alleviates the problem," Kellman states. "The symptom is transferred from the thyroid to the psyche. Then it becomes amenable to change." The next step is making the actual change that is required. That might mean giving up a 9:00 to 5:00 job to follow your life calling as an artist, or it might just mean changing your approach to life so that each day becomes more meaningful. It may be difficult at first, but, "all of a sudden you look back, and the thyroid deficiency went away."

Supplemental Thyroid Hormone. Some holistically oriented physicians give patients a natural form of thyroid hormone replacement therapy using Armour thyroid (porcine or pig thyroid). They consider this a natural and effective way to replace some of the thyroid hormone that the body has lost. The synthetic version of this hormone is Synthroid, which contains T4, the inactive form of thyroid hormone. T4 must be converted to T3 before the body can utilize it, and many people with thyroid problems are unable to do that properly or fully. For some people, therefore, taking Synthroid will have little effect on improving thyroid health.

Other physicians rely less on hormone therapy because they feel that replacement therapy fails to address the true causes of thyroid disease itself. They prefer to address diet, stress relief, detoxification, and psychological issues, feeling that, in time, energy, mental health, and correct rate of metabolism will all return.

THE ADRENAL GLANDS

The body has a feedback system that, ideally, regulates the amount of calories taken in each day to match its actual metabolic requirements. But this system may be thrown out of balance, and when the feedback loop is disturbed, the amount of calories consumed exceeds the amount of calories the body requires to function. These extra calories turn into fat, which is stored in various parts of the body.

One of the ways homeostasis, or bodily balance, may be disturbed is by a condition known as glucose instability syndrome, or what in more common parlance is called a hypoglycemic tendency. Control over the glucose level in the blood is multifactorial, involving the adrenal glands; the pancreas; the liver; the minerals chromium, zinc, and manganese; and the B complex vitamins, among others. The adrenal glands are important because they play a role in the production of glucocorticoid hormones, which normal adrenal glands produce when the blood's glucose level is too low. These adrenal-produced hormones will correct the low glucose level. But when this mechanism isn't working as well as it should, hypoglycemia results.

Hypoadrenalism, or low adrenal function, can create a host of other health problems, including weight gain, fatigue, allergies, sleep disturbances, and panic attacks. Also, as the adrenal glands are needed to convert the inactive thyroid hormone, T4, to its active state, T3, poorly functioning adrenal glands will result in a less effective thyroid gland and a subsequent slowdown of metabolic processes. Because the standard battery of medical tests does not usually pick up markers for adrenal exhaustion, the person who complains usually is told that the problem is imaginary.

This is unfortunate because, to handle stress, whether physical, mental, or emotional, people need good adrenal function. When your sugar levels are low, many things you could ordinarily have handled get blown out of proportion. You feel tense and anxious, with a sense of impending doom. Also, when the adrenal glands are depressed, a person has less energy and is not as likely to exercise. A person who, before, would follow a structured exercise regimen, spending x number of minutes on the treadmill or power walking, for example, is likely to reduce these activities once energy begins to falter. This adds to a weight problem, as a diminished output of energy means fewer calories burned.

Overstressed adrenal glands also will cause the kidneys to produce an excess of the hormone aldosterone. Initially this results in sodium retention and bloating. Over time an inability to produce aldosterone and a subsequent sodium deficiency develops. Symptoms can include wrinkles and sunken eyes from tissue dehydration as well as flatulence, diarrhea, nausea, vomiting, confusion, fatigue, low blood pressure, irritability, breathing difficulties, and heightened allergies.

Diagnosis

How do doctors diagnose suboptimal adrenal function? First, a medical history is taken, with particular attention paid to low-energy states, particularly in the morning. Typically, a person with low adrenal function will sleep eight, nine, or even more hours, and then, upon awakening from a good night's sleep, will still feel tired in the morning.

Another sign of subpar adrenal function is low blood pressure. Specifically, the Raglan blood pressure test is used. The patient lies down on a table for approximately five minutes and rests, and the blood pressure is taken in this horizontal position. The patient then rapidly stands up, and the blood pressure is retaken in the vertical position. In the normal, healthy person, the systolic blood pressure (the upper number) will rise. But the person with suboptimal adrenal function will have blood pressure that stays the same. And if the adrenals are severely suboptimal, the systolic number will actually decrease. Also, on occasion, a patient will get dizzy and need to rest for a period of time.

Blood tests also can be performed to check adrenal function. Or salivary levels of adrenal hormones can be taken, a method that allows for a more exact diagnosis of hypoadrenal function. The salivary analysis technique also enables multiple samples to be taken throughout the day, week, or month, and can be used to reveal other hormone levels as well.

Complementary physician Martin Feldman of New York City notes that in our culture, those with lowered adrenal function tend to reach for caffeine. A common cry is "I need my coffee to get me going in the morning!" While people with suboptimal adrenal glands may get by on coffee for years, in the long run this substance will only exacerbate an adrenal problem. Caffeine is irritating to the adrenal glands and, thus, prevents them from healing properly. A greater problem with coffee is one of chemical dependency. Caffeine is a chemical that causes addiction to the extent that those giving it up can be in withdrawal for weeks. As Feldman explains, "People with coffee addictions are getting the immediate energy, but in the long run this is going to lead to suboptimal adrenal function and eventually hypoglycemic tendencies, as well as potential food allergy problems, and thyroid problems." Part of obesity prevention, then, is getting off coffee. While coffee has many deleterious effects, the most pertinent one for obesity is its relationship to hypoadrenal function.

Supporting Adrenal Function

When you need a pick-me-up, rather than habitually reaching for coffee and sweets, items that ultimately increase stress, take something that's good for you. Pantothenic acid (500–1,000 mg daily) and vitamin C

(2,000–3,000 mg daily) are extremely important building blocks for the adrenal glands. Also important for normalizing blood sugar levels are zinc and other trace minerals, such as chromium. The proper mineral balance is essential for alleviating such hypoglycemic symptoms as irritability, fatigue, and dizziness. Licorice root supports adrenal function as well, although people taking it should check with their physician if they have blood pressure problems, as this herb is known to elevate blood pressure.

There are other important steps you can take to support adrenal function: Avoid environmental toxins when possible, minimize stress where you can, and cut down on your consumption of simple-sugar foods. This last factor in particular can make a big difference in your adrenal wellness.

OTHER HORMONES AFFECTING OBESITY

"There's so much new information coming out on hormones and their effect on fat," notes Michael Rosenbaum, a medical doctor from northern California and the author of several books on nutrition, including *Super Supplements*. "The number of puzzle pieces in obesity has increased, and you have to look at the entire spectrum." Aside from subclinical thyroid deficiencies, too much insulin, and too little DHEA (the body's master hormone), other hormones that may impair the ability to lose weight include growth hormone and estrogen.

Growth Hormone

Our levels of growth hormone, which is secreted by the pituitary gland, gradually decline with age. This slowdown is our body's way of telling us that we've reached the end of our reproductive years. In addition to a diminished libido and sexual performance, we see changes in body composition. Most notably, fat increases, and lean muscle mass decreases. In fact, each year after the age of forty a pound of fat replaces a pound of muscle. This means that by the time a person is fifty, ten pounds of muscle have been replaced with ten pounds of fat.

Experts disagree on the benefits of supplementing with growth hormone. Some are excited by the antiaging benefits seen in scientific studies. In these studies, senior citizens given growth hormone experienced increased lean muscle mass, decreased body fat, increased energy, stronger immune systems, sharper eyesight, and better mental functioning. Other experts, however, caution that more research into safe amounts is needed. We most certainly need to keep up with new studies on this potential "fountain-of-youth" hormone.

Estrogen

A woman's tendency to develop a pear-shaped body is often the result of estrogen's penchant for fat and water retention. Birth control pills and hormonal supplements are culprits here, as are foreign estrogens (called xenoestrogens) from soft plastics, such as Baggies, and pesticides that leach into our foods. Because there is far more exposure to estrogen today than ever before, we see higher incidences of weight gain and weight-loss difficulties. Other than becoming pear-shaped, signs of too much estrogen may include tender breasts, swollen fingers, and bloating as well as other symptoms that mimic pregnancy. Menopausal women should look into safer varieties of the hormone, such as estriol. Eating more soy products also may help. Soy contains special phytochemicals called isoflavones that studies have shown to balance estrogen levels. This may be why women who follow traditional Asian diets that are high in soy exhibit far fewer menopausal symptoms than those who eat standard American fare.

Chapter 4

Eating Disorders

I n the early 1980s singer Karen Carpenter died of anorexia nervosa, and the media began to focus attention on this growing problem among American women. Today eating disorders—anorexia nervosa, bulimia nervosa, food addiction, and binge eating disorder—have reached alarming proportions in all segments of the population. To what can we attribute this epidemic, and, more important, what can we do about it?

The reasons for eating disorders are not clear, in part because research in this field is new—less than two decades old—and in part because of the way investigations have been conducted in the past. Kelly Brownell, Ph.D., director of the Yale Center for Eating and Weight Disorders and coauthor of *Eating Disorders and Obesity: A Comprehensive Handbook,* notes that up until recently, eating disorder researchers have worked apart from scientists investigating obesity, and the two groups have not communicated. Brownell explains, "The issue of what governs hunger and satiety, for example, would be very important to know in the eating disorders field, but almost all of the study on that goes on in the obesity field. There's a lot of important work on body image that goes on in the eating disorders field, and the obesity field doesn't study it very much."

Fortunately, more sharing is starting to take place, and our understanding of these issues is becoming enriched. Current thinking attributes eating disorders to a combination of physiological, psychological, and sociological factors. There is also a genetic component: New research—specifically, investigations of identical twins raised apart—supports the hypothesis that eating disorders are, to an extent, inherited. While such studies may seem to take the emphasis off cultural factors, our culture obviously plays a large role in the development of eating disorders, as evidenced by the increasing incidences of anorexia and bulimia in the past ten years.

THE MIXED MESSAGES OF OUR MEDIA

Our mass media do more than spread information and promote products; they influence how we feel about ourselves. Magazines, television, and movies tell us that we must look a certain way in order to be accepted. Although more research needs to be done in this area, magazine ads appear most persuasive, perhaps due to their pervasiveness and to the fact that the models used are extremely thin. In fact, some studies suggest that the smaller the models used in a magazine, the more young women favor that magazine.

Television adds to this pressure in overt and subtle ways. During the Clinton/Lewinsky scandal, for instance, late-night television jokes about Monica Lewinsky and Linda Tripp made fun of their appearance, as opposed to examining their actions. Commercials are constantly trying to sell people on a particular look, and this can make viewers feel depressed about their current self-image. In one experimental study, ads focusing on appearance were shown to produce an immediate negative effect on the self-image of undergraduate female subjects. At best, the media are giving women mixed messages, telling them to try a rich recipe, for example, and in the same magazine including an article on how to get rid of that "disgusting" cellulite. Ultimately, what women are hearing is that their self-esteem comes from the way they look, while other values that go into each person's uniqueness take a distant second place. The feminist movement also has suggested that judging females by appearance alone is a means of controlling women in a male-dominated society. Because men feel threatened by women who want equal salaries and competitive jobs, they put women down for their appearance to make them feel less welcome in the workplace and other venues.

Social worker Carol Bloom, the author of *Eating Problems: A Feminist Psychoanalytic Treatment Model,* notes that while women are hardest hit, men and children are being increasingly affected: "The sociological trends are that we need new markets now to exploit. As long as products are being sold that have to do with image, you are going to have people in this very bizarre relationship to their bodies. They are going to try to transform their outer selves so that they can accomplish these culturally sanctioned goals about human identity. Women are the grossest example of this—as long as self-esteem and identity are tied together, women will be trying to get control over their food and their bodies so that they can gain acceptability."

Clothes Make the Mind-Set

Not only can ads and models be demoralizing, but so can a lot of the clothing being sold today. If you look around a "juniors" department, where teenagers and young women traditionally have shopped, you'll notice that much of what's available is extremely flimsy and skimpy— even more so than during the miniskirt era—so that any young woman with even the slightest bit of extra padding is going to feel self-conscious in a lot of the garments. Reports one parent of a teenager: "The skirts available are either very long, as in evening wear, or very short, as in women-of-the-night wear, with no easy-to-move-around-in middle ground. If a girl wants a comfortable dress to wear to school, forget it."

The next size category up, "misses" clothing, also offers women a lot of body-baring items, such as cropped or tank tops and garments made out of stretchy or thin material. Some fashion writers feel that this trend is a result of clothing manufacturers trying to cut costs; it's cheaper to use thin material and less of it. In addition, by relying on stretchy synthetic material rather than something like linen, the manufacturer can get away with offering only a few sizes of an item—small, medium, and large—rather than a more extensive collection of numbered sizes. Whatever the reason, the fashion trends today are not kind to women looking for clothes that are forgiving to a less-than-perfect body. Says one person connected with the fashion industry: "You currently have a lot of women going around feeling bad because they look bad in clothes. It never occurs to them that the problem is the shoddy clothes!"

Even children's departments are selling a lot of skimpy, "sexy"-type clothing for little girls. Parents report having to resort to catalog shopping, particularly from European catalogs, for functional and appropriate clothing for girls and teenagers.

A Hundred Years of Hating Our Bodies

When did the obsession with slimness start? Peter N. Stearns, author of *Fat History: Bodies and Beauty in the Modern West,* has studied the history of dieting in Western nations and traces it to the 1890s, when fashion began to dictate the desirability of slenderness (although the meaning of "slim" then would seem heavy by comparison with today's standards). As corsets went out of fashion and women's clothing began to reveal more of the body's natural shape, the premium on slenderness grew. Each decade has seen some oscillations in the ideal, although the overall trend has been toward a greater exposure of the body and greater thinness. While women have been affected most by fashion's dictates, in recent years men's fashions have emphasized a move in this direction as well.

Further pressure to lose weight began in the 1940s and 1950s, when the connection between cardiovascular disease and weight became more apparent and family physicians started to urge their overweight patients to go on diets. Ongoing studies correlating obesity with illness and with shorter life expectancy have resulted in doctors and insurance companies prodding people toward the goal of leanness.

The problem is, meeting rigid weight requirements in Western societies, where food is plentiful and of central importance in so many situations, is no easy task. As Stearns notes: "Modern American history, in this area, is something of a civil war between injunctions for dieting, which lots of people take seriously on the one hand, and the increasingly available attractive presentations of food on the other. And food often wins."

The French, who also place an emphasis on being small and who have the same love of food, have been more successful in keeping their relationship to food healthy, possibly due to a difference in outlook. In America, being overweight has moral implications, while in France it does not. As Stearns explains, "Overweight people are not seen as merely unhealthy or even unattractive, though they are seen this way, but also as somehow immoral." In this country, weight is taken to be indicative of a flawed character, one characterized by laziness, lack of self-discipline, or slovenliness. Sadly, for many men and women, this belief may become a self-fulfilling prophecy. It has other unfortunate consequences as well. Stearns elaborates: "Various campaigns at different points in time have tried to exclude overweight people from certain job categories, partly on grounds that they were health risks, but more on grounds that they had bad character, that the weight was something that was an index of flaws that would carry over into work."

Ruth Raymond Thone, author of *Fat: A Fate Worse Than Death*, asserts that if you're a fat woman in America, you are essentially a second-class citizen: "Studies show that women do not get hired, do not get promoted, do not get grants. . . . There's a prejudice against women who do not fit whatever the current description of attractive is. And it does mean sexually attractive. The other thing is people feel free to come up to you and say, 'Look at that tummy. Don't you think you better do something about that?' People say terrible things to large women."

Thone talks about her own struggle to live up to American standards of beauty and how far she and other women will go to meet the cultural ideal of attractiveness. She says that for most of her life she did feel attractive, but only because she managed to stay thin by chronically dieting. Dieting, it seemed, was automatically part of a woman's life. "What I have done and what women do is very, very destructive to health, and, in fact, sometimes results in death, as you will find with anorexia and bulimia."

Thone recalls the time a doctor told her that she needed to quit smoking. "I stopped for two weeks and started to gain weight. So I immediately went back to smoking. That is blatantly a choice to die of either lung cancer or emphysema rather than be heavy. That's a really stupid choice. But it's a clear choice that millions of women make every day. Stomach stapling, jaw wiring, surgery that's conducted on faces and bodies—there's a lot of life-threatening stuff that goes on in the name of what you look like. So it's a life-and-death issue for women. It's a huge issue that I don't believe will be over in my lifetime. In fact, I think it's getting worse."

For many, being overweight in our society clearly becomes a paramount concern and a significant source of worry. Some find that this fear makes the task of losing weight too overwhelming even to begin, while for others it creates a willingness to take extreme measures. Stearns and others concerned with the issue wonder if whether a change in the way doctors, insurance companies, and the media approach weight loss might be helpful.

Says Stearns: "I think there are at least two obvious suggestions. One would be to encourage doctors and insurance experts to get their act together and push more realistic models of body types. Some doctors will come out saying that adherence to the most rigorous weight standards does not demonstrably improve health, that oscillation in weight is possibly more dangerous than a certain degree of overweight. I think most people hear diversity of opinion from medical and insurance sources, and the easiest voices to spot are the ones that say 'Just get the weight off. If you're ten pounds under your desired weight you'll be healthier.' I don't deny the possibility that that's scientifically true, but I think in terms of human impact it's proving counterproductive. It makes the game seem too difficult while keeping the pressure on.

"The second source would be the media. A larger array of body types in the media should be seen as effective and desirable. Unfortunately, television and the movies compound the problem by the fact that these media add ten pounds to the frame, so that even to look normal actual stars have to be pretty damn skinny. Again, if we eased up here, if we simply applied the message that we like to apply in other respects—that is, a welcoming of diversity—we might see a certain relaxation of the pressure. Whether we would choose to do this, given our fascination with these types and our insistence that our role models be particularly thin . . . I really don't know."

Eating Disorders in the Gay Community

While in the heterosexual world women are the most profoundly affected by body-image disturbances and eating disorders, the opposite appears to be true in the gay community, reports Dawn Atkins, author of *Looking Queer: Body Image* and founder of the Body Image Task Force, a group with a mission to educate people on dieting, eating disorders, and appearance discrimination. Atkins speculates on the complexity of the problem: "Before coming out, before coming to accept their sexuality, lesbian and bisexual women probably have higher rates of eating disorders or at least rates as high as the general population. They're raised in the same culture with the same messages that all other women get. And it might be more so because of their insecurities around their sense of identity. If you're feeling insecure about your sexuality, you're going to feel insecure about your body. But once they've come to some sort of resolution with who they are sexually, they're more likely to come to some sort of resolution around their body.

"Gay men, unfortunately, from what I've seen, are usually worse off after coming out. At this point in time, gay men's culture has taken on some of the worst aspects of 'looksism.' . . . In some ways it's worse than straight women or at least on par with them. They not only have to look good for their partner (with a very narrow ideal of what looking good means), but they're expected to want someone who looks like a particular stereotype and to be that stereotype in order to be wanted."

Atkins attributes the problem to the internalization of homophobia in our society. Men, believing that gay means less masculine, feel the need to look like he-men so as not to be labeled effeminate. In addition, gay men have fewer opportunities for meeting socially than do heterosexuals. A primary place for socializing is the gay bar, where meeting people is based on looks, not substance. In contrast, straight people have more occasions in everyday life, outside of bar scenes, for meeting potential partners—through church or work, for example, where people have more of a chance to get to know each other. Finally, AIDS has complicated the problem, in that a particular look signifies health, regardless of whether the person is truly healthy or not.

ANOREXIA AND BULIMIA

It appears that almost everybody in America—regardless of race, ethnic background, class, or income—wants to be slim. When this desire becomes an overriding obsession with achieving bone thinness, it can translate into the distorted eating patterns of anorexia or bulimia. Estimates of the scope of these disorders necessarily involve guesswork, but some say that more than 35 percent of American women and over 75 percent of American teenage girls have at least flirted with either bulimia or anorexia. The incidence among males has not been adequately studied, but it appears to be rising.

Anorexia nervosa is a condition of self-induced starvation tied in to a fear of becoming fat, poor body image, mental stress, and biochemical imbalances. A person loses a minimum of 20 percent of her or his body weight and still perceives her- or himself as fat. Every pound lost is seen as a victory and gives the person a feeling of greater control over his or her life.

The effects of anorexia go far beyond a person's looking emaciated. Starvation, whether involuntary or self-inflicted, affects mental function, so that the person can no longer think clearly. This does not help the person deal with or comprehend the seriousness of the physical problems that develop. These include fatigue, loss of menstruation, constipation, and hormonal changes, including increased levels of cortisol, the stress hormone. One of the many problems of this progressive condition is that when the person's electrolyte balance, particularly in relation to sodium and potassium, becomes disturbed, it can lead to life-threatening complications, including kidney failure, heart rhythm abnormalities, and cardiac arrest.

Bulimia nervosa, which describes a binge-purge cycle, is not as obvious a disorder as anorexia. Here a person eats uncontrollably and then purges the food in one of several ways. She or he may vomit; take laxatives, purgatives, diuretics, or enemas; sit in a sauna; or even cover her- or himself in plastic wrap. Whatever the method, the goal is the same: to avoid the consequence of eating too many calories. After a person takes several laxatives a day—and in rare instances as many as 100—over a period of time, the body loses its ability to eliminate on its own. Other serious medical consequences of bulimia include loss of tooth enamel and tooth decay, rupturing of the esophagus and stomach, throat muscle enlargement, dehydration, low blood sugar, and personality changes. As with anorexia, bulimia can result in severe chemical imbalances, leading to abnormal heart rhythms and even death.

Physiological/Biochemical Roots

Are there physical and chemical imbalances that predispose us toward anorexia or bulimia? Many researchers think so.

The Zinc Link. The relationship between eating disorders and zinc deficiency was initially discovered in the 1930s, when animals experimentally placed on diets missing only this mineral developed anorexia (a word that, by itself, simply means lack of appetite). More recently, zinc deficiencies have been associated with three types of eating disorders in humans: morbid obesity, anorexia nervosa, and bulimia. In the first instance, an inverse relationship has been noted between obesity and zinc.

In other words, on average, the more overweight the obese individual, the less zinc he or she has in his system. Anorexics and bulimics are almost always zinc-deficient as well. Zinc is one of the most important minerals for overall good health, and is essential for a healthy immune system.

Zinc deficiency seems to be both symptomatic and causative of eating disorders, which means that a vicious cycle of increasing zinc deficiency can result. Individuals prone to eating disorders are often anxiety ridden, and zinc diminishes during periods of psychological stress. Once lost, it is hard to replace sufficient amounts of this essential nutrient. Add to that a lack of nutrients from purging or starvation and you see the magnitude of the problem.

Once zinc is lost, various symptoms arise as a result of the body's attempt to replace it. For example, in the anorexic individual, the body will leach zinc from muscle tissue in its struggle to survive. This results in a devastating symptom of the illness—muscle wasting. If the heart muscle is attacked, any number of heart conditions, and even death, can result. It is also important to note that research studies correlate low zinc levels in eating-disorder patients with lowered rates of treatment success. The crucial relationship between zinc and eating disorders also may explain why more women suffer from these disorders than men. As this nutrient is essential to sperm development, males have high concentrations of zinc in their prostate gland.

The positive aspect of the zinc link to eating disorders is that a majority of individuals with these disorders respond to a simple solution— the addition of liquid zinc to the diet. Prominent eating disorders researcher Dr. Alexander Schauss, of Tacoma, Washington, is part of a research team that has carefully studied the zinc–eating-disorder connection for years. In the following case history, Schauss illustrates why he is convinced of the value of this nutrient in the treatment of bulimia:

"We were doing blinded studies, which means that neither I nor the patient were aware of whether they were receiving a placebo or liquid zinc. [One of our subjects] was a forty-seven-year-old psychotherapist with a doctoral degree in psychology who had been treating patients with eating disorders for the past fifteen years and who herself had bulimia—about five binge-purge episodes per day for the past thirty-four years. She could hardly recount a single day in the last thirty-four years when she did not engage in bulimic activity. She was referred to us by a local hospital because of a particular risk factor for chronic bulimia—the esophageal flap can tear and result in a person choking to death.

"We give a small amount (about 5 or 10 milliliters [ml], which is less than a tablespoon) of liquid zinc to a person, ask them to swirl it around the mouth for a few seconds and tell us what they taste. The inability to detect any taste is evidence of a systemic zinc deficiency. [This woman] couldn't taste anything. The protocol consisted of giving her 120 ml of the solution spaced throughout the day in 30- to 40-ml doses on an empty stomach.

"A few days later the woman called back to say that she had no desire to binge or purge that day. It was the first time she could recall feeling that way in thirty-four years. This was very interesting to us. When you've engaged in an obsessive/compulsive behavior for thirty-four years, you have to wonder how it would be possible for it to disappear in a few days.

"It has been five years now, and she has never gone back to bingeing and purging. More important, she was provided no therapy. This is very similar to the experience of hundreds of bulimics that we've studied. We're quite convinced that it was the liquid zinc that was effective."

Why *liquid* zinc? Individuals with eating disorders usually have a difficult time absorbing the nutrient any other way. This is because zinc in powder, tablet, or capsule form must first be absorbed by the small intestine before it can do any good. And if the zinc is combined with another element (as it is in zinc sulfate, gluconate, or picolinate, for example), first the complex has to be broken down in the stomach to liberate the zinc, then it must be absorbed by the small intestine. People with eating disorders usually have digestive difficulties; therefore, these products are relatively useless. Liquid zinc, on the other hand, will bypass the stomach and small intestine and directly enter the blood and liver. Once the liver recognizes zinc's presence, a positive chain of events will be set into motion.

It may take some time, anywhere from three days to three weeks, before the effects of liquid zinc are seen. This is because zinc depends on a protein carrier, and it generally takes several days for zinc to facilitate its production. Once the protein carrier is synthesized, zinc is transported to where it needs to go. The nutrient begins to saturate brain tissue and effect a positive shift in perceptions. As zinc is involved in over 200 enzyme reactions in the brain, this influx begins to correct the underlying mechanisms that contribute to the eating disorder.

Schauss is not the only researcher to praise the benefits of liquid zinc. Its value has been confirmed worldwide in several studies performed since the 1980s. Placebo-controlled, double-blind experiments do confirm that most eating-disorder patients are zinc-deficient and that administering liquid zinc is highly beneficial. Further, five years after initial treatment with liquid zinc, follow-up studies find that nearly 65 percent of bulimics and 85 percent of anorexics remain fully recovered. Additionally, liquid zinc has been correlated with mood improvement. The latter findings have implications not just for people with eating disorders but for a wider population with mental health concerns.

Clearly then, liquid zinc should be a first line of defense in any eating disorders program. Available in the United States since 1984, the product is safe, effective, and easy to use. A problem, however, is that most eating-disorder treatment facilities have been slow to recognize zinc's importance. This is unfortunate for a number of reasons, including financial ones. Institutional costs of programs that combat eating disorders can add up to nearly $30,000 a month. By contrast, liquid zinc costs $2 to $5 a day and promises good results.

It should be remembered that, even if you don't have an eating disorder, zinc is an important nutrient for appetite regulation as well as for bolstering the immune system and maintaining optimum skin condition. Some good food sources of this mineral include wheat germ, lima beans, lentils, almonds, split peas, tuna, and pumpkin seeds.

Searching for Serotonin. Dr. Leo Galland, an internist practicing integrated medicine in New York City and author of *The Four Pillars of Healing,* reports a possible relationship between bulimia and the hormone serotonin. Specifically, carbohydrate cravings in bulimics may represent an attempt to build serotonin levels in the brain. "Serotonin depletion is associated with depression," notes Dr. Galland, "and bulimics tend to have a terrible self-image. Physiological and psychological factors feed into each other continuously."

Galland adds that bulimia is also associated with food allergies brought on by cravings for endorphin-producing foods. Bulimic individuals appear to require high levels of beta endorphins, substances released from the pancreas when insulin is produced. Often they crave foods that create an endorphinlike effect—dairy products, wheat, and sugar, for example. Bulimic people become addicted to these substances and develop food allergies.

In Galland's practice, treatment for bulimia includes removal of these druglike foods and addition of supplements, such as 5-hydroxytryptophane or tryptophane taken at night to increase serotonin, chromium to help overcome hypoglycemia, and the amino acid DL-phenylalanine during the day to slow down the body's breakdown of endorphins.

Mineral Deficiency Alert. Not surprisingly, people with anorexia and bulimia have a suboptimal supply of a long list of nutrients. This is due to both a lack of nutritional intake as well as to digestive problems that routinely develop. Ironically, the first to go are often the minerals that are not only essential for good health but necessary to keep our bodies naturally thin. The following list describes some of the important minerals, other than zinc, that are commonly lost and their effects on the body.

- Calcium loss can add a complication to eating disorders—a loss of bone density that eventually can cause osteoporosis. Furthermore, since calcium is a natural tranquilizer, not having enough of it can lead to nervousness, irritability, insomnia, and depression.

- Chromium has been found to help remove excess fat from the blood. When there is a chromium deficiency, fat is not removed adequately, and atherosclerosis can develop. In addition, the liver becomes unable to make lecithin, which is needed to break down cholesterol. Not only will cholesterol levels remain high, but fatigue, overweight, and premature aging can result. The adrenal glands suffer as well, making it more difficult to cope with stress. And as if these problems were not bad enough, with chromium deficiency the immune system easily wears down and sickness is more frequent.

- Iodine is needed to stimulate the thyroid, which, in turn, keeps the metabolic rate up so that calories can be burned efficiently. Iodine also is needed to make the hormone thyroxine, which is needed for childhood growth and the maintenance of healthy adult tissue, resistance to infection, cholesterol level control, and protection from heart disease.

- Magnesium, found in dark, leafy vegetables and whole grains, has a calming effect on the nerves. A range of digestive processes depend on magnesium; a lack of this mineral is associated with many symptoms experienced by those with eating disorders—vomiting, indigestion, flatulence, abdominal pain, cramps, and constipation.

- Manganese is needed by the brain and nerves to protect against mental disorders. In addition, it keeps the blood sugar in balance and is important for fat metabolism. This trace mineral also plays a major role in protection against cancer, neuromuscular diseases such as Parkinson's, and other degenerative illnesses. One such disease, lupus, usually attacks young women, the same group most likely to develop eating disorders.

- Potassium assists iodine in the creation of thyroid hormones, needed to increase metabolism and regulate glucose metabolism. Potassium is needed by the muscles, nerves, and brain cells.

- Selenium is an antioxidant that protects against degenerative diseases, such as cancer and heart disease. In addition, selenium stimulates the immune system to protect against bacteria and viruses. It is vital to eyesight and needed to keep the blood sugar balanced.

As you can see, inadequate amounts of even one mineral can have serious consequences. That's why, for individuals with eating disorders, a complete nutritional workup is vital to address mineral needs. Treatment programs should always include concentrated sources of minerals, such as those found in sea vegetables, including dulse, kelp, sea palm, and nori. Such foods are excellent aids for overcoming malnutrition. For people not yet able to eat solid food, pieces of seaweed can be added to soup. Other sources of condensed minerals are the so-called superfoods, such as spirulina, blue-green algae, barley grass, and alfalfa. Just a small amount added to water or juice will replenish missing nutrients. These foods are easy for people with eating disorders to digest, and when taken with liquids they help to rehydrate the person, which is important because people with eating disorders often are dehydrated without realizing it. In addition, the superfoods are low in calories and therefore nonthreatening to the recovering individual.

Carbohydrate Intolerance. Advocates of high-protein diets talk a lot about carbohydrate intolerance, and I want to elucidate the reality behind this concept. There are two kinds of carbohydrates—refined carbohydrates, such as simple sugars and white flour, and complex carbohydrates, such as fruits and vegetables in their natural state and whole grains. In all my years of experience, I have never seen anyone with an intolerance to complex carbohydrates, unless you are talking about a specific food allergy. On the other hand, *everyone* has an intolerance to refined carbohydrates because these processed products affect us all adversely. Some people are just more negatively affected by these foods than others, and these are the people who are said to have a true carbohydrate intolerance.

Dr. Shari Lieberman, author of *The Real Vitamin and Mineral Book,* views bulimia as an extreme version of carbohydrate intolerance. Lieberman explains, "If I ask a bulimic, 'Will you binge on bread?' the answer is yes. If I ask, 'Will you binge on cold cereal?' the answer is again yes. If I say, 'Will you binge on beans?' they will reply no. 'Will you binge on a baked potato?' Again, no. . . . This is a person who has far more clarity on her illness than anybody gives her credit for. . . . It is mostly a chemical imbalance and an inability to deal with a very serious blood sugar problem. They can't handle their food."

A key to overcoming bulimia permanently, Lieberman says, is learning to avoid foods that trigger binge episodes. Lieberman has her patients eat complex carbohydrates, such as potatoes and yams, and not eat foods that trigger binges, such as rice cakes, cold cereals, and other highly refined, or processed, carbohydrates. Patients are guided toward other healthful food choices—lentils and beans, for example—and asked to keep a food diary.

Lieberman reports outstanding success and says that many of her patients have been eating normally for ten years. After a time, former bulimics become less carbohydrate-sensitive and can tolerate a piece of bread or a bowl of pasta now and then without losing control. But they must remember to keep these occasions to a minimum to avoid having to start over from square one.

Psychological Roots

As important as physiological factors may be in the genesis and treatment of eating disorders, the psychological component lies at the heart of these conditions. Central questions are how a person sees him- or herself and whether he or she is satisfied with what is seen.

Self-Image/Body Image Disturbances. Many studies have focused on the relationship between body-image disturbances and the onset of eating disorders and have discovered a close connection between the two. Body-image disturbances can be defined as feelings of extreme dissatisfaction with one's appearance that result in an obsession with the way one looks. People with body-image disturbances imagine themselves to look different from the way others see them. They may be rail thin, for example, and picture themselves as being extremely overweight.

Researchers studying body-image disturbances look for factors that lead to eating disorders in the hope of intervening before a problem begins. Dr. J. Kevin Thompson, editor of *Exacting Beauty: Theory, Assessment, and Treatment of Body Image Disturbance,* is one such investigator who has studied the relationship between negative verbal feedback and poor body image. He reports that people with a strong history of having been teased about their appearance are the ones most likely to feel unacceptable and that the onset of body-image problems tends to surface about three years later. Other researchers looking at the impact of negative remarks from parents and peers agree that various degrees of disparaging remarks, from mild teasing to severe criticism, have negative consequences.

Body-image disturbances in women may affect their behavior in various ways. Extreme self-consciousness may cause a woman to cover up areas with presumed deficits, such as the hips or buttocks. Feelings of insecurity may manifest in assurance-seeking behaviors, such as when a woman asks a friend or spouse over and over again such questions as "Does this make me look fat?" Repetitive weighings and mirror checks become a part of her daily routine. There may be a tendency to overreact to benign comments, for instance, "Did you hear about the gym opening up across the street?" Feelings of physical inadequacy may lead to the canceling of planned engagements in order to stay at home. Depression and greater insecurity may result. In extreme instances, a woman may acquire dysmorphic disorder, a disturbance characterized by an obsessive focus on a certain part of the body. The problem can become so severe as to keep the woman housebound.

Men's body-image disturbances are usually different from women's in that while women generally want to be smaller, most men want to be larger and more muscular. Their role models are usually sports greats and musclemen, such as Michael Jordan and Arnold Schwarzenegger. Research on male body image relates the desire to be muscular to the type of teasing that takes place in the locker room. Other research into popular culture may shed some light on future problems. A recent study by Harvard psychiatrist Dr. Harrison Pope showed that a popular doll, or "action figure," played with by boys, G.I. Joe, has gone from a relatively normally proportioned representation of the male body in

1964 to a ridiculously large-muscled figure today. Like the Barbie doll for girls, G.I. Joe and other similar male action figures now embody an ideal that is difficult or impossible to achieve, and it will be interesting to see if there is a rise in the number of young men with eating disorders several years down the line. As of now, it is estimated that up to 10 percent of those suffering from eating disorders are men, although accurate statistics on this population are lacking. For more information on this topic, read *Males with Eating Disorders* by Arnold Anderson or *The Source Book* by Carolyn Costin.

Improving Body Image. Being completely comfortable with one's body is ideal but perhaps not fully possible in a society such as ours, in which people are brought up to have a narrow view of what constitutes beauty. Still, we can take steps to counter the negative messages around us and within. One thing we can work on is self-acceptance—looking in the mirror, for instance, and making positive affirmations about our appearance. Rather than saying to ourselves "You're so fat," we need to treat ourselves the way we would want to be treated by a very good friend.

One method for achieving this is cognitive therapy. In studies using this technique, obese women learned to change their perceptions of themselves. Results suggest that a person's level of self-satisfaction or dissatisfaction need not be dependent on her or his appearance.

Such a program teaches people to desensitize themselves to the part of the body they are having difficulty with. In front of a mirror or in the imagination, they make positive statements about the body site to overshadow the irrational and anxiety-provoking thoughts that usually fill the mind. Another part of the treatment engages people in positive activities, such as working out at the gym or buying a new outfit. Activities are also chosen to show individuals that their fears are greatly exaggerated. A woman who is self-conscious about her shape, for example, may be asked to wear a form-fitting outfit in public so that she can see for herself that no one particularly notices. Such activities help to counter previous avoidance behaviors and, further, help the individual become less egocentric.

The Role of Role Models. Anorexia nervosa was initially blamed on overcontrolling mothers, but this association may be too simplistic. Rather, what seems to be happening, says Carolyn Costin, author of *The Dieting Daughter* and *The Eating Disorder Sourcebook*, is that young girls are watching their mothers obsess about food and weight and following in their footsteps. Costin explains:

> When you have statistics showing that 80 percent of fourth-grade girls are dieting and that 10 or 11 percent of those report that they're vomiting in these diets, you've got to look at what's happening with their role models. A six-year-old in my waiting room said she was really excited to have the chicken pox. I asked her, 'What's so good about that?' and she said, 'It means I won't have any calories.' Kids are little sponges. Her mother was a binge eater seeing me for treatment. She heard her mother say that calories were in food and that calories were bad. So, she learned that part of being female is trying not to have too many calories.

Costin adds that fathers play an important part in their daughters' lives and can do much to prevent body image and dieting problems. First, fathers need to be conscious of what they say about female bodies in the presence of their daughters. Second, they should give their daughters validation by praising them for who they are, not merely for how they look. And finally, fathers need to show interest by spending quality time with their daughters.

Activity Disorder. Just as unhealthy as excessive control of food intake is excessive exercising. While moderate exercise is physically, emotionally, and mentally beneficial, some people jeopardize their health by exercising to the extreme. These people put their lives on hold in order to work out hours a day, even if they're sore, injured, or in pain. One result can be breakdown of muscle tissue. Activity disorder—or an emotional addiction to exercise—affects people who eat normally as well as those with eating disorders. Although there is increasing recognition of this condition, as it is surfacing more and more in our culture, it is not yet an officially classified disorder.

OVERCOMING EATING DISORDERS

Recent studies show that it *is* possible to overcome eating disorders— nearly 76 percent of anorexics fully recovered in one study at the University of California at Los Angeles—and to have a healthy relationship with food once again. Bulimics report full recovery too. But getting to that point takes time, sometimes years, as individuals first need to recognize their problem. Eating disorders are ego syntonic, meaning that patients like the illness or feel ambivalent about it and do not want to give it up. Some anorexics actually will seek treatment because they are *not* losing weight, not because they are harming themselves. The illness is complex, and eating-disorder therapists require great patience to be able to help their clients.

When individuals get to the point of being ready to receive help, some can function as outpatients while others will require around-the-clock inpatient care. The Eating Disorder Academy criteria for inpatient treatment include the following:

- The patient weighs less than 75 percent of normal body weight.
- Electrolytes are unbalanced.
- The patient is unable to control multiple binges and purges each day.
- There is no support system.
- Blood pressure is too low.

The eating-disorder therapist must understand that the individual suffers from feelings of depression and confusion. The act of keeping weight off is an attempt to be perfect and masks a sense of confusion about who the person really is. A good therapist always has to keep in mind that the eating disorder is just a symptom of a deeper underlying problem and that the disorder is, in fact, the patient's way of dealing with that problem. So the therapist may help patients understand how the illness is serving them by asking questions such as "What's good about this? How has it helped you? What are the advantages of it?" Patients need to understand how their sickness serves them, to understand that it helps them to feel special and that it may be a way to deal with anger.

At the same time, eating-disorder patients need to work with nutritionists to become reeducated about healthful foods and serving sizes. Often anorexics think actual healthful servings are way too large and bulimics think they are way too small. Nutritionists also attempt to help anorexics to find "safe" foods that they feel are low in calories and yet contain valuable nutrients, such as egg whites. In addition, people guiding those with eating disorders need to dispel many myths surrounding food. In this fat-phobic culture, for example, people need to learn that all fat is not bad and that, in fact, some fats are essential to good health. Patients also can be guided into good habits by learning to exercise regularly and eat healthfully. But these practices should be approached with the right attitude. A person should exercise because it feels good, improves stamina, and helps memory, not for fear of gaining weight. And people should eat right because it's nutritious and the body needs good food, not to eliminate calories and fat.

To help with the biological components of healing, supplements may be necessary. As mentioned earlier, serotonin and zinc are of primary importance. In addition, many patients are able to successfully replace medications with amino acids, such as phenylalanine and tyrosine, to overcome the depression that so often accompanies these illnesses. The herb St. John's wort has been proven beneficial to that end as well. Tryptophane helps counter sleeping problems and is especially good for bulimics.

Utmost care must be taken to protect patients against further harm. A bulimic who depends on seventy laxatives a day, for instance, can't just stop cold turkey, or severe constipation and edema may result. The eating-disorder therapist will have to guide the person in cutting back on laxatives before completely eliminating them. Another problem is that anorexic patients can develop what is called refeeding edema if food is reintroduced to the system too quickly. This can place undue strain on the heart and result in death. The trained expert will slowly raise calorie levels and carefully monitor patients to make sure their body can handle the stress that comes from increasing food intake.

Toward Full Recovery

Former anorexic and present eating-disorders counselor Carolyn Costin stresses that individuals with eating disorders need to learn the concept of moderation, and feels that programs designed for people with addictions and chemical dependencies can be counterproductive.

"I learned about people who say 'Once bulimic always bulimic.' They think you should go to Overweight Anonymous–type meetings and say, 'Hi, I'm Carolyn, and I'm a recovering bulimic' for the rest of your life. I think that's too much of a self-fulfilling prophecy. . . . Anorexics and bulimics are pretty much all-or-nothing thinkers anyway. They think, 'I'm either perfect or a failure, either fat or thin.'

"I try to get anorexics back to a more positive relationship with food. New studies show that people can fully recover from these illnesses, but it takes a long time, approximately five to eight years. We're talking about becoming recovered, which takes the addiction part out of it. It's different than the twelve-step notion of chemical dependency where you have to admit that you're an addict for the rest of your life."

Recovered bulimic Jane Latimer, author of *Living Binge Free*, would agree. Living with bulimia from the age of eleven until her late twenties, Latimer finally found her way back to total health. The process was one of trial and error in which, at first, attendance at the traditional type of support group meetings taught her to believe that full recovery wasn't possible. However, an inner feeling compelled her to search actively for a way back to normalcy. A turning point in her life came with the discovery of integrative body psychotherapy such as positive guided imagery, an approach she incorporates into her practice to help others on the road to full recovery.

How Families Can Help

Years ago families were blamed when daughters developed eating disorders. Today specialists admit that they don't know what, if anything, families do to cause these illnesses; however, there are ways of responding to the conditions that can help or cause harm.

Trying to take total charge of the person's diet is not generally helpful, according to Judith Brisman, the director of the Eating Disorder Resource Center in Manhattan and coauthor of *Surviving an Eating Disorder: Strategies for Family and Friends.* Brisman says that this is something that should not be attempted, because while the eating-disordered person may comply initially, this can end up being a battle of wills. A mother wants her daughter to stop overeating, for example, and the daughter begins to eat secretly. Such an approach also keeps the person from becoming responsible for her or his own behavior and can create an overdependence on someone else. Brisman notes that giving up control is not easy for family members, and it's an issue she helps them face in counseling sessions. She may ask, for example, "What do you fear if you stop trying to control this?" She advises that it's better to deal with underlying feelings than to try to control a battle while being constantly angry.

What Brisman does advocate is that families take an indirect approach that encourages self-reflection and responsibility: "If your daughter is clearing out the refrigerator, instead of saying 'No, you're not allowed to eat,' you might say 'Look, if you're going to eat, this is your responsibility. Either pay us back for the food or replenish the refrigerator. If that means being late for school, then you will have to pay the consequences.'" Such an approach helps the person with the eating disorder to realize "It's up to me whether I want to eat or not."

Confronting an anorexic individual can be even more difficult, but it must be done. Brisman recommends a three-part process, beginning with the right environment. It's important to sit down together for a talk when you both have time and are feeling calm. You can approach the subject by saying first what you are noticing: "I've noticed that you've lost a lot of weight," you can say, or some words to that effect. The second step is to say how this is affecting you. A sister, for example, might say "I'm really worried about you," or "I'm really worried about this." Third, you want to advise the person to seek professional help. Here you might say "I want you to talk to me about this, and afterward, I want you to get some help," or "Perhaps I can go with you to find a counselor." Again, you're not trying to control the person's eating but to help the person take responsibility for his or her own eating disorder.

It's quite possible that the person with the eating disorder will be in a state of denial. In such a scenario, the family member will have to use leverage. A sister, for instance, might need to say that "I'm going to talk to Mom and Dad if you don't," while parents might have to insist on their going to a professional to decide whether a problem exists or not. It's important for parents to realize that they *do* have the right to insist, Brisman stresses: "I've had parents of little, skinny, ninety-pound fifteen-year-olds say, 'I can't do it. I'm too upset.' Well, you *can* do it. You can literally, with support—whether it's another family member or a friend—or alone, pick up the kid and get them in a car and take them to a professional, even if they're kicking and screaming all the way. You want to be in a position where someone else who's an expert in this is saying 'You know what? There really is a problem. And this is what you need to do.'"

Counseling for an eating disorder is an opportunity for families to grow closer. Rather than focus just on food, the relationship between family members can be explored. Relationships always need to be reevaluated, and a crisis such as this can be the perfect opportunity to explore issues of communication, control, and other problems.

BINGE EATING

We sit down with the intention of having one piece of bread and end up eating the whole loaf. Or we mean to taste only a spoonful of ice cream and find ourselves finishing the container. This loss of control around food is called bingeing. It's an activity usually done in secret, one that generates a tremendous amount of guilt and shame afterward, not to mention a consequent weight gain.

In 1994 the American Psychiatric Association recognized recurrent binge eating as a new type of eating disorder. In its diagnostic manual the group lists binge eating disorder under "Eating disorders not otherwise specified," meaning that more study needs to be done in this field.

The vast majority of people with a binge eating disorder are overweight or obese—approximately 30 percent of obese patients seeking treatment are binge eaters—yet not everyone who is overweight can be classified as having a binge eating disorder. The differences between individuals who have a binge eating disorder and those who are overweight but do not experience a loss of control around food are currently under investigation. It seems that those in the binge eating disorder group often eat for emotional reasons. And researchers are finding an increased psychopathology in the binge eating disorder group. In other words, many times there are other psychiatric disorders, such as major depression and personality disorders.

An important question is whether adherence to rigid diets precedes the onset of a binge eating disorder. For some people who binge, this is indeed the case. (With bulimia nervosa, researchers note, unhealthy or rigid dieting almost always precedes the condition.)

One person for whom dieting led to a binge eating disorder is social worker Carol Bloom, who remembers this of her college days in the 1960s and 1970s: "I was a compulsive eater who was dieting all the time and hating my body. But it was a kind of secret, private experience which was common to most women. At that time, women were always dieting. They were going from bingeing to dieting to bingeing to dieting. We didn't actually have bulimia in those days, and very few people were anorexic. But a lot of women were compulsive overeaters and living this private hell."

As part of a consciousness-raising women's group, Bloom and others came to the realization that they weren't alone in their anguished relationship to food. That's when they decided to stop dieting and get more in tune with their bodies. A feeling of relaxation and acceptance resulted in an end to dieting and bingeing cycles and a natural return to their normal weight. "By letting go of a diet," Bloom says, "by really tuning in to my body's hunger and to satiety, by really questioning and challenging my myths and all my beliefs about what I thought was true about health and feeding and food, I got my eating under control."

Today, as a counselor for people with eating disorders, Bloom urges her clients to give up dieting, which she believes will always end in failure, and to learn to trust in themselves instead. She states, "It has been proven that dieting causes binges. As long as something is based on restriction, psychologically speaking, it's an absolutely natural setup for not being able to do it, for failure, for self-hatred, for becoming alienated from your own body. Most women have dieted their way up to large body sizes. Anything that provides an external regime is going to be part of the problem. You've got to do it from the inside. You've got to make peace with your own desires and needs."

Depression as Both Cause and Effect

Many times people turn to food because they don't feel they have the power to run their lives the way they want. The only thing in their lives over which they feel they have control is what goes into their mouths. Food also carries with it powerful associations from our childhood. If we feel that as children we did not receive the emotional attention we needed from our parents, we look to food for comfort. Of course, as we can never adequately substitute food for love, we feel more depressed when the binge is over.

It is important to get to the root of personal issues if we are going to make any lasting life changes. Before we can successfully change our physical system through exercise and nutrition, we need to reexamine our belief systems. One effective way to do this is through journal writing.

Binge Journals

Psychotherapist Jane Latimer helps her patients control binges by getting in touch with the feelings that spark them and then redirecting that energy: "I always say, instead of going to the kitchen, sit down in a comfortable chair and feel what's happening to you. And you'll feel that in your body. Usually what's felt is a high level of anxiety. It's kind of a panicky place. And that's where the eating comes from. If I'm able to get people to stay away from the food so they can feel that panic, then they can start writing. That's where a binge journal is very, very powerful. Then they are able to start making connections between those feelings of panic underneath. And maybe that's where the childhood wounding is."

Latimer adds that, frequently, obese patients are eating to cover a sense of vulnerability: "Sometimes it has to do with sexual abuse. Other times there's a feeling that it's not safe to feel attractive in one's body. Or there's a sense of fragility or vulnerability that they don't want to have. The weight makes them feel strong and grounded. And that's a lot of the reason why people will not take the weight off and keep it off." Again, a journal can be a powerful tool in breaking a behavior pattern by enabling a person to stop, right in the middle of the behavior, and think about why it's happening.

Chapter 5

False Promises— and True Ones

New diet programs are always surfacing, with advocates of each different technique assuring consumers that their plan is the key to weight-loss success. Many programs gain popularity because they promise to help you lose a lot of weight quickly. Others take a more sensible approach, guaranteeing the loss of a pound or two weekly. But as just about anyone who has ever dieted knows, for the majority of people most of these approaches don't work. They may give the illusion of success at first, but in the long run the pounds come back and the diet regimen itself can be damaging to both the body and spirit.

WHY THE TRADITIONAL DIET IS DOOMED

The problem with most weight-loss programs is that they encourage us to curb calories in an attempt to lose weight through what is essentially starvation. Unfortunately, all this approach does is trigger a hunger mechanism located in the hypothalamus of the brain. This center regulates weight much like a thermostat in that it is set to the level of fat it has become used to and strives to maintain it. That level is what is known as the setpoint. If your body is used to being 150 pounds and you then lose 10 pounds through dieting, your internal thermostat is going to become activated to return you to your established setpoint of 150 pounds. The body does this by sending out signals to eat.

Feelings of hunger can become overpowering, causing cravings for forbidden foods that lead to bingeing. This happens with each new diet attempt and often leads to a vicious cycle, the end result of which is that more weight is gained than lost. You may initially lose five pounds, for instance, only to gain ten back. Very few people can spend the rest of their lives fighting their appetite. In the end, restrictive weight-loss programs are nothing more than the bait that lures people into the destructive cycle of Yo-Yo dieting.

Other diets promote a high-protein, no-carbohydrate intake. Although calories are not restricted, you are still eliminating an entire food group, and this imbalance leads to carbohydrate cravings. Mood swings, depression, and fatigue often go along with these cravings, and we usually opt for the less-healthful type of carbohydrate to satisfy them, reaching for the white flour and refined sugar products, which ultimately results in weight gain.

The no-carbohydrate approach to losing weight can also pose a danger to your health, because of the excessive consumption of animal protein. These programs overtax the body's organs of detoxification, specifically the liver and kidneys, which struggle to deal with the growth stimulating hormones, antibiotics, and other chemicals found in meat and dairy products. Also, because the digestion of animal protein requires large amounts of water, this type of program has a diuretic effect and can dehydrate the dieter. People do lose weight, but this is often due mainly to water loss rather than to healthy fat-burning. And as with any restrictive diet, the results are usually temporary.

Dr. Dallas Clouatre an esteemed alternative physician and a critic of high-protein diets, elaborates: "You should be suspicious of any diet that causes you to lose four or five pounds in a week, because no human body can sustain that. Typically you can only lose this amount of weight if most of it is water. A pound of fat is about 3,500 calories, and most people will, under ordinary circumstances, consume roughly 2,000 calories a day. If you starve yourself for a few days you may eliminate enough calories to equal roughly a pound of fat. But it simply isn't possible to rid yourself of more than a pound of actual fat a week. Given the way the body functions, you can't burn enough calories in order to do this."

Dieting also has a psychological downside that can set off an entire cycle of negative effects. As author and diet expert Jane Hirshman puts it: "Diets also make people obsessive about the foods forbidden to them. Cake can become the center of your life if you're denied it. Diets make people depressed because they don't work, leading the dieter to think there's something wrong with him or her." The end result is that diets end up making people fatter because they create a deprivation-binge syndrome. Hirshman asserts, "Dieting is very dangerous to your health—your psychological health as well as your physical well-being."

The Individuality Element

Another problem with traditional diets is their assumption that all people are biochemically equal. Traditional weight-loss programs fail to address various imbalances and sensitivities that contribute to overweight conditions and obesity. As we explained in Chapter 2, nutritional deficiencies, food allergies, and candida prompt overeating and, at best, limit a diet's effectiveness.

Our Prehistoric Ancestors, Ourselves

One reason why diets that limit caloric intake result in weight gain has to do with our genetic link to the past. For our prehistoric ancestors, losing weight was potentially lethal because, living in the wild, they never knew when they would have their next meal. When food was scarce, only the fittest survived, and they were the ones who were better able to conserve energy by slowing down their metabolism.

This survival mechanism has been passed down and is still at work today, which is why dieting makes it harder to lose weight. We are predisposed to deal with threatened famine or limited caloric intake by burning our fat stores slowly in order to maintain our baseline weight as long as possible. Combine this with another holdover from prehistoric times—our urge to gorge ourselves whenever food becomes available—and you can see why so many of us are overweight. These days most of us certainly aren't threatened by famine, but we're still eating like cave people! Thus calorie-counting diet plans where we starve ourselves in order to lose weight actually work *against* us rather than for us.

THE PROBLEMS WITH PILLS

Although weight-loss medications originally were designed as a temporary adjunct to be used along with diet and lifestyle changes, our desire for a simple solution has resulted in their serious misuse and overuse. Even people looking to lose only a few pounds have no problem obtaining prescriptions for pharmaceuticals. If one doctor refuses to write a prescription, another doctor surely will. This was evidenced in the mid-1990s, when the phenomenally popular appetite suppressant drug combination known as fen-phen (fenfluramine-phentermine) was being dispensed, in the United States alone, at the rate of nearly 20 million pills a year. The fen-phen fest came to an abrupt end, however, when the *New England Journal of Medicine* found its use to be associated with valvular heart disease. Wyeth-Ayers Laboratories, the manufacturer of diet drugs containing these compounds, which were sold under the brand names Redux and Pondimin, voluntarily removed them from the market.

Valvular heart disease is a serious disorder. The damaged heart valve fails to open or close properly, causing a backward blood flow. This can result in blood pressure and circulatory changes, an unsteady heartbeat, and ultimately even heart failure. Weight-loss medications containing fen-phen also have been linked to pulmonary hypertension, a condition in which an abnormally high blood pressure within the arteries and veins of the lungs proves fatal for nearly half of those afflicted.

Recently a new diet drug has replaced fen-phen as the magic bullet for fighting obesity. Orlistat, sold under the brand name Xenical, is sold by prescription only but, like fen-phen, is easily accessible. One company even dispenses the medication over the Internet, where all an interested party has to do is fill out an electronic application. After reviewing the data, the online company's doctor prescribes the drug. Eye-catching advertisements on the World Wide Web help lure new consumers with the promise of obtaining a cure-all that will "solve all their weight loss problems."

Such false promotions and ethically irresponsible drug-dispensing practices directly contradict recommendations from Xenical's manufacturer, Hoffman-LaRoche, that indicate the product should be used only by very obese individuals and only under a doctor's direct supervision. As with all prescribed medications, a physician is needed to monitor patients and be on the lookout for any adverse side effects. Another caveat that some of Xenical's promoters ignore is that no drug alone will cure obesity. Drug therapy is only one component of a weight-loss program that also should include a nutritional makeover, an exercise protocol, and counseling. Otherwise, once the drug is stopped, the excess weight undoubtedly will return. What's more, results from studies contradict some of the grander claims made by some of the drug's proponents. One study showed that after a year on Xenical and a low-calorie diet, patients lost just 5 to 10 percent of their body weight.

Further concern is being expressed by health professionals who worry about yet-to-be-discovered side effects. Digestive upsets are commonly seen, including bloating, flatulence, an oily stool, and diarrhea. However, the treatment is generally well tolerated. Furthermore, as Xenical works by blocking fat absorption, its use is associated with decreased levels of the fat-soluble vitamins—A, D, E, K, and beta-carotene, although such vitamins often remain within the normal range. There is additional concern that people with eating disorders will be attracted to the drug or that adverse effects might occur when Xenical is taken in combination with other drugs.

Considering this drug's limited effectiveness and unknown risks, one would be wise to think long and hard before using Xenical—or any other antiobesity medication, for that matter. For several decades now, obesity drugs have been enthusiastically marketed and later found to be unsafe—diuretics, human chorionic gonadotrophin (HCG), amphetamines; even natural products containing ephedrine and caffeine have all followed this pattern. More are sure to follow, each with new promises. But, if history is any guide, one should always beware of the advertisers' claims.

It should be noted that not all diet drugs are obtained via the legal prescription route—which should be an immediate tip-off to their dangers. Some, such as certain types of amphetamines and cocaine, are obtained illegally, and despite, or perhaps because of, that, they've been extremely popular. In the 1970s and into the 1980s, many people intent on a partying lifestyle used amphetamines as a way of helping them stay up all night and carouse. Some users found that these metabolism-quickening drugs helped them lose weight as well, especially when amphetamine use was combined with a calorie-restricted diet. But this kind of weight-loss approach has terrible side effects. Amphetamines overstimulate the neurons in the brain and disrupt normal brain function, causing people to become emotionally destabilized, in some cases to the point of becoming psychotic. Those with high blood pressure run additional risks, and those combining amphetamines with amyl nitrate, a drug used to enhance sexual pleasure, run even more risks. Today, thankfully, amphetamine abuse has lessened, although it is still around.

Finally, concerning drugs, you should know that "natural" is not always benign. Specifically, Chinese ephedra, also called ma huang, is an ancient herb known as a thermogenic agent. Thermogenic agents increase body temperature, which results in increased calorie burnoff. The herb also may reduce appetite cravings. But as with so many drugs, there are problems. Excessive or improper use may cause nervousness, rapid heartbeat, and other heart irregularities. You would be wise to avoid this herb and should definitely not take it if you are on antidepressants or drugs for high blood pressure, or are pregnant, nursing, or under eighteen years of age.

IF NOT A DIET, OR DRUGS—WHAT?

Rather than look for a "magic" weight-loss remedy, or risk gaining weight on more trendy "Hollywood diets," why not turn to a clinically proven way of healthful eating?

When a person chooses a diet, he or she is never quite certain whether that particular eating program has been proven safe and effective. The person generally bases his or her opinion on word of mouth, what's currently being advertised, the claims made on infomercials or endorsements. But one thing people generally don't do is turn to the scientific literature to see whether this type of eating program has been tested scientifically. As a result, depending on the amount of promotion, the promoter's personality, and the advertising campaign, unhealthy, unproductive diet programs can become national best-sellers and stay at the top of the best-seller list for months or even years because there is no shortage of people desperate for their promise. Then one day someone finally decides to do a careful examination of their protocol and finds out that (a) the diet doesn't sustain a weight loss, or (b) it is toxic. But by the time the message that a diet is ineffective or dangerous gets out, people shrug their shoulders and say, "Oh, well," and look around for the next surefire plan or diet guru on the horizon.

In fact, there has been an amazingly effective, surefire diet around all the time, although you haven't seen it on an infomercial. I'm referring to the vegetarian way of eating. Vegetarianism refers to more than restricting your diet to fruits and vegetables—it's an entire philosophy of eating that encourages us to choose foods that supply us with healing energy and nutrients while avoiding dead foods, such as meat, sugar, and processed carbohydrates. Rather than getting our protein from animal sources, we get it from grains, legumes, nuts, and seeds. In the next section of the book we'll be looking at how a sensible vegetarian—or mostly vegetarian—diet that includes juicing can help you lose weight in a sustainable way when combined with an appropriate exercise program. You'll see the results for yourself when you try it.

But does such an eating program have side effects? The answer is yes—and they're all good. These side effects are the many health benefits of vegetarianism, which have been extensively documented in peer-reviewed scientific literature. People who are not doctors or scientists do not generally read such literature; it's dry and sometimes hard to understand. But it's the gold standard for evaluating dietary recommendations, which is why I've included Appendix D with capsule descriptions of articles supporting vegetarianism as well as some that warn against the high-protein way of eating. Take a look and decide for yourself. But before we move on to the heart of our weight-loss program, let's look at some of the research on vegetarianism, so that you'll understand the basis of my recommendations.

What the Literature Tells Us About Vegetarianism

Consider, for example, the article titled "Rapid Reduction of Serum Cholesterol and Blood Pressure by a Twelve-Day, Very Low Fat, Strictly Vegetarian Diet." Published in the *Journal of the American College of Nutrition* in October 1995, it reports that in a group of 500 people, just twelve days of a vegetarian, very-low-fat diet lowered cholesterol levels an average of 11 percent and blood pressure an average of 6 percent. What's more, men experienced a weight loss averaging 2.5 kilograms (5.5 pounds) and women lost 1 kilogram (over 2 pounds) on this regimen.

A lot of the research conducted on plant-centered eating looks at the lives and health of Seventh-Day Adventists, because this religious group advocates vegetarianism as part of its belief system, and most of its members do abstain from meat. Another article that examines this group appeared in the April 1999 issue of the *Journal of the American College of Nutrition*. In this article, the authors assert that risk factors for two major modern scourges—cardiovascular disease and diabetes—are both lowered by eating in the vegetarian style. Specifically, this study found that Hispanic Seventh-Day Adventists eating a plant-based diet had significantly lower body mass index and waist-to-hip ratios compared to Hispanic Catholic omnivores. (Omnivores are those who include meat in their diets.) The Seventh-Day Adventists also showed significantly lower systolic blood pressure, lower cholesterol and triglycerides, and higher levels of high-density-lipoprotein (HDL) cholesterol (the good kind).

Seventh-Day Adventists were also the subject of a May 1994 article in the *American Journal of Clinical Nutrition*, which reported on a study of almost 28,000 members of their group. While most members are vegetarians, some are not, and this study found that those who ate meat had a significantly higher incidence of hospitalizations and surgeries than did the vegetarian group. In addition, the study found that use of medication was more than double in the nonvegetarian males and increased by 70 to 115 percent in the nonvegetarian females. An omnivorous diet also was associated with an increased prevalence of chronic diseases, including asthma.

In "Vegetable Consumption and Risk of Chronic Disease," a study published in the journal *Epidemiology* in March 1998, the connection between lowered chronic disease rates and plant-based eating was again emphasized. In the research reported on here, over 46,000 individuals were evaluated. Those who ate the most vegetables had appreciably lower risks—compared to those who ate the least vegetables—for a variety of ailments: myocardial infarction, peptic ulcers, angina pectoris, chronic bronchitis, chronic asthma, cirrhosis of the liver, kidney stones, and arthritis.

A review article is one that takes a survey of other literature and makes conclusions based on that wide-ranging view. Because of this methodology, a review article is less likely to be swayed by biases than an article based on one research study only. Such an article appeared in the journal *Digestive Diseases* in the May–June 1994 issue. It said that vegetarians have longer life expectancy and lower incidences of gastrointestinal cancer, gallstones, diverticular disease, and constipation than do meat-eaters and that meat-eating is associated with increased mortality from all causes.

I could go on and on citing studies, but my point should be clear by now: When you use a vegetarian diet to lose weight, chances are very good that you'll be reaping the additional benefits of improved health and longevity. You certainly won't be courting the negative side effects of restrictive fad diets and weight-loss pills.

Besides scientific literature on vegetarianism, one other thing I'd like to share with you is a long list of names of famous vegetarians. I do not intend to imply that because a lot of famous people do something, you should do it too; rather I want to show that this kind of eating is not an exotic or "fringe" fad but a way of life embraced by many people through the ages.

HISTORICAL FIGURES WHO WERE VEGETARIANS

Louisa May Alcott
Buddha
Clara Barton
Jesus Christ
Charles Darwin
Leonardo da Vinci
Thomas Edison
Albert Einstein
Benjamin Franklin
Mahatma Gandhi
John Harvey Kellogg
Mohammed
Ovid
Plato
Pythagoras
Albert Schweitzer
George Bernard Shaw
Mary Shelley
Percy Bysshe Shelley
Upton Sinclair
Socrates
Leo Tolstoy
Lao Tzu
John Wesley

SOME VEGETARIANS OF OUR TIME

Hank Aaron, baseball player

Maxine Andrews, of the Andrews Sisters singers

Bob Barker, TV personality

Kim Basinger, actress

Surya Bonaly, Olympic figure skater

David Bowie, rock musician

Martin Buber, existential philosopher

Roger Brown, football player

Ellen Burstyn, actress

Andreas Cahling, champion bodybuilder

Peter Falk, actor

Henry Heimlich, inventor of the Heimlich maneuver

Dustin Hoffman, actor

Desmond Howard, football player

Mick Jagger, rock musician

Billie Jean King, tennis champion

Marv Levy, coach, Buffalo Bills

Steve Martin, comedian and actor

Michael Medved, film critic

Edwin Moses, Olympic gold medalist in track

Martina Navratilova, tennis champion

Dean Ornish, physician and author

Bill Pearl, four-time Mr. Universe

Phylicia Rashad, actress

Fred Rogers, TV's Mr. Rogers

Rabbi David Rosen, former Chief Rabbi of Ireland

Dave Scott, six-time Ironman triathlon winner

Isaac Bashevis Singer, writer and Nobel Prize winner

Tina Turner, rock singer

Lindsay Wagner, actress

In the next section, after we examine how changing your day-to-day behavior can help you achieve your weight-loss goals, we'll explore how a plant-centered diet enters into the weight-loss equation.

Part 2

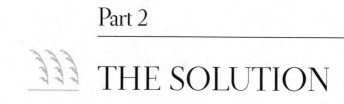

THE SOLUTION

Chapter 6

The Beauty of Behavior Modification

As we discussed in Chapter 5, in our culture the word "diet" has come to signify a pattern of eating that you read about in a magazine, follow for a few weeks, and then quit because the regimen feels too restrictive or doesn't work. The majority of diets ask us to pay close attention to the number of calories or grams of fat we consume, and these are also doomed to failure. One reason is that they are time-consuming, and who needs one more thing to keep track of? Second, such programs are based on the premise that the body is a machine, when in reality it's a miraculous organism responsive to a whole variety of factors, some of which we can't quantify. In beginning our weight-loss program, instead of searching for a panacea, we need to realize that the only time a diet can ever really work is when it is an eating plan that we can live with comfortably every day. In fact, the word "diet" comes from the Latin *diaeta*, which means "a way of life." The best diet, therefore, teaches us new eating behavior—a whole new way of life that feeds our body what it needs and that we can feel comfortable with over the long term.

105

WHAT SHOULD YOU WEIGH, ANYWAY?

Most of us compare our scale readings with the height and weight charts put out by insurance companies. But this is not the best measure of fitness. Because muscle weighs more than fat, it's possible for a fit, muscular athlete to be "overweight" according to the charts and for an individual who is in reality overfat to weigh the "right" amount. Ideally, men's bodies should be composed of between 8 and 14 percent fat, and women should have between 12 and 20 percent. The average man, however, has 15 to 25 percent and the average woman, 22 to 27 percent. To find out where you fit in terms of these body fat ranges, take a painless test called an impedance test. An impedance test is a simple machine that attaches an electrode to your finger or toe. Information about your age, ideal weight, and height are fed into the computer, which then sends a nonperceivable electrical current throughout the body. Based on the feedback from this current as it passes through your bone, body water, muscle, and fat, the computer is able to discern what percentage of your body is lean muscle, fat, and water. You may be surprised by the results—even if you don't look overweight, you may find that you have a higher percentage of body fat than is healthy. Another even simpler "test" that should not be underestimated: Look at yourself nude in a full-length mirror.

If you're still psychologically tied to actual weight measurement as a way of gauging your level of fitness or fatness, you might want to use body mass index (BMI), the latest and most sophisticated chart system. This is now the generally accepted system for detecting obesity levels and their associated health risks in a population. Note that, in addition to the fat-versus-muscle issue, one shortcoming of the system is that it does not take into account how fat is distributed in a person, a factor that may impact our health. Specifically, fat that is concentrated in the abdomen poses a greater health risk than fat that is evenly distributed over the body.

To calculate your BMI, follow this formula: Determine your weight in kilograms (1 kilogram equals roughly 2.2 pounds). Then divide that number by the square of your height in meters (m). If you weigh 75 kilograms, for example, and are 1.85 m in height, your BMI is 23.1.

Then, to see what your final number means, refer to the following chart.

INTERPRETING YOUR BMI

Category	BMI
Underweight	Less than 18.5
Normal	18.5 to 24.9
Overweight	25 or greater
Obese	30 or greater

A WAY OF LIFE FOR EACH DAY OF LIFE

Making the right food choices becomes a matter of developing new habits. As I'm sure you know, it takes time as well as persistence to create a new habit, but the results are well worth the effort. Each time you go to the movies, for example, you may routinely make a dash for the refreshment counter. Stopping that behavior takes conscious effort at first, but in time not eating at the movies will become second nature. Witnessing these changes in yourself is a great confidence-booster and a motivator. "Nothing succeeds like success," the saying goes, and that certainly applies to the realm of dietary improvement.

How can we learn to enjoy healthier foods and eating habits? Simply by exposing ourselves to them—repeatedly. You may be in the habit of adding salt to your meals, for instance, but if you start eating a low-salt diet, in time your taste buds will become accustomed to less salty fare and, in fact, become sensitive to too much salt. Learning to overcome temptations of advertisers and supermarket displays, and surrounding ourselves, instead, with more wholesome choices, consisting of mostly fresh fruits, vegetables, grains, and legumes, is key to staying healthy and slim. This needn't be boring, as many creative recipes teach us how to spice up salad dressings using balsamic vinegar, lemon juice, fresh garlic, cayenne, and other seasonings instead of salt; create enzyme-rich, delicious juices and smoothies from fresh fruits and vegetables; and make baked goods from a variety of non–allergy-producing grains and the herbal sweetener stevia instead of sugar. Chapter 8, on creating your own "recipe revolution," will get you started in this direction.

Staying flexible is very important because the best outcomes are derived from plans that allow room for some variation. Otherwise, you will feel that you need to give up after the slightest deviation. Say you find yourself celebrating a birthday with a piece of cake. Rather than feeling that all is lost and "going off the deep end" by abandoning your new healthful eating plan, you should remain positive and stay focused on your long-term goal.

When you do deviate from your planned intake, it's best, whenever possible, to diverge quantitatively, not qualitatively. In other words, it's better to eat a second helping of whole-grain pasta or air-popped popcorn than to eat any cream-filled pastries or potato chips. And when you're under duress, it's okay to look for comfort foods, as long as you turn to those that offer optimal nourishment. Soups are an especially good choice for their soothing effect on digestion.

Remember, it's only natural to fall back occasionally after making strides forward, so don't let slipups rattle your confidence. Realize that, and then get back on track. Think of your weight-loss program as a process. Even small improvements will help you to reach your goal—one step at a time. After all, isn't the loss of a pound a month better than a pound-a-month gain?

Make It a Family Affair

If you are a parent altering your diet to lose weight, you have the opportunity to help your children at the same time. Since today more than ever, youngsters are running the risk of becoming overweight—one in three American children weighs too much—what could be better than the gift of sound health? This will not only help to prevent or correct many diet-related disorders, including attention deficit disorder and asthma, but it will do much to bolster a child's sense of self-esteem, as overweight children are often shunned by peers and made fun of, experiences that can leave emotional scars well into adulthood.

Children are naturally receptive to proper guidance. In fact, a child's whole world is learning. The earlier good eating habits are acquired, the easier it is. In fact, immediately after birth is the best time to begin because an infant will learn to like whatever foods he or she is given. We all tend to have an innate preference for sweets, but studies have found that babies given a sugar-water solution in the first weeks of life had more of a preference for sugar later on than did children who were not given the solution. As children get a little older, they take longer to develop a liking for certain foods. If you have not constantly included certain foods in children's diet, and then suddenly introduced them to that taste, there's a high probability that they will reject it if it does not mirror the tastes they liked previously. Often it helps to disguise the foods children are rejecting, especially if they are healthful ones. For example, if your child likes bananas but doesn't like carrots, you could puree the carrot into the banana. You can also try creative substitutions. If your child likes potato chips—deep fried, highly salted, refined carbohydrate potato chips—clearly this is not in the child's best interest. However, you might try thinly slicing fresh, organic potatoes, dressing them with a healthful seasoning (like a garlic or onion flavor, turmeric or curry, or cayenne), and then baking them. You would then have something that actually looks and tastes like a regular potato chip but provides much more nutrition. If children like ice cream, switch to a rice dream ice cream, which does not contain dairy or processed sugars and tastes great. The same goes for cheese. Your child may love grilled cheese sandwiches, but wheat bread and American cheese slices are frequently allergenic. Try using spelt bread with 100% dairy free soy American cheese—it provides the smell, the taste, and the feel of a grilled cheese sandwich, but without the overprocessed, highly allergenic components.

Older children, although they may balk at first, are actually fairly open to dietary improvement and can be especially fun to work with.

Children love receiving attention and praise from their parents and can be surprisingly responsible when it comes to following a healthful diet. Make it a game not only to keep each other on track but to find new foods that fit within established guidelines. Youngsters love demonstrating their new knowledge and become especially motivated as food-related ailments vanish and both energy and appearance improve. It may surprise—and even inspire—a parent to learn how positive their children can be.

Take advantage of your child's abundant energy by encouraging him or her to form good exercise habits. In fact, the whole family can play a game of basketball, go bike riding, or take a walk together. Whenever possible, choose active types of recreation. Instead of seeing a movie, go bowling or play miniature golf. If possible, encourage your children to walk to school and accompany them part of the way. You need not spend a lot of time on exercise; even a half hour together each day is a great way to add quality time to your relationship and foster physical health.

TAKE TIME FOR YOUR FOOD

There was once a time when families made time to enjoy meals together. Dining was an experience, something to be savored. It wasn't just food that was appreciated, but everything related to it—the ambience, the conversation, the guests, and the music. Few of us nowadays make mealtime an event. Rather, we squeeze a meal into our day, grabbing a burger at a fast-food restaurant on the way to a meeting, or stopping for pizza on the way home because it's quick and we have Little League practice. Outside activities take precedence over family time.

When we eat on the go, we can't help but overeat. This is because we're not paying attention to our food but just grabbing something and shoving it into our mouths. The pace is so fast we're not giving our body the requisite time to send our brain the I'm-full feeling—a signal that takes about twenty minutes from the beginning of a meal to become operational. Also, our fast-food choices are more likely to have a higher fat, salt, and sugar content than home-cooked fare.

Most people eat until their stomach feels full and pushes against them, until they can't eat anymore. It may be surprising to learn that the stomach holds only a cup or two of food. (One cup will hold about one medium-size apple; you need two cups for a slice of pizza and probably three if you include the crust.) After that the stomach starts to expand like a rubber bag. It will stretch to hold a lot more, but it isn't necessary to have that much to feel satisfied.

One approach to achieving a satisfying feeling of fullness sooner is to eat more slowly in a systematic way. Dr. Nan Katherine Fuchs, a nutritionist from northern California and the author of *Overcoming the Legacy of Overeating*, suggests the following technique: Prepare meals in advance whenever possible, and do not eat the food right away. Rather, the meal should be divided into quarters, and the first quarter should be eaten ten or fifteen minutes after the first twinge of hunger appears. Chewing slowly—twenty-five to thirty chews per bite—will not only make the food last longer, it also will allow us really to taste our food. Moreover, when we thoroughly chew our food, the brain signals us to feel full sooner. Once that quarter portion has been eaten, wait another ten to fifteen minutes, and repeat the process. Fuchs calls this type of eating "grazing" and notes that when we eat slowly, our blood sugar level remains steady, which prevents cravings, and helps optimize concentration, mood, and our overall sense of well-being.

It's important to recognize the sensation of fullness that your body sends you. Since most of us are not used to paying much attention to our body, this may be difficult at first. But once this is an established way of life, it will become second nature. The result: The amount of food you require to be satisfied will be dramatically lessened.

MOVE IT AND LOSE IT

Those who are overweight or overfat may believe that overeating is the cause of their condition. That's the common view. But lack of exercise is a factor that's every bit as culpable. And inactivity doesn't just mean that you burn fewer calories. It causes muscle fibers to decrease in size and to fill up with and become surrounded by fat. This, in turn, diminishes the muscle's ability to burn fat. Metabolism slows down.

The upside of all this is that anyone can decrease his or her body fat by exercising more. A combination of aerobic and anaerobic exercise (see Chapter 11) will increase lean muscle and keep fat deposits from forming. The result is more lean muscle that's better at burning calories. In addition to working out, make some adjustments to your daily routine. Walk instead of ride, whenever possible, and take the stairs instead of the escalator.

When you start exercising, don't be disheartened if you maintain your weight at first or even notice a slight gain. Since muscle weighs more than fat, initial improvement may be seen on your body but not on the scale. Rest assured that you are helping yourself to get rid of intramuscular fat and gaining muscle volume, and let a tape measure and a mirror, not a scale, be your guide.

BIG BREAKFAST, SMALL DINNER

Think of the word "breakfast" as the time to break your overnight fast, and don't fall into the habit of skipping or skimping on the first meal of the day and eating too much at night. Follow the adage "Eat breakfast like a king, lunch like a prince, and supper like a pauper." This way you'll be eating the most in the morning, when your digestive system and metabolism are up and ready to go. With an entire day of activity ahead of you, far more calories will be burned than at night, when your digestive system is preparing to retire.

Another eating pattern that works for some is to eat four to six small meals during the day instead of the conventional three. That helps to distribute calories evenly throughout the day and keep blood sugar levels balanced so that there is less possibility of overeating late in the day and having nighttime cravings. This is a great way to start a weight-loss program. After one or two months, when your body has become used to eating smaller amounts, you can work your way back to just three meals a day.

Snacks should be kept to a minimum, and your choices should be low-calorie fare that wards off hunger. Eating a fruit a half-hour before a meal is a good way to curb cravings. Beware of unhealthful, calorie-laden snacks and the heavy late-night meals that have become easily available with the advent of the twenty-four-hour diner and the all-night supermarket. Also, avoid the strategically located vending machine that has found its way into our workplace, school, shopping mall, and travel environments.

FORGET FAT AND SUGAR

We tend to like fatty foods, more so when those foods contain sugar, like ice cream. One of the reasons that we crave fat is to create a feeling of satiety—fat allows our appetite to feel satisfied. And we all know how addicted Americans are to the energy boost we get from sugar—we guzzle heavily sugared coffee at the office to keep us awake in those long afternoon meetings, or reach for a candy bar when we need a pick-me-up. However, one of the reasons we constantly feel fatigued is—you guessed it—because we eat too much sugar. Sugar depletes the body's natural adrenaline by causing it to be oversecreted, and causes a "Yo-Yo" syndrome in our blood sugar levels. Foods like sodas or candy give us an instantaneous kick for about five minutes, but afterward, our blood sugar level plunges down below what it normally should be, putting us in a low blood sugar state that can continue for an hour or two. We again feel fatigued, so we reach for another round of sugar.

If, however, you eat complex carbohydrates and quality starchy foods, such as rice, beans, nuts, seeds, and legumes, your blood sugar will stay level for most of the day and won't have those severe spikes. If you don't have a big sugar up, you won't have a big sugar down. One way to break the habit of eating fat and sugar is to resolve to eat as little of this fare as we possibly can. Instead of saying "I will eat 30 grams of fat every day," or "I will eat only 10 grams of sugar," you should avoid fatty foods and those with refined sugars altogether. In doing so you will be developing brand-new eating habits that you can live with every day.

The daily consumption of sugar, especially in combination with saturated fats and chemical additives, does more than add pounds; it can have serious health consequences, leading to such problems as cholesterol buildup and coronary heart disease. Sugar is also associated with candidiasis and digestive tract weakness and contributes to tooth decay by creating plaque, on which bacteria thrive. Similarly, sugar exacerbates diabetes by constantly raising the sugar level beyond what the body's normal metabolism can handle. In time, you simply exhaust the pancreas—which secretes digestive enzymes that facilitate digestion and regulate blood sugar levels—by overloading the body with so much sugar that the pancreas cannot compensate. Moreover, sugar is a primary contributor to menstrual irregularities and mood swings and is associated with alcohol abuse. I also feel that problem behaviors in children would lessen if more care were taken to decrease or eliminate sugar in their diet.

As you begin to revise your diet, beware of hidden sugars. Today, to improve taste and boost their sales, manufacturers add sugar to almost everything. On food labels, where ingredients are listed in order of amount, sugar may be listed as the third ingredient. However, the list also may include sucrose, corn syrup, glucose, and fructose, which are all processed sugars and should be avoided at all costs. So when you add it all up, sugar is actually the number-one ingredient. The separate categories mislead unwary consumers into believing that a product contains less sugar than it really does. This is one reason why the consumption of sugar has risen dramatically over the past few decades. The average person eats up to 33 tablespoons of sugar a day, or 150 pounds per year. Too much sugar not only spoils our taste for natural foods; it can deplete the body of essential nutrients, such as zinc and B vitamins. The vegetarian diet that I am advocating here is great for eliminating excess sugar and will give you more energy, less peaks and valleys moodwise, and a greater feeling of satiety.

Another major health threat comes from trans fatty acids, which are in the hydrogenated oils found in everything from baked goods and chips to margarine. Hydrogenation, a process used to increase the shelf life of products, does the reverse to human life. The negative effect occurs at the cellular level, where these harmful fats clog our cell walls. As a result, cellular membranes become less capable of taking in oxygen and nutrients and of eliminating toxins.

When fat begins accumulating in the arterial walls, it acts as an adhesive, collecting other debris, including cholesterol, and bonding it onto the surface. In time, the accumulation begins to limit the amount of blood that's able to flow at a normal pace through the arteries and veins. Then it starts to harden the surface, killing the artery cells, since blood and nutrients are not able to get in through the cell surface to provide nourishment. When people gain weight, their heart needs to beat harder to supply all the excess fat cells with blood. At some point the heart simply will become unable to maintain the output of blood that is demanded of it, particularly if blood flow is restricted by increasingly narrow arteries and blood vessels. At this point, the heart will either develop arrhythmias or undergo an ischemic heart attack.

Commercial oils (corn oil, cottonseed oil, soy oil, and canola oil) sold in supermarkets have the highest percentage of these trans fatty acids, but many vegetable oils from health food stores are not much better. There are problems in both processing and packaging. While health food store oils are superior to supermarket oils in that they're not processed with heavy solvents, they are exposed to oxygen in processing, which creates trans fatty acids. Also, many of these oils are heated to above the safe 118-degree level—up to 500 degrees—thereby creating trans fatty acids. The moment you heat an oil that is unstable at a high temperature, you change its chemical configuration. That can lead to what we call "unhealthy fats."

Most people do not refrigerate their oils. Instead they're left on a stove, generally in a kitchen with some exposure to oven heat. That means that the bottle is subject to high heat, which can cause oxidative damage. Exposure to air also causes oxidative damage, which can turn the oil rancid in a hurry. What's more, 90 percent or more of oils sold today come in clear plastic bottles. Light also has a powerful oxidizing effect, which can result in more trans fatty acids.

It's easy enough not to buy oils in clear containers. But checking for other measures of quality takes a bit more detective work, as even the words "cold-pressed" can be meaningless in an industry where there is no regulatory board to check company claims. If you want to go the extra step and be sure that your oil is all it's supposed to be, write the manufacturer, requesting assays, test results, manufacturing procedures, proof the product is from organic seeds, and evidence that it has been processed under 118 degrees. A legitimate manufacturer will provide a response.

VARIETY'S THE KEY

Trendy diets that ask us to eliminate an entire food group are bound to fail because they create a physiological imbalance that eventually must be rectified. If we completely remove carbohydrates from the diet, for example, sooner or later we will give in to our natural need for carbohydrates and, in all likelihood, reach for the simple sugars found in bagels, pasta, cake, and other refined foods that cause us to gain back every pound we've lost, plus a few more. Also, when we starve ourselves or eat nutrient-deficient foods, our bodies go into a starvation mode and actually start to *conserve* fat; it's part of our innate survival mechanism. By eating a variety of nutritious foods, we ensure that the body does not perceive starvation and that we can experience a normal metabolic rate, which allows for the shedding of extra pounds.

Another advantage of including a variety of wholesome foods in the diet is that doing so helps to keep the body's pH levels balanced. The human body likes to be mostly alkaline, in the approximate ratio of 80 percent alkalinity to 20 percent acidity. Eating too much protein creates an acid state that is associated with poor health; fruits and vegetables, however, are alkaline foods that promote health as well as weight loss. As you restructure your eating habits, be sure to include lots of lemons, green leafy vegetables, carrots, apples, melons, celery, tomatoes, berries, plums, almonds, sesame seeds, seaweeds, asparagus, cabbage, and grapes in your diet. Balancing these complex carbohydrate foods with quality amounts of protein and healthy fats will keep the body in top form. By "quality" protein, I mean protein that does not contain growth stimulating hormones, antibiotics, pesticides, and other toxic residues that can end up in animal protein. Some good examples are tofu; tempeh; nuts, such as soy nuts or sunflower seeds; beans, such as black beans or turtle beans; and grains, such as brown rice.

Lean on Lean Protein

You do need to include some protein in your diet, and one of the best ways to prevent hunger is to have some protein at every meal. Complete protein does not have a high glycemic index (meaning that it does not digest quickly), so when you eat a piece of broiled fish, for example, you slowly release sugar into your bloodstream and maintain insulin stability. Because of the complexity of the molecular structure of amino acids found in protein, it must be broken down slowly by special protein-splitting acids and enzymes. In contrast, when you eat a candy bar, the sugar in the candy bar requires no digestion in the stomach or in the intestine. It is immediately absorbed—in as little as ten minutes—giving you that familiar sugar rush. Digesting quality protein, however, may take anywhere from an hour to five hours, depending on the type of food you eat, how relaxed you are when you consume it, how well you chew it, and how it is prepared.

Proteins are the building blocks of life, and so it is extremely important that they remain in your diet. The building blocks are called amino acids, and eight amino acids are essential for adults. Many of us have been led to believe that only animal sources contain these essential amino acids, but this isn't the case—they can be found in all vegetarian sources. Good sources of lean protein to incorporate into your diet include fish and legumes, especially soybeans and soy products, such as tofu, tempeh, and soy milk. Nuts, grains, and seeds, such as fresh almonds and organic sunflower seeds, are rich in protein too and make excellent midday snacks. Organic eggs are another great protein source.

GET INTO THE ORGANIC HABIT

Food appearance can be deceptive. For instance, you could look at two fields of lettuce, one greener than the other, and conclude that the greener field contained the better lettuce. But the facts could be just the opposite, because the bright green field could have gotten that way through the use of artificial fertilizer, and the lighter-hued field could be filled with organic lettuce that contains more vitamins and minerals than the conventionally grown produce. Numerous studies have shown that organic food does indeed contain more nutrients than its nonorganic counterpart, without the addition of toxic chemicals.

The sad reality is that today, many foods we expect to be fresh are enzyme-dead and robbed of vitamins and minerals thanks to the addition of fungicides, pesticides, and herbicides. Other harmful practices, such as irradiation, long-term storage, canning, freezing, and drying, destroy active enzymes and thus contribute to obesity and its related health problems.

The body requires two types of enzymes: *exogenous* and *indogenous.* Exogenous enzymes are the ones that come from outside of the body, from sources such as fruits, vegetables, grains, seeds, nuts, legumes, and herbs. Each food requires its own specific set of enzymes to be fully and healthfully digested and utilized; therefore, foods that are highly processed and stripped of their enzymes and fiber are more difficult to digest. People who are eating an enzyme-rich diet are almost always going to be losing weight and feeling more energetic, simply because their digestion is working well. If, however, you are eating a highly processed, animal-based diet, you will be relying solely on the enzymes produced by the body (primarily by the liver and the pancreas) to help you digest and process your food. Usually this is not adequate for optimal well-being and leads to an incomplete utilization of the food's nutrients. The unused food may then be deposited in the body's tissue as fat.

Fresh organic foods are extremely important because of their ability to supply our bodies with the vital nutrients needed for a long, healthful life. Most health food stores and more and more supermarkets carry a wide array of organic fruits and vegetables. One good way to start the organic habit is by purchasing organic sprouts or, for just pennies, sprouting organic seeds on your own. Sprouting breaks foods down to their simplest components—proteins become amino acids, fats become fatty acids, and carbohydrates become simple sugars—making them easily digestible. Moreover, these high-quality, low-calorie foods become a nutritional powerhouse through the germination process. A regular chickpea cannot be eaten raw, for example—it has to be cooked. However, a sprouted chickpea *can* be eaten raw, because the sprouting makes it easily digestible. In addition, the vitamin C in a sprouted chickpea will increase eightfold.

Historically, cultures have sprouted foods as a way of enhancing live enzymes and nutrients. In the last thirty years, sprouting has gained great popularity in the United States. Many seeds and herbs can be put into a dish, soaked overnight, drained, put into a bowl with a little cheesecloth over it, twice a day rinsed in a colander, and then put back in the dish. After about three or four days, you will begin to see tiny little sprouts coming out of the seeds. In about five to six days, you have a full bowl of sprouts. Chlorophyll, plentiful in sprouts, is the richest single source of enzymes and the highest-level nutrient that we know of. And believe it or not, calorie for calorie, sprouts give you more protein than steak. By including sprouts in your diet, you are enhancing your overall well-being tremendously. Over thirty different seeds or beans can be sprouted safely and healthfully, and you can juice certain sprouts, such as those from sunflower seeds. Sprouts add variety to salads and casseroles, and are very high on my daily must-eat list.

One word of caution: There have been recent reports of salmonella found in sprouts, due either to contaminated seeds or contaminated water used in growing. Be sure to rinse your sprouts, as well as all other fresh foods, before eating.

EAT A LOT—AND LOSE

Most of us view dieting as a test of will. We struggle to see how long we can go without eating, cut back on portion sizes, and feel guilty after every bite. Contrary to what we've been taught, though, there is no reason we shouldn't eat a lot. Eating is a part of our nature, not something to fear. In other cultures—Asian and Mediterranean ones, for example—people are just as involved with food as we are, if not more so, and yet they're significantly slimmer. Yes, people in these cultures tend to be less sedentary than we are, but something else comes into play, and it's the type of food being eaten.

You actually can increase your food intake and get slimmer at the same time if you choose the correct foods. The key is to adjust your diet so that you get the most value for your calorie. This means cutting back on or eliminating fatty animal proteins and refined carbohydrates, on foods that contain no fiber or phytochemicals, and making room for more fruits and vegetables.

Fiber, of which we need thirty to fifty grams per day, comes in two forms, soluble and insoluble. Soluble fibers are those that actually can go into the bloodstream; insoluble fibers are too large to penetrate the cell wall of the intestine and, therefore, remain there and act as a natural cleanser. Fruit fibers are very soft while grain and legume fibers are stronger. Grain fibers hold more water and thus can clear more debris out of the intestine. So you need to have a combination of nut, seed, bean, and fruit and vegetable fibers in your diet.

The term "phytochemical" refers to a plant-based chemical. Any given fruit or vegetable can contain 150 or more different chemicals that play an important part in maintaining human health. Some phytochemicals help protect us from cancer, others help stop viral infection, others attack bacteria, others protect us from the effects of radiation, while still others repair damage to our DNA. Many Americans are sick, overweight, and unhealthy because their diet is completely lacking in phytochemicals and healthy fibers.

Dr. Joel Furhman, a physician specializing in nutritional medicine, elaborates: "If the average American male, who consumes 2,400 calories on average, were to eat like a gorilla, he'd be consuming over 20 pounds of leaves a day, because green leafy vegetables are only about 100 calories per pound. Since the human stomach is only designed to hold a liter, you wouldn't even be able to fit this much food into it all at once, and you'd be chewing and eating all day long, getting lots of phytochemicals, vitamins, minerals, and essential fatty acids. Such a diet would be nutrient-dense but low in calories, the ideal for anyone trying to lose weight."

This, of course, is an extreme example. You wouldn't want to eat one food all day long. Nor would you want to eat that much food. The point is that you can eat more, fill up, feel satisfied, and still lose weight if you eat the right foods. In the process, you will transform an overweight, malnourished body into one that is leaner, stronger, and healthier.

So what should you eat more of? Choose carbohydrates with a low glycemic index—that is, those that are digested more slowly and won't rapidly increase your blood sugar levels—or those with more water and less starch. In fact, you can eat as much of the following low-glycemic, low-starch foods as you want:

LOW-GLYCEMIC FOODS

Beverages
Soy milk

Breads
Oat bran bread
Barley kernel bread

Breakfast Cereals
Rice bran
Kellogg's All-Bran Fruit 'n' Oats
All-Bran

Dairy
Yogurt
Milk

Fruits

Apples

Apricots

Blackberries

Cantaloupe

Cherries

Cranberries

Grapefruit

Guavas

Kiwis

Lemons

Limes

Melons (all types)

Oranges

Papayas

Peaches

Plums

Raspberries

Tangerines

Tomatoes

Grains

Barley, pearled

Brown rice

Buckwheat

Bulgur wheat

Rye

Wheat kernels

Legumes

Black beans

Butter beans

Chickpeas

Kidney beans

Lentils

Lima beans

Navy beans

Pinto beans

Soy beans

Split peas

Nuts

Peanuts

Pasta

Fettuccine

Pastina

Spaghetti, protein enriched

Vermicelli

Vegetables

Asparagus

Bean sprouts

Beet greens

Beets

Broccoli

Brussels sprouts

Cabbage

Cauliflower

Celery

Cucumber

Dandelion greens

Eggplant

Endive

Kale

Kohlrabi

Leeks

Lettuce

Mustard greens

Okra

Onion

Pimiento

Red pepper

Spinach

String beans

Swiss chard

Turnip

Watercress

Foods with a higher glycemic index—those that are rapidly digested—even whole foods such as carrots, corn, potatoes, bananas, and dried fruits, will raise your blood sugar rapidly and may result in a buildup of abdominal fat if you are insulin-resistant or eat too many of these foods. Here are some key, and very popular, high-glycemic foods you should avoid:

HIGH-GLYCEMIC FOODS

Bakery Products
Angel food cake

Croissants

Doughnuts

Flan

Waffles

Beverages
Soda

Breads
Bagels

Bread stuffing

French baguettes

Melba toast

Wheat bread

White bread

Breakfast Cereals
Cheerios
Cocoa Puffs
Cornflakes
Crispix
Golden Grahams
Rice Chex
Rice Krispies
Total

Dairy
Ice cream

Fruits
Dates

Grains
Instant rice
Tapioca
White rice

Legumes
Fava beans

Pasta
Brown rice pasta

Vegetables
Parsnips
Potatoes
Pumpkin
Rutabaga

TIPS ON USING THESE LISTS

- Obviously, you're not going to go on a watercress or pimiento binge, but these low-glycemic fruits and vegetables can be combined into an endless variety of salads that not only taste great but make perfect nutrient-dense, low-calorie dishes that you can consume in large amounts. Just remember not to drown your salads in creamy dressing. Opt instead for a simple olive oil and vinegar dressing perhaps with a dash of lemon juice, and use only a small amount. Remember, a salad bowl isn't a swimming pool!

- For best results, eat fruits separately from the rest of your meal; fifteen to twenty minutes before a meal is okay.

- To prevent allergic responses, eat a variety of fruits and vegetables, rotating foods so as not to eat the same fare every day. Particularly observe any reactions to citrus and melon. In some people, these foods provoke allergic responses.

- Most grains, legumes, and dairy products also have a low-glycemic index.

REBALANCING METABOLISM

In earlier chapters, we looked at the many factors responsible for people being overweight. We saw that problems may arise from poor digestion and absorption, food allergies that create "addictions," eating too much and exercising too little, ingesting poor-quality foods, hormonal imbalances, and psychological issues. We also saw that many times, an overweight condition stems from metabolic instabilities, where the body machinery is seriously out of balance. While there is no quick-and-easy way to rebalance your metabolism, by adopting the dietary practices outlined here, you will be able to jump-start your metabolism over the long haul.

You probably will do best to move slowly into your new way of eating, starting with a transitional diet and gradually growing into a healthier lifestyle. A transitional diet allows you to make small changes that ultimately help you to rebalance your metabolism. Chapter 8 presents a thirty-one-day transitional diet for you to use. When you are revamping your diet, grossly unsound practices, such as smoking cigarettes and drinking alcohol, should be the first to go. You also will want to gradually wean yourself off coffee, sugar, salt, and white flour, dairy products, chicken, and meats. At the same time, introduce more fruits and vegetables into the diet, with a small amount of raw foods at first. If you don't already have a juicer, purchase one as soon as possible. Start your day with freshly made apple juice, which is a good liver cleanser, or a citrus juice for its vitamin C content, and drink two to three glasses of other juices (see Chapter 9) throughout the day. You'll be sure to feel a difference, because fresh juices, unlike the store-bought variety, are rich in oxygen and filled with nutrients.

Initially, your body may have an uncomfortable reaction to raw foods in the diet. If they promote gas, stay away from other gas-producing foods until your digestion improves. Also, too much green juice at first may cause people who are toxic to feel sick. Go slowly with green juices, blending a little bit with apple or tomato and a little water. And don't eat too much fruit at first, to prevent wide fluctuations in your blood sugar level.

Remember to acknowledge and reward yourself for every small change on your road to a new way of life and a better you.

Chapter 7

Don't Diet— Detoxify!

I magine that you want to make improvements to your house. Before you call in the architect, the contractors, or the decorators, what's the very first thing you do? You make sure your house has a solid foundation. You know it would make no sense to build on an unsound foundation, so you try to get the basic structure as shipshape as possible before you go further.

Likewise, it doesn't make sense to start a body improvement program, including—and especially—a weight-loss program, without detoxifying first. What exactly is detoxification? It's a broad term referring to the removal of substances that do not belong in the body. A detox program can mean anything from a diet high in alkaline foods to juice fasting, to increased exercise, to saunas. The immediate goal is not only to help the organs of detoxification—the liver, skin, kidneys, and intestines—do their job better but to increase the ability of each cell to release toxins. The ultimate goal is to get all body processes working at an optimal level of efficiency. With digestion, metabolism, and elimination all working as they should, weight loss will be much easier than when your body was in a sluggish, predetoxed state.

An unfortunate fact of modern life is that toxins surround us. They are in the air we breathe, the water we drink, the food we eat, and the metals placed in our mouths. Rather than poison us all at once, these toxins accumulate in our bodies and, over time, cause increasingly serious problems. As pollutants build up in our bodies, they deplete our systems of potassium, a mineral essential to the activation of enzymes. Since enzymes are needed to activate most digestive and energy-producing activities, inhibited enzyme function results in our gastrointestinal systems slowing down and thus in poor fat and protein digestion. The liver and kidneys, in turn, become overworked, and fat begins to deposit in the arteries, leading to cardiovascular illnesses. So detoxification is important for a whole range of health concerns. I'd actually call it the key to health, to feeling good, and to weight loss.

SPRING CLEANSING

Just about all holistic health practitioners emphasize detoxification for the reasons I've outlined, although they've all got their own particular take on it. Some like to connect the one-week detoxification process to the seasons. In March and April, they say, when we get the urge to clean our closets, we should be cleansing our bodies too. During the spring (and fall as well), the weather begins to change and we are more likely to experience congestive problems—allergies, sluggish intestines, a rise in blood pressure, higher cholesterol levels—and weight gain. Following a detoxification program can help restore balance to our systems. Dr. Elson Haas, author of *The Detox Diet*, has been doing a spring cleanse for twenty-five years and states that such a program "works better therapeutically than almost anything else I can do."

Generally, a detoxification diet is one that eliminates sugar, nicotine, alcohol, caffeine, and chemicals, and focuses on fresh fruits and vegetables, whole grains, and lots of pure water. The body will benefit from the focus on alkaline foods, as these restore that all-important potassium to the system, which can then reactivate digestive enzymes. As acids are released through the kidneys, bladder, intestines, and skin, toxins are eliminated too. I've provided a nine-step program to help you through the detoxification process and start you down the road to long-term weight loss.

In time, you may be ready to engage in a deeper cleanse—a one-to-four-day juice and water fast—to clear deeper physical problems and renew the spirit. The fast should include plenty of pure water and a variety of juice combinations. Also excellent are cleansing teas, such as red clover, burdock, and dandelion.

Always consider your current state of health when starting a detoxification program. If you are extremely toxic, you are going to experience more uncomfortable symptoms and you should work with a professionally trained health practitioner and even consider going to a health facility where you will be carefully guided and monitored. People who are ill always should consult their physicians before beginning a cleanse. Fasting can exacerbate certain medical conditions, such as kidney stones, low blood pressure, and irregular heartbeat, for which you need to be on the lookout. Whether working alone or under supervision, remember to take your time with each of the steps. Wait at least a week before moving on to the next step, especially if you are a beginner. Do not fast if you are pregnant.

The Healing Crisis

On the road to good health, you may endure a short transition period, known as a healing crisis, when you feel headachy, cold, irritable, and tired. Don't get scared; this is actually a good sign. When you begin to purify your body, particularly if you're on a juice fast, the organs of elimination release unwanted debris. A healing crisis and its symptoms mean that your body is working to get rid of toxic waste products that have accumulated over the years.

Have faith and stay with the program because in a few days' time your weakness will be replaced with a feeling of radiance and strength. Another benefit, particularly important to weight-loss aspirants, is that most likely you will require less food, as the food you do eat will be assimilated more easily. That's because the walls of the intestines will have become cleaner and better able to absorb nutrients.

STEP 1: CLEANSE YOUR LIVER

Do you ever think about your liver? You should. Multifaceted, the liver serves as a blood filter and cleanser, breaking down substances such as drugs, alcohol, nicotine, and caffeine. This organ helps to reduce the work of the immune system, and when it becomes overloaded and unable to function as it should, your health probably will suffer. A poorly performing liver will have a ripple effect on the immune system, increasing the likelihood of allergies, sinus problems, asthma, autoimmune diseases, and recurrent infections. Analysis of your blood can indicate if your liver is functioning properly; liver enzyme levels of SGOT, SGPT, and GGTP may be elevated if there is a problem. Your physician can get you set up with this and other blood tests to help you fine-tune an individualized health program.

According to Dr. Sandra Cabot, author of *The Liver Cleansing Diet: Love Your Liver and Live Longer,* petrochemicals in the food chain build up in the liver and are a major contributor to immune system problems: "I tell people that the greatest asset they can have in this day and age is a healthy immune system. But look at everyone out there with chronic fatigue syndrome, autoimmune diseases, and inflammatory problems. Their immune system is overloaded. What conventional medicine often does is suppress symptoms without thinking about the cause."

In her book, Cabot talks about how to improve liver function by listening to the body and learning to make healthy choices that respond to its needs. She recommends lots of water and an abundance of fresh, raw foods for their liver-cleansing effect. Vitamin C and other antioxidants also help to rid the body of dangerous chemicals. At the same time, it's important to stop bingeing on refined sugars, which the liver converts into triglycerides and which can lead to a fatty liver. If dairy and gluten products are a problem, they should be avoided as well.

To detoxify your liver, consider the following cleansing formula daily for one week every four months.

LIVER DETOXIFYING DRINK

3 glasses of cabbage juice
4 oz. apple juice
3 oz. juice from dark green vegetables, such as spinach or kale
1 oz. aloe vera

1. Separately juice the cabbage, apples, and green vegetables.
2. Combine juices and mix in the aloe vera.
3. Drink immediately.

You also should take milk thistle supplements in the recommended dosage daily.

STEP 2: CLEANSE YOUR SKIN

The skin is our largest organ of detoxification. Good care must be taken of the skin so that pores remain unclogged. Otherwise, the lungs, the liver, the kidneys, and the large intestine may become overloaded. One excellent method of sloughing off dead skin is dry skin brushing. This method involves using a soft luffa or vegetable bristle brush before showering, and brushing up the legs toward the abdomen, up the back, and down the arms, avoiding the delicate neck and face skin. In addition to opening up pores, this technique will help get toxins unstuck so that the lymphatic circulation can move them out.

Exercise also helps the detoxification process because it induces sweating. In addition, exercise gets the lymphatic system moving, and the flow of lymph throughout the body is vital to clearing out debris from our systems. Some people, however, feel worse after exercise because their systems are overly acidic. They can't release toxins fast enough to feel good from exercising. According to Linda Berry, author of

Internal Cleansing: Rid Your Body of Toxins and Return to Vibrant Good Health, people with chronic fatigue or fibromyalgia who find it difficult to exercise but want to cleanse their skin can benefit from more magnesium. This mineral feeds mitochondria, the powerhouses of our cells, so that more toxins are pushed out through the skin. One of the best ways to get magnesium, Berry states, is by taking a bath in Epsom salts. These are available in supermarkets and drugstores, and what you do is simply add one to four cups to bath water. You can add equal parts of baking soda for a more alkalizing effect. Soaking in this solution helps to move out toxins, and at the same time, it relaxes muscles. This is a great way to end a tension-ridden day.

Drinking sufficient amounts of pure water is also excellent for the skin. When you are in the process of detoxifying, it is good to drink half your body weight in ounces of water. If you are a 140-pound person, for example, drinking seventy ounces of water would be optimal for detoxification. While this is not a lifetime recommendation, it's an important part of your detoxification program.

STEP 3: THREE-DAY BOWEL CLEANSE

According to Berry, there are five critical components to bowel health: water, fiber, essential fatty acids, listening to the body, and exercise. I recommend using these components to develop your bowel cleansing program.

Water

Sufficient water prevents the feces from drying up and getting stuck in the intestines.

Fiber

Fiber is an important aspect of diet, with fresh, live foods being the best sources. We need a great deal of fiber for good health, and most of us don't get nearly enough. While the recommended daily allowance for fiber is twenty-five grams, Americans generally get between ten and twenty grams. According to scientific research, however, what we want for optimal health, not just to get by, is forty to sixty grams.

Although many people claim to be on a high-fiber diet, often they are getting less fiber than they need to maintain good health. Some people add a teaspoon of fiber to sugary, fatty foods, believing that they are eating healthfully when what they are doing is actually counterproductive to good health. To make a difference, increased fiber intake must be part of an overall change in eating habits, although fiber supplements, such as psyllium and bran, can be helpful additions to any diet. However, a tablespoon of psyllium husk, for example, contains only about seven grams of fiber. To get the needed amounts, people should eat between five and ten servings of fruits and vegetables daily. (One serving equals one cup of raw fruits and vegetables or a half cup of cooked fruits and vegetables.)

Beyond that, fiber helps by decreasing the transit time of fecal matter so that it leaves the body in a timely manner. Otherwise, it gets stuck in the intestinal tract. On the standard American diet, the usual transit time is between forty and sixty-five hours, which is much too long. About three-and-a-half days of digested food impacts the intestines, creating an environment that is not conducive to good health. Berry states, "Some food rots, so instead of becoming a nourishing substance it becomes toxic for your body. Also, carcinogenic substances are produced. Colon cancers are one of the major causes of death in this country. We therefore want to make sure that we get enough fiber in our colons to help us eliminate. People who eat a high-fiber diet have a transit time of between twenty and forty-five hours, which is much healthier."

In addition, fiber softens the feces, reducing pressure on the colon walls. Thus bowel movements become easier. Fiber also helps to normalize blood sugar levels, lower cholesterol, and bind and release toxic chemicals that we ingest. Remarkably, it also helps to convert carcinogenic substances into safe elements.

Essential Fatty Acids

Americans also need to be taking in more essential fatty acids (EFAs). "We're on a fat-reducing craze," Berry comments, "but, in reality, as Americans are reducing fat they're getting fatter." Essential fatty acids are called that because they *are* essential. Good sources include fish, primarily saltwater fish, and nuts, such as walnuts and pumpkin seeds. Flaxseeds are another good source, although if you have liver trouble, it may be difficult for you to metabolize the fat in flax. Eating fish two to three times a week and a handful of nuts on a regular basis along with some flax fiber will help the body to nourish itself so that you're lubricated and better able to eliminate toxins. Also oil of evening primrose— 1,000 to 2,000 mg daily will help.

Listening to Your Body

It is important to listen to your body when it tells you that you've got to go to the bathroom. Ignoring your body's signals will only make elimination more difficult.

Exercise

Bodies were meant to move, and exercise is something everyone can do. Exercise is the fifth component important for cleansing the bowel. Even if you're in a wheelchair you can exercise—move your arms, move your body back and forth, or get into a pool. Those of us who can walk should take every opportunity to do so. Says Berry, "One of my favorite remedies for constipation was popular in the old days: Eat a carrot and go for a walk. That helps in a number of ways. There are some good oils in carrots as well as fiber. Exercise helps to stimulate your system and get your metabolism going. It warms your body up so that you have better elimination."

STEP 4: ELIMINATE YOUR ALLERGIES

Although most of us dismiss them as simply annoying and uncomfortable, chronic allergies are actually one of the prime contributors to poor health and overly toxic bodies. You may not even be aware that you are allergic to a particular food or substance, but over time the effects of the allergens can place tremendous stress on your immune system and health. One of the most important steps in detoxification is to closely examine eating and lifestyle habits and observe how your body reacts when it encounters a particular food or substance. If you have always noticed that you have gas after eating a specific food, or that snuggling with your dog makes you sniffle, you may have allergies that are quietly wreaking havoc on your body and health. Furthermore, allergies do not always manifest themselves in typical ways; rather than developing a runny nose or itchy hives, your allergies may cause mood swings, arthritis flare-ups, sensitive breasts, distention of the belly, or brain fatigue or fog.

If you suspect you are allergic to something you're eating, keeping a diet notebook is a way of pinning down exactly what it is. Divide notebook pages into two columns. In one column write down what and when you eat, and in the other list your symptoms and when they occur. After a few days, patterns may begin to appear. Then, if a particular food jumps out at you, you can do a food challenge. What this means is simply eliminating that food in any form from your diet for four days and then, on the fifth day, eating that food alone. If a reaction appears when you reintroduce the food, you're on the right track. You also can use the test we discussed in Chapter 2, where you take your pulse first thing in the morning and then sample certain foods.

Note that sometimes it takes longer, more detailed tests to determine what's going on. If you suspect that you have allergies but have not been successful in pinpointing them on your own, make an appointment with your doctor or an allergist for a more complete exam. A doctor of environmental medicine can help you discover your allergy and then decide how to deal with it.

Rotating Your Foods

If your problem is not severe and you want to go it alone, I generally recommend a four-day rotation diet as a good way of minimizing food allergy problems. What you do is simply what you *don't* do: Once you've identified your potential allergen, you don't eat that food more than once every four days. Say you eat peanuts on Sunday. Thursday, then, will be the soonest that you can eat this food again. This doesn't mean you should go hog-wild over peanuts every four days—keep it moderate. By not eating a food constantly, you're cutting down on the chance that you'll develop an allergic or addictive reaction to it. Plus you won't get in a food rut where, for instance, you're eating nothing but wheat-based products all the time and gaining weight in the process. Food rotation is also a great way to ensure that you're getting a wide range of vitamins and other nutrients.

STEP 5: USING VITAMIN C

Some holistically oriented doctors like to use vitamin C as a major component of a detoxification protocol, particularly for those patients experiencing withdrawal symptoms as they give up a particular food or chemical. They explain that C helps with withdrawal because addictive and allergic reactions are acidifying to the body, and a buffer is needed against the acid. Vitamin C, in the form of sodium ascorbate, serves this function. Also, the vitamin binds with toxins, aiding in their removal. And as an antioxidant, vitamin C does the important work of stopping free radicals from destroying cell membranes.

Some physicians administer the vitamin intravenously, giving as much as twenty-five to fifty grams. I usually recommend that people using C at home for detoxification purposes take bowel-tolerance doses orally. Every three to four hours they should take a teaspoon of vitamin C powder up to the point of diarrhea. Then they should back off to a dose just below that amount. You don't want to do this for more than one week, but during a primary period of cleansing, it can be very helpful. Doctors remind us to be sure to drink a lot of water as we take the vitamin C. That's a good idea at any time, particularly if we're detoxifying.

STEP 6: IN WITH THE LIVE FOOD . . .

Losing weight has less to do with counting calories than with what you eat. Vegetables, fruits, and whole grains not only help you lose weight; they also make you healthier because of their high vitamin, mineral, and fiber content. Dr. Agatha Thrush, author of *Nutrition for Vegetarians* and *The Animal Connection,* a doctor who encourages vegetarianism, says, "We have confidence in vegetarianism as a preventer of disease. If we can predict the likelihood that a person might develop a disease later in life, let's say twenty years down the line, and we can arrange a kind of lifestyle for them at a point where they first begin to show signs of that disease, we feel that we can assist a person in avoiding their appointment with the disease."

Diet is a complex subject, and other doctors favor lean animal protein in health regimens. But all holistically oriented doctors agree on this: Dietary emphasis should be on whole foods—fruits, vegetables, grains, legumes, and the right kinds of fats and oils.

Fruits and Vegetables, Your Phytochemical Factories

Fruits and vegetables are great for warding off hunger. These foods fill you up and are low in calories. Be aware, however, that diabetics must limit some fruits.

Furthermore, fruits and vegetables are rich in phytochemicals, or plant chemicals, powerful disease preventers that evolved to shield plants from harm. Dr. Stephanie Beling, author of *Power Foods: Good Food, Good Health with Phytochemicals, Nature's Own Energy Boosters,* explains, "Plants stand in the sun all day long and need to protect themselves against the damaging effects of ultraviolet light. They are also subject to drought, freezing, insects, parasites, and viruses, just as humans and animals are." In order to survive, plants have their own chemicals to counter these dangers, and those phytochemicals can benefit us too—*if* we eat plant foods in as natural a state as possible.

Phytochemicals express themselves as rainbow colors, and we get the most benefit from eating a variety of these pigments. As Beling reminds us, "It's important to have color in our food: red, yellow, orange, purple, and green. Green is important because it contains chlorophyll, while orange foods are rich in carotenoids. Most people know of beta-carotene, but there are many carotenoids that have been identified in foods. This is why taking a supplement is not the ideal. Food is finally being recognized as a very important part of health."

The phytochemicals found in cruciferous vegetables, so named for the cross-shaped flower that forms on these plants, are powerful cancer fighters. They work with our enzymes to make our cells more resistant to certain cancer-causing chemicals. Everyone knows these foods—broccoli, broccoli rabe, Brussels sprouts, cauliflower, kale, and cabbage. Beling explains, "It's our own bodies doing the protection and healing, but the foods we eat give us the raw material and the stimulus to allow our bodies to do this."

Other cancer-fighting foods contain lycopene. These foods have a red pigment, and include tomatoes, watermelon, beets, and pink grapefruits. Citrus fruits contain the phytochemical turpine. Besides having anticancer properties, these foods help to protect against dental decay and ulcers. Garlic, onions, leeks, chives, scallions, and shallots are anti-inflammatory, antiviral, and antibacterial. They help to ward off infection and boost the immune system. Fruits and vegetables, like grains, are also vitally important for their high fiber content.

We'll be discussing phytochemicals in greater detail in Chapter 9.

Sea Vegetables

Sea vegetables, such as sea palm, nori, kelp, wakame, and dulse, are available in natural food and Asian markets. They are loaded with minerals, especially iodine, which is important for thyroid functioning and something we often don't get enough of. Sea vegetables also provide magnesium, a nutrient beneficial to the heart, and calcium in a form that is more easily usable than that in dairy products, which many people are allergic to. Did you know that sea vegetables contain more calcium by dry weight than milk? It is time that these superb food sources, used widely throughout the world, became more known in the United States.

Grains and Legumes

In parts of the world where whole grains and legumes are dietary staples, people do not experience the chronic health problems that are so common in America. In this country, people eat an abundance of highly processed grains, such as white pasta and bread—foods that in large quantities cause sluggishness, weight gain, and poor health. It is far better to concentrate on healthful whole grains and legumes. Whole grains include whole wheat berries, bulgur wheat, brown rice, millet, spelt barley, quinoa, amaranth, and teff, and are widely available in health food stores and supermarkets. Legumes—or beans—come in all shapes and sizes; there are black beans, adzuki beans, red beans, kidney beans, black-eyed peas, lentils, and nearly eighty more varieties.

Soy is the king of all beans. Eaten as a bean or as tofu, tempeh, or soy milk, soy helps to lower levels of the so-called bad cholesterol and raise levels of the good kind. It also has been found to protect us from prostate, breast, and ovarian cancer. In fact, in Asia, where a lot of soy is consumed, incidences of these cancers are much lower than in the United States.

When you are detoxifying, you should have at least three servings of grains and beans every day. First try grains that you normally wouldn't have, such as teff and amaranth. Then add to your diet some of the more common ones, like buckwheat, rye, oats. Leftover grains are perfect warmed up for breakfast—sweet rice is wonderful mixed with ground cinnamon and pureed bananas, for example, or you can make a rice pudding with sweet rice and soy milk. It tastes like a sweet dessert but has the vital vitamins and minerals you need.

Most people avoid beans because they occasionally cause gas. They are less likely to do so if you soak them overnight in water before you cook them, then change the water before cooking. Improper food combining also can cause gas. For example, eating foods that are digested quickly, such as fruit, after eating beans, which are a complete protein and don't leave the stomach as quickly, may cause gas. To eliminate the problem, try eating foods that are digested the quickest first. Canned beans are fine if you don't have the time to make them from scratch. Just rinse them off and add them to soups and salads to enrich your diet. You'll find plenty of recipes for grains and legumes in Chapter 8.

Fats and Oils

"Low-fat" and "no-fat" have generally been considered positive buzzwords among people trying to lose weight, which seems to include most of us. But that's really too simplistic an approach to how we should be eating. If you want to win at the weight-loss and health game, you have to be a little more sophisticated in your understanding of fats and oils.

"Fat is our friend, not our enemy," asserts Ann Louise Gittleman, former director of nutrition at the Pritikin Longevity Center in Santa Monica, California, and author of *Eat Fat, Lose Weight.* "I truly believe that the secret to maintaining permanent weight loss and health from head to toe lies in the fats known as the omegas." While most vegetable oils, margarine, and shortening are rightfully considered unhealthful and connected to weight gain, health problems, and fast aging, omegas have the opposite effect and are a prerequisite to good health and appearance.

Omega-3s, 6s, and 9s are found in essential fatty acids (EFAs), and as the name suggests, they are essential for optimal functioning. Good fats will not only promote weight loss and maintenance, they can help alleviate a variety of health conditions. Some of their many abilities include the breakup of cholesterol, the transportation of fat, and the regulation of hormones. They promote weight loss, boost immunity, relieve depression and fatigue, heal skin conditions and improve dry skin, control

PMS and other menstrual problems, and even help to prevent breast and prostate cancer. New research even suggests that the omega-3s may be helpful in controlling migraines and fighting multiple sclerosis. Essential fatty acids are also excellent for optimal brain function, as the brain is 80 percent fat.

Nutritionally oriented physician Dr. Majid Ali, of Denville, New Jersey, adds that one other crucial role of essential fatty acids is their ability to carry electrical charges to cells: "Cells talk to each other through electromagnetic signals, and the electromagnetic signals are primarily created by polar moieties of fatty acids. That means it's the fats in the cell membranes that carry electrical charges. We tend to think of hormones carrying messages, and that's very true. But at a deeper level, the fatty acids are responsible. Cell membranes contain phospholipids, or fats, which are the body's electrical wiring system. Fats are absolutely critical for cell function."

Excellent sources of EFAs are flaxseed oil, extra-virgin olive oil, sesame oil, and pumpkin oil. These cold-pressed, uncooked oils will increase thermogenesis, a process that revs up fat-burning cells. They also send a message of satiety to the brain to create a feeling of fullness so that there is less of a desire to eat. According to Dr. Ali, the listed oils should be rotated in the diet to prevent an allergic reaction to any one of them. Additional good sources are wheat germ; pumpkin, sesame, and safflower seeds; and fatty fish, such as mackerel and salmon. In supplement form, evening primrose and borage oil can be taken.

How much of an essential oil to take varies from individual to individual. Generally, a tablespoon of the uncooked oil twice a day is recommended, although some people need to start with a teaspoon twice a day and gradually increase the amount to avoid loose stools. For weight management, Gittleman usually recommends between four and six 500-mg capsules of evening primrose or borage oil and one tablespoon of olive oil or half an avocado. The primrose and borage oils contain omega-3s and the olive oil and avocado are comprised of omega-9s; together they provide a healthful balance of nutrients that get fat engines burning. "We've seen that demonstrated in clinical studies," Gittleman states, "where individuals who didn't do anything else but include eight 500-mg capsules of evening primrose oil each day lose a total of five to ten pounds." She says that you can eat fat and lose weight simply by taking advantage of the metabolism-raising factors of the healthy and essential fats.

The right fats should be included at every meal. Gittleman recommends mixing a tablespoon of flaxseed oil with soy yogurt for breakfast. At lunch you can use a tablespoon of flaxseed oil on a salad, and at dinner add a tablespoon of olive oil to stir-fries; twice a week eat salmon or mackerel. In between meals, eat a handful of omega-rich almonds or pumpkin seeds to ward off hunger. ("Handful" is the operative word; don't go overboard on nuts if you want to lose weight.) Gittleman states, "There are lots of colorful and tasteful ways to incorporate essential fats into food and not feel deprived at all. So eat fat, lose weight, and know that it is your greatest ally."

STEP 7: ... OUT WITH THE DEAD

Detoxifying and taking in healthy substances are vital processes, but not sufficient to promote good health on their own. At the same time, we need to eliminate harmful eating practices that run our bodies down and set the stage for illness. Cumulative bad habits eventually take over our lives and ruin us. We get hooked on stimulating poisons, such as caffeine and sugar, for the short-term energy jolt they provide, and end up depleting our own natural energy sources. Or we sedate ourselves with alcohol or nicotine, which in time paralyze the brain or destroy the lungs. Contaminated and devitalized foods rob us of nutrients rather than supply them, adding to the burden. The following sections present some of the deadening foods that you should give up in order to look and feel your best and assist the detoxification process.

Processed Foods: Too Much of a Bad Thing

As we've discussed, nothing contributes more to the degeneration of mind and body than a diet of overly processed foods. Unfortunately, the

food industry and its advertisers have swayed people to want these substances from an early age. Dr. Kelly Brownell, director of the Yale Center
for Eating and Weight Disorders, describes the situation:

"If you want to explain the epidemic of obesity, all you need to do is
point to the environment. You'll find that over 5,000 schools serve fast
foods in their cafeterias. You'll find that every service station has been remodeled to include a minimarket that sells high-fat and sugar snack
foods. You'll find three new McDonald's popping up every day somewhere in the country. And you know how effective McDonald's is at advertising when your typical American recognizes 'supersize' as a verb.
And what do you get when you 'supersize'? You get 900 calories from a
meal that's mainly sugar and fat. It's been promoted heavily, and it's a
huge problem."

Brownell goes on to describe the recent trend of soft-drink companies forging financial deals with schools whereby the companies get exclusive rights to sell their beverages there. "A soft drink company paid a
Colorado school district millions of dollars for an agreement saying that
the cola company would be their exclusive bottling company. Allegedly,
the contract read that the school district had to sell a certain number of
cases of cola in order to 'meet their numbers.' When they weren't doing
it, supposedly the superintendent's office sent out letters to the princi-
pals mandating them to move cola machines to the highest-traffic areas
of the schools. A letter even went out saying that teachers should be permitted to let kids drink cola in the classrooms . . . this is why we're fat;
it's not biology."

It's not just the obvious junk foods we eat that cause problems. Many
so-called healthful foods—such as bread, muffins, crackers, soup, and
canned and frozen fruits and vegetables—contain refined starch,
bleached flour, saturated fat, hidden sugar, excess salt, and a chemical
soup of additives and preservatives. Companies routinely strip foods of
their nutrient and fiber content, replacing them with unwholesome substances that promote taste and a long shelf life. Because such food is devoid of its natural enzyme content, the body is forced to work much
harder by using its own enzymes to break down pollutants and chemi-

cals and to pass them through the body. These foods provide little more than empty calories and are a major reason why our nation is overweight and plagued with degenerative diseases.

The Wicked Whites: Sugar, White Flour, and Salt

Not only is sugar a leading cause of obesity, it is associated with a host of health problems. For one, it's habit-forming and can lead to hypoglycemia, a condition whose symptoms may include weakness, headaches, vision problems, loss of coordination, anxiety, and other personality changes—and eventually diabetes. Moreover, sugar is one of the leading contributors to tooth decay and menstrual irregularities.

Foods made from refined white flour also add to the problem. Unlike complex carbohydrates, which are high-fiber foods that generally do not raise blood sugar levels, refined carbohydrates have a negative impact on people with carbohydrate sensitivities. Eliminating refined carbohydrates may help put an end to Yo-Yo dieting and keep you naturally thin.

Excess sodium in the diet causes the body's tissues to retain water, which can lead to edema. This excess of fluid can lead to inflammation of the connective tissues in the joints, which inhibits motion and causes pain similar to that of arthritis. Once the inflammatory process begins, you gradually lose full mobility in the ankles, wrists, knees, elbows, and other joints. By lowering the salt content of your diet, you can avoid the strain that too much salt puts on the body. Beware of soy sauce and miso, by the way, because they're loaded with sodium.

Meat, and Why You Don't Need It

In 1993 we heard the frightening news that 700 people had been poisoned and 4 children had died after eating bacterially contaminated fast-food hamburgers in a West Coast franchise. In the past twenty-five years, incidences of food-borne illnesses have almost doubled, with 81 million Americans suffering from reactions to various pathogens in food. In fact, what we often think is the flu could actually be a case of food poisoning.

Although meat is not the only food subject to microbial contamination, it has a high potential for making us sick, largely because of modern agricultural practices. The majority of today's livestock are raised in environments based on industrial models. Often animals are crowded together, routinely given antibiotics, exposed to dirty food and water, and raised in unclean surroundings. Another serious problem results from breeding practices. While the production of near-identical animals may ensure rapid growth, it also makes for animals that are equally susceptible to the same diseases. So it's not uncommon to find salmonella or some other pathogen in an entire flock of chickens, for example. Further stress plagues the animal until slaughter, when their meat plus whatever microbes it carries is distributed nationwide.

The pollution of chickens presents yet another problem, the creation of tainted eggs. It is no longer safe to add a raw egg to your Caesar salad, thanks to salmonella. Many times the bug gets transported from the chicken ovary to the egg and thus becomes part of the package.

Perhaps the most serious problem is with today's beef, as a new pathogen, *E. coli* 015787, is seeping into the supply. The microbe originates from the toxic shigella bacterium and can cause severe illness and death. Ground beef products are most susceptible. Years ago beef was freshly ground at a local butcher shop. In today's world, meat from hundreds of cattle, from different states and countries, is sent to huge processing plants where the meat from different animals gets combined. Thanks to modern, more "efficient" methods, one contaminated cow can now pollute 16 tons of meat. Investigative journalist Nicholas Fox, the author of *Spoiled: Why Our Food Is Making Us Sick and What We Can Do About It*, comments on the impossibility of ensuring purity: "The USDA is doing very few spot checks on hamburger, and occasionally they come up with a positive. Oftentimes, that's when we see a massive recall. But are they checking all of it? They can't. All you do when you check one little, tiny sample of hamburger is to guarantee that you do or do not have *E. coli* in that sample. Obviously, that doesn't say anything else for the vast amount that was probably in that day's lot. So all hamburger must be considered highly suspect and must be cooked very thoroughly." Even under the best conditions, though, eating beef can open us up to the risk of developing serious health problems. High in saturated fat and cholesterol, beef increases our risk for hardening of the arteries, heart disease, and a variety of cancerous conditions, including colon, rectal, and breast cancer. Too much animal protein puts stress on two important organs of detoxification: the kidneys and the liver. Also, the uric acid contained in the meat may settle in the joints, causing painful gouty arthritis over time. Numerous gastrointestinal disturbances may result from the ingestion of meat, starting with gas and constipation and leading to more serious illnesses down the road.

There are many people, myself included, who would suggest that we avoid meat completely. They argue that we have been brainwashed into believing that meat is essential to good health and point to the design of our bodies as proof of the unnaturalness of humans eating flesh. Our teeth are flat as opposed to pointy and sharp and thus are better at grinding plants and grains than tearing meat, and our long digestive tracts resemble those of herbivores. We secrete a special enzyme designed to break down plant foods. Carnivores, on the other hand, have no such enzyme and possess short digestive tracts for getting rid of meat quickly before it putrefies. Plus their teeth are sharp, not flat.

And going beyond these considerations, many people find it unethical to kill another creature for food when it is not necessary to do so. Indeed, our nonanimal sources of nourishment are both abundant and more healthful than meat. Then too, the earth's resources—both land and water—are much less strained when we obtain nutrients directly from plants, as opposed to the roundabout way of getting them through the animals that eat the plants. It's a matter of planetary efficiency.

The health benefits of vegetarianism are being documented all the time in the peer-reviewed scientific literature, and more and more physicians are seeing the light in this area. Vegetarianism advocate Dr. Agatha Thrash mentions just two of the mountains of articles that have come out supporting plant-based eating:

"It was back in the '70s that *The Lancet*, probably the most prestigious medical journal, reported on four cases of angina cured by very simple things: a vegetarian diet, a small amount of exercise, and reducing free fats. . . . The vegetarian diet contained no animal protein. About two years later, *The Journal of the Medical Association* reported forty-two cases of angina treated in this very same way, thirty-eight of which were entirely cured. Four were not cured, but there was a question as to their compliance with the program. We began looking in earnest for patients who had angina and tried to treat them in this way. We now have over a dozen cases of angina totally cured by the use of just a simple vegetarian routine, no animal protein, a great reduction in free fats, and moderate exercise as the patient can tolerate. We expect to never have a failure with angina."

Thrash adds that for many people, the realization that meat is anything other than a food to make one strong and robust is a new and perhaps difficult-to-comprehend concept. She suggests that in order to protect themselves from disease, people should learn to create tasty meatless recipes that promote good health. Some doctors do recommend that their patients have some meat. However, if you do decide to follow such advice, remember that meat should be eaten sparingly and obtained from organically raised sources.

The Case Against the Dairy Case

Although dairy foods have significant amounts of calcium, they are unhealthful in other ways. Cheeses are high in fat and contain casein, a coagulator that gives cheese its bendable, rubbery quality. We pay a price for ingesting a substance that is also used in glue. Cheese can lead to hardening of the arteries, gallbladder problems, and gallstones. Listeria, a bacterium that actually likes refrigerator temperatures, may find its way into soft cheeses and other prepared foods; this organism can have devastating effects on pregnant women, causing miscarriage and even death.

Milk consumption can have unwelcome consequences as well.

While raw milk has more available nutrients than the sterile homogenized, pasteurized variety, it may be loaded with dangerous pathogens, such as *E. coli* and campylobacter. Also, the antibiotics and synthetic hormones given to cows find their way into much of the commercially produced milk on the market today. In addition, milk becomes difficult to digest after infancy, and allergies or malabsorption problems are common.

"But what about my need for calcium?" you may wonder. Consider mineral-rich sea vegetables and a good supplement with the correct ratio of calcium, magnesium, and vitamin D.

Caffeine

We like the taste; we're even willing to spend extra at coffee bars on fancy lattes and capuccinos. The irony of it is that while we're drinking coffee and other caffeinated beverages to relax, in reality we're putting our body into overdrive and placing undue stress on ourselves. Caffeine is an addictive stimulant that we have come to depend on daily. Once you're hooked, it's hard to go a day without it because of the symptoms of withdrawal that start to appear—moodiness, headaches, fatigue, and sometimes cramps.

Scientists have demonstrated conclusively that caffeine can have a number of negative effects on the body. First, caffeine is a diuretic that contributes to the body's loss of a number of important minerals, such as calcium, magnesium, and potassium. Children hooked on soft drinks who turn into coffee-loving adults are bound to have mineral deficiencies as they get older. Second, in studies of women, caffeine has been correlated with a greater frequency of fibrocystic breasts and uterine fibroids. In addition, caffeine places added stress on our adrenal glands and adversely affects our nervous system, resulting in anxiety, hyperactivity, and insomnia. Researchers are also looking into possible links between regular caffeine consumption and increased incidences of cancer and prostate problems. The consumption of caffeine is not only unnecessary, it is hazardous to your health.

Alcohol

Well-documented dangers are associated with drinking. As with caffeine, drinking alcohol results in the loss of valuable nutrients through urination. Depleted are such essentials as the B vitamins, vitamin C, calcium, magnesium, and manganese. Alcohol also causes irritation and inflammation of the liver and may ultimately lead to cirrhosis of the liver, which can be deadly. Additionally, as a sugar, alcohol causes the blood sugar to rise rapidly. Over time, this can lead to blood sugar disorders.

It seems that not all the news regarding alcohol is bad; recent evidence supports a single daily serving of wine as a way of preventing heart disease. But what you don't hear the wine industry shouting about is other research showing a link between small amounts of alcohol and increases in breast cancer. Additionally, new studies link moderate alcohol consumption to colon cancer. Drinking diminishes folic acid, and low levels of this essential B vitamin are associated with higher incidences of the disease.

When stopping the alcohol habit, as you begin to detoxify, give your body the extra support it needs. Be sure to include the B vitamins folic acid and niacin as well as vitamin C, calcium, magnesium, and manganese. Additionally, a minimum of 200 micrograms of chromium picolinate can help normalize sugar metabolism. Between 500 and 1,000 mg of the amino acid L-glutamine will do the same as well as stop your alcohol cravings. Further, you should take milk thistle daily, as the herb's active component, silymarin, promotes recovery from liver damage.

Nicotine

Fear of gaining weight is the reason that many smokers won't even try to give up this health-robbing habit. But studies reveal that smoking does not prevent age-related weight gain. Perhaps knowing this, along with more publicity concerning recent reports of nicotine's relationship to impotence, might prevent young people from picking up the habit.

While the dangers of smoking are both well documented and well publicized, nicotine addiction remains one of the hardest habits to kick. In large part, the problem may be that while people know intellectually how harmful it is to smoke, they don't feel strongly enough about the issue until it is too late.

Dr. J. Barton Cunningham, author of *The Stress Management Handbook*, notes that in order to give up smoking, lose weight, or make any life-affirming change, we must first feel passionately about the new person we want to create: "When a doctor says, 'Clean up your act and stop smoking,' very few of us respond—only 6 percent. But when we're on our deathbed, 43 percent stop. [In order to change] we have to create a burning platform within us. We have to seriously want a new life."

STEP 8: DETOXIFY YOUR ENVIRONMENT

While you're cleaning up your insides, don't forget to clean your surroundings. Getting toxins and allergens out of your home will make the air you breathe and the water you drink cleaner, which can make a real difference in your long-term health.

"But I live in the middle of the city!" you may say. "It's a losing battle!" Not so. You can get an air filter for your apartment or house that will remove a significant amount of dust and other allergens and a water filter that will block chlorine, lead and other metals, and bacteria. After that, you can do a clean sweep of your house, starting literally with the floor. Get rid of dust-collecting wall-to-wall carpeting and heavy draperies that aren't easy to take down and wash. Exile toxic household cleaners for which you can substitute more natural products, such as baking soda and vinegar. If particleboard in new furniture or kitchen cabinets is giving off fumes, you can shellac it to stop the outgassing.

An important change you may want to make in your home is to set up an area near your entranceway that people can use to leave their shoes before they enter it. Shoes bring in an enormous, if invisible, load of street filth and automotive exhaust, which includes lead, every time you or a visitor cross the threshold. Whether you make a no-shoe rule or not, get a good vacuum cleaner with a HEPA-type filter. And as you clean your home, remember to wipe down, with alcohol, frequently touched objects, such as doorknobs, keyboards, cabinet handles, and remote controls. This will cut down on the number of germs to which you're exposed.

Another thing to cut down on in your home is clutter. It's amazing how easy it is to accumulate all manner of stuff over the years—and how difficult it is to sort through it all and give or throw things away. But I believe it's worth the effort, even if you have to resort to hiring a personal organizer. The benefits actually go beyond the fact that you have fewer dust- and germ-cultivating surfaces. For one thing, you can think more clearly with less clutter. For another, decluttering aids weight loss, not just because you'll be carrying all those heavy garbage bags out to the street, but because if your house is lighter, *you're* going to want to be lighter. The feeling is contagious.

Finally, as you detox your home, cut down on close-up sources of electromagnetic pollution, such as digital alarm clocks that stay near your head as you sleep and old computer monitors that do not meet current emissions guidelines.

STEP 9: DETOXIFY YOUR RELATIONSHIPS

Say you've gone on a juice fast, cleaned up your environment, eliminated processed foods, given up smoking and drinking, and started an exercise program. Does this mean you've done everything important for detoxing? Not quite. If you've still got toxic relationships in your life, you haven't done a complete job. You are still undermining your health.

You also could be undermining your weight-loss plans. If those close to you project negative attitudes—saying, for example, that you can't possibly lose weight because you've failed so many times before, or that if you don't eat and drink the way they do, you won't be part of the crowd—this could damage your resolve and set you up for failure. This is why I always advise people in my health support groups to examine their relationships and recognize those that aren't honoring who they are and what they are striving to accomplish.

Granted, you're not going to be able to get all the negative people out of your life. You're probably related to some of them, or you may work for some of them. What I recommend is that when you get negativity thrown at you, calmly respond with an explanation of why your own outlook is a positive one.

THE EXTRAS

Following are two alternate detoxification methods that can be extremely useful if you are undergoing an extensive detoxification program. However, I don't recommend these for beginners. When attempting a juice fast or using a sauna, seek the advice of your physician first.

Juice Fasting

Get your physician's go-ahead before you do this, but a couple of days of not eating and of drinking only freshly squeezed organic juice, pure water, and perhaps some herbal tea and two to three high-quality protein drinks, with approximately fifty grams of high-quality vegetable-based protein per day can do detoxifying wonders for your system.

You won't be undernourished on a juice fast; you'll be drinking about eight ten-ounce glasses of vegetable and fruit juice a day, flooding your body with a highly usable mix of antioxidant vitamins and minerals, chlorophyll, enzymes, and phytochemicals. Yes, you will be cutting down on calories, but that's part of the point. The other part of the point is to jump-start the detox process, and there's no better way of doing this than a juice fast. I recommend doing a juice fast for two days every two months.

Before you start on this project get a good juice extractor, an investment that's going to serve you well. Read the machine's instructions and suggestions for combining juices. (See Chapter 9 for more juice recipes.) Basically, watery juices should form the major part of your juice combinations; cabbage, celery, and cucumber are three high-water-content vegetables. Dark green vegetables, by contrast, are very concentrated, and their juices need to be diluted with the more watery ones or simply with water or aloe vera. The dark green sources include parsley, spinach, arugula, and watercress.

Another thing to remember when you're on a juice fast is not to gulp down your drinks; consume them slowly to facilitate digestion and savor the tastes.

When you come off a juice fast, do so slowly. Easing your way back into the world of solid food will help you avoid stomach upset. It will also enable you to mindfully establish a more healthful eating pattern than what you were used to, before your fast.

The Sauna Detoxification Process

The sauna detoxification process often is the best method for releasing deeply embedded chemicals from the body. A temperature of about 130 degrees Fahrenheit will heat deep tissues so that the chemicals housed in fat tissue start moving. Then these substances enter the bloodstream, pass through the liver, and leave the body through the stool, the urine, or sweat. Medical practitioners who use this method monitor individuals closely to see that their organs of detoxification are in good working order to eliminate poisons. They also supplement the procedure with nutrients to further promote detoxification, such as phosphatidyl-choline, B vitamins, and vitamin C. You should *not* do a sauna if you are pregnant, have high blood pressure, heart disease, or are taking medications. It's an absolute must to consult with your physician before considering a sauna as a method of detoxification. If you are a good candidate for this type of cleansing, I recommend that you do two saunas a week, once every two months.

Once you have thoroughly cleansed your body and removed toxins and other harmful substances, you will have given yourself a clean slate. The dietary changes you make now will be that much more effective. So let's take a closer look at what you're actually going to eat as you strive to lose those unwanted pounds.

Chapter 8

Creating Your
Recipe Revolution

Probably the most important step in your weight-loss program is changing the way you eat. But to do this, you first have to change the way you buy and prepare food, and even the way you eat out at restaurants, dinner parties, and other venues. First we'll take a look at these preliminary steps, and then I'll show you how to develop a revolutionary new meal plan and repertoire of recipes.

CHANGING THE WAY YOU BUY FOOD

Have you ever gone to the supermarket with one food item in mind only to walk out with ten other foods? Do you ever shop while hungry and find yourself snacking on the way home? Do you buy foods simply because the label says "all-natural" or "fat-free"? If you identify with any of these scenarios, you may be setting yourself up for weight-loss failure. After all, a successful program of healthy eating begins at the market with the foods that you buy, and developing healthy shopping habits.

Here are some tips to help you make sure that you purchase the right foods for the right reasons.

• *Prepare yourself.* Before you even get to the grocery store, put yourself into a frame of mind that will enable you to make healthy, sensible choices. Begin by setting aside some time to determine the specific ingredients you will need for the meals you'll be creating. Then make a list to help you stay on target as you shop.

• *Do not go to the supermarket hungry.* This is very important. Eat a satisfying sensible meal before you go so that you won't look at the cakes and pies in the bakery section or be tempted by the candy at the checkout aisle. Remember, a supermarket is a business that is trying to make money off you, and marketing people put those candies by the cash register on purpose. Don't let them derail your shopping agenda or your weight-loss program.

• *Shop when you are feeling relatively content.* It's also a good idea to shop when you are feeling positive and upbeat about your health and weight-loss plan. If you are feeling depressed, lonely, or worthless, you will tend to fill your cart with worthless junk food or fattening comfort foods. Try exercising before you go. This is a terrific way to stimulate your endorphins and feel good about yourself and positive about your future. You might also want to do some self-hypnosis or visualization so that you actually can hold on to the image of the ideal you while you shop. For more on these techniques, see Chapter 12.

• *Become an educated consumer.* Learn to discriminate between what's good and what's not, and don't expect food stores to do it for you. If stores were to create such labels, it would only suggest that the rest of the store is unhealthy, which would conflict with business. Never assume that everything sold in markets is okay to eat either. Scores of special interest groups lobby the Food and Drug Administration so that their products can be sold. Read labels carefully and don't be swayed by false advertising. Many companies, aware of the growing desire for more natural fare, try to fool the consumer into believing their products are healthy when they actually are not. Products described as "all natural" or "fat-free," for instance, are often loaded with sugar.

• *Opt for real foods.* Food stores love to tempt dieters with imitations of the favorite foods they can no longer have. You can find everything from artificially sweetened sodas and cookies to instant mashed potatoes and chips made with the fake fat Olestra. Our bodies are not designed to process such chemicals, and these additives do nothing to support good health. Learn to bypass these manufactured offerings and instead fill your cart with real foods. And since even natural foods are often tampered with—many are picked before they are ripe, for example, and forced to ripen in transit with the help of chemicals—you should try to buy foods that are locally grown and in season. A good rule to keep in mind is that if our ancestors didn't eat it, then neither should we.

• *Keep it balanced.* Be sure to buy foods from all of the food groups— proteins, carbohydrates, and fats—to get the greatest range of nutrients. As we've discussed, you will want to differentiate between good and bad sources—complex versus simple carbohydrates, protein from plant sources and fish rather than meat and dairy, and unsaturated versus saturated fats.

CHANGING THE WAY YOU PREPARE FOOD

People who are switching from a high-fat diet to one that's more nutritionally oriented often worry that they will be forced to endure bland-tasting dishes, but this needn't be the case. The foods you eat should be delicious as well as nutritious, and delicious meals are easy to accomplish with so many health-minded cookbooks available that provide countless tasty recipes using whole foods. Meals can be prepared to please the palate with sour, sweet, salty, bitter, and spicy tastes that keep us satisfied. And by using a variety of colors and textures, you can make meals aesthetically delightful. Let's look at some basics of food preparation.

Vegetables should never be overcooked, as this will deplete them of nutrients as well as taste and crunch. Lightly steaming vegetables, never allowing the water actually to touch them, will preserve the texture and natural taste. While some vegetables are good raw in salads or dips, others, such as cauliflower, broccoli, asparagus, Brussels sprouts, and carrots, are better if you first steam them very lightly, then rinse them in cold water, and keep them refrigerated. This technique will keep them crisp and fresh while making them more digestible.

Grains such as brown rice and barley should be rinsed well before cooking and can be prepared in different ways. All grains can either be sprouted for optimal nutrition or cooked until tender. To create a crunchier texture, try dry-toasting grain and sautéing it before cooking. Start with a cold skillet, preferably of cast iron. Heat the skillet, then evenly coat it with canola oil. (If the oil smokes, it's too hot.) Stir the grain until a few kernels pop and a delicious aroma begins to arise. Add just enough water to cover the grains, then, after the water boils, lower the flame, cover, and cook until tender. Grains at least double in size after cooking; one cup will feed two or three people.

Since regular commercial grains are heavily processed with chemicals, buy organic grains when you can. Be sure to clean grains before preparing them by rinsing them first in a strainer or colander, then transferring them to a pot of water and lifting out bits of debris, such as dirt and husks that float to the surface. Of course, use fresh water to cook the grains in.

Beans must be properly rinsed and soaked so as not to produce gas and digestion problems. Soak the beans in cold water overnight for best results. (Note: You do not have to soak lentils.) In the morning, change the water and cook the beans slowly to allow the gas to escape before you eat them. This will make them easy to digest. Usually one cup of dry beans makes about two and a half cups of cooked beans, enough for four servings.

Sprouting beans, as discussed in Chapter 6, makes them even easier to digest and will increase their nutrient content many times. Sprouts are a great taste and texture addition to salads and sandwiches. Some popular types of bean sprouts, including alfalfa, mung, soy, and broccoli sprouts, are known for their anticarcinogenic properties. Always wash sprouts before eating them.

Sea vegetables, which are actually seaweeds, can be an acquired taste for many Americans but are important sources of trace minerals that should be eaten at least weekly. The high calcium content of seaweeds makes them a good mild substitute for those who are allergic to dairy. Common seaweeds, such as the jet-black hijiki (or hiziki), the iodine-rich, brown kombu (or kelp), the purple nori, and the transparent agar, can be found at health food stores and food co-ops. Most seaweeds are easy to prepare, requiring just a short soak before cooking. Hijiki, for instance, should be soaked in water for twenty minutes, then strained in a colander and lightly pressed to squeeze out extra moisture. Then it is ready to sauté with other vegetables and grains for an excellent meal.

Herbs and spices can transform any bland dish into a uniquely flavorful one. Be creative with your herbs and spices, and learn how to season instead of salt your food. The flavors of cumin, cardamom, garlic, dill, oregano, and thyme will help you forget your cravings for salt.

A Word About Microwaving

Because of their convenience, microwave ovens have become an integral part of the typical modern kitchen. Almost anyone who can afford a microwave wouldn't think of being without one. But it's important to stop and think about what you are doing when you cook by microwave. You are, basically, overheating the inside of the food, which in turn causes genetic damage through molecular rearrangement of and destruction to cells. Also, by using radiation, you are destroying important antioxidants, which are vital to a properly functioning body. What's more, microwaves can disrupt your body's natural electromagnetic balance if you are close by when they are at work or if your microwave should leak. It is best to cook the old-fashioned way and set aside the time needed to prepare healthful, tasty meals instead of relying on the microwave to quickly zap everything on the table.

CHANGING THE WAY YOU EAT OUT

Did you ever notice that fast food restaurants decorate their interiors in loud, obnoxious colors, have uncomfortable seating, and often play noisy music? They are obviously not attempting to create the kind of environment where people want to linger over their meals, savoring every bite. On the contrary, they are in the business of getting you out as fast as possible. This is not a healthy situation for you to be in digestion-wise, and it certainly doesn't promote weight loss, because it makes you eat faster and eat more.

When you eat out, try to choose restaurants that are comfortable and that allow you to sit and enjoy your meal with soothing music and a pleasant interior. Make certain that they serve foods that you feel good about eating—fresh vegetables, steamed rice and other grains, fish, and foods that are not greasy or overly sweetened. There are many health-conscious restaurants around these days, and a large number are vegetarian or offer a variety of meatless dishes. Never be afraid to tailor a dish to suit your needs. You can ask the waiter what is in the dish you would like to order and then request that the cream sauce be omitted or that the dressing be brought on the side. If you are going to drink water, make sure it's bottled, not tap water.

As we've discussed, part of relaxing at a meal means eating slowly, savoring the taste sensations, and enjoying the company of others. A quality mealtime also involves appreciating the care that went into preparing the dishes and respecting what the food will be providing your body. Eating too quickly and under stressful circumstances is not good for your body and, more particularly, for your weight. The faster you eat, the less you chew, and the more food you can take in at one sitting without feeling full. Eating "fast and furious" also causes great stress on your organs and makes it more difficult to digest your food. A restaurant is a wonderful place to take your time, enjoy yourself, and respect the power that the food holds to nourish you.

When attending dinner or cocktail parties, remember: The main purpose of the gathering is to socialize with friends and family; food is secondary. If you are not certain about what will be served and suspect that it might be something you will not feel good about, eat before you leave your house. At the gathering there will most likely be something you can munch on, such as vegetables or fruit; this way you won't have to worry about embarrassing yourself, your host, or your friends.

On occasion, you may choose to diverge from your program to enjoy a meal out. If you are eating well most of the time and have developed enough self-control to return to your program, it's good to be flexible and allow yourself a treat. On the other hand, it may be too difficult for you to deal with. If, for example, you have a blood sugar imbalance and are just beginning a program that requires you to avoid all sugar, eating any sugar at all might set you back. You need to be the judge of your particular situation and act in your own best interests. You need never be confrontational—you can always compliment your host by asking to take some food home, and then give it to a neighbor or throw it away to avoid temptation.

Making the choice to lose weight and to take on a healthy eating lifestyle requires determination and courage, and the support of others is always an added bonus. However, if you are not finding the support you need from your friends, simply refrain from eating around them. Sometimes friends and family will pressure you to eat or drink what you don't want because they are feeling bad about their own choices or they simply don't understand why you have made yours. Changing your diet is a very personal decision that you have made, and you should not be affected by your friends' opinions, just as you should not feel it necessary to force your eating choices on them.

AN INTRODUCTION TO THE RECIPES

The foremost question on your mind is probably "What am I actually going to eat?" The following meal plan and recipe sections will help you to answer this question, and I imagine that many of you are going to find this the most useful part of the book. This is probably especially true for those readers who are not familiar with the vegetarian way of eating but rather have a history of three square meals a day, a meat-and-potatoes diet, or the pattern of starving themselves all day and then gorging themselves at night. To those people in particular I would like to say "Welcome to a totally new way of eating, feeling—and looking."

Let me give you a general introduction to the meal plan and recipes by saying, first, that this eating program is not designed to be exact. It's not meant to be a one-size-fits-all regimen but rather a general guide that outlines what has worked for thousands of people, each of whom has modified it to fit his or her individual needs. I myself follow this general model and have for twenty-five years. I know it's worked for me because, without ever dieting or counting calories, I've stayed healthy and energetic and maintained the same weight and percentage of body fat over the years. This can be your experience too.

A HEALTHY DAY OF EATING

First, let's look at what I consider a healthy day of eating. We're not going to be counting calories, because there's no need to with this plan. However, you may want to count your dietary grams of protein, especially at the beginning of your new eating program. Let's begin by examining the role of protein in your new diet.

Be a Protein Pro

Savvy eaters know that it's best to distribute protein intake throughout the day, so that you're getting approximately one-third of your daily protein requirement at each of your three meals. The reason is simple: The body cannot store protein. Your body uses the protein you eat to meet your immediate needs, then it generally stores the excess as fat. So when people gorge and put all their protein into one meal—eating, for instance, a big steak at dinner—the body cannot use all of that protein at once, and what is left over is converted into fat. You obviously want to avoid that, and the way to do so is to divvy up your protein intake throughout the day.

How much protein do you need? Women generally require 45 to 65 grams daily, although if you're pregnant, highly athletic, or recovering from illness, you may need more. Men generally need 50 to 80 grams; but again, needs are individual, so if you're bulking up, large framed, highly active, or convalescing, you could need more. There's a formula you can use too. You need .9 of a gram of protein per kilogram of your ideal body weight. (You can multiply your ideal weight in pounds by 0.453 to get the kilogram value.)

Breakfast Is Basic

The first thing you should remember about breakfast is: Don't skip it. You need quality fuel to get yourself functioning well in the morning, and you don't want to set yourself up for the weight-gain trap of consuming most of your calories in the evening. The second thing you should remember about breakfast is, as I've just explained, to try to eat about a third of your protein at that time.

I generally have one juice meal a day, and very often breakfast is that meal. I take a large glass (ten to twelve ounces) of a juice combo (see recipes later in this chapter) and spike it with a heaping tablespoon or scoop of a protein powder supplement. There are many such supplements on the market. I recommend using those that are nondairy in source, meaning that they have no whey powder. A good supplement could be based on rice protein, which has very low allergenic activity, or it could have a soy protein base. It should also contain branched chain amino acids, which will be listed on the label. The heaping tablespoon of protein powder that I use contains about 30 grams of protein, but you may want to modify this amount downward, depending on your daily protein needs as explained in the previous section.

Having this kind of breakfast works extremely well because you're getting, in addition to the protein, an array of health-promoting phytochemicals in the juice, which helps to detox and rejuvenate your system. But you do not have to restrict yourself to a juice meal if it doesn't appeal to you. You might want to take that same protein powder and blend it into a hot cereal; millet, oatmeal, or rice cereals are all good choices. Other good cereal add-ins include bananas; fresh berries; rice, almond, or soy milk; or apple juice. This breakfast gives you complex carbohydrates, protein, B vitamins, and quality fiber. With either the juice or cereal breakfast you'll enjoy the advantage of not feeling hungry for the next four hours, during which time you should be optimally energized.

Lunch — When Bigger May Be Better

Are you sometimes so busy that you skip lunch? Or do you skimp on this meal with the idea that doing so will allow you to eat a giant dinner? If so, neither of these is a good idea, either energy-wise or weight-wise.

Unless I'll be socializing in the evening, I generally make lunch my largest meal of the day; if you can, I recommend that you do the same thing. You don't have to make a big production out of it, but, as with breakfast, give yourself a third of your daily protein needs at this meal. A great lunch would be fish, served with some vegetables, grains, and a salad. Or you could have a pasta-based casserole with these same side dishes, or a large glass of juice.

Alternatively, lunch, rather than breakfast, could be your juice meal, into which you'd incorporate protein powder equal to about a third of your day's requirement. You could even make a smoothie instead of plain juice, adding a banana and some vitamin C. Smoothies are more filling than just juice, and some people prefer that. Go with your own preferences in adapting this basic pattern, because you'll be more likely to stick with it that way.

Downsize Your Dinner

Other advisors on health and I recommend having a dinner that's smaller than your lunch, but we also need to be realistic. Because of the way American society is organized, with people on the run or working nonstop during the day, and families coming together for meals only in the evening, dinner is still going to be the most important meal for many. If that's the case for you, don't feel guilty. Keep dinner as your main meal. But downsize it. If you're used to eating until you're full, which frequently means you're overeating, try to cut back gradually. Over a period of two months, for example, decrease the size of your portions. If you're a big meat eater, used to eating a twelve- or sixteen-ounce steak for dinner, cut back first to a steak of half that size. Then make a shift from steak to chicken, and eventually from chicken to fish. Yes, you can go cold turkey and shift abruptly to a more healthful eating pattern, if that's your style. However, the gradual approach, removing one unhealthful item per week from your diet—and keeping that item out permanently—seems to work better for most people in terms of achieving lasting change.

As you create your dinners and other meals, remember that it's sometimes what you put *on* a food rather than the food itself that's fattening. For instance, pasta makes a good dinner; it's a complex carbohydrate that gives you protein, fills you up, and is not high in calories. But a problem comes in if you top that pasta with a cream-based sauce. Instead, opt for marinara-style sauce. Or use an olive-oil-based garlic sauce, adding onions, other vegetables, and herbs to taste.

The same idea holds for salads. Centering meals around large salads is a great idea for those concerned with weight control, but you have to forgo creamy dressings if you want this approach to work. Instead, create something more healthful with balsamic vinegar, olive oil, garlic, and herbs. Also, remember that good bread, which often is served with salads, doesn't need anything on it. But if you must use something, forget butter or margarine. Instead, dip the bread in a little olive oil, as people in the Mediterranean region do. This region, by the way, is often held up as a dietary model not only because olive oil is a staple there, but because the people eat their large meal in the early afternoon rather than at night, and because they eat more fresh vegetables and fruits than we do. Another factor that cannot be underestimated is that they spend more time at meals than we do, savoring the food and reconnecting with their families and friends in an unhurried way.

Develop Snack Strategies

A lot of people do well at mealtimes in terms of eating sensibly but find that snacks are their dietary downfall. Even if you eat as little as 300 extra calories a day in unhealthful fatty foods, in less than two weeks you will have gained a pound. And over time, that will add up to numbers you don't even want to think about.

The best snack strategy I can give you is embodied in one word: juices. The more juices you have, the less hungry you are going to be between meals. This snack strategy involves having juices as meals and as snacks, midmorning and midafternoon, as the need arises. By turning to juice you will get valuable nutrients unaccompanied by fat.

Another snack strategy you should adopt is to never snack close to bedtime. To be more precise, don't eat within at least two or three hours of going to bed. When you sleep, your body's in a catabolic state, meaning that it's slowly breaking down what you've taken in that day and that it's recovering, detoxifying, and cleansing. It doesn't need any last-minute fuel, and it certainly isn't equipped to deal with anything like pizzas, hamburgers, cookies, or ice cream. These foods may raise your blood sugar, keeping you awake, and add on more pounds.

Respect Your Own Individuality

Because everyone is physiologically unique, each individual using this book is going to lose weight at a different rate. Some people, using the thirty-one-day meal plan and conscientiously trying to do everything I suggest in the rest of the book, may lose weight at a slower rate than they'd anticipated. Others, adopting only some of the practices I recommend, may find the pounds rolling off. In this category I think back to a man who came up to me a few months after my December 1998 PBS appearances. He'd seen me on TV, read *Gary Null's Ultimate Anti-Aging Program*, and followed just some of my recommendations for healthful eating. He did not buy organic food, he did not juice, and he did not take any of the suggested supplements. But he did eliminate beef, chicken, dairy products, sugars, caffeine, carbonated beverages, and wheat. The upshot was that he lost thirty pounds in just a few months and said he felt terrific, better than he ever had. And this was just with a straight elimination diet—and nothing else.

Such a change in lifestyle would be a great start for anyone. Then, as a second phase, if you could gradually begin including juices and nutritional supplements into your diet, that would be even better. But, like the man I spoke with, you may not be motivated to take this next step. And that's okay. Each person has to implement change at a level he or she feels comfortable with.

Sometimes, with lifestyle change, you actually may find yourself losing weight at a faster rate than you want. This happens particularly to people who give up foods to which they've been allergic. The pounds melt off quickly, and you see it reflected in their face and neck, which are the first areas to show weight loss, and which can appear gaunt. If you find yourself losing weight too quickly, modify your diet: Eat more! If you find yourself needing more calories and energy, it is a good idea to add some nut butter to your diet. In addition to peanut butter, almond or walnut butter are delicious and nutritious additions to hot cereal or health drinks. Or be traditional and use them on whole grain bread for a lunch or midafternoon snack.

The thirty-one-day meal plan and recipes that follow are designed to help everyone:

- Eat a relatively large volume of food
- Get a feeling of satiety after each meal
- Not feel starved between meals
- Lose weight
- Feel energized
- Get healthier

If you find after eating one of these meals that it provided you with too much food or too little, then please adjust them to meet your individual needs. These menus are designed to be flexible. Please experiment, using different seasonings and amounts to your taste. Additional recipes can be found in my books, *The International Vegetarian Cookbook, The Joy of Juicing,* and *Vegetarian Cooking for Good Health* (just exclude the dairy and wheat recipes). Have fun, and eat well.

YOUR THIRTY-ONE-DAY EATING PLAN

As you begin, remember that these recipes are only suggestions. They can be adjusted in terms of both seasonings and quantities of ingredients to accommodate your individual tastes. I've provided you with different breakfast, lunch, and dinner recipes for each day of the month as well as one protein shake recipe. The basic format of the menus is as follows:

BREAKFAST

A juice drink

or

A breakfast cereal

LUNCH

A juice drink (if you did not have one for breakfast)

or

A luncheon meal of fish and a salad

DINNER

A juice drink (if you did not have one for breakfast or lunch

or

A dinner meal of pasta, or a casserole, or any combination of grains, beans, and starchy vegetables

A salad (if you did not have one for lunch)

A dessert dish

You should substitute the protein shake for one of the three meals throughout the day. Some of you may want to adopt a more aggressive approach and have two shakes and one full meal a day. That's fine—just make sure that the meal you eat is big enough to meet all your nutritional requirements and satisfy your appetite. You also should have at least one salad a day, at either lunch or dinner, as you prefer. And if you've decided to keep to a strict vegetarian diet, you may eliminate fish entirely.

Any meal recipe may be substituted for another comparable recipe—you'll find all the recipes grouped by meal and listed in alphabetical order at the end of the chapter. Many of these recipes are intended to serve two or three individuals, making them ideal for family meals or dinner parties. You can also save the extra portion or adjust the amounts of ingredients to make an individual serving.

Concerning Dessert

Remember that dessert is not for everyone. If you are losing weight and feeling great and want to reward yourself with a healthful, tasty treat, then you can select from the desserts in our eating plan. Most people, however, should skip the desserts, at least for the first several months.

DAY 1

Breakfast
Tropical Paradise Amaranth Cereal
or
Carob Nut Milk Shake

Lunch
Tuna with Sesame-Orange Sauce
Endive Salad
or
A juice drink if you did not have one for breakfast

Dinner
Mushroom Broccoli Quiche
Salad if you did not have one for lunch

Mandarin Cream Pudding

or

Substitute a juice drink if you did not have one today

DAY 2

Breakfast
Banana-Coconut Walnut Millet Rice Cereal

or

Pecan Protein Shake

Lunch
Grilled Salmon with Tomato and Basil
Herbed Tomato Salad

or

A juice drink if you did not have one for breakfast

Dinner
Cumin Chickpeas
Salad if you did not have one for lunch
Mixed Melon/Strawberry Pudding

or

Substitute a juice drink if you did not have one today

DAY 3

Breakfast
Raspberry Oat-Soy-Banana Pancakes

or

Strawberry Delight

Lunch
Tangy Lemon Tofu-Vegetable Kebobs
Raw Spinach Salad

or

A juice drink if you did not have one for breakfast

Dinner

Eggplant Soy Mozzarella

Salad if you did not have one for lunch

Zesty Mango Lime Pudding

or

Substitute a juice drink if you did not have one today

DAY 4

Breakfast

Cream of Maple Barley

or

Watermelon Pineapple Gerfingapoken

Lunch

Broiled Sole with an Herb Vinaigrette

Raita Salad

or

A juice drink if you did not have one for breakfast

Dinner

Pesto and Tomatoes on Fettuccini

Salad if you did not have one for lunch

Tropical Blend Pudding

or

Substitute a juice drink if you did not have one today

DAY 5

Breakfast

Old-Fashioned Oatmeal Breakfast

or

Frosty Pear and Carrot/Celery Juice

Lunch

Orange Roughy or Sea Bass with Teriyaki Sauce

Endive Salad

or

A juice drink if you did not have one for breakfast

Dinner

Rice Noodle Fantasy

Salad if you did not have one for lunch

Mango Pineapple Lime Pudding

or

Substitute a juice drink if you did not have one today

DAY 6

Breakfast

Sweet Spice Rice

or

Zesty Papaya Shake

Lunch

Tofu Stew

Cucumber and Tomato Salad

or

A juice drink if you did not have one for breakfast

Dinner

Stir-Fried Tempeh with Broccoli and Lemon Threads

Salad if you did not have one for lunch

Cherry/Berry Pudding

or

Substitute a juice drink if you did not have one today

DAY 7

Breakfast

Nutty Quinoa

or

Tangerine Pineapple and Kiwi Cocktail

Lunch

Broiled Halibut Steaks with Mustard Glaze

Hot Dulse and Potato Salad

or

A juice drink if you did not have one for breakfast

Dinner

Spring Scalloped Vegetables

Salad if you did not have one for lunch

Spelt Crisps

or

Substitute a juice drink if you did not have one today

DAY 8

Breakfast

Nutty Morning

or

Exotic Pineapple Shake

Lunch

Stewed Salmon with Tomatoes and Herbs

Fancy Vegetable Combo Salad

or

A juice drink if you did not have one for breakfast

Dinner

Potato Chowder

Salad if you did not have one for lunch

Chewy Macadamia Treats

or

Substitute a juice drink if you did not have one today

DAY 9

Breakfast
Rice and Nuts
or
Carob Orange Twist

Lunch
Spicy Sea Bass and Tofu Delight
Potato and Herb Salad
or
A juice drink if you did not have one for breakfast

Dinner
Japanese Rice Noodles with Shiitake Mushrooms
Salad if you did not have one for lunch
Fruity Carob Bars
or
Substitute a juice drink if you did not have one today

DAY 10

Breakfast
Blueberry Breakfast Treat
or
Celery Apple Juice

Lunch
Fillet of Sole with Dill
Spicy Cucumber and Tofu Salad
or
A juice drink if you did not have one for breakfast

Dinner
Lentil Burgers
Salad if you did not have one for lunch

Coconut Date Paradise

or

Substitute a juice drink if you did not have one today

DAY 11

Breakfast

Sweet Cinnamon Quinoa

or

Citrus Delight

Lunch

Tasty Bass with Spices

Pasta Tomato and Garlic Salad

or

A juice drink if you did not have one for breakfast

Dinner

Parsley and Mushroom Lasagna

Salad if you did not have one for lunch

Raspberry and Spelt Crust

or

Substitute a juice drink if you did not have one today

DAY 12

Breakfast

Fluffy Raisin Amaranth

or

Mixed Vegetable Juice

Lunch

Herbs and Brook Trout

Caesar Salad with Thyme Croutons

or

A juice drink if you did not have one for breakfast

Dinner

Spicy Texas Chili

Salad if you did not have one for lunch

Peach in a Pumpkin Crust

or

Substitute a juice drink if you did not have one today

DAY 13

Breakfast

Quinoa Mango Delight

or

Sunflower Sprout Apple Juice

Lunch

Fish Sticks with Gary's Salsa Sauce

Red Potato Salad

or

A juice drink if you did not have one today

Dinner

Zesty Soy Chunks with Rice and Vegetables

Salad if you did not have one for lunch

Gary's Fruity Kazootie Cocktail

or

Substitute a juice drink if you did not have one today

DAY 14

Breakfast

Amaranth Decadence

or

Strawberry Banana Split

Lunch

Nori-wrapped Soy Fish

Salad if you did not have one for lunch

Raw Spinach Salad

or

A juice drink if you did not have one for breakfast

Dinner

Potato Pancakes

Salad if you did not have one for lunch

Strawberry Carob Pudding

or

Substitute a juice drink if you did not have one today

DAY 15

Breakfast

Cream of Spelt

or

Romaine Lettuce and Apple Refresher

Lunch

Spicy Manhattan Tofu Chowder

Endive Salad

or

A juice drink if you did not have one for breakfast

Dinner

Ratatouille

Salad if you did not have one for lunch

Raspberry Cinnamon Pudding

or

Substitute a juice drink if you did not have one today

DAY 16

Breakfast

Spelt Vitality

or

Almond-Flavored Watermelon Shake

Lunch

Cayenne Flounder

Fancy Vegetable Combo Salad

or

A juice drink if you did not have one for breakfast

Dinner

Olive and Rice Pasta

Salad if you did not have one for lunch

Mango Cream

or

Substitute a juice drink if you did not have one today

DAY 17

Breakfast

Quinoa Brown

or

Coconut Cherry and Melon Shake

Lunch

Tuna Delight

Cucumber and Tomato Salad

or

A juice drink if you did not have one for breakfast

Dinner

Sea Vegetable and Cabbage over Linguine

Blackberry Pudding

or

Substitute a juice drink if you did not have one today

DAY 18

Breakfast
The Ancient Cereal
or
Sunflower Coconut Papaya Shake

Lunch
Spring Stew
Fancy Vegetable Combo Salad
or
A juice drink if you did not have one for breakfast

Dinner
Vegan Spring Rolls
Salad if you did not have one for lunch
Peaches and Cream
or
Substitute a juice drink if you did not have one today

DAY 19

Breakfast
Carob Sunflower Oats
or
Gingery Orange Splash

Lunch
Macaroni Marconi
Herbed Tomato Salad
or
A juice drink if you did not have one for breakfast

Dinner
Green Pea Pilaf
Salad if you did not have one for lunch

Raspberry Gelatin

or

Substitute a juice drink if you did not have one today

DAY 20

Breakfast
Maple Brown Rice

or

Leafy Beet Vegetable Juice

Lunch
Hawaiian Tuna
Raw Spinach Salad

or

A juice drink if you did not have one for breakfast

Dinner
Vegetable Chili
Salad if you did not have one for lunch
Nutty Cream

or

Substitute a juice drink if you did not have one today

DAY 21

Breakfast
Almond Cinnamon Barley

or

Blueberries and Pear Macadamia Shake

Lunch
Salmon Quiche
Caesar Salad with Thyme Croutons

or

A juice drink if you did not have one for breakfast

Dinner

Vatapa

Salad if you did not have one for lunch

Cranberry Pudding

or

Substitute a juice drink if you did not have one today

DAY 22

Breakfast

Power Oats Breakfast

or

Cranberry Ginger Spritzer

Lunch

Pumpkin Cream Soup

Spicy Cucumber and Tofu Salad

or

A juice drink if you did not have one for breakfast

Dinner

Orzo Turanerole

Salad if you did not have one for lunch

Orange Cream and Granola

or

Substitute a juice drink if you did not have one today

DAY 23

Breakfast

Cream of Oats

or

Juicy Carrot and Swiss Chard

Lunch
Pochee
Fancy Vegetable Combo Salad
or
A juice drink if you did not have one for breakfast

Dinner
Gary's Vegetable Pan
Salad if you did not have one for lunch
Fruit Salad in Cream
or
Substitute a juice drink if you did not have one today

DAY 24

Breakfast
Barley Brown
or
Date Pineapple Nut Shake

Lunch
Pasta and Black Bean Soup
Endive Salad
or
A juice drink if you did not have one for breakfast

Dinner
Mushroom Broccoli Quiche
Salad if you did not have one for lunch
Blackberry Pudding
or
Substitute a juice drink if you did not have one today

DAY 25

Breakfast
Maple Amaranth
or
Apple Plum and Cherry Surprise

Lunch
Fish and Chips
Fancy Vegetable Combo Salad
or
A juice drink if you did not have one for breakfast

Dinner
Cumin Chickpeas
Salad if you did not have one for lunch
Banana Cream
or
Substitute a juice drink if you did not have one today

DAY 26

Breakfast
Cream of Quinoa
or
Kiwi Lemon Melon Tonic

Lunch
Popeye Loves Olive
Endive Salad
or
A juice drink if you did not have one for breakfast

Dinner

Aromatic Vegetable and Noodles

Salad if you did not have one for lunch

Apple and Cinnamon Pudding

or

Substitute a juice drink if you did not have one today

DAY 27

Breakfast

Cream of Rice

or

Celery Purple Cabbage Surprise

Lunch

The Original Broccoli Stir-Fry

Potato and Herb Salad

or

A juice drink if you did not have one for breakfast

Dinner

Gary's Favorite Casserole

Salad if you did not have one for lunch

Almond Balls

or

Substitute a juice drink if you did not have one today

DAY 28

Breakfast

Breakfast in Peru

or

Strawberry Banana Split

Lunch

Gary's Veggie Stew

Raw Spinach Salad

or

A juice drink if you did not have one for breakfast

Dinner

Gary's Food for the Soul

Salad if you did not have one for lunch

Mango Pineapple Lime Pudding

or

Substitute a juice drink if you did not have one today

DAY 29

Breakfast

Cream of Amaranth

or

Tangy Strawberry Carrot Shake

Lunch

Eggplant Parmigiana Sandwich

Hot Dulse and Potato Salad

or

A juice drink if you did not have one for breakfast

Dinner

Olive and Rice Pasta

Salad if you did not have one for lunch

Nutty Cream

or

Substitute a juice drink if you did not have one today

DAY 30

Breakfast

Rice 'n' Strawberries

or

Pineapple Cranberry Twist

Lunch

Fava Salad with Cashews and Dill

Endive Salad

or

A juice drink if you did not have one for breakfast

Dinner

Zesty Cauliflower with Garlic Sauce

Salad if you did not have one for lunch

Mixed Melon/Strawberry Pudding

or

Substitute a juice drink if you did not have one today

DAY 31

Breakfast

Raspberry Oat-Soy-Banana Pancakes

or

Almond Flavored Watermelon Shake

Lunch

Broiled Tuna with Herb Vinaigrette

Cucumber and Tomato Salad

or

A juice drink if you did not have one for breakfast

Dinner

Zesty Soy Chunks with Rice and Vegetables

Salad if you did not have one for lunch

Zesty Mango Lime Pie

or

Substitute a juice drink if you did not have one today

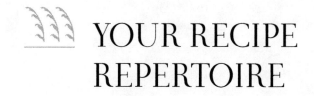

YOUR RECIPE REPERTOIRE

BREAKFAST CEREALS

TIPS

Grains cooked in advance may be reheated by steaming.

Grains are more flavorful when cooked with 1/2 teaspoon sea salt per cup of dry grain.

Although unhulled barley is most desirable because it is the whole grain, it has a longer cooking time than "pearled" barley; look for the darker varieties of pearled barley, found in health food stores, as they are minimally processed.

Grade B or C maple syrup is less processed than Grade A, retaining more of its natural minerals.

Rice milk and soy milk may be used interchangeably, with slight taste variation; however, soy milk adds a protein complement to grains.

ALMOND CINNAMON BARLEY

1 cup cooked pearled barley
1 1/2 ounces almonds, blanched and chopped
2 tablespoons protein powder
Pinch of cinnamon

Combine barley in a medium-size saucepan with water. When water comes to a boil, lower heat and cook until water is absorbed, stirring occasionally. Add remaining ingredients and mix well. Serve immediately.

SERVES 1

AMARANTH DECADENCE

1/2 cup amaranth
1 1/4 cups (approximately) filtered water for the amaranth
3 tablespoons filtered water for the carob powder
3 tablespoons carob powder
1/2 cup raspberries
2 tablespoons pure maple syrup
1 tablespoon protein powder

1. Bring amaranth and 1 1/4 cups water to a boil and cook covered over low heat for 25 minutes, or until tender.
2. In a saucepan, stir carob powder into 3 tablespoons of filtered water. Add raspberries and maple syrup. Let simmer for 5 minutes.
3. Pour carob sauce over amaranth. Sprinkle protein powder over sauce and serve immediately.

SERVES 1

THE ANCIENT CEREAL

1/2 cup amaranth
1 1/4 cups filtered water
1/4 teaspoon sea salt
4 dates
1/2 tablespoon pure maple syrup
1 tablespoon protein powder

1. Bring amaranth and salted water to a boil. Lower heat, cover, and cook until tender, about 25 min. Then let stand 5 minutes.
2. Dice dates and add with maple syrup to cooked amaranth.
3. Sprinkle protein powder over cereal and serve immediately.

SERVES 1

BANANA-COCONUT WALNUT MILLET RICE CEREAL

1/2 cup millet
1 1/2 cups filtered water
1 cup mashed banana
1/4 cup coconut flakes
5 tablespoons monukia raisins
2–3 tablespoons pure maple syrup
3 tablespoons chopped walnuts
1/2 cup rice or soy milk

1. Combine millet and water in a medium-size saucepan. Bring to a boil over medium heat. Lower heat and cook 3 to 7 minutes, or until tender.
2. Add the remaining ingredients and 1 to 2 minutes.
3. Serve with rice or soy milk on top.

SERVES 2

BARLEY BROWN

3 tablespoons carob powder
3 tablespoons filtered water
1/2 cup raspberries
2 tablespoons pure maple syrup
1 cup cooked pearled barley
1 tablespoon protein powder
Handful of slivered almonds
Vanilla soy milk

1. In a small saucepan, stir carob powder into water. Add raspberries and maple syrup. Let simmer 5 minutes.
2. Pour raspberry carob sauce over cooked barley. Sprinkle protein powder and slivered almonds over sauce and serve immediately with vanilla soy milk on the side.

SERVES 1

BLUEBERRY BREAKFAST TREAT

1 cup cooked brown rice (at room temperature)
1/2 cup blueberries, cut in half
2 tablespoons sunflower seeds
2 figs, chopped
sprinkle of unsweetened, flaked coconut

Combine all ingredients. Mix well.

SERVES 1

BREAKFAST IN PERU

1/2 cup quinoa
1 1/2 cups filtered water
1 ripe bosc pear, quartered and sliced
dash sea salt
handful of chopped cashews
1/2 tablespoon pure maple syrup
1 tablespoon protein powder

1. Cook quinoa in 1¼ cups of the water with the sea salt.
2. Cook pears with maple syrup and remaining water over low heat until tender, about 3–5 minutes.
3. Spoon pear mixture over cooked quinoa.
4. Sprinkle protein powder and cashews on top and serve immediately.

SERVES 1

RICE 'N' STRAWBERRIES

1 cup soy milk
1 tablespoon pure maple syrup
⅛ to ¼ teaspoon pure vanilla extract
½ cup raw cashews
pinch sea salt
½ cup sliced strawberries
1 cup cooked brown rice, hot

1. In a blender, combine soy milk, vanilla extract, maple syrup, cashews, and salt.
2. Sprinkle strawberries over hot rice.
3. Pour cashew sauce over all.
4. Serve immediately.

SERVES 1

CAROB SUNFLOWER OATS

½ cup oats
¾ cup filtered water plus 3 tablespoons
3 tablespoons carob powder
½ cup raspberries
2 tablespoons pure maple syrup
1 tablespoon protein powder
¼ cup ground or handful raw sunflower seeds
salt to taste

1. Bring oats and ¾ cup water to a boil, cover, lower heat and cook until tender, about 15 minutes.

2. In a small saucepan, stir carob powder into 3 tablespoons filtered water. Add raspberries and maple syrup. Let simmer for 5 minutes.
3. Pour carob sauce over oats. Sprinkle protein powder and sunflower seeds over sauce and serve immediately.

SERVES 1

CREAM OF AMARANTH

1/2 cup amaranth
1 1/4 cups filtered water
1/4 teaspoon sea salt
1/2 cup silken tofu
1 palmful cashews
1 palmful raisins
1 tablespoon pure maple syrup
2 tablespoons protein powder

1. Bring amaranth and salted water to a boil. Lower heat and cook covered until tender, about 25 minutes. Let stand for 5 minutes.
2. Mix in the rest of the ingredients until creamy.
3. Sprinkle protein powder on top and serve immediately.

SERVES 1

CREAM OF BARLEY

1/2 cup cooked pearled barley
1/2 cup silken tofu
2 tablespoons chopped walnuts
1 banana, mashed
1 tablespoon pure maple syrup
2 tablespoons protein powder

1. In a saucepan, combine all of the ingredients except barley and protein powder over low heat until creamy.
2. Add barley, stirring until hot.
3. Sprinkle protein powder on top and serve immediately.

SERVES 1

CREAM OF MAPLE BARLEY

1/2 cup barley
11/2 cups filtered water
3 tablespoons pure maple syrup
1/2 teaspoon cinnamon
1/4 teaspoon ground nutmeg
2 tablespoons protein powder
1 banana
4 strawberries

1. Simmer barley in water with maple syrup for about 11/4 hours, until tender.
2. Sprinkle with spices and protein powder. Add fresh fruit and serve immediately.

SERVES 1

CREAM OF OATS

1/2 cup rolled oats
3/4 cup filtered water
1/4 teaspoon salt
1/2 cup silken tofu
2 tablespoons almonds
1 peach, diced
1 tablespoon pure maple syrup
2 tablespoons protein powder

1. Bring oats and salted water to a boil. Lower heat and cooked, covered, until tender, about 15 minutes.
2. Mix in the rest of the ingredients, except protein powder, stirring until creamy.
3. Sprinkle protein powder on top and serve immediately.

SERVES 1

CREAM OF QUINOA

1/2 cup quinoa
1 cup filtered water
1/4 teaspoon sea salt
1/2 cup silken tofu
2 tablepoons walnuts
1 orange, chopped
1 tablespoon pure maple syrup
2 tablespoons protein powder

1. Bring quinoa and salted water to a boil. Cover and cook over low heat until tender, about 15 minutes.
2. Mix in the rest of the ingredients, except protein powder, stirring until creamy.
3. Sprinkle protein powder on top and serve immediately.

SERVES 1

CREAM OF RICE

1/2 cup short-grain brown rice
1 cup filtered water
1/4 teaspoon sea salt
1/2 cup silken tofu
3 tablespoons toasted almonds
1/2 cup chopped apple
1 tablespoon pure maple syrup
2 teaspoons protein powder

1. Bring rice and salted water to a boil. Cook, covered, over low heat until tender, about 40 minutes.
2. Mix in the rest of the ingredients, except protein powder, stirring until creamy.
3. Sprinkle protein powder on top and serve immediately.

SERVES 1

CREAM OF SPELT

1/2 *cup spelt*
1 1/4 *cups filtered water*
1/4 *teaspoon sea salt*
1/2 *cup silken tofu*
2 *tablespoons Brazil nuts*
1/4 *fresh pineapple, diced*
1 *tablespoon pure maple syrup*
2 *tablespoons protein powder*

1. Bring spelt and salted water to a boil. Cover and cook over low heat until tender, about 1 1/4 hours.
2. Mix in the rest of the ingredients, except protein powder, stirring until creamy.
3. Sprinkle protein powder on top and serve immediately.

SERVES 1

FLUFFY RAISIN AMARANTH

1 *cup cooked amaranth (at room temperature)*
handful of raisins
1 *tablespoon honey*
pinch of cinnamon

Combine all ingredients. Mix well.

SERVES 1

MAPLE AMARANTH

1/2 *cup amaranth*
1 1/4 *cups filtered water*
3 *tablespoons pure maple syrup*
1/2 *teaspoon cinnamon*
1/4 *teaspoon ground nutmeg*
2 *tablespoons protein powder*
1 *banana, sliced*
4 *strawberries, sliced*

1. Bring amaranth and salted water with maple syrup to a boil. Cover and cook over low heat until tender, about 25 minutes. Let stand 5 minutes.
2. Sprinkle with spices and protein powder. Add fresh fruit and serve immediately.

SERVES 1

MAPLE BROWN RICE

1/2 cup short-grain brown rice

1 cup water

1/4 teaspoon salt

3 tablespoons pure maple syrup

1/2 teaspoon cinnamon

1/4 teaspoon ground nutmeg

2 tablespoons protein powder

1 banana

4 strawberries

1. Bring brown rice in salted water and maple syrup to a boil. Lower heat and cook covered, about 45 minutes, until tender.
2. Sprinkle with spices and protein powder. Add fresh fruit and serve immediately.

SERVES 1

NUTTY MORNING

1 cup cooked short-grain brown rice (at room temperature)

1/2 banana, mashed

1/4 cup pecans, chopped

2 tablespoons barley malt

Combine all ingredients. Mix well and serve immediately.

SERVES 1

NUTTY QUINOA

1 cup cooked quinoa (at room temperature)
1/2 pear, cut into bite-size pieces
1/4 cup walnuts, chopped
1 tablespoon pure maple syrup

Combine all ingredients. Mix well and serve immediately.

SERVES 1

OLD-FASHIONED OATMEAL BREAKFAST

3/4 cup rolled oats
1 1/2 cups filtered water
1/4 teaspoon sea salt
1 tablespoon pure maple syrup or raw honey
1 tablespoon protein powder
1 banana, mashed

1. Cook oats in salted water for 10–15 minutes over medium heat, stirring occasionally.
2. Sprinkle with protein powder. Add banana and mix well. Serve immediately.

SERVES 1

QUINOA MANGO DELIGHT

1 cup cooked quinoa (at room temperature)
3/4 cup unsweetened dried mango, chopped
1/4 cup pecans, chopped
pinch of ground cloves
pinch of allspice

Combine all ingredients. Mix well and serve immediately.

SERVES 1

RASPBERRY OAT-SOY-BANANA PANCAKES

2 tablespoons egg substitute
2 tablespoons vanilla extract
1 banana, mashed
¼ cup rice milk
¼ cup whole spelt flour
1 cup oat flour
½ cup soy flour
1 teaspoon baking powder
1 teaspoon baking soda
4 tablespoons raisins
3 tablespoons unsweetened flaked coconut (optional)
¼ cup raspberries
Canola oil

1. In a medium-size mixing bowl, combine egg replacer, vanilla, banana, and rice milk. Mix with fork until well blended.
2. In a separate bowl, combine flours, baking powder, and baking soda. Mix well. Add flour mixture to banana and milk mixture, blending well with a spoon. Stir in raisins, coconut if desired, and raspberries.
3. Heat oil in a large skillet over medium heat. Pour in 2 to 3 tablespoons of batter at a time. Cook each pancake for 3 to 5 minutes on each side until light brown. Re-oil skillet as necessary to prevent sticking.

YIELDS 14 PANCAKES

RICE AND NUTS

¾ cup cooked brown rice (at room temperature)
¼ cup flaked unsweetened coconut
¼ cup pecans, chopped
¼ cup chopped dried apples
2 dried apricots, chopped
¼ cup filtered water
flaxseeds for garnish

1. Combine brown rice with coconut, pecans, apples, and apricots.
2. Puree half the mixture in blender with water until coarsely ground.
3. Add ground mixture to the rest of the rice. Sprinkle with flaxseeds for garnish and serve immediately.

SERVES 1

RISING IN THE TROPICS

1 cup cooked short-grain brown rice (at room temperature)
1/3 cup fresh pineapple, cut into bite-size pieces
1/3 cup fresh mango
1 tablespoon pure maple syrup
pinch of cinnamon

Combine all ingredients. Mix well and serve immediately.

SERVES 1

SWEET CINNAMON QUINOA

1 cup cooked quinoa (at room temperature)
1–2 dried apricots, chopped
pinch of cinnamon

Combine all ingredients. Mix well and serve immediately.

SERVES 1

SWEET SPICE RICE

1 cup cooked short-grain brown rice (at room temperature)
1/2 large peach, cut into bite-size pieces
1 tablespoon pure maple syrup
pinch of nutmeg
pinch of allspice

Combine all ingredients. Mix well and serve immediately.

SERVES 1

POWER OATS BREAKFAST

3/4 cup rolled oats
1/4 teaspoon sea salt
1 cup filtered water
4 dates
1/2 tablespoon pure maple syrup
1 tablespoon protein powder

1. Cook oats in salted water for 10–15 minutes over medium heat, stirring occasionally until tender.
2. Dice dates. Add with maple syrup to cooked oats and mix well.
3. Sprinkle with protein powder and serve immediately.

SERVES 1

QUINOA BROWN

1/2 cup quinoa
1 cup filtered water plus 3 tablespoons
1/4 teaspoon sea salt
3 tablespoons carob powder
1/2 cup raspberries
2 tablespoons pure maple syrup
1 tablespoon protein powder

1. Bring quinoa to boil in 1 cup of salted water. Lower heat and cook, covered, 10–15 minutes until tender.
2. In a small saucepan, stir carob powder into 3 tablespoons water. Add raspberries and maple syrup. Let simmer for 5 minutes.
3. Pour carob sauce over quinoa. Sprinkle protein powder over sauce and serve immediately.

SERVES 1

SPELT VITALITY

1/2 cup spelt
1 1/4 cups filtered water
3 tablespoons pure maple syrup
1/4 teaspoon sea salt
1/2 teaspoon cinnamon
1/4 teaspoon ground nutmeg
2 teaspoons protein powder
1 banana, sliced
4 strawberries, sliced

1. Bring spelt in water with maple syrup and salt to a boil. Lower heat and cook, covered, about 1 1/2 hours or until tender. Add more water if necessary.
2. Sprinkle with spices and protein powder. Add fresh fruit and serve immediately.

SERVES 1

TROPICAL PARADISE AMARANTH CEREAL

Note: To toast nuts, preheat over to 375 degrees F. Place nuts on an ungreased cookie sheet and bake for 10 to 15 minutes, or until light brown.

2 cups coconut milk

1 banana, sliced

1/2 cup pitted dates

1/2 cup chopped pineapple

1/4 cup unsweetened, flaked coconut

2 cups cooked amaranth

1 tablespoon chopped macadamia nuts, toasted (see note below)

1 tablespoon almond extract

2 teaspoons vanilla extract

1. In a medium-size saucepan, combine coconut milk, banana, dates, and pineapple. Cook over medium-low heat for 2 to 3 minutes.
2. Add the remaining ingredients and mix well. Cook an additional 2 to 3 minutes. Serve hot.

SERVES 2

VERMONT MAPLE PUMPKIN

1 small whole pumpkin

filtered water

1 tablespoon maple syrup

1 tablespoon protein powder

pinch of allspice

1. Preheat oven to 400 degrees F.
2. Cut pumpkin in half, remove the seeds, and discard them.
3. Place pumpkin halves in baking dish cut side down. Add enough filtered water to measure 1/3 inch. Bake for 40 minutes.
4. When cooled, spoon out pumpkin and place in a bowl.
5. Add remaining ingredients. Mix well.

SERVES 1

JUICES AND SHAKES

Note: As you know, I recommend using juices and shakes as liquid breakfasts. However, if these are not sufficient for your appetite, you may have a piece of fruit not less than one hour after your drink.

ALMOND-FLAVORED WATERMELON SHAKE

3 cups watermelon chunks, peeled (1 cup juice) with seeds
1 banana
1/4 cup plain soy milk
2 tablespoons protein powder
1/2 teaspoon pure almond extract
1/2 teaspoon cinnamon
1 cup ice

1. Juice watermelon.
2. In a blender or food processor, combine 1 cup watermelon juice with remaining ingredients. Blend for 2 minutes, or until smooth.
3. Serve immediately.

YIELDS 2 CUPS

APPLE PLUM AND CHERRY SURPRISE

5 apples (1 1/4 cups juice)
3 plums (1/2 cup juice)
1 lemon (2 tablespoons juice)
1/4 cup pitted cherries, frozen
1 heaping tablespoon protein powder
1 cup ice

1. Separately juice apples, plums, and lemon. Set aside.
2. In a blender or food processor, combine 1 1/4 cups apple juice, 1/2 cup plum juice, and 2 tablespoons lemon juice with the remaining ingredients. Blend for 2 minutes, or until smooth.
3. Serve immediately.

YIELDS 3 CUPS

AVOCADO AND STRAWBERRY DELIGHT

Note: May have 6 whole strawberries one hour after this breakfast drink if necessary.

1 apple (¼ cup juice)
¼ cup avocado
¼ banana
½ cup strawberries, fresh or frozen
½ cup plain soy milk
½ teaspoon pure almond extract
2 teaspoons protein powder
1 cup ice

1. Juice apple.
2. In a blender or food processor, combine ¼ cup apple juice with remaining ingredients. Blend for 2 minutes, or until smooth.
3. Serve immediately.

YIELDS 2½ CUPS

BLUEBERRIES AND PEAR MACADAMIA NUT SHAKE

2 pears (½ cup juice)
½ cup blueberries
½ cup ground or whole white macadamia nuts, unsalted
1 banana, mashed
¾ cup unsweetened soy milk
2 heaping tablespoons protein powder
½ teaspoon pure lemon extract
1 cup ice

1. Juice pears.
2. In a blender or food processor, combine ½ cup pear juice with remaining ingredients. Blend for 2 minutes, or until smooth.
3. Serve immediately.

YIELDS 3 CUPS

CAROB NUT MILK SHAKE

4 apples (1 cup juice)

2 bananas

4 tablespoon ground or whole walnuts or walnut butter, unsalted

1 cup plain soy milk

1¹/₂ tablespoons pure unsweetened carob powder (pure unsweetened cocoa may be substituted)

1 teaspoon pure almond extract

1 heaping tablespoon protein powder

1 cup ice

1. Juice apples.
2. In a blender or food processor, combine 1 cup apple juice with remaining ingredients. Blend for 2 minutes, or until smooth.
3. Serve immediately.

   YIELDS 3 CUPS

CAROB ORANGE TWIST

1–2 oranges (¹/₃ cup juice)

1 tangerine (¹/₄ cup juice)

¹/₄ banana

1 tablespoon unsweetened carob powder (or pure unsweetened cocoa powder)

¹/₂ teaspoon pure vanilla extract

¹/₄ teaspoon ground cinnamon

2 teaspoons protein powder

1 cup ice

1. Separately juice orange and tangerine.
2. In a blender or food processor, combine ¹/₃ cup orange juice and ¹/₄ cup tangerine juice with remaining ingredients. Blend for 2 minutes, or until smooth.
3. Serve immediately.

   YIELDS 2¹/₂ CUPS

CELERY PURPLE CABBAGE SURPRISE

2 stalks celery (¹/2 cup juice)
¹/2 head purple cabbage (¹/2 cup juice)
2 apples (¹/2 cup juice)
1 beet (¹/4 cup juice)
1¹/2 lemons (1 tablespoon juice)
2 teaspoons protein powder

1. Separately juice celery, cabbage, apples, beet, and lemons.
2. In a blender or food processor, combine ¹/2 cup celery juice, ¹/2 cup cabbage juice, ¹/2 cup apple juice, ¹/4 cup beet juice, and 1 tablespoon lemon juice.
3. Combine the juices with protein powder in a blender. Serve immediately.

YIELDS 1³/4 CUPS

CRANBERRY GINGER SPRITZER

4 carrots (1 cup juice)
4 pears (1 cup juice)
¹/4 cup cranberries (1 tablespoon juice)
1-inch piece gingerroot (1 teaspoon juice)
2 tablespoons protein powder

1. Separately juice carrots, pears, cranberries, and ginger.
2. In a blender or food processor, combine 1 cup carrot juice, 1 cup pear juice, 1 tablespoon cranberry juice, and 1 teaspoon ginger juice with protein powder.
3. Serve immediately.

YIELDS 2 CUPS

CELERY APPLE JUICE

4 stalks celery (1 cup juice)
4 apples (1 cup juice)
2 heaping tablespoons protein powder

1. Separately juice celery and apples.
2. In a blender combine 1 cup celery juice and 1 cup apple juice, with protein powder.
3. Serve immediately.

YIELDS 2 CUPS

CITRUS DELIGHT

Note: May have a whole grapefruit 1 hour after this breakfast drink if necessary.

4 oranges (1 cup juice)
1/2 grapefruit (1/3 cup juice)
1 lemon (2 tablespoons juice)
1/2 cup club soda
1 heaping tablespoon protein powder
1 cup ice

1. Separately juice oranges, grapefruit, and lemon.
2. In a blender or food processor, combine with club soda, protein powder, and ice. Blend for 2 minutes, or until smooth.
3. Serve immediately.

   YIELDS 2½ CUPS

COCONUT CHERRY AND MELON SHAKE

2 cups honeydew melon chunks, peeled (1/2 cup juice)
1 banana
1/4 cup pitted cherries, frozen
1 tablespoon unsweetened flaked coconut
2 tablespoons ground or whole almonds or almond butter, unsalted
1/2 cup unsweetened soy milk
2 tablespoons protein powder
1 cup ice

1. Juice melon.
2. In a blender or food processor, combine 1/2 cup melon juice with remaining ingredients. Blend for 2 minutes, or until smooth.
3. Serve immediately.

   YIELDS 2½ CUPS

DATE PINEAPPLE NUT SHAKE

3/4 pineapple (3/4 cup juice)

2 tablespoons chopped dates

1 tablespoon unsweetened flaked coconut

1 tablespoon ground or whole unsalted pecans or pecan butter

1/4 cup plain soy milk

1/2 teaspoon ground nutmeg

2 tablespoons protein powder

1 cup ice

1. Juice pineapple.
2. In a blender or food processor, combine 3/4 cup pineapple with remaining ingredients. Blend for 2 minutes, or until smooth.
3. Serve immediately.

   YIELDS 2 CUPS

EXOTIC PINEAPPLE SHAKE

1 apple (1/4 cup juice)

1 slice peeled pineapple (2 tablespoons juice)

1 slice papaya (1 tablespoon juice)

1/2 lemon (1 teaspoon juice)

1/4 cup mashed avocado

1/2 cup rice milk

1 heaping tablespoon protein powder

1/8 teaspoon pure lemon extract

1/8 teaspoon ground nutmeg

1 cup ice

1. Separately juice apple, pineapple, papaya, and lemon.
2. In a blender or food processor, combine 1/4 cup apple juice, 2 tablespoons pineapple juice, 1 tablespoon papaya juice, and 1 teaspoon lemon juice with remaining ingredients. Blend for 2 minutes, or until smooth.
3. Serve immediately.

   YIELDS 2 1/4 CUPS

FROSTY PEAR AND CARROT JUICE

6 pears (1 1/2 cups juice)
3 carrots (3/4 cup juice)
2 bananas
2 tablespoons protein powder
1 1/2 cups ice

1. Separately juice pears and carrots.
2. In a blender or food processor, combine 1 1/2 cups pear juice and 3/4 cup carrot juice with remaining ingredients. Blend for 2 minutes, or until smooth.
3. Serve immediately.

YIELDS 3 1/2 CUPS

GINGERY ORANGE SPLASH

6 oranges (1 1/2 cups juice)
1-inch piece ginger root (1 teaspoon juice)
1/4 cup cranberries (1 tablespoon juice)
2 heaping tablespoons protein powder
1 cup ice

1. Separately juice oranges, ginger, and cranberries.
2. In a blender or food processor, combine 1 1/2 cups orange juice, 1 teaspoon ginger juice, and 1 tablespoon cranberry juice. Blend for 2 minutes, or until smooth.
3. Serve immediately.

YIELDS 2 CUPS

JUICY CARROT AND SWISS CHARD

4 carrots (1 cup juice)
2 apples (1/2 cup juice)
1 cucumber (1/4 cup juice)
1 stalk celery (1/4 cup juice)
1 small bunch Swiss chard (1 tablespoon juice)
2 heaping tablespoons protein powder

1. Separately juice carrots, apples, cucumber, celery, and Swiss chard.
2. Combine 1 cup carrot juice, 1/2 cup apple juice, 1/4 cup celery juice, and 1 tablespoon of the Swiss chard juice in a blender or food processor with protein powder.
3. Serve immediately.

   YIELDS 2 CUPS

LEAFY BEET VEGETABLE JUICE

2 apples (1/2 cup juice)
2 carrots (1/2 cup juice)
1 small bunch beet greens (1 tablespoon juice)
1 beet (1/4 cup juice)
2 heaping tablespoons protein powder
1 1/2 cups ice

1. Separately juice apples, carrots, beet greens, and beet.
2. In a blender or food processor, combine 1/2 cup apple juice, 1/2 cup carrot juice, 1 tablespoon beet greens juice, and 1/4 cup beet juice.
3. Serve immediately.

   YIELDS 2 1/4 CUPS

KIWI LEMON MELON TONIC

4 cups watermelon chunks, peeled (1 1/3 cups juice)
3 carrots (2/3 cup juice)
8 kiwis with skins (2/3 cup juice)
1 lemon (2 tablespoons juice)
3 heaping tablespoons protein powder
1 1/3 cups ice

1. Separately juice watermelon, carrots, kiwis, and lemon.
2. In a blender or food processor, combine 1 1/3 cups watermelon juice, 2/3 cup carrot juice, 2/3 cup kiwi juice, and 2 tablespoons lemon juice with remaining ingredients. Blend for 2 minutes, or until smooth.
3. Serve immediately.

   YIELDS 3 1/2 CUPS

MIXED VEGETABLE JUICE

2 apples (¹/₂ cup juice)
4 pears (¹/₂ cup juice)
2 carrots (¹/₂ cup juice)
1 cucumber (¹/₂ cup juice)
1 beet (¹/₄ cup juice)
1 small bunch Swiss chard (1 tablespoon juice)
1 red bell pepper (1 tablespoon juice)
1-inch piece ginger root (1 teaspoon juice)
1 heaping tablespoon protein powder

1. Separately juice apples, pears, carrots, cucumber, beet, Swiss chard, red pepper, and ginger.
2. Combine ¹/₂ cup apple juice, ¹/₂ cup pear juice, ¹/₂ cup carrot juice, ¹/₂ cup cucumber juice, ¹/₄ cup beet juice, 1 tablespoon red pepper juice, and 1 teaspoon ginger juice with protein powder in a blender or food processor.
3. Serve immediately.

YIELDS 2¹/₄ CUPS

PINEAPPLE CRANBERRY TWIST

1 pineapple (1 cup juice)
2 cups watermelon chunks, peeled (²/₃ cup juice)
¹/₂ cup cranberries (2 tablespoons juice)
1 lemon (2 tablespoons juice)
²/₃ cup seltzer
2 heaping tablespoons protein powder
¹/₂ cup ice

1. Separately juice pineapple, watermelon, cranberries, and lemon.
2. In a blender or food processor, combine 1 cup pineapple juice, ²/₃ cup watermelon juice, 2 tablespoons cranberry juice, and 2 tablespoons lemon juice with remaining ingredients. Blend for 2 minutes, or until smooth.
3. Serve immediately.

YIELDS 3¹/₄ CUPS

PECAN PROTEIN SHAKE

1 apple (¹/₄ cup juice)
¹/₄ banana
¹/₃ cup ground or whole pecans or pecan butter, unsalted
3 tablespoons protein powder
¹/₂ teaspoon pure lemon extract
1 cup seltzer
1 cup ice

1. Juice apple.
2. In a blender or food processor, combine ¹/₄ cup apple juice with remaining ingredients. Blend for 2 minutes, or until smooth.
3. Serve immediately.

YIELDS 2¹/₂ CUPS

ROMAINE LETTUCE AND APPLE REFRESHER

6 apples (1¹/₂ cups juice)
2 carrots (¹/₂ cup juice)
3–4 leaves romaine lettuce (¹/₄ cup juice)
¹/₂ lemon (1 tablespoon juice)
2 tablespoons protein powder

1. Separately juice apples, carrots, lettuce, and lemon.
2. Combine 1¹/₂ cups apple juice, ¹/₂ cup carrot juice, ¹/₄ cup lettuce juice, and 1 tablespoon lemon juice with protein powder in blender or food processor.
3. Serve immediately.

YIELDS 2¹/₄ CUPS

STRAWBERRY BANANA SPLIT

2 apples (¹/₂ cup apple juice)
1 pear (¹/₄ cup juice)
2 cups strawberries (¹/₄ cup juice)
2 stalks celery (¹/₂ cup juice) or ¹/₂ cup water
¹/₂ banana
2 tablespoons protein powder
1 cup ice

1. Separately juice apples, pear, strawberries, and celery (if desired).

2. In a blender or food processor, combine 1/2 cup apple juice, 1/4 cup pear juice, 1/4 cup strawberry juice, and 1/2 cup celery juice (or water) with remaining ingredients. Blend for 2 minutes, or until smooth.
3. Serve immediately.

YIELDS 2 1/2 CUPS

SUNFLOWER COCONUT PAPAYA SHAKE

1 papaya (1/2 cup juice)
2 tablespoons unsweetened flaked coconut
2 tablespoons hulled sunflower seeds, unsalted
1 teaspoon pure almond extract
1/2 cup rice milk
2 heaping tablespoons protein powder
1 cup ice cubes

1. Juice papaya.
2. In a blender or food processor, combine 1/2 cup papaya juice with remaining ingredients. Blend for 2 minutes, or until smooth.
3. Serve immediately.

YIELDS 2 1/4 CUPS

SUNFLOWER SPROUT APPLE JUICE

6 apples (1 1/2 cups juice)
4 carrots (1 cup juice)
1/2 cup sunflower or alfalfa sprouts (1 tablespoon juice)
1 heaping tablespoon protein powder

1. Separately juice apples, carrots, and sprouts.
2. Combine 1 1/2 cups apple juice, 1 cup carrot juice, and 1 tablespoon sprout juice with protein powder.
3. Serve immediately.

YIELDS 2 1/2 CUPS

TANGERINE PINEAPPLE AND KIWI COCKTAIL

1 tangerine (¼ cup juice)
1 kiwi (¼ cup juice)
¼ pineapple (¼ cup juice)
1 heaping tablespoon protein powder
¾ cup ice

1. Separately juice tangerine, kiwi, and pineapple.
2. In a blender or food processor, combine ¼ cup tangerine juice, ¼ cup kiwi juice, and ¼ cup pineapple juice with remaining ingredients. Blend for 2 minutes, or until smooth.
3. Serve immediately.

YIELDS 1½ CUPS

TANGY STRAWBERRY CARROT SHAKE

3 carrots (⅔ cup juice)
2 apples (½ cup juice)
½ cup cranberries (2 tablespoons juice)
1 cup strawberries, fresh or frozen
½ cup plain soy milk
3 heaping tablespoons protein powder
1 teaspoon ground nutmeg
1 cup ice

1. Separately juice carrots, apples, and cranberries.
2. In a blender or food processor, combine ⅔ cup carrot juice, ½ cup apple juice, and 2 tablespoons cranberry juice with remaining ingredients. Blend for 2 minutes, or until smooth.
3. Serve immediately.

YIELDS 3 CUPS

TROPICAL FRUIT AND TOFU PUDDING

2 tangerines (¹/₄ cup juice)
2 mangoes (¹/₂ cup juice)
¹/₄ pineapple (¹/₄ cup juice)
1¹/₂ cups silken tofu
¹/₄ cup pure maple syrup
2 teaspoons pure almond extract
¹/₄ teaspoon ground nutmeg
1 small banana, mashed
¹/₂ cup unsweetened flaked coconut
¹/₄ cup mashed raisins
3 tablespoons blanched slivered almonds
1 tablespoon protein powder

1. Separately juice tangerines, mangoes, and pineapple.
2. In a blender or food processor, combine ¹/₄ cup tangerine juice, ¹/₂ cup mango juice, and ¹/₄ cup pineapple juice with tofu. Blend for 2 to 3 minutes, or until smooth.
3. Add maple syrup, almond extract, and nutmeg, and continue to blend.
4. Transfer mixture to a small mixing bowl. Stir in banana, coconut, raisins, and almonds.
5. Chill for at least 1 hour before serving. Top with protein powder when serving.

SERVES 2–4

WATERMELON PINEAPPLE GERFINGAPOKEN

1¹/₂ cups peeled watermelon cubes (¹/₂ cup juice)
¹/₂ peeled pineapple (¹/₂ cup juice)
4 kiwis
¹/₂ cup rice milk
2 tablespoons protein powder
¹/₂ cup ice

1. Separately juice watermelon and pineapple.
2. In a blender or food processor, combine ¹/₂ cup watermelon juice and ¹/₂ cup pineapple juice with remaining ingredients. Blend for 2 minutes, or until smooth.
3. Serve immediately.

YIELDS 2 CUPS

ZESTY PAPAYA SHAKE

1 apple (¹/₄ cup juice)
1 slice papaya (1 tablespoon juice)
¹/₂ lemon (1 tablespoon juice)
¹/₂ lime (1 teaspoon juice)
¹/₂ cup rice milk
1 heaping tablespoon protein powder
¹/₈ teaspoon pure lemon extract
¹/₈ teaspoon ground nutmeg
1 cup ice

1. Separately juice apple, papaya, lemon, and lime.
2. In a blender or food processor, combine ¹/₄ cup apple juice, 1 tablespoon papaya juice, and 1 tablespoon lime juice with remaining ingredients. Blend for 2 minutes, or until smooth.
3. Serve immediately.

   YIELDS 2 CUPS

LUNCH

BLACK BEAN PASTA AND SOUP

6 cucumbers (1½ cups juice)
½ head cauliflower, steamed and chilled (½ cup pulp)
¼ cup diced yellow onions
3 tablespoons extra-virgin olive oil
¼ cup unsweetened soy milk
1½ cups chopped tomatoes
¾ cup cooked black beans
½ cup chopped escarole or kale
¼ cup chopped celery
¼ cup sliced carrots
2 teaspoons chopped fresh dill
2 teaspoons chopped fresh basil
½ teaspoon sea salt
½ teaspoon white pepper
1 clove garlic, crushed
1 cup uncooked whole-grain macaroni

1. Separately juice cucumbers and cauliflower.
2. In a large saucepan, sauté onion in oil for 2 to 3 minutes.
3. Add 1½ cups cucumber juice, cauliflower pulp, and soy milk. Bring to a boil over high heat, then reduce the heat to medium. Add remaining ingredients except for macaroni, and simmer, uncovered, for 15 minutes.
4. Boil macaroni, drain, and add to mixture. Serve hot or cold.

SERVES 3–4

CAYENNE SWORDFISH

Sauce

2 tablespoons olive oil

2 scallions

1 tablespoon tamari

1 teaspoon cayenne

1/2 cup silken tofu, processed until creamy in blender or food processor

1 tablespoon mustard

1 tablespoon horseradish

2 teaspoons lemon juice

yellow, red, orange, purple pepper slices for garnish

1/2 pound spelt noodles, cooked

2 tablespoons extra-virgin olive oil

1 pound swordfish, cubed

1. To prepare the sauce: In a saucepan, heat oil over medium heat. Brown scallions, then add tamari, cayenne, tofu, mustard, horseradish, and lemon juice. Heat through.
2. To prepare the fish: In a sauté pan, heat oil over medium heat. Cook swordfish until it is opaque and flakes when tested with a fork, about 15 to 17 minutes.
3. Toss fish with the sauce. Serve with noodles and garnish with fresh pepper slices.

SERVES 2–3

EGGPLANT PARMIGIANA SANDWICH

4 (1/4-inch-thick) circular slices eggplant

3 tablespoons olive oil

1 clove garlic

3 plum tomatoes

1/2 cup filtered water

1/4 teaspoon oregano

1/4 teaspoon sea salt

2 slices spelt bread (any kind)

2 ounces soy mozzarella

1. Preheat oven to 375 degrees F. Oil pan with 2 tablespoons of the oil. Bake eggplant slices in oiled pan for 20 minutes or until tender. Set aside.

2. In a saucepan sauté garlic in remaining 1 tablespoon of the oil for 2 minutes.

3. Dice tomatoes. Add to saucepan with water, oregano, and sea salt. Simmer for 20 minutes, stirring frequently.

4. Toast spelt bread. Place eggplant on 1 slice bread and cover with tomato sauce. Top with sliced soy cheese. Cover with another slice of bread and bake for 5 minutes. Remove and serve immediately.

SERVES 2

FAVA SALAD WITH CASHEWS AND DILL

2 cups steamed fava beans
¼ cup soy mayonnaise with dill to flavor
¼ cup raw cashews
1 tablespoon poppy seeds
¼ cup fresh dill sprigs for garnish

1. In a medium-size mixing bowl, toss beans with mayonnaise.

2. Sprinkle cashews and poppy seeds on top of bean mixture.

3. Serve cold or at room temperature, garnished with the dill sprigs.

SERVES 2

FISH 'N CHIPS

1 Salmon filet, cubed (swordfish or blackfin shark may be substituted)
4 carrots, sliced
¼ cup thinly sliced celery
¼ cup shredded red cabbage
2 Vidalia onions, chopped
6 cloves garlic, diced
6 peppercorns
1 plantain, sliced
2 tablespoons macadamia oil
⅛ teaspoon ground ginger
¼ teaspoon cumin
¼ teaspoon thyme
pinch of fresh oregano
1 tablespoon fresh chopped basil
1 tablespoon chopped Italian parsley
½ teaspoon soy sauce

1. In a steamer, steam salmon until thoroughly cooked, about 5 minutes, or until fish flakes when tested with a fork.
2. Steam carrots 10 minutes, until thoroughly cooked. Add celery and red cabbage and cook 2-3 minutes more.
3. Sauté onions, garlic, peppercorns, and plantain in macadamia oil until lightly browned.
4. Add spices, cook 2 minutes more, and combine all ingredients.

SERVES 2

GARY'S VEGGIEBALL STEW

1 teaspoon sea salt
1/8 teaspoon white pepper
1 tablespoon Worcestershire sauce
1 teaspoon grated lemon peel
1/2 teaspoon dried thyme
1 tablespoon curry powder
1 teaspoon tamari sauce
1 stalk celery, chopped
1 scallion, chopped
2 tablespoons egg substitute
1 tablespoon Bragg's liquid aminos
4 ounces seitan, chopped
1/4 cup spelt flour
1 tablespoon extra-virgin olive oil
4 cups filtered water
1 cup yellow squash, sliced
1 small turnip, boiled and cubed
1 medium red potato, boiled and shredded
1 cup fresh tomato, peeled, cored, and chopped
1 leek with top sliced off
vegetable broth bouillon, for 1 quart
1 tablespoon chopped fresh dill

1. In a medium-size bowl, combine salt, pepper, Worcestershire, lemon peel, thyme, curry, tamari, celery, scallion, egg substitute, Bragg's aminos, and chopped seitan. Shape into 1-inch balls and roll in spelt flour.
2. Heat oil in a skillet and brown the balls, turning gently between a fork and a spoon. Set aside. Save any drippings.

3. In a large saucepan, with 4 cups water, place squash, turnip, potato, tomato, leek, and vegetable bouillon. Boil on medium heat for approximately 30 minutes.

4. Add veggieballs to soup and reheat for 5 to 7 minutes. Sprinkle dill on top. Serve with homemade bread.

SERVES 3–4

HAWAIIAN TUNA

1 pound fresh tuna
1 lemon
¹/₂ cup pineapple chunks
2 tablespoons pure maple syrup
¹/₂ cup agar agar
¹/₂ cup blueberries
1 blood orange, sliced
1 kiwi, peeled
2 tablespoons extra-virgin olive oil
Brown rice

1. Preheat oven to 400 degrees F. Bake tuna in an oiled baking pan for 20 minutes. Turn over and bake other side until fish is cooked and flaky.

2. Begin Hawaiian stew by grating lemon skin. Combine with pineapple chunks, maple syrup, agar agar, blueberries, blood orange slices, and kiwi in a saucepan. Simmer on low heat for 10 minutes.

3. Pour Hawaiian stew over tuna. Enjoy with short-grain brown rice.

SERVES 2–3

MACARONI MARCONI

1/2 pound quinoa pasta

10 artichoke hearts

1/4 teaspoon sea salt

1/4 teaspoon cayenne

1/2 lemon

2 tablespoons extra-virgin olive oil

3 cloves garlic, minced

2 ounces sun-dried tomatoes

1/2 pound salmon filets, cubed

1 sprig fresh basil, chopped

15 green olives, pitted and sliced

1/4 cup grated soy or rice Parmesan, optional

1. Cook pasta. Steam artichoke hearts until tender.
2. Season salmon with salt, cayenne, and lemon.
3. In a skillet sauté garlic with sundried tomatoes in the olive oil, 3 minutes.
4. Add salmon, basil, and olives and cook until salmon flakes when tested with a fork, about 5 minutes more.
5. In a large bowl, toss salmon mixture with the pasta, and Parmesan and serve.

   SERVES 2

THE ORIGINAL BROCCOLI STIR-FRY

1 cup firm tofu

2 cups broccoli florets

2 tablespoons hot sesame oil

2 tablespoons tamari sauce

1/4 teaspoon hot cayenne pepper

1 teaspoon grated fresh ginger

3 cloves garlic, minced

1. In a medium-size saucepan, sauté tofu and broccoli in oil for 3 minutes over medium heat. Remove from pan and place mixture in a bowl.
2. Combine remaining ingredients in the saucepan. Cook on medium heat until mixture simmers for 1 minute. Add broccoli mixture and cook, covered, for 2 minutes.
3. Stir well. Serve with short-grain brown rice or Far East rice noodles.

   SERVES 1

POCHEE

2 tablespoons extra-virgin olive oil

1 cup sliced mushrooms

1 cup cubed red potatoes

1 cup chopped dandelion greens

1/2 cup tofu, diced and baked (optional)

2 tablespoons chopped fresh dill

1 tablespoon chopped fresh rosemary

2 cups grated soy cheese

1/4 cup grated soy parmesan cheese

1. Preheat oven to 350 degrees F.
2. Add oil to a large saucepan. Sauté mushrooms, potatoes, dandelions, tofu, parsley, and rosemary over medium-high heat for 5 minutes.
3. Lightly grease a large loaf pan or baking dish, and pour vegetable mixture into it. Top with cheeses. Cover with aluminum foil and bake for 35 to 40 minutes.

SERVES 2–3

POPEYE LOVES OLIVE

3/4 cup uncooked orzo

1 cup distilled water

3/4 teaspoon fresh oregano, finely chopped (or 1/2 teaspoon dried)

2 tablespoons finely chopped Italian parsley

3 tablespoons extra-virgin olive oil, divided

1 tablespoon balsamic vinegar

1/2 clove garlic, pressed

1 tablespoon hazelnuts, finely chopped

sea salt to taste

freshly ground black pepper to taste

5–6 Greek olives, green and black, pitted and chopped

4 soy sausage links

6 cups (9 ounces) spinach leaves, washed, dried, and steamed until just wilted

1/4 cup crumbled tempeh

parsley for garnish

1. Cook orzo according to package directions.

2. In glass jar, mix water, oregano, parsley, 1³/₄ tablespoons olive oil, vinegar, garlic, hazelnuts, salt, and pepper. Cover tightly and shake well.
3. Combine chopped olives and cooked orzo in a bowl. Pour dressing over mixture and toss.
4. Lightly brown sausage links in remaining olive oil.
5. Arrange steamed spinach leaves with soy sausages on two plates. Fill with orzo and olive mixture and sprinkle tempeh on top. Garnish with parsley.

SERVES 3–4

PUMPKIN CREAM

2 tablespoons walnut oil
1 small onion, chopped
1 scallion, chopped
1 clove garlic, chopped
¹/₂ cup apple, peeled, cored, and chopped
¹/₂ cup pumpkin flesh, grated
¹/₂ cup chopped celery
1 cup silken tofu
1 teaspoon mild curry powder
¹/₄ teaspoon ground turmeric
¹/₄ teaspoon ground cumin
1 tablespoon chopped basil
1 tablespoon chopped arugula
1 tablespoon rice flour
1 teaspoon arrowroot powder
3 cups vegetable broth or 3 cups water plus 2 vegetable bouillon cubes
2 tablespoons protein powder

1. In a saucepan, heat oil and sauté onion, scallion, garlic, apple, pumpkin, and celery for approximately 5 minutes.
2. Stir in tofu and cook for 2 minutes. Add remaining ingredients except broth and cook, stirring, an additional three minutes.
3. Slowly add broth and bring to a boil. Cover, lower heat, and simmer for 15 minutes.
4. Place half the soup in a blender with the protein powder and puree. Return puree to the pot. Cook an additional 3 minutes. Serve hot.

SERVES 2

SALMON QUICHE

1/2 pound salmon

2 tomatoes (1/2 cup juice)

1 large bunch fresh basil (1/2 cup pulp)

1 cup silken tofu

1 cup mashed avocado

3/4 cup grated soy Parmesan

2 tablespoons extra virgin olive oil

1/8 teaspoon sea salt

1/8 teaspoon black pepper

2 cups broccoli florets

1 1/4 cups thinly sliced mushrooms

1 Spelt Crust (recipe follows) or use pre-baked spelt crust (available at health food stores)

1. Preheat oven to 375 degrees F. Bake salmon in an oiled pan for 10 minutes.
2. Juice tomatoes and basil separately.
3. In a blender or food processor, combine salmon, avocado, cheese, oil, salt, and pepper. Blend for 1 minute, or until creamy. Add tofu, juice, and pulp and blend until mixed.
4. Arrange broccoli and mushrooms on bottom of prepared basic Spelt Crust. (Recipe follows.) Pour tofu mixture over vegetables.
5. Bake quiche at 375 degrees for 30 minutes, until lightly browned.
6. Remove and let cool before serving.

SERVES 2–4

SPELT CRUST

1/2 cup whole spelt flour

1/2 teaspoon ground allspice

1/3 cup cold nonhydrogenated soy mayonnaise

1/4 cup plus 3 tablespoons cold water or plain soy milk

1. In a small mixing bowl, combine spelt flour and allspice.
2. With a fork, cut soy margarine into flour mixture until mixture is moist and fine. Add cold water (or rice milk) by the tablespoon until the dough has a smooth, even consistency.
3. Roll dough into a ball, and place it in a bowl. Cover bowl with plastic wrap, and chill for 1 hour.
4. Lightly flour a smooth, clean surface and rolling pin. Place chilled dough on floured surface. Roll dough from the center out until it is ½ inch larger than a 9-inch pie plate. (Check by placing empty pie plate on top of rolled dough.)
5. Loosen dough by gently sliding a floured spatula underneath it toward the center and moving around the entire area of the dough until it can be lifted. Transfer dough to a lightly greased 9-inch pie plate.
6. Preheat oven to 350 degrees F. Bake for 30 minutes, or until crust is light brown.

MAKES 1 9-INCH CRUST

TUNA DELIGHT

1 vegetable bouillon cube
½ cup filtered water
2 (8-ounce) tuna steaks
1 cup chopped fresh plum tomatoes
¼ cup chopped fresh dandelion greens
2 tablespoons chopped scallions
1 clove garlic
1½ teaspoons dried oregano
½ teaspoon sea salt

1. In a large saucepan, dissolve bouillon cube in water. Lay tuna steaks in bouillon and place remaining ingredients on top. Cook, covered, over medium heat for 15 minutes.
2. Serve hot.

SERVES 2–3

TUNA WITH RICE AND PEPPERS

1/2 pound canned tuna

1 1/2 cups cooked brown rice (warm or at room temperature).

3/4 tablespoon chopped fresh marjoram

1/2 teaspoon chopped fresh tarragon

1–2 tablespoons diced red bell pepper

1–2 tablespoons diced yellow bell pepper

1–2 tablespoons diced green bell pepper

1 teaspoon sea salt

1/4 teaspoon cumin

1 1/2 tablespoons extra-virgin olive oil

1. Steam peppers 1 minute only, to keep them crisp.
2. Combine all ingredients in a bowl and mix well.

   SERVES 1–2

SALADS

CAESAR SALAD WITH THYME CROUTONS

3 carrots (3/4 cup pulp)

4 1/2 cups chopped romaine lettuce

3/4 cup thyme croutons (recipe follows)

1 1/2 tablespoons grated soy cheese

natural Dijon salad dressing (available at health food stores)

1. Juice carrots.
2. In a large mixing bowl, toss 3/4 cup carrot pulp with lettuce.
3. Toss salad with the desired amount of Dijon salad dressing, thyme croutons, and cheese. Serve cold or at room temperature.

   SERVES 2

THYME CROUTONS

2–3 slices whole-grain bread, cut into 3/4-inch cubes (1 cup)

2–4 tablespoons extra-virgin olive oil

1 1/2 tablespoons finely chopped fresh thyme

dash sea salt

1. Preheat oven to 375 degrees F.
2. In a small mixing bowl, combine all ingredients and toss.
3. Spread bread cubes on an ungreased cookie sheet. Bake for 15 to 20 minutes, or until light brown in color.
4. Toss with salads.

YIELDS 1 CUP

CUCUMBER AND TOMATO SALAD

For the Salad

1 large cucumber

1 large tomato, diced

1 tablespoon diced onion

1 tablespoon diced green pepper

1 tablespoon diced red bell pepper

1 tablespoon chopped scallion

For the Dressing

1/2 teaspoon prepared stone-ground mustard

1/2 teaspoon apple cider vinegar

1 tablespoon plain soy milk

sea salt to taste

freshly ground pepper to taste

1 1/2 tablespoons canola oil

1. Peel cucumber and cut in half. Remove seeds and cut into very thin slices.
2. Cut tomato into 1/4-inch chunks.
3. In a bowl, combine tomatoes and cucumber with onion, peppers, and scallion.
4. In a small bowl, stir together mustard, vinegar, and soy milk. Pour over vegetable mixture. Add canola oil and mix well. Season to taste with sea salt and pepper.

SERVES 2

ENDIVE SALAD

1/2 pound endive, washed
1 medium red onion
olive oil for sautéing and dressing
2 large cloves garlic
1 teaspoon grated fresh or powdered ginger
alfalfa or mung bean sprouts
1/4 teaspoon turmeric
sea salt to taste

1. Place dried endive in a bowl and spread the leaves out.
2. Cut onion into rings, and mix into endive.
3. In a lightly oiled pan over medium heat, sauté garlic cloves until slightly brown. Allow a few minutes for garlic to cool, then cut into strips or rings and add to dish.
4. Add sprout, and sprinkle on turmeric and sea salt to taste.
5. Sprinkle on olive oil, as desired. Serve immediately, or refrigerate and serve later.

SERVES 2–3

FANCY VEGETABLE COMBO SALAD

For the Salad
1/2 cup broccoli florets
1/2 cup arugula, chopped
1/2 cup cherry tomatoes, chopped
1/2 red pepper, diced
1/2 yellow pepper, diced
1/4 cup artichoke hearts, chopped
1/2 pound mushrooms, sliced
1 gherkin
8 green and black pitted olives
1/2 cup peas
1 teaspoon fresh oregano, chopped
1 1/2 tablespoon capers
1 cup cannelloni beans, canned
sea salt to taste
freshly ground black pepper to taste

For the Dressing

1 teaspoon lemon juice

1/4 cup extra-virgin olive oil

2 tablespoons balsamic vinegar

1. Toss broccoli, arugula, tomatoes, peppers, artichoke hearts, mushrooms, gherkin, olives, peas, oregano, capers, and beans in a salad bowl. Season with sea salt and pepper.
2. Add lemon juice, oil, and balsamic vinegar, and toss lightly.
3. Serve immediately.

SERVES 2

HOT DULSE AND POTATO SALAD

3 large potatoes or 7 baby new potatoes

1 tablespoon diced white or yellow onion

2 tablespoons chopped dulse leaves

1 teaspoon extra-virgin olive oil, plus extra oil for sautéing

1 1/2 tablespoons Bragg's liquid aminos

1/3 cup hot filtered water

1 garlic pickle or cucumber, diced

1 tablespoon ground fennel seeds

1/2 teaspoon lemon juice

2 sprigs fresh parsley, chopped

sea salt

freshly ground pepper

1. If larger potatoes are used, cut into quarters. Boil potatoes in their skins until tender but firm, about 15–18 minutes. Discard the skins (or leave organic potato skins on, if desired), and slice potatoes into a large bowl.
2. Sauté onion and dulse in a few drops of oil over medium-high heat.
3. Mix aminos with water and pour over cooked potatoes.
4. Add onion, dulse, pickle, and fennel. Mix well. Add 1 tablespoon olive oil and sprinkle with lemon juice and parsley. Add small amount of water if dry. Serve hot, adding salt and pepper to taste.

SERVES 2

PASTA, TOMATO, AND GARLIC SALAD

4 cups cooked whole-grain or green spinach pasta (bow ties, shells, or ziti)
3 cups tomato salsa
1 cup broccoli florets, steamed
1 cup whole pine nuts

1. In a large bowl, toss pasta with the remaining ingredients.
2. Serve cold as a main dish or salad.

   SERVES 2

POTATO AND HERB SALAD

1/2 pound red potatoes
1 medium celery stalk, minced
1/2 small onion, minced
1/4 cup finely chopped green and red bell peppers
1 tablespoon minced parsley
1 tablespoon minced dill
1/4 teaspoon sage
1/2 cup soy mayonnaise
2 tablespoons sweet pickle relish (optional)
sea salt to taste
freshly ground pepper to taste

1. Steam potatoes until cooked but firm, about 15 to 18 minutes. Drain, peel, and allow to cool.
2. Place celery, onion, and peppers in a large bowl. Add parsley, dill, and sage.
3. When potatoes have cooled, dice them and add to celery and onion mixture.
4. Add mayonnaise a little bit at a time until mixture is well coated but not too wet. Add relish, sea salt, and pepper to taste and mix well. Cover with plastic wrap and refrigerate.
5. Serve cold.

   SERVES 2

RAW SPINACH SALAD

1/2 pound washed spinach
1 medium-size red onion
8 dandelion leaves
olive oil for sautéing and dressing
2 large cloves garlic
1 teaspoon grated fresh or powdered ginger
alfalfa or mung bean sprouts
1/4 teaspoon turmeric
sea salt to taste

1. Place dried spinach into a bowl and spread the leaves out.
2. Cut onion into rings, and mix into the spinach.
3. Cut up dandelion leaves into 1-inch strips and add to dish.
4. In a lightly oiled frying pan over medium heat, sauté garlic cloves until slightly brown. Allow a few minutes for garlic to cool, then cut into strips or rings and add to dish.
5. Add sprouts, and sprinkle on turmeric and sea salt to taste.
6. Sprinkle on olive oil. Serve immediately, or refrigerate and serve later.

SERVES 2–3

RED POTATO SALAD

1/2 carrot (1 tablespoon juice, 2 tablespoons pulp)
2 teaspoons chopped fresh dill
1 teaspoon celery seeds
2 cups diced red potatoes, steamed
1 teaspoon sea salt
1/2 teaspoon black pepper
1/2 cup chopped celery
1/8 –1/4 cup soy mayonnaise
2 tablespoons chopped red onion
2 tablespoons extra-virgin olive oil

1. Juice carrot.
2. In a medium-size mixing bowl, toss 1 tablespoon carrot juice and 2 tablespoons carrot pulp with remaining ingredients.
3. Serve cold or at room temperature.

SERVES 2

SPICY CUCUMBER AND TOFU SALAD

1 large cucumber, sliced

1 1/2 teaspoons Spectrum's Mediterranean Oil or olive oil blend

1 teaspoon sea salt

1 dash Mrs. Dash Table Salt

1 clove garlic, cut in half

2 tablespoons chopped fresh dill

1 cup silken tofu

2 tablespoons chopped fresh mint

1 teaspoon freshly squeezed lemon juice

1/4 teaspoon jalapeño or Tabasco sauce

2 teaspoons apple cider vinegar

dash paprika

1. Combine all ingredients except cucumber and paprika in a blender.
2. In a serving bowl, mix together cucumber slices and blender mixture.
3. Garnish with paprika and serve immediately.

SERVES 2

DINNER

\\|//

ALMOND CHOP SUEY

For the Sauce

1 teaspoon honey
1 cup vegetable broth or 1 vegetable bouillon cube
1 teaspoon tamari
1 tablespoon rice vinegar
3/4 cup diagonally sliced celery
1 1/2 tablespoons arrowroot powder
1 tablespoon apple cider vinegar

For the Vegetables

4 leaves bok choy
2 teaspoons sesame oil
1 clove garlic, minced
1/2 cup canned bamboo shoots, rinsed, drained, and sliced diagonally
1 cup cauliflower
1 celery stalk, sliced
1 cup sliced straw mushrooms
1 cup bean sprouts, preferably mung beans, rinsed
1/2 cup tamari almonds, sliced for garnish

1. To prepare the sauce: In a small saucepan, heat honey, broth, tamari, and rice vinegar.
2. In a bowl, whisk together arrowroot and cider vinegar.
3. To prepare the vegetables: Separate bok choy leaves from stems. Heat sesame oil in wok. Add garlic, bamboo shoots, bok choy stems, cauliflower, and celery, and stir-fry 4 minutes. Add mushrooms, bean sprouts, and bok choy leaves. Stir-fry 2 more minutes. Empty wok into a large bowl.
4. Combine honey-tamari mixture with arrowroot sauce in middle of wok. Stir constantly until sauce thickens and loses its cloudiness.
5. Gently stir in vegetables and reheat for 2 minutes.
6. Garnish with tamari almonds.

SERVES 2

CUMIN CHICKPEAS

12 ounces or 1 can chickpeas
1 cup filtered water
3 tablespoons sesame oil
1/2 cup finely chopped onion
4 cloves garlic
1 scallion
1/4 teaspoon freshly grated ginger
3 tablespoons lemon juice
1/4 cup roasted pecans
4 tablespoons ground cumin
1 teaspoon sea salt or to taste
finely chopped radicchio or cilantro for garnish (optional)
fresh green salad (premix available in grocery)

1. Simmer chickpeas in water with sesame oil, onion, garlic, scallion, ginger, and lemon juice for 15 to 20 minutes, until chickpeas are soft.
2. Add pecans, cumin, and salt. Let cook 5 more minutes. Be careful not to over-cook, or it will become mushy. Drain.
3. Garnish with radicchio or cilantro and serve with a fresh green salad. Serve immediately.

SERVES 2

EGGPLANT SOY MOZZARELLA

2 small to medium eggplants, peeled
sea salt to taste
2 tablespoons extra-virgin olive oil blended with 2 sprigs chopped saffron
2/3 cup tofu cream cheese
1/4 pound fresh soy mozzarella, thinly sliced
1 (8-ounce) can tomato sauce
1 teaspoon dried oregano
1/4 teaspoon cayenne pepper
2 tablespoons fresh chopped basil
1/4 cup rice or soy parmesan cheese

1. Cut eggplants into slices 1/4 inch thick. Sprinkle slices with salt, and weight them down with a heavy plate.

2. Let stand for 1 hour or overnight. Drain and rinse slices and pat them dry.
3. Mix chopped basil into tofu cream cheese.
4. In a heavy skillet, heat oil over medium-high heat. Sauté eggplant slices until golden brown on both sides. Drain on paper towels.
5. Preheat oven to 350 degrees F.
6. In a round casserole dish, layer eggplant, tofu cream cheese mixture, soy mozzarella, tomato sauce, oregano, and cayenne. Continue to build layers until you have used up all of the ingredients. The final layer should be tofu cream cheese mixture sprinkled with parmesan.
7. Bake for 20 minutes, until top is golden brown and bubbly.
8. Serve warm.

SERVES 2

GARY'S FOOD FOR THE SOUL

1 cup finely chopped chard, steamed 5 minutes
1 cup diced pears
1 cup sliced mushrooms
1/2 cup sliced leeks
1 teaspoon sea salt
1 teaspoon freshly ground black pepper
2 tablespoons extra-virgin olive oil
4 1/2 teaspoons apple juice
1/2 cup black-eyed peas, steamed 15 minutes
1/2 teaspoon paprika (preferably Hungarian)
3 tablespoons ground allspice
1 teaspoon ground nutmeg
1/2 cup cashews

1. In a large saucepan, sauté chard, pears, mushrooms, leeks, salt, and pepper in oil over medium-high heat for 7 minutes.
2. Add remaining ingredients and cook an additional 10 minutes.
3. Serve hot.

SERVES 3 TO 4

GARY'S FAVORITE CASSEROLE

2¹/2 *tablespoons sesame oil, divided*
¹/4 *cup oat flour*
¹/2 *cup cooked split peas*
¹/3 *teaspoon curry powder*
¹/4 *teaspoon minced garlic*
¹/4 *teaspoon sea salt*
¹/4 *teaspoon oregano*
¹/4 *cup filtered water*
¹/2 *cup coarsely chopped kale*
¹/2 *cup bite-size broccoli pieces*
1 *cup cooked brown short-grain rice*
¹/2 *avocado, sliced*

1. Preheat oven to 375 degrees F. Lightly grease 4-by-8 baking pan with sesame oil.
2. In a blender, combine oat flour, split peas, oil, curry, garlic, sea salt, oregano, and water.
3. In a separate bowl, combine kale, broccoli, and brown rice. Mix well.
4. Transfer to covered baking pan, top with flour and peas mixture. Bake for 15 minutes. Place avocado slices on top for garnish.
5. Serve hot.

SERVES 2

GARY'S VEGETABLE PAN

2 tomatoes (1/2 cup juice)

1 pound extra-firm tofu, cut into 1-inch cubes

2 tablespoons canola oil

3/4 cup chopped yellow onions

2 cups frozen peas

1 cup chopped tomatoes

3/4 cup plain soy milk

3 teaspoons apple cider vinegar

1/2 cup finely chopped arugula

2 green chili peppers, finely chopped

3 cloves garlic, crushed

2 teaspoons grated ginger root

1 teaspoon ground coriander

1 teaspoon ground turmeric

1/4 teaspoon chili powder

1 1/2 teaspoons sea salt

Spinach or other leafy green salad

1. Juice tomatoes. Set aside 1/2 cup of the juice.
2. In a large frying pan, brown tofu in oil over high heat.
3. Add onions. Sauté for 2 to 3 minutes, or until onions are soft.
4. Reduce heat to medium-low. Add the 1/2 cup of tomato juice and remaining ingredients except the salad, and simmer, uncovered, for 5 minutes.
5. Serve with fresh green salad.

SERVES 4

GREEN PEA PILAF

2 tablespoons walnut oil

2 shallots, finely chopped

1 clove garlic, minced

3/4 cup white jasmine basmati rice, rinsed and drained

1 1/3 cups vegetable broth (optional) or filtered water

1/3 cup chopped fresh spearmint

1/2 cup frozen peas

1 tablespoon Bragg's liquid aminos, or to taste

spinach or cooked arugula

1 tablespoon extra-virgin olive oil

1. In a stockpot, heat walnut oil over low heat. Sauté shallots and garlic for 3 minutes.
2. Add uncooked rice and stir 1 minute.
3. Add vegetable broth or water, spearmint, peas, and aminos. Bring to a full boil, then reduce heat to a simmer. Cover and cook over low heat for about 15 minutes, or until water is absorbed and rice is tender.
4. Remove from heat. Release steam by angling lid away from face and hands. Cover the pot with a towel to absorb excess water vapor without losing heat.
5. Serve on a bed of spinach or arugula sprinkled with olive oil.

SERVES 2

HERBED TOMATO SALAD

1 teaspoon sea salt
1/8 teaspoon cayenne
1/2 teaspoon freshly ground black pepper
2 tablespoons lime juice
2 tablespoons fresh dill
1/2 tablespoon chopped fresh thyme
3 ripe tomatoes
1 bunch arugula
1 bunch watercress

1. In a small bowl, combine salt, cayenne and black pepper, lime juice, dill, and thyme.
2. Cut tomatoes into thick slices; toss with arugula and watercress. Pour dressing over salad, and let marinate for 1 hour in the refrigerator.
3. Serve chilled.

SERVES 2

JAPANESE RICE NOODLES WITH SHIITAKE MUSHROOMS

2-inch piece ginger root (2 tablespoons juice)
1¹/2 cups sliced stemmed shiitake mushrooms
1 cup sliced zucchini
3 tablespoons safflower or other light oil
1 cup mung bean sprouts, drained
3 teaspoons tamari
3 teaspoons sliced scallions
³/4 pound rice noodles, cooked

1. Juice ginger.
2. In a large frying pan, sauté mushrooms and zucchini in oil over high heat until soft.
3. Reduce heat to medium-low. Add 2 tablespoons ginger juice, bean sprouts, soy sauce, and scallions. Simmer for 1 to 2 minutes, or until mixture has thickened.
4. Spoon the vegetable mixture over rice noodles and serve hot.

   SERVES 2

LENTIL BURGERS

4 carrots (¹/2 cup pulp)
1 cup cooked red lentils
¹/4 cup lentil sprouts
¹/4 cup ground unsalted cashews or cashew butter
2 tablespoons chopped unsalted almonds
1 tablespoon diced yellow onion
2 teaspoons curry powder
¹/2 teaspoon ground coriander
¹/2 teaspoon sea salt
¹/2 cup whole-wheat bread crumbs
2 pita bread pockets

1. Preheat oven to 425 degrees F.
2. Juice carrots.
3. In a small mixing bowl, combine ¹/2 cup carrot pulp with remaining ingredients except bread crumbs and pita. Mix well.
4. Shape mixture into 2 patties. Coat patties with bread crumbs, and place them on ungreased cookie sheet.

5. Bake patties for 10 minutes. Turn patties over, and bake an additional 10–15 minutes.
6. Serve hot in pita bread pockets (add hummus flavored with lemon for a more exotic taste).

SERVES 2

MUSHROOM BROCCOLI QUICHE

2 tomatoes (¹/₂ cup juice)
1 large bunch fresh basil (¹/₂ cup pulp)
1 cup silken tofu
1 cup avocado, crushed with 3 tablespoons lemon juice
¹/₄ teaspoon finely chopped jalapeño peppers
¹/₄ cup finely chopped tomatoes
¹/₄ cup finely chopped Bermuda onion
³/₄ cup grated soy cheese
2 tablespoons extra-virgin olive oil
¹/₈ teaspoon sea salt
¹/₈ teaspoon black pepper
1¹/₂ cups broccoli florets
1¹/₄ cups thinly sliced mushrooms
1 Spelt Crust (use recipe from p. 225) (or use pre-baked available at health food stores)

1. Preheat oven to 375 degrees F.
2. Separately juice tomato and basil. Set aside ¹/₂ cup of the tomato juice and ¹/₂ of the basil pulp.
3. In a blender or food processer, combine tofu, avocado jalapeños, onion, cheese, oil, salt, black pepper and tomato juice and basil pulp mixture. Blend for 1 minute, or until creamy.
4. Arrange broccoli and mushrooms in the bottom of Spelt Crust. Layer the chopped tomatoes on top. Pour tofu mixture over vegetables.
5. Bake quiche, uncovered, for 25–30 minutes, or until the top has set and begun to turn light brown. Remove quiche from the oven. Let stand for 5 minutes before cutting.
6. Serve hot with a salad.

SERVES 4–6

OLIVE AND RICE PASTA

3/4 *teaspoon fresh oregano*
1/8 *cup finely chopped Italian parsley*
1 3/4 *tablespoons extra-virgin olive oil*
2 *tablespoons balsamic vinegar*
1 *clove garlic, pressed*
1 *tablespoon finely chopped hazelnuts*
sea salt to taste
freshly ground black pepper to taste
12 *ounces–1 pound rice pasta*
5 *or* 6 *Greek black olives, pitted and chopped*
4 *cups (about* 1/2 *pound) spinach leaves, washed, dried, and steamed until*
   just wilted
1/2 *pound medium-firm tofu, cubed*
1/4 *cup crumbled tempeh*
parsley for garnish

1. In a glass jar, mix oregano, Italian parsley, olive oil, vinegar, garlic, hazelnuts, salt, and pepper. Cover tightly, shake well and set aside for flavors to meld.
2. Cook rice pasta in filtered water according to package directions.
3. Combine pasta and chopped olives in a bowl. Pour dressing over mixture and toss.
4. Divide pasta onto 2 plates. Arrange steamed spinach leaves on top, fill with cubed tofu and olive mixture and sprinkle tempeh on top. Garnish with parsley.

SERVES 2

ORZO TURANEROLE

1/4 pound orzo pasta
1/3 cup cooked and then diced into 1/2-inch cubes spaghetti squash
filtered water
1/2 cup chopped Swiss chard
1/4 cup chopped onion
1/4 cup chopped green pepper
25 almonds, blanched and chopped
1 teaspoon minced garlic
2 teaspoon thyme
1/2 teaspoon sea salt

1. Cook the orzo pasta, according to package directions. Drain and set aside.
2. Steam Swiss chard for 6 minutes.
3. Combine Swiss chard with squash, orzo, garlic, thyme, and sea salt in a baking dish.
4. Bake at 375 degrees F for 15 minutes. Serve hot.

SERVES 1

PARSLEY AND MUSHROOM LASAGNA

4 carrots (1 cup pulp)
4 cups soy ricotta cheese
2 teaspoons soy egg replacer
3 1/2 cups shredded soy or rice mozzarella cheese
1/2 cup grated soy or rice Parmesan
1/4 cup fresh chopped parsley
1/2 teaspoon sea salt
1/4 teaspoon black pepper
2 cups broccoli florets
2 cups sliced mushrooms
3 tablespoons extra-virgin olive oil
2 cups tomato sauce (seasoned, if desired)
1 pound whole-grain lasagna noodles, cooked according to package directions

1. Preheat oven to 425 degrees F.
2. Juice carrots.
3. In a medium-size mixing bowl, combine 1 cup carrot pulp, soy ricotta cheese, egg replacer, soy mozzarella cheese, parsley, salt, and pepper. Mix well with a whisk.
4. In a large saucepan, sauté broccoli and mushrooms in oil over high heat for 3 to 5 minutes.
5. Spread 1 cup tomato sauce on the bottom of an ungreased 12-by-17-inch baking dish. Then arrange a layer of cooked lasagna noodles, a layer of broccoli and mushrooms, a layer of the ricotta cheese mixture, and another layer of the noodles. Repeat the layers, ending with additional layers of sauce and cheese, and Parmesan sprinkled on top.
6. Cover lasagna with foil. Bake for 45 to 55 minutes. Let stand for 5 minutes before cutting.
7. Serve hot with a green salad and whole-grain bread.

SERVES 4-6

PESTO AND TOMATOES ON FETTUCCINI

1 cup sliced mushrooms
1 cup broccoli florets
3 tablespoons extra-virgin olive oil
1/2 pound whole-grain fettuccini, cooked according to package directions
1 cup prepared pesto sauce
1 cup chopped tomatoes
1/4 cup grated soy or rice Parmesan, as garnish

1. In a large saucepan, sauté mushrooms and broccoli in oil over high heat for 3 to 5 minutes.
2. Reduce heat to low. Add fettuccini and pesto sauce, and toss.
3. Add tomatoes, and toss.
4. Serve immediately, garnished with soy or rice Parmesan.

SERVES 2

RICE NOODLE FANTASY

2 teaspoons tamarind pulp

1 cup sunflower oil

6 ounces thin rice noodles

1 clove garlic, minced

1/3 cup chopped yellow onion

fresh diced red chili peppers, slivered

1/2 cup egg substitute

8 ounces dulse or nori seaweed, thinly chipped into bits

1/2 pound extra-firm tofu, cut into 1/4-inch-thick slices

2 teaspoons arrowroot powder

2 teaspoons tamari plus 2 tablespoons hot water

1 tablespoon honey (tupelo preferred)

1/4 teaspoon cumin

1/4 teaspoon dried marjoram

1 teaspoon grated lemon zest

1 tablespoon canned yellow bean sauce

1 pickled garlic clove, sliced

1/2 cup mung bean sprouts

2 teaspoons chopped fresh parsley for garnish

orange rind for garnish

1. Strain and discard tamarind pulp, reserving juice.
2. Preheat oil in wok over high heat. Working a small handful at a time, fry noodles for approximately 30 seconds, turning frequently with spatula to ensure uniform cooking.
3. Remove noodles with a slotted spoon before they turn brown, and drain. Strain and reserve hot oil from wok.
4. Return 2 tablespoons of oil to wok, and heat on medium heat until hot. Stir-fry garlic for 1 minute, then remove and set aside. Repeat with onion and chili peppers, and add to garlic.
5. Cook egg substitute in wok until scrambled and golden brown. Remove and add to garlic/onion mixture.
6. Stir-fry seaweed for 1 minute, being careful not to overcook. Remove and set aside.
7. Add a bit more oil if needed. Stir-fry tofu 2 minutes. Remove and set aside.
8. In a bowl, combine arrowroot powder, tamari sauce, honey, cumin, marjoram, and lemon zest. Pour into center of wok. Heat and stir until simmering and slightly thickened. Add tamarind juice, bean sauce, pickled garlic, tofu,

egg substitute/garlic/onion/chili pepper mix, mung beans, and noodles. Gently mix until combined and heated.

9. Serve on platter topped with parsley and orange rind as garnish.

SERVES 2

POTATO CHOWDER

2 tablespoons extra-virgin olive oil

1 medium onion, chopped

2 stalks celery, minced

4 cloves garlic, minced

1 yellow pepper, diced

2 scallions, white only, chopped

1 tablespoon sherry (optional)

3 cups filtered water

1 cup plain soy milk

1/2 cup diced carrots

1 pound golden potatoes, peeled and cut into 1/2-inch cubes

1/2 pound purple potatoes, peeled and cut into 1/2-inch cubes

1 bay leaf

1 small jalapeño pepper

1/4 teaspoon freshly ground black pepper

1 teaspoon sea salt

1/4 teaspoon dried thyme seeds

1 teaspoon ground sage

1/2 teaspoon dried basil

1/2 teaspoon Pick a Pepper or Tabasco Sauce

1 tablespoon mustard seeds

1 tablespoon fennel seeds

1 tablespoon honey

parsley and Hungarian paprika, for garnish

1. Steam potatoes for 10 minutes.
2. In a stockpot, heat oil over medium heat and sauté onion, celery, garlic, yellow pepper, scallions, and optional sherry.
3. Add soy milk, carrots, and steamed potatoes to the sautéed vegetables. Add bay leaf, jalapeños, pepper, salt, thyme, sage, basil, pepper sauce, mustard seeds, fennel seeds, and honey. Stir and simmer an additional 15 minutes.
4. Garnish with parsley and Hungarian paprika.

SERVES 2

POTATO PANCAKES

3 new potatoes, peeled
1/2 cup rice milk
1/8 teaspoon sea salt
1/4 cup egg substitute
1/4 teaspoon cinnamon
2 tablespoons canola oil

1. Boil potatoes until tender, then mash them.
2. Add milk, salt, and egg substitute to mashed potatoes, and sprinkle on the cinnamon.
3. Shape into individual cakes. Sauté in medium-hot oil until golden brown.
4. Serve with Ratatouille (recipe follows).

SERVES 2-4

RATATOUILLE

4 tablespoons plus 1/4 cup extra-virgin olive oil
1 small eggplant, peeled and cubed
1 small yellow squash, cubed
1/4 cup minced shallots
1 scallion, chopped
2 cloves garlic, pressed
1 small zucchini, cubed
1/4 teaspoon thyme
1/4 teaspoon dried basil
1 small onion, chopped
2 tablespoons minced dulse leaves
1/2 stalk celery, chopped
1/3 cup sun-dried tomatoes, reconstituted in 1/3 cup water
1 teaspoon curry powder
sea salt to taste
freshly ground black pepper
1/4 cup raw sunflower seeds

1. Heat olive oil in a large skillet over medium heat. Add eggplant, yellow squash, shallots, scallion, garlic, and zucchini. Cook, stirring 3 minutes. Add thyme, basil, onion, dulse, and celery, and cook another 3 minutes.

2. In a blender, puree reconstituted sun-dried tomatoes, remaining 1/4 cup olive oil, and curry powder.
3. Preheat oven to 35 degrees F.
4. Transfer contents of skillet and blender to a lightly oiled quart baking dish or Dutch oven. Toss lightly. Season with salt and pepper.
5. Sprinkle top with sunflower seeds and bake for 35 minutes. Serve hot.

SERVES 2

SEA VEGETABLE AND CABBAGE OVER LINGUINE

2 tablespoons extra-virgin olive oil
1 small red onion, diced
4 cloves garlic, chopped
1 ounce kombu or arame seaweed, soaked in water for about 20 minutes to reconstitute
1/4 teaspoon date sugar or 2 tablespoons maple syrup or honey
1/4 pound red cabbage, shredded
1/2 pound green cabbage, shredded
1 Granny Smith apple, diced
1/4 cup white wine (Chardonnay is ideal)
1/4 cup filtered water
sea salt to taste
1 tablespoon white wine vinegar
1/2 pound whole-grain linguine, prepared according to package directions

1. Heat oil in a large pan over medium heat. Sauté onion, garlic, and seaweed until onions are golden.
2. Stir in sugar and add cabbages and apples. Mix well, cover, and cook over low heat for 20 minutes.
3. Add wine and water. Cover and cook for about 20 minutes more. Season with salt and vinegar.
4. Serve over whole-grain linguine.

SERVES 2

SPICY TEXAS CHILI

4 carrots (1 cup juice)
3 red or green bell peppers (¼ cup juice)
½ cup finely chopped yellow onions
1 cup extra-virgin olive oil
½ eggplant, chopped
½ cup cooked red kidney beans
½ cup sliced patty pan squash or zucchini
⅓ cup stewed tomatoes
¼ cup chopped green bell peppers
¼ cup corn kernels, fresh or frozen
¼ cup tomato puree
2½ teaspoons chopped green chili peppers
1 clove garlic, crushed
½ pound whole grain penne

1. Separately juice carrots and peppers.
2. In a large saucepan, sauté onions in oil over high heat, until onions are soft.
3. Add 1 cup carrot juice, ¼ cup pepper juice, and the remaining ingredients to the saucepan, and bring to a boil. Reduce heat to medium-low, and simmer, uncovered, for 15 to 20 minutes, or until vegetables are tender.
4. Serve hot over whole-grain penne.

SERVES 2–4

SPRING SCALLOPED VEGETABLES

10 parsnips (½ cup juice and 2 tablespoons pulp)
1½ cups plain soy milk
2 tablespoons chopped fresh parsley
1 tablespoon cold-pressed flavorless oil (sunflower, safflower, or canola)
½ teaspoon sea salt
1 teaspoon chopped fresh thyme or ½ teaspoon dried thyme
½ teaspoon chopped fresh rosemary or ¼ teaspoon dried rosemary
1 clove garlic, crushed
1½ cups sliced parsnips
1 cup sliced white potatoes
1 cup sliced acorn squash
½ cup chopped leeks
2 cups grated Swiss cheese or soy cheese (optional)

1. Preheat oven to 425 degrees F.
2. Juice parsnips.
3. In a small mixing bowl, combine ½ cup parsnip juice and 2 tablespoons pulp with soy milk, parsley, oil, salt, thyme, rosemary, and garlic. Mix well.
4. In a medium-size mixing bowl, toss together the sliced parsnips, potatoes, squash, and leeks.
5. Arrange vegetables on the bottom of a greased 9-by-12-inch baking dish. Pour sauce over vegetables, and sprinkle on cheese, if desired. Cover and bake for 25 minutes, or until vegetables are tender.
6. Serve hot with a salad or whole-grain pasta dish.

SERVES 4

STIR-FRIED TEMPEH WITH BROCCOLI AND LEMON THREADS

5 cups fresh basil (1 cup pulp)
2 lemons (¼ cup juice) plus 1 lemon
4 cloves garlic (1 teaspoon pulp)
¼ cup tamari
1–2 tablespoons whole spelt flour
1 tablespoon apple cider vinegar
1 teaspoon chopped red chili peppers
1 teaspoon grated ginger root
2 cups tempeh, cut into 1-inch cubes
1 tablespoon sesame oil + 1 tablespoon canola oil
¼ cup sliced scallions
1 pint cherry tomatoes
3–4 cups cooked brown rice

1. Separately juice basil, 2 lemons, and garlic.
2. Peel remaining lemon, and slice peel into threads. Set aside 1 tablespoon of the threads.
3. In a blender or food processor, combine 1 cup basil pulp, ¼ cup lemon juice, and 1 teaspoon garlic pulp with soy sauce, flour vinegar, peppers, and ginger. Blend for 2 minutes.
4. Transfer basil mixture to a small saucepan. Stir in lemon peel threads, and heat for 4 to 5 minutes, or until warm.
5. In a large frying pan, brown the tempeh in oil over medium to high heat.

6. Reduce the heat to medium-low. Add broccoli and scallions. Cover and cook for 2 minutes.
7. Add tomatoes, and cook, uncovered, for 1 minute.
8. Arrange tempeh mixture on a serving platter and pour heated sauce over mixture.
9. Serve hot with brown rice.

SERVES 3–4

VATAPA

3 slices rice bread or almond bread (available at health food stores)
¹/₄ cup coconut milk
¹/₂ cup chopped onion
1 clove garlic, minced
¹/₂ teaspoon paprika
1¹/₈ teaspoons cayenne
¹/₂ teaspoon chopped cilantro
¹/₂ teaspoon sea salt
¹/₂ teaspoon minched fresh ginger
¹/₂ pound dulse seaweed
filtered water
¹/₂ cup Brazil nuts, toasted and finely chopped
¹/₃ cup cashews, finely chopped
Peanut oil for greasing pan

1. Trim crusts from bread and discard. Break bread into pieces in a bowl.
2. Pour coconut milk over the bread and allow to soften.
3. Mash the softened bread mixture with a fork until fine. Add onion, garlic, paprika, cayenne, cilantro, salt, and ginger. Mix well.
4. Soak seaweed in enough water to cover, until fluffy looking and drain. Marinate with other ingredients for 20 to 30 minutes.
5. Preheat oven to 325 degrees F. Oil 9-inch square baking pan. Add mixture, sprinkle cashews on top and bake for 25 minutes.
6. Serve warm.

SERVES 2

VEGAN SPRING ROLLS

For the Marinade

1/8 teaspoon minced fresh ginger

2 tablespoons finely chopped carrot

1/4 cup green cabbage, finely chopped

1/4 teaspoon minced garlic

1/4 teaspoon minced scallion

2 teaspoons tamari sauce

1 tablespoon lime juice

For the Filling

1 tablespoon minced garlic

1 cup textured vegetable protein

2 teaspoons honey

1 tablespoon protein powder

1/2 teaspoon minced jalapeño pepper

2 tablespoons mung bean sprouts, freshly rinsed

1/2 teaspoon chili paste

2 teaspoons chopped roasted peanuts

1–2 teaspoons egg replacer

6 egg roll wraps

1. To prepare the marinade: Combine marinade ingredients in a small bowl. Mix well.
2. To prepare the filling: In a separate bowl, combine all filling ingredients except egg roll wraps. Add marinade, and mix well.
3. To form spring rolls: Follow directions on the egg roll wrap package by rolling up the filling in the wraps.
4. In a separate bowl, except peanuts. Sprinkle chopped peanuts on top. Serve remaining marinade in a small bowl.

SERVES 3

VEGETABLE CHILI

2 cups small dried navy beans

2 tablespoons extra-virgin olive oil

1 medium onion, finely chopped

1 scallion, finely chopped

1½ small red dried chiles

8 cloves garlic, minced

½ teaspoon ginger powder

½ tablespoon sweet paprika

½ teaspoon freshly ground black pepper

1 tablespoon minced green bell pepper

1 tablespoon curry powder

2 teaspoons ground cumin

5 sun-dried tomatoes, reconstituted and pureed to generate ½ cup tomato paste

1 tomato, coarsely chopped

3½ cups filtered water or vegetable broth

1 bay leaf

pinch of cayenne

1¼ tablespoons sea salt

10 fresh flat-leaf parsley sprigs tied together with kitchen string

5 fresh cilantro sprigs, chopped

1. Soak dried beans overnight. Drain and set aside.
2. Heat oil in a saucepan over medium heat. Cook onion and scallions, stirring occasionally, until tender, 6 to 8 minutes.
3. Add chiles, garlic, ginger powder, paprika, pepper, green pepper, curry powder, and cumin. Cook, stirring, for 2 to 3 minutes. Add sun-dried tomato paste and cook, stirring, until the mixture thickens, 1 to 2 minutes. Stir in fresh tomato and 1 cup water or broth, and bring to a boil.
4. Add beans and remaining water or broth, bay leaf, cayenne, sea salt, and parsley bundle. Lower heat to medium-low. Cover and cook until the beans are tender, 1 to 2 hours.
5. Discard chiles, bay leaves, and tied parsley before serving. Stir in the minced parsley and cilantro.
6. Serve warm.

SERVES 2

ZESTY CAULIFLOWER WITH GARLIC SAUCE

3 tablespoons tahini
1 cup chickpeas (precooked and pureed)
1 cup cauliflower florets
1 cup broccoli florets
1 cup sliced red bell peppers
1 teaspoon lemon juice
1/4 teaspoon turmeric
1/2 cup unsalted whole cashews
1/2 cup diced red bell peppers as garnish
4 sprigs fresh parsley, as garnish

1. Preheat oven to 425 degrees F.
2. In a medium-size mixing bowl, combine tahini, chickpea puree, cauliflower, broccoli, sliced red pepper, lemon juice, turmeric, and cashews. Toss to mix.
3. Pour mixture into a greased 9-by-12-inch baking dish. Cover with foil. Bake for 25 to 30 minutes, or until cauliflower is just tender. (Other vegetables should still be crunchy.)
4. Garnish with diced red pepper and parsley. Serve hot or cold with a rice dish or green salad.

SERVES 2

ZESTY SOY CHUNKS WITH RICE AND VEGETABLES

1 pound soy chunks
filtered water
1/2 cup Bragg's liquid aminos
2 tablespoons extra-virgin olive oil
1/4 yellow onion, chopped
1 clove garlic, minced
1/4 green bell pepper, chopped
1/4 cup chopped, stewed tomatoes
1 tablespoon tamari
1/4 teaspoon freshly ground black pepper
1 bay leaf
1/4 cup sliced black olives
3 tablespoons chopped fresh dill
1 tablespoon chile pepper
1 teaspoon sea salt
1 teaspoon cumin
1/2 teaspoon lemon juice
1/4 tablespoon paprika
2 cups dry white wine (optional)
1/2 lb. basmati white rice noodles, cooked
3 tablespoons green peas
1/2 onion, chopped, for garnish
orange and pepper slices and carrot peels for garnish

1. Soak soy chunks in water to cover for about 2 hours, or until puffed up. Drain, then marinate in Bragg's liquid aminos for about 1 hour.
2. Heat oil in skillet. Shake off any excess liquid from soy chunks, and sauté soy with onion, garlic, and green pepper until onion is golden.
3. Add tomatoes, tamari, black pepper, bay leaf, olives, dill, chile pepper, salt, cumin, lemon juice, and paprika. Simmer for 10 minutes.
4. Add wine and rice noodles and simmer for 20 minutes, until rice is tender.
5. Sprinkle peas on top and cook 5 minutes more.
6. Serve hot garnished with orange and pepper slices and carrot peels.

SERVES 2

DESSERTS

APPLE AND CINNAMON PUDDING

1 cup silken tofu
1/2 cup agar agar
1 apple, peeled and cored
1 teaspoon cinnamon plus extra for garnish
1/4 cup pure maple syrup

1. In a blender, combine all ingredients until smooth and creamy.
2. Garnish with bit of cinnamon, and serve warm or cold.

SERVES 2

ALMOND BALLS

3/4 cup dates, pitted
1/2 cup almonds

1. In a blender or food processor, grind dates until mashed.
2. Grind almonds in a nut or coffee mill, or place them in a paper or wax bag, fold in a towel and pound with a mallet.
3. Shape dates into small balls. Roll date balls in ground/crushed almonds.

SERVES 1

BANANA CREAM

1 cup silken tofu
1/2 cup agar agar
1 banana, peeled
1 teaspoon cinnamon plus extra for garnish

1. In a blender, combine all ingredients until smooth and creamy.
2. Garnish with dash of cinnamon.

SERVES 1

BLACKBERRY PUDDING

1 cup silken tofu

1/2 cup agar agar

3 tablespoons all-natural blackberry syrup (or 1/4 cup blackberries) plus extra for garnish

1. In a blender, combine all ingredients until smooth and creamy.
2. Garnish with a few drops of blackberry syrup or blackberries.

SERVES 1

BLUEBERRY PUDDING

1 cup silken tofu

1/2 cup agar agar

3 tablespoons all-natural blueberry syrup (or 1/4 cup blueberries) plus extra for garnish

1. In a blender, combine all ingredients until smooth and creamy.
2. Garnish with a few drops of blueberry syrup or blueberries.

SERVES 1

CHERRY-BERRY PUDDING

1 lemon (2 tablespoons juice)

3 cups pitted frozen cherries (or any other frozen berries)

1 1/2 cups silken tofu

1 tablespoon protein powder

1/4 cup pure maple syrup

1. Juice lemon.
2. In a blender or food processor, combine 2 tablespoons lemon juice, cherries, tofu, protein powder, and maple syrup. Blend for 2 minutes, or until smooth.
3. Serve chilled.

SERVES 2–3

CHEWY PECAN-ALMOND TREATS

6 parsnips (1 cup pulp)
1 1/2 cups sweet rice syrup
1/2 cup raw almond butter
3 teaspoons pure vanilla extract
2 cups coarsely chopped unsalted pecans
1 cup blanched slivered almonds

1. Preheat oven to 375 degrees F.
2. Juice parsnips.
3. In a medium-size mixing bowl, combine sweet rice syrup, almond butter, and vanilla extract. Add 1 cup parsnip pulp, pecans, and almonds. Mix well.
4. Pour the mixture into a greased 9-inch square baking dish. Bake for 10 minutes, or until nuts begin to turn light brown in color.
5. Cool for about 5 minutes before cutting into 6 squares.

SERVES 6

COCONUT DATE PARADISE PIE CRUST

3 carrots (1/2 cup pulp)
3 cups whole pitted dates
1 cup unsweetened flaked coconut
1 1/2 cups unsalted pecans, soaked and drained

1. Juice carrots.
2. In a blender or food processor, combine 1/2 cup carrot pulp with remaining ingredients. Blend until smooth.
3. Press the mixture into a lightly greased 9-inch pie plate (or a 9-by-12-inch baking dish).
4. When a recipe calls for a baked crust, put the crust in a 350 degree F. oven for 15 minutes, or until light brown in color.

SERVES 3–4

FRUITY CAROB BARS

4 apples (1 cup pulp)

3/4 cup pure maple syrup

1 teaspoon pure vanilla extract

2 teaspoons egg replacer

1/2 teaspoon ground allspice

1 cup mashed banana

1 cup unsweetened flaked coconut

3/4 cup unsweetened carob chips

1 cup coarsely chopped cashews or pecans, unsalted

4 tablespoons (1/2 stick) nonhydrogenated soy or safflower margarine, softened

1/4 cup light-colored honey (clover, tupelo, or wildflower)

1/2 cup whole spelt flour

2 tablespoons protein powder

1. Preheat oven to 375 degrees F.
2. Juice apples.
3. In a medium-size mixing bowl, whisk together maple syrup, vanilla extract, egg replacer, and allspice. Add 1 cup apple pulp, banana, coconut, carob chips, cashews or pecans, and stir well.
4. In another medium-size mixing bowl, blend margarine, honey, flour, and protein powder. Blend until a dough forms.
5. Press dough into a greased 9-by-12-inch baking dish. Pour maple syrup mixture over crust, and bake for 15 to 20 minutes.
6. Allow to cool and set for 10 minutes before slicing into 12 bars.

YIELDS 12 BARS

CINNAMON PUDDING

1 cup silken tofu

1/2 cup agar agar

3 tablespoons all-natural raspberry syrup (or 1/4 cup raspberries)

1 teaspoon cinnamon

4 peppermint leaves

1. In a blender, combine all ingredients until smooth and creamy.
2. Garnish with peppermint leaves.

SERVES 1

CRANBERRY PUDDING

1 cup silken tofu

1/2 cup agar agar

3 tablespoons all-natural cranberry syrup

4 peppermint leaves

1. In a blender, combine all ingredients until smooth and creamy.
2. Garnish with peppermint leaves.

SERVES 1

FRUIT SALAD IN CREAM

2 cups silken tofu

1 cup agar agar

1/2 peach

1/2 orange

4 strawberries or 3 tablespoons all-natural strawberry syrup plus extra for garnish

10 blueberries or 3 tablespoons all-natural blueberry syrup plus extra for garnish

1. In a blender, combine all ingredients until uniform but not smooth.
2. Garnish with a few blueberries or strawberries.

SERVES 2

GARY'S FRUITY KAZOOTIE COCKTAIL

2 tangerines (1/4 cup juice)

2 papayas (1/2 cup juice)

1/4 pineapple (1/4 cup juice)

1 1/2 cups silken tofu

1/4 cup pure maple syrup

2 teaspoons pure almond extract

1/4 teaspoon ground nutmeg

1 banana, mashed

1/3 cup unsweetened flaked coconut

3/4 cup mashed raisins

3 tablespoons blanched slivered almonds

2 tablespoons red fruit powder

2 tablespoons protein powder

2 tablespoons concentrated aloe vera juice

1. Separately juice tangerines, papayas, and pineapple.
2. In a blender or food processor, combine ¼ cup tangerine juice, ½ cup papaya juice, and ¼ cup pineapple juice, with silken tofu. Blend for 2 to 3 minutes, or until smooth.
3. Add maple syrup, almond extract, and nutmeg, and continue to blend.
4. Transfer mixture to a small mixing bowl, and stir in banana, coconut, raisins, remaining ingredients.
5. Chill for at least 1 hour before serving.

SERVES 2–4

MANDARIN CREAM PUDDING

8 mandarins (2 cups juice)
½ cup plain soy yogurt
3 tablespoons unsweetened flaked coconut
3 tablespoons ground almonds or almond butter, unsalted
1 teaspoon pure vanilla extract
1½ cups silken tofu
¼ cup pure maple syrup

1. Juice mandarins.
2. In blender or food processor, combine 2 cups juice with remaining ingredients. Blend for 2 minutes, or until smooth.
3. Serve chilled.

SERVES 1–2

MANGO CREAM

1 cup silken tofu
½ cup agar agar
1 mango
1 teaspoon cinnamon
dash of ground nutmeg for garnish

1. In a blender, combine all ingredients except nutmeg until smooth and creamy.
2. Garnish with dash of nutmeg.

SERVES 1

MANGO PINEAPPLE LEMON PUDDING

8 mangos (2 cups juice)
1 1/2 pineapples (1 1/2 cups juice)
1 1/2 lemons (3 tablespoons juice)
4 cups silken tofu
1 tablespoon protein powder
1/2 cup pure maple syrup

1. Separately juice mangoes, pineapples, and lemons.
2. In a small mixing bowl, combine 2 cups mango juice, 1 1/2 cups pineapple juice, and 3 tablespoons lemon juice with remaining ingredients, mixing well with a spoon.
3. Serve chilled.

   SERVES 6

MIXED MELON STRAWBERRY PUDDING

2 cups peeled red or yellow watermelon chunks (1/2 cup juice)
1 cup peeled honeydew melon chunks (2/3 cup juice)
1 lemon (2 tablespoons juice)
1/2 teaspoon stevia extract
3/4 cups strawberries, frozen
1 teaspoon lemon extract
2 cups silken tofu
1/4 cup pure maple syrup

1. Separately juice the watermelon, honeydew melon, and lemon.
2. In a blender or food processor, combine 1/2 cup watermelon juice, 2/3 cup honeydew melon juice, and 2 tablespoons lemon juice with remaining ingredients. Blend for 2 minutes, or until smooth.
3. Serve chilled.

   SERVES 2–3

NUTTY CREAM

1 cup silken tofu
1/2 cup agar agar
1 palmful almonds plus extra for garnish
2 tablespoons pecans
2 tablespoons macadamia nuts

1. In a blender, combine all ingredients until smooth and creamy.
2. Garnish with finely chopped almonds.

SERVES 1

ORANGE CREAM AND GRANOLA

1 cup silken tofu
1/2 cup agar agar
1 orange, peeled
1 teaspoon granola for garnish

1. In a blender, combine all ingredients except granola until smooth and creamy.
2. Garnish with dash of granola.

SERVES 1

PEACHES AND CREAM

1 cup silken tofu
1/2 cup agar agar
3 tablespoons all-natural peach syrup (or 1 peach)
1 teaspoon cinnamon plus extra for garnish

1. In a blender, combine all ingredients until smooth and creamy.
2. Garnish with a dash of cinnamon.

SERVES 1

RASPBERRY GELATIN

1 cup agar agar
1/2 cup raspberries
1/4 cup all-natural raspberry syrup
1/4 cup silken tofu, whipped
2 tablespoons pure maple syrup

1. In a blender, combine agar agar, raspberries and syrup.
2. Whip tofu separately with maple syrup in blender or beat together by hand.
3. Serve gelatin with whipped silken topping.

SERVES 1

PEACH IN A PUMPKIN CRUST

Filling

6 medium peaches, pitted and peeled

1/2 pound silken tofu

Crust

1 medium pumpkin, steamed and chilled (2 cups pulp)

1 teaspoon egg replacer

1/4 cup finely chopped dates

1/2 teaspoon pure vanilla extract

1. Preheat oven to 350 degrees F.
2. To prepare the filling: In a food processor, puree peaches with tofu.
3. To prepare the crust: In a small mixing bowl, combine 2 cups pumpkin pulp with remaining ingredients. Mix together well.
4. Press the crust mixture into a lightly greased 9-inch pie plate (or 9-inch square baking dish). Fill crust with peach-tofu blend.
5. Bake for 40 minutes, or until golden brown in color.
6. Let cool to room temperature before serving.

SERVES 4–6

RASPBERRY SPELT PIE

1 cup fresh raspberries

1/2 cup whole spelt flour

1/2 teaspoon ground allspice

1/3 cup cold nonhydrogenated soy margarine

1/4 cup plus 3 tablespoons cold water or plain soy milk

1. Puree raspberries in a food processor or blender. Set aside.
2. In a small mixing bowl, combine spelt flour and allspice.
3. With a fork, cut soy margarine into flour mixture until mixture is moist and fine. Add cold water (or soy milk) by the tablespoon until the dough has a smooth, even consistency.
4. Roll dough into a ball, and place it in a bowl. Cover bowl with plastic wrap, and chill for 1 hour.
5. Lightly flour a smooth, clean surface and rolling pin. Place chilled dough on floured surface. Roll dough from the center out until it is 1/2 inch larger than 9-inch pie plate. (Check by placing empty pie plate on top of rolled dough.)

6. Preheat oven to 350 degrees F.
7. Loosen dough by gently sliding a floured spatula underneath it toward the center and moving around the entire area of the dough until it can be lifted Transfer dough to a lightly greased 9-inch pie plate.
8. Drain excess water, if any, from raspberry puree. Spoon into crust and bake for 30 minutes, or until crust is light brown.
9. Fill with Rice Dream or soy ice cream, chill and serve.

MAKES 1 9-INCH CRUST

SPELT CRISPS

1 parsnip (1/4 cup pulp)
1/2 cup plus 2 tablespoons sweet rice syrup
1/4 cup organic peanut butter
1 1/2 teaspoons pure almond extract
3 cups unsweetened spelt flakes
1/4 cup chopped figs

1. Juice parsnip. Keep.
2. In a 2-quart saucepan, combine rice syrup, peanut butter, and almond extract. Bring to a simmer.
3. Immediately remove the mixture from the heat, and stir in parsnip pulp, spelt flakes, and figs. Mix together well.
4. Spoon mixture into a greased 9-by-12-inch baking dish, and press down firmly.
5. Cool completely before slicing into 9 bars.

YIELDS 9 BARS

STRAWBERRY CAROB PUDDING

1 cup silken tofu
1/3 cup filtered water
1/2 cup agar agar
3 tablespoons all-natural strawberry syrup (or 1/4 cup strawberries) plus extra for
  garnish
3 tablespoons carob powder
1/4 cup pure maple syrup

1. In a blender, combine all ingredients until smooth and creamy.
2. Garnish with a few drops of strawberry syrup.

SERVES 2

TROPICAL BLEND

6 apples (1¹/2 cups juice)

3 carrots (²/3 cups juice)

2 bananas, frozen without peel (1 cup pulp)

3 tablespoons chopped dates

3 tablespoons unsweetened flaked coconut

3 tablespoons ground almonds or almond butter, unsalted

1 teaspoon ground nutmeg

1 teaspoon pure almond extract

1¹/2 cups silken tofu

¹/4 cup pure maple syrup

1. Separately juice apples, carrots, and frozen bananas.
2. In a blender or food processor, combine 1¹/2 cups apple juice, ²/3 cup carrot juice, and 1 cup banana pulp with remaining ingredients. Blend for 2 minutes, or until smooth.
3. Serve chilled.

YIELDS 4 CUPS

ZESTY MANGO LIME PUDDING

4 cups peeled honeydew melon chunks (1¹/3 cups juice)

2 lemons (3 tablespoons juice)

6 mangoes (1¹/2 cups juice)

2 limes (3 tablespoons juice)

2 tablespoons protein powder

1¹/2 cups silken tofu

¹/4 cup maple syrup

1. Separately juice melon, lemons, limes, and mangoes.
2. In a blender or food processor, combine 1¹/3 cups honeydew melon juice, 3 tablespoons each lemon and lime juice, and 1¹/2 cups mango juice with protein powder, silken tofu, and maple syrup. Blend well.
3. Serve chilled.

SERVES 4

Chapter 9

Reduce with Juice

One of the easiest and tastiest ways to slim down is to forget calorie-free diet sodas with their harmful side effects and switch to juice instead. Juicing foods is a fantastic way to eat light and healthful meals without sacrificing essential nutrients. You can use juiced fruits and vegetables as a beverage, a snack between meals, or—if the juice contains some added protein—a meal in itself. As a low-calorie, filling addition to the diet, juice is a real boon to those seeking to lose weight.

WHY JUICE?

Because it is concentrated, freshly made juice floods the system with far more nutrients than eating healthful foods alone ever could. You would have to eat about two carrots and three celery stalks, for example, to get the amount of nutrients in one glass of carrot/celery juice. To get the equivalent of three glasses of juice daily, you'd have to eat 15 of those vegetables, a difficult task. Indeed, although the National Cancer Institute recommends five servings of vegetables and three of fruits daily, the typical American eats only one-and-a-half servings of vegetables and, on average, half a serving of fruit per day. This is a serious problem that's associated, along with other bad nutritional habits, with America's high levels of obesity and chronic health problems, including arthritis, intestinal problems, and cancer.

Even if you do have better eating habits than most, unless you juice, you might not be getting the best benefit from your food. The process of juicing takes full advantage of all the nutrients in the produce by separating them out from the fiber, which can trap nutrients and keep them from being absorbed into your body. Fiber is, of course, a vital part of a healthy, well-rounded diet, but it can be eaten separately in whole vegetables, fruits, grains, and nuts after the nutrients from the juice are hard at work in your system.

Juiced produce contains hundreds of vitamins, minerals, and phytochemicals that are essential for maintaining a healthy body. These chemicals are vital to healthy organs and cells as well as to a strong immune system. In addition, they keep us looking our best. Beta-carotene and vitamin A found in carrots, for example, help optimize our metabolism so we can burn more fat.

Raw fruits and vegetables are enzyme-rich foods. Enzymes are proteins that are catalysts; that is, they cause or speed up chemical reactions. Enzymes make it possible for you to convert food into body tissue and fuel to keep you going. In fact, enzymes help us carry out virtually every life process, from breathing and respiration to digestion and absorption. Eating an enzyme-rich diet is a must for overcoming or preventing health challenges—and for remaining slim. It is interesting to note that in Asian cultures, even though food is an important social focal point, most people remain naturally slim. That's because the traditional Asian diet consists largely of fresh, raw fruits and vegetables, lightly cooked fare, fermented foods, and rice—all enzyme-rich choices.

Here in the West, though, our diets can be enzyme-poor, because enzymes are largely destroyed by the heat of cooking and processing, things that we do a lot of in our culture. Juicing, on the other hand, keeps produce enzyme-rich. When the juice is consumed promptly or after a brief period of storage in the freezer or a vacuum bottle, you still benefit from the enzymes.

Following is a list of some of the enzymes that function as digestive aids and the foods that contain them. Juicing and eating these foods may help to prevent or overcome overweight conditions:

- Bromelain, found in pineapple
- Esterase, found in many plant foods (starchy vegetables, such as peppers, and leafy vegetables, such as lettuce)
- Hemicellulase, in seeds and green plants (spinach, lettuce, arugula, broccoli, cauliflower, kale, Swiss chard, parsley)
- Invertase, in cucumber, green plants
- Lactase, in tomato, persimmon, apple, peach
- Lipase, in green plants, wheat germ, flaxseed
- Maltase, in beet leaves, green plants, banana, mushroom
- Nuclease, in mung beans
- Papain, in papaya
- Sucrase, in green plants, beet leaves and stems, banana

Plants also produce chlorophyll, a substance with a structure very similar to that of hemoglobin, the compound that transports oxygen in the bloodstream. Consuming fruits and vegetables, or their juices, can improve the efficiency of oxygen transport in the body, which aids in cleaning out toxins and thinning the blood to prevent clotting and heart disease. Oxygen transport is also necessary for a successful exercise program because the body needs oxygen to develop muscles and to burn fat.

In addition to vitamins, minerals, enzymes, and chlorophyll, fruits and vegetables contain a vast range of other ingredients, known as phytochemicals or phytonutrients ("Phyto" simply means "plant.") A single fruit or vegetable may contain up to several hundred phytochemicals, many of which have been proven to promote health. For example, studies have found that lycopene, the red phytochemical found in tomatoes and watermelon, and indoles, found in broccoli and other cruciferous vegetables, contain anticancer properties.

There is still much to learn regarding the value of specific plant chemicals as well as the effects of phytonutrients working together. From a scientific standpoint, we may never comprehend the full benefit derived from combined phytonutrients, but we are learning that nature, in its wisdom, has combined ingredients that complement one another and work synergistically. Thus in the health field we have the saying: "The whole food is greater than the sum of its parts." And for speedy healing and overall well-being, juicing is better yet.

THE JUICY DETAILS

With all the essential nutrients found in raw fruits and vegetables, the quick and easy process of juicing should be a mainstay in everyone's routine. Here are some tips for making the best juices possible.

First, the major part of your juices should come from watery fruits or vegetables, such as cucumber, tomato, celery, apple, and cabbage. Dark green vegetables, such as spinach, are valuable additions, but use less of these, as they are more concentrated. Add sprouts into your juicing mix by all means, for their enzymatic and other nutritional benefits. If you're using carrot juice, dilute it with water or other juices, to avoid excessive sugar. And of course if you have diabetes or another health condition, are pregnant, or are on a medication, consult your healthcare professional before you start a new dietary routine such as juicing, because you don't want to be using foods that are contraindicated.

One other reminder I always like to give to juice novices is that you should not gulp. We Americans tend to gobble our food and practically pour our drinks down our throats, but this is not good for the digestion or the psyche. It's not good for the waistline either, because, as we've discussed, quick eating doesn't give you a chance to have the feeling of satiety register before you overconsume. Especially if you're adding protein powder, a glass of juice is like a meal, so try this: Enjoy it for as long as you would a delicious meal—in an elegant setting, with company!

Go for Organic

For juicing, as for eating, you should use organically grown produce when it's possible. A fruit or vegetable that is labeled organic means that it is grown in compliance with laws certifying that the products have been grown and handled according to strict procedures without toxic chemical input. The types of chemicals that might be used on nonorganically grown produce are herbicides (weed killers), fungicides (mold killers), and insecticides. Many of these have been found to be potential cancer-causers, according to the Environmental Protection Agency. Another consideration is that pesticides and other toxins reduce a food's enzyme levels. By eating and juicing organically you're avoiding any of those nutritional pitfalls.

What's more, organic farmers focus on maintaining healthy soil through proper tillage and crop rotation. Healthy soil contains thousands of microorganisms, which helps retain water and provide nutrients to the plants, nutrients that are then passed on to you. Healthy soil also produces strong, healthy plants that are better able to resist insects and disease on their own, without toxic chemicals. Because juiced produce is not cooked or boiled, it is even more important that these foods be free of toxins.

The Way We Wash Our Fruit

All fruits and vegetables should be washed properly before juicing, even organically grown produce, which does, after all, grow in dirt. If you are unable to get organically grown produce, then you must certainly wash, or, in some cases, peel and discard the skin to get rid of some of the toxic chemicals. The best way to wash produce effectively is to hold it under running water while scrubbing it with a vegetable brush. Later you can use this brush to clean the stainless steel strainer found in most juicers.

To Peel or Not to Peel?

Many fruits and vegetables should be juiced with their peels on. Others, however, must be peeled because they are either too thick for the machine to grind up or have been found to contain toxic substances. Fruits that should always be peeled are kiwis, papayas, oranges, grapefruits, tangerines and bananas. But with oranges and grapefruits, make sure that you keep the bitter, white skin on the inside of the rind because it contains many nutrients that you do not want to lose. Watermelon rind also contains a great deal of nutrients; although it is thick, it can be juiced quite easily. (You may not want to juice the rind unless you are looking for a natural diuretic, as the juice is not as sweet as the juice of the fruit's flesh.) Waxed fruits and vegetables such as apples or turnips should always be peeled, as wax may be carcinogenic.

Why Seeds and Pits Are the Pits

Remove all pits before juicing because they are too large and too solid to go through the juicer. Also, most seeds should be taken out because they might create an unpleasant, bitter taste. Note that apple seeds in particular *must* be removed because they have been found to contain toxic substances. Some seeds, however, such as watermelon and cantaloupe seeds, can be juiced and are in fact a dietary aid because of their natural diuretic properties, which means that they can aid the body in getting rid of excess water.

When Raw Is a Raw Deal

Juicing vegetables raw will provide you with the maximum amount of nutrients, including live enzymes. However, a few vegetables need to be lightly steamed (and then chilled) before juicing: asparagus, broccoli, Brussels sprouts, and cauliflower. Remember to drink your juice as soon after juicing as you can, or the vitamins, minerals, and enzymes will not be as potent. However, if you juice in the morning and refrigerate the drink, it will still be fine in the evening.

When the Blender Is Better

Juicing recipes often call for nuts, but their hard consistency makes it impossible to throw them in the juicer as is. Instead, use a blender, food processor, or food mill to grind nuts down before adding them to the rest of the juice mixture. Also, if a recipe calls for ice, make sure to juice the produce in the juicer and then combine it with the ice in a blender or food processor. (Note: Ice is never really necessary in a juice; it's fine to use water instead and have a warmer drink.) Bananas are best juiced in the blender, unless you first peel and freeze them, in which case the juicer will give you a lumpless and creamy blend.

Protein Powder Power

You may want to add extra nutrients to your juices by mixing in some vegetable protein powder to increase not only protein content but complex carbohydrates, fiber, and vitamins and minerals as well. Protein powders can be found in health food stores and will help to complete your balanced diet. They generally consist of rice, sesame seeds, egg whites, or soy blends. You also can add protein powder to hot cereal or to supplement foods on a road trip to maintain the balanced diet that often gets ignored when we travel. When you're using juice as a meal, as I often do, add two scoops of protein powder to ensure that you are not leaving out any important nutrients.

YOUR BIOCHEMICAL MAKEOVER

Once you start juicing, in a sense you're giving yourself a biochemical makeover in that juices make you beautiful from the inside out. In fact, the health benefits of juicing cannot be overstated. Many everyday ailments as well as life-threatening diseases can be avoided or ameliorated through juicing on a daily basis.

Many arthritis sufferers, for instance, have turned to juicing to try to alleviate their symptoms and have found positive results. A drink that would be beneficial to arthritis sufferers is one that contains a large amount of vitamin C and bioflavinoids to strengthen collagen, which is part of the protein fibers that support joints. Kale, parsley, spinach, and citrus fruits provide these nutrients. Pineapple and ginger root also would help because pineapple contains the enzyme bromelain, which has anti-inflammatory properties.

Someone who suffers from prostate enlargement needs to consume lots of zinc. Ginger, parsley, and carrots contain amounts of this essential mineral. Vitamin B6 is also recommended for this condition and can be found in the dark, leafy greens, such as kale, spinach, and turnip greens.

People who suffer from water retention, also known as edema, may be pleasantly surprised to learn that juice can work to reverse this condition. In fact, a juice drink that is high in potassium, to help counteract the effects of sodium in the body, and vitamin B6, to boost the kidneys' ability to secrete sodium, can be as effective as diuretic pills, which actually leach potassium from the body. Some natural diuretics are watermelon or cantaloupes, juiced with their seeds.

It is important to realize the impact that stress has on our bodies and to replenish nutrients that are lost when we're experiencing tension. Does stress bring out your "chocoholic" tendencies? A chocolate craving may stem from a deficiency in magnesium, and it can be relieved by a magnesium-rich juice made with apples, celery, or beets. Because of stress, immune overreaction, and the constant input of sugar, we easily lose many B vitamins, including pantothenic acid, which is needed to strengthen the body. Pantothenic acid can be found in broccoli and kale, among other veggies. We also tend to lose vitamin C and need to replenish our supply as well as add more zinc to keep us from becoming vulnerable to colds and diseases. It is also important to increase our intake of beta-carotene, which is at the top of the list when it comes to cancer protection and can be found in carrots, parsley, and collard greens.

Of course, disease conditions or excess stress may not be your prime concerns; you may simply be looking to lose some extra pounds. The biochemical makeover that juice provides your body is going to help you too in a way that's actually a "double whammy." First, as I said at the outset, juice is both low in calories and filling. But you also get an unparalleled energy boost with juice, as it floods your body with easily accessible nutrients in a way that solid food—which has to be broken down first—can't. With this added energy, you're going to feel more like exercising than you ever have before. Go with that feeling and—voilà— you burn yet more calories! In Chapter 11 we'll be looking at some aerobic exercise goals that juicing can help you work toward.

JUICE RECIPES

Following are some juice recipes. But first, when you wish to create more or less juice than a recipe suggests, or when you're inventing a juice combination of your own, it may be helpful to refer to the following conversion table for amounts to use. Use these measures as a general guideline only; these are not exact, as the exact number will depend on the size and type of produce and your individual juicer. As you begin to juice on a routine basis, you will become more familiar with the amounts that you require.

JUICE CONVERSION TABLE

Produce	For 1/4 Cup Juice, Use . . .	For 1/2 Cup Juice, Use . . .	For 1 Cup Juice, Use . . .
Apple	1 apple	2 apples	4 apples
Beet	1 beet	2 beets	4 beets
Cabbage	1/4 cabbage	1/2 cabbage	1 cabbage
Carrot	1–2 carrots	2–3 carrots	4–6 carrots
Cauliflower	1/4 cauliflower	1/2 cauliflower	1 cauliflower
Celery	1 stalk	2 stalks	4 stalks
Cranberry	1 cup	2 cups	4 cups
Cucumber	1 cucumber	2 cucumbers	4 cucumbers
Honeydew melon	1/4 melon	1/2 melon	1 melon
Kiwi	3 kiwis	6 kiwis	12 kiwis

JUICE CONVERSION TABLE (cont.)

Produce	For 1/4 Cup Juice, Use . . .	For 1/2 Cup Juice, Use . . .	For 1 Cup Juice, Use . . .
Leek	5 leeks	10 leeks	20 leeks
Lemon	2 lemons	4 lemons	8 lemons
Mango	1 mango	2 mangos	4 mangos
Nectarine	3 nectarines	6 nectarines	12 nectarines
Orange	1 orange	2 oranges	4 oranges
Papaya	1 papaya	2 papayas	4 papayas
Parsnip	5 parsnips	10 parsnips	20 parsnips
Peach	2 peaches	4 peaches	8 peaches
Pear	2 pears	4 pears	8 pears
Pepper, Green	4 green peppers	8 green peppers	16 green peppers
Pepper, Red	4 red peppers	8 red peppers	16 red peppers
Pineapple	1/4 pineapple	1/2 pineapple	1 pineapple
Plum	3 plums	6 plums	12 plums
Squash, Acorn	1 1/2 squash	3 squash	6 squash
Squash, Butternut	1 1/2 squash	3 squash	6 squash
Squash, Yellow	1 squash	2 squash	4 squash
Strawberry	2 cups	4 cups	8 cups
Tangerine	2 tangerines	4 tangerines	8 tangerines
Tomato	1 tomato	2 tomatoes	4 tomatoes
Watermelon	3/4 cup	1 1/2 cups	3 cups
Zucchini	2 zucchini	4 zucchini	8 zucchini

MORE RECIPES—THIS TIME, JUST JUICE!

Here are some of my favorite juicing recipes that you can use for delicious snacks or as substitutions for entire meals. A great way to become and stay slim is to have just juce for breakfast—and then solid meals for lunch and dinner.

VERY VEGETABLE JUICE WITH BEET GREENS

2 apples (1/2 cup juice)
3 carrots (1/2 cup juice)
1 beet (1/4 cup juice)
1 small bunch of beet greens (1 tablespoon juice)
1 1/2 cups ice

1. Separately juice the apples, carrots, beets, and beet greens.
2. In a blender or food processor, combine 1/2 cup apple juice, 1/2 cup carrot juice, 1/4 cup beet juice, and 1 tablespoon beet greens juice with the ice. Blend for 2 minutes, or until smooth.
3. Serve immediately.

YIELDS 2 1/4 CUPS

SPROUT 'N' APPLE JUICE

6 apples (1 1/2 cups juice)
4 carrots (1 cup juice)
1/2 cup sunflower or alfalfa sprouts (1 tablespoon juice)

1. Separately juice the apples, carrots, and sprouts.
2. Combine 1 1/2 cups apple juice, 1 cup carrot juice, and 1 tablespoon sprouts juice.
3. Serve immediately.

YIELDS 2 1/2 CUPS

PINEAPPLE MELON SUMMERTIME SPRITZ

2 cups peeled watermelon chunks (2/3 cup juice)
2/3 pineapple (2/3 cup juice)
1/2 cup seltzer
3/4 cup ice

1. Separately juice the watermelon and pineapple.
2. In a blender or food processor, combine 2/3 cup watermelon juice and 2/3 cup pineapple juice with the seltzer and ice. Blend for 2 minutes, or until smooth.
3. Serve immediately.

YIELDS 2 3/4 CUPS

SWEET AUNT MABEL'S MIXER

2 apples (1/2 cup juice)
4 pears (1/2 cup juice)
3 carrots (1/2 cup juice)
2 cucumbers (1/2 cup juice)
1 beet (1/4 cup juice)
1 red bell pepper (1 tablespoon juice)
1 small piece ginger root (1 tablespoon juice)

1. Separately juice the apples, pears, carrots, cucumber, beet, red pepper, and ginger.
2. Combine 1/2 cup apple juice, 1/2 cup pear juice, 1/2 cup carrot juice, 1/2 cup cucumber juice, 1/4 cup beet juice, 1 tablespoon red pepper juice, and 1 tablespoon ginger juice.
3. Serve immediately.

YIELDS 2 1/4 CUPS

STRAWBERRY BANANA BOAT

2 apples (1/2 cup juice)
2 pears (1/4 cup juice)
2 cups strawberries (1/4 cup juice)
1/2 banana
3/4 cup ice

1. Separately juice the apples, pears, strawberries.
2. In a blender or food processor, combine 1/2 cup apple juice, 1/4 cup pear juice, and 1/4 cup strawberry juice with the banana and ice. Blend for 2 minutes, or until smooth.
3. Serve immediately.

YIELDS 2 1/2 CUPS

HONEY BLUE MOON

1 pear
1/2 lemon (with 1/2 inch skin)
2 tablespoons raw (unheated) honey
1 cup filtered water
1 cup ice
1/4 cup blueberries

1. In a blender or food processor, combine all the ingredients. Blend until smooth.
2. Serve immediately.

SERVES 2

GREEN MONSTER

2 kiwis
1 pear
2 apples
1 bunch dandelion greens
4 stalks celery
1/2 cup blueberries
1-inch piece ginger root

1. Separately juice kiwis, pear, apples, dandelion greens, celery, and ginger.
2. In a blender or food processor, combine the juice with the blueberries. Mix until smooth.
3. Serve immediately.

SERVES 2

PURPLE POWER

3 cups watermelon (rind included)
3 stalks celery
1 cup grapes

1. Juice watermelon with rind, celery, and grapes.
2. Serve immediately.

SERVES 2

THIRST QUENCHER

3 cups watermelon (without the rind)
1/4 pineapple
2 cups grapes

1. Juice watermelon, pineapple, and grapes.
2. Drink immediately or serve chilled for a refreshing drink.

SERVES 2

TROPICALITE

1/2 pineapple
1 kiwi
1 mango
2 tangerines
1 1/2 cups ice

1. Separately juice the pineapple, kiwi, mango, and tangerines.
2. In a blender or food processor, combine the juices with the ice. Blend for 2 minutes, or until smooth.
3. Serve immediately.

SERVES 2

GREEN APPLE

1/2 bunch Swiss chard
1 cup sunflower or alfalfa sprouts
1 bunch watercress
3–4 leaves romaine lettuce
1 cucumber
4 stalks celery
1-inch piece ginger
2 apples

1. Juice all the ingredients together.
2. Serve immediately.

SERVES 2

CRAZY BEET

4 stalks celery
1/2 bunch kale
1/2 bunch arugula
1/2 bunch parsley
1 cucumber
3 beets
1-inch piece ginger

1. Juice all the ingredients together. (You may want to add a little flaxseed oil. If so, put the juice and oil in a blender or food processor and blend for 1 to 2 minutes.)
2. Serve immediately.

   SERVES 2

VERY BERRY BLUE

3 stalks celery
1/2 head purple cabbage
1 bunch parsley
1 red bell pepper
2 beets
1-inch piece ginger
1 cup blueberries

1. Juice all the ingredients together except blueberries.
2. In a blender, combine the juice with the blueberries. Blend for 2 minutes, or until smooth.
3. Serve immediately.

   SERVES 2

PAPAYA BLUE

2 apples
2 slices pineapple
2 slices papaya
1/2 cup blueberries
1 cup ice

1. Juice the apples and pineapple together.
2. In a blender or food processor, combine the juice with the remaining ingredients. Blend until smooth.
3. Serve immediately.

   SERVES 2

SWEET DANDELION

2 apples
3 cups honeydew melon chunks (without the rind)
4 dry dates
1/2 bunch dandelion greens
1/2 head broccoli
1-inch piece ginger root

1. Juice all the ingredients together.
2. Serve immediately.

   SERVES 2

HAPPY CAMPER

1/2 bunch watercress
1 medium fennel
1 medium parsnip
3 stalks celery
1 cup alfalfa or sunflower sprouts
1 cucumber
1/2 bunch parsley
2 carrots

1. Juice all the ingredients together.
2. Serve immediately.

   SERVES 2

WILD WORLD

1 bunch dandelion greens
1/2 head cabbage
3 beets with tops
1 medium parsnip
1/2 bunch parsley
2 carrots
1-inch piece ginger root
1/2 cup raspberries

1. Juice all the ingredients together.
2. Serve immediately.

SERVES 2

SOME LIKE IT HOT

2 red peppers
1 head lettuce
1/2 cup radish sprouts
1 cup clover sprouts
4 stalks celery
4 leaves turnip greens
1 bunch spinach
2 radishes
2 apples
1-inch piece ginger root

1. Juice all the ingredients together.
2. Serve immediately.

SERVES 2

PAPAYAN MANGO

1 mango
1 papaya
½ pineapple
2 cups ice
2 bananas

1. Juice together the mango, papaya, and pineapple.
2. In a blender or food processor, combine the juice with the remaining ingredients. Blend for 2 minutes, or until smooth.
3. Serve immediately.

SERVES 2

ORANGE PASSION

1-inch piece ginger
2 oranges
2 grapefruits
1 lemon
1 lime
2 tablespoons raw honey

1. Pass the ginger through a juicer. Then pass the oranges, grapefruits, lemon and lime through.
2. Combine with honey and serve immediately.

SERVES 2

WHY YOU OUGHT TO DRINK WATER

Not everything you drink has to be nutrition-packed. Water is the best thirst-quencher and detoxifier there is, as well as a zero-calorie beverage that can fill you up somewhat. For all of these reasons you should make some of your daily liquid intake—which should be, by the way, at least eight glasses, of eight to ten ounces of liquid each—pure filtered water.

FOR ADDITIONAL INFORMATION

When they used to talk about eating an apple a day to keep the doctor away, they didn't know what was in the apple. They just knew that it was important for health. Well, now we know that there are over a hundred different chemicals in that apple, as there are in every fruit and vegetable, and that these do a lot of good things. These plant nutrients can help repair damage to our DNA, help prevent cancer, and ward off viral and bacterial infections. They are essential to good health and can play an important role in your journey toward a leaner, healthier body. Appendices A, B, and C of this book contain a glossary of phytochemicals and their health benefits as well as a complete listing of the phytochemicals found in common fruits and vegetables. I include this information so you can tailor-make juices with attention to particular healing properties. You also can peruse these sections to get an idea of the wonder that is "nature's medicine cabinet"—the produce aisle!

Chapter 10

Nutrient News You'll Need

W hen we seek to lose weight and gain energy, whole foods should be our first, but not our only, source of nutrition. All of us need extra support from vitamin supplements in today's world, where modern farming practices result in depleted soils and foods fall short of their nutrient potential. Of course we should not rely solely on supplements; rather we should integrate them into a holistic weight-loss protocol.

This chapter talks about the role of vitamins, minerals, herbs, and amino acids in helping us to reach and maintain our ideal weight. Some supplements address the problem directly. Certain nutrients, for instance, reduce food cravings and decrease appetite. Then there are the nutrients that enhance thermogenesis, the body's ability to burn fat. Still others enhance insulin receptivity so that sugar is processed properly before it has the chance to turn into fat. In addition, supplements that regulate metabolism less directly may be taken. For example, blood-cleansing teas made from dandelion, burdock, nettles, and cleavers help liver function, which in turn improves metabolism.

Supplements are not a magic bullet, and there is no one formula that will benefit everyone. Rather, a combination of nutrients should be individually determined with the help of a health practitioner. Dr. Ronald Hoffman, a leading alternative physician in New York City, explains the need for an individualized program.

"It's a little bit like a broken computer. There are so many circuits in a computer and a millionfold more in the human body. Many diverse reasons cause people to have a metabolic slowdown. One person might have a zinc deficiency, another might have a magnesium deficiency, and yet another might be low or deficient in B vitamins to the point where they can't get their engines to turn over and burn calories. . . . We individualize our approach by doing vitamin and mineral profiles. That helps us see what that person's critical link in their metabolic chain might be."

While exact nutrient protocols should vary according to individual needs, to give you a grounding in the area of supplementation vis-à-vis weight control, I have listed several important vitamins, minerals, herbs, and other supplements for trimming down, along with an explanation of their role in weight management and overall health. The supplements I have suggested are the general preventive dosages; you should use the information here as a jumping-off point for developing your personalized program with a health practitioner.

VITAMINS

Vitamins are organic compounds that help regulate metabolism and assist us in forming bone and tissue. There are two categories of vitamins: oil soluble, which are stored in body fat, and water soluble, which are not stored in the body and need to be replenished daily. The following are the most important vitamins for everyone to be familiar with, particularly those who may be cutting down on their food intake in order to lose weight.

• *Vitamin A.* Your skin, your teeth, and your hair depend on it, so you need this one to look your best. But actually, vitamin A's benefits extend to every cell of your body, because this antioxidant works to fight off disease and the effects of psychological stress. A is a fat-soluble vitamin. If you are following a low-fat diet, you may be reducing your vitamin A intake as well. Be sure to include "good" fats in the diet and to take vitamin A—even better, take it with zinc—to help lower cholesterol levels. For women of childbearing age, beta-carotene is recommended in place of vitamin A. Vitamin A can be found naturally in fish oils, fruits, and vegetables. The recommended dosage is 5,000 International Units (IU) per day.

• *B Complex.* Among its many vital functions, the B complex plays an important role in normalizing appetite, maintaining a healthy metabolism, and helping digestion. B vitamins activate our enzymatic system, converting glucose and fatty acids into energy, and help the adrenal glands control how fat is deposited in the body. B12 helps prevent the accumulation of fatty deposits in the liver and plays a key role in the creation of methionine and choline, two substances needed to move fats. Niacin, or vitamin B3, improves metabolic activity, helping to transform sugar and fat into energy. B complex comes only in supplement form and should be taken in dosages of 50 mg per day.

• *Vitamin C.* Also called ascorbic acid, this all-important antioxidant detoxifies and supports the cells, prevents sickness, and promotes fast healing. It works to build collagen, which physically supports the tissues in the body. Furthermore, vitamin C is necessary for the secretion of thyroid and adrenal hormones. Thyroxin from the thyroid gland and adrenaline and noradrenaline from the adrenal cortex are not only essential in helping us cope with stress, they play vital roles in the management of sugar and weight. When combined with vitamins B5, B6, zinc, and selenium, C helps the body overcome food allergies. The recommended dosage is 1,000 to 20,000 mg a day, depending on the state of your health and your immune system.

• *Vitamin E.* Vitamin E is a protector against pollution, a natural energizer, and essential to good health and a beautiful appearance. If you don't get enough E, you could experience edema, or swelling, poor skin condition, circulatory problems, and even abnormal heartbeat. Conversely, being well supplied with this vitamin is a prudent step for those who intend on staying energetic and youthful. E is a prime component of antiaging protocols and should be taken in dosages of 200 to 1,200 IU per day, depending on your specific requirements.

Vitamin Protocol for Children

When helping children and teenagers learn to follow a good diet, be sure to include, at the very least, these extras every day: a basic multivitamin, 100 to 200 IU of vitamin E, and 500 mg of vitamin C. The exact amount to be given will depend on the child's weight and age; smaller children should take less.

MINERALS

Minerals serve as building materials for bones, teeth, tissue, muscle, blood, and nerve cells. They also serve as catalysts for many biological reactions in the body and help to maintain the fragile balance of body fluids.

• *Chromium.* To curb a sweet tooth, try chromium. It can help to reduce sugar cravings and enhance insulin receptivity. In fact, studies show chromium to be exceptionally effective in helping to prevent and reverse type 2 (non–insulin-dependent) diabetes. Often when people become insulin-resistant, their blood sugar goes up; once the condition improves, blood pressure naturally lowers. This mineral is also important to fat loss; experiments show that when we take chromium picolinate supplements, we lose body fat and tend to keep it off. In addition, when we exercise, chromium helps us develop muscle. Don't expect to lose weight instantly, though—it may take two to three months to see results.

This gradual lowering of body fat will be accompanied by more sustained energy levels, and there will not be the cravings to eat everything in sight. Further, chromium picolinate has been associated with lowering total and LDL (bad) cholesterol and raising HDL (good) cholesterol. This mineral not only enhances good health in a variety of ways; it appears, from recent research, that chromium picolinate may have a direct link to life extension. Recommended amounts for adults are from 400 to 600 mcg—that's micrograms—per day. It is naturally found in green and sea vegetables. For insulin-resistance problems you might need up to 800 mcg.

• *Magnesium*. Highly underrated, magnesium works throughout the body and plays a crucial role in weight management. Magnesium breaks up fat globules into fatty acids and transforms glucose into glycogen, both of which become sources of energy. Magnesium also acts as a coenzyme that stimulates the digestion and absorption of foods. Inadequate amounts of the mineral can lead to constipation and other digestive problems. Magnesium also controls insulin production. It too is found naturally in green and sea vegetables and should be taken in 1,200-mg dosages per day.

• *Manganese*. Manganese will help to control insulin reactions and blood sugar levels. The mineral also seems to improve thyroid function and aids in the production of sex hormones. Like chromium and magnesium, manganese can be found in green and sea vegetables. It should be taken in 10-mg dosages per day.

HERBS

Herbs are whole foods that help to detoxify and rebuild the system as you lose weight. In addition, certain herbs help to lessen appetite or increase metabolism. A practitioner skilled in herbal use can not only guide your selection but instruct you on how much of an herb to use, when to use it, and in what form. Some of the herbs you may be advised to include are listed below. As with all your food, you should buy organically grown herbs when possible. Be aware that some herbs are counterindicated with different medications, or pregnancy. Always consult your physician and pharmacist first.

Herbs for Cleansing and Rebuilding

Detoxifying herbs gently improve liver function. As the liver is the main regulator of metabolism, these herbs pave the way for improved metabolic function. Additionally, they encourage the immune system to purify tissues and thus contribute to better overall health.

Herbs for Cleansing the Blood, and More

• *Red clover.* This common purple-flowering herb provides a powerhouse of benefits. Used alone or in combination with other cleansing herbs, red clover will purify the blood, soothe the stomach, calm the nerves, and help the liver and lymph glands. Herbalists also recognize red clover as an important plant for combating cancerous growths. Recommended dosage: 100 mg per day.

• *Dandelion.* It may be known as a weed, but this common plant provides extraordinary value to the kidneys, liver, spleen, pancreas, and gallbladder. For hygienic reasons, do not use dandelion found on the streets. I recommend a two-ounce serving of fresh dandelion every day.

• *Burdock.* This earthy root is one of the best blood cleansers, making it of special value for the clearing of skin conditions like boils, sties, and sores. Burdock also helps the kidneys eliminate wastes and uric acid and is a tonic for indigestion. I recommend eating one ounce of fresh burdock every day.

• *Echinacea.* Once popular among Native Americans and early immigrants, the beautiful purple coneflower has made a strong comeback in recent years for its ability to ward off colds and the flu in their early stages. Also of note is echinacea's benefit to the blood and lymph. Plus it is a wonderful digestive tonic and acts to eliminate poisons, pus, and abscess formations. Recommended dose: 100 mg per day for one week per month for 6 months.

• *Sarsaparilla.* Taken sparingly, sarsaparilla can help many conditions, including arthritis and gout. It helps heal skin outbreaks, promotes urine flow, and expels gas. Recommended dose: 25 mg per day. A combination of yellow dock, another herb, and sarsaparilla makes an excellent spring weight-loss tonic. Combine the following ingredients and take for one week:

> 1-inch piece ginger
> Juice from 2 apples
> Juice from 1 lemon
> 1 ounce aloe vera
> 1 cup filtered water
> 100 mg echinacea tincture
> 25 mg sarsaparilla
> 50 mg yellow dock

• *Alfalfa.* Mineral- and vitamin-rich, alfalfa aids in the metabolism of proteins, fats, and carbohydrates. Recommended dose: 100 mg per day.

Herbs for the Bowels. Constipation is a distressing symptom of modern lifestyles brought on by devitalized, low-fiber diets; too much meat, coffee, and alcohol; and too little exercise. When accompanied by a correction of these habits, herbs can play an important role in getting the bowels to move again. Consider chickweed, ginger, fennel seed, psyllium, elder, Oregon grape, rhubarb root, licorice, and aloe. These work best at a very low dosage—I recommend 25 mg doses for all of these herbs, but you should not use more than one at a time. One word of caution: Regular use of certain bowel-stimulating herbs, such as cascara sagrada, will have a laxative effect that can hinder your body's ability to have a bowel movement on its own.

Herbs for Rebuilding the Body. Some good strengthening herbs include ginkgo, astragalus, and ginseng. One of ginseng's many benefits is its ability to reduce blood sugar. An alternative to ginseng would be a digestive tea made from equal parts of peppermint, chamomile, fennel seed, and licorice root. For many, drinking the tea for four to seven days results in improved digestion and greater energy. If you choose to take them as supplements, take them in the following dosages: Try each dosage for one week and see how your body responds.

Astralagus: 100 mg
Chamomile: 50 mg
Fennel: 25 mg
Ginkgo: 100 mg
Ginseng: 100 mg
Licorice Root: 25 mg
Peppermint: 50 mg

Herbs for Slimming Down

The following herbs, which can be purchased in supplement form at a health food store, have fat-fighting properties. They should be taken one at a time in the recommended dosages. Try each for a week and see what works best for you.

- *Coleus* helps increase fat breakdown and boost thyroid function. Recommended dose: 50 mg per day.
- *Fennel* is a kitchen spice that helps decrease appetite, increase urine flow, and quicken recovery from food poisoning. Recommended dose: 50 mg per day.
- *Kava-kava* promotes calmness and is better to turn to than an antidepressant or comfort food when the little stresses of life begin to get to you. Recommended dose: 50 mg per day.

THERMOGENIC AIDS:
SUPPLEMENTS THAT FIGHT FAT

If you find yourself unable to burn fat even after consistent intense workouts at the gym, you might want to give thermogenic aids a try. These supplements activate the body's brown fat, typically found along the central nervous system and in the back. (Most fat is an off-white or yellowish color, but the brown variety gets its color from being filled with blood cells.) Brown fat is loaded with mitochondria, and thermogenic aids stimulate these energy-producing organelles.

While certain thermogenic aids, like coenzyme Q10 and omega-3-containing oils, are safe and extremely beneficial to overall good health, others, such as ma huang and ephedra, may prove dangerous to people with arrhythmias, mitral valve prolapse, hypertension, and other heart conditions and should not be used.

Additionally, some of these stimulants increase the production of neurochemicals, which, in turn, speeds up free radical damage. Free radicals are molecules that can damage normal cells and tend to glom on to fatty acids. People with more fatty acids in thier body thus retain more free radicals. Dr. Dallas Coulatre, author of *Anti-Fat Nutrients* and *Reduce Body Fat in 15 Days with Vitamins and Herbs*, confirms, "You're taking something that radically speeds up the body, plus you're releasing greater amounts of adrenaline and noradrenaline. Too much of these neurochemicals can cause damage from free radicals at the nerve sites throughout the body." To minimize the effects of free radical damage from thermogenic aids, Coulatre recommends taking three grams of vitamin C daily as well as L-tyrosine (an amino acid supplement that will be discussed later) to prevent adrenal exhaustion.

When following a weight-loss program, consider these thermogenic aids, which can be taken together or separately.

• *Coenzyme Q10.* This nutrient is not only safe but vital to good health and high energy. Known mostly for its association with a healthy heart and gums, coenzyme Q10 (coQ10) also may have implications for weight loss in some individuals, according to experimental results. The body naturally produces small amounts of coQ10, and some people produce less of it than others. Most people need between 100 and 150 mg daily as a supplement.

• *Omega-3 oils* found in evening primrose oil, borage oil, blackcurrant seed oil, and flaxseed oil work somewhat more slowly than do most thermogenic aids but are far safer for turning the body's brown fat into fuel. One 300- or 500-mg capsule, or one to three tablespoons a day, are generally effective, although I recommend starting lower and working up to that amount. A little with each meal is recommended because when too much is taken at once, the oil is eliminated by the body. Omega-3 oils have been proven to help insulin receptors work more effectively, thus aiding carbohydrate digestion. Additionally, studies have found that when children are given omega-3 oils, their bodies make fewer fat cells.

• *Carnitine* is a favorite of bodybuilders for increased energy before workouts. It helps transport fat to the cells' mitochondria, where it can be burned more efficiently. Between 500 and 1,000 mg a day are recommended.

• *Alpha-lipoic acid* is a powerful antioxidant that protects cells against aging and disease and makes the mind more lucid. It also improves our ability to handle stress and promotes the Krebs cycle, a process that quickly converts fat and sugar into energy. The nutrient also improves the body's insulin response, which lowers blood sugar and reduces fat. In fact, some studies suggest that by supplementing with lipoic acid, sugar metabolism can increase by up to 25 percent. With proper medical supervision, lipoic acid may be an adjunctive treatment of choice for diabetes and the neuropathies caused by the disease. While 50 to 100 mg a day are recommended for antioxidant purposes, up to 600 mg daily may be needed for diabetes and insulin resistance. As one dose will last just two to three hours, take three divided doses throughout the day.

• *Chitosan* is a natural dietary fiber from the skeletons of shellfish that its proponents say attracts fat like a magnet attracts iron. Taken before meals, chitosan binds with a certain percentage of fat eaten and removes it from the body before it has the chance to become absorbed. I recommend a dose of 25 mg per day before each meal.

• *Pyruvate* has the ability to aid fat loss and increase the noticeable effects of exercise. Double-blind studies performed on the effects of pyruvate suggest that its use contributes to the loss of body fat and the gain of lean muscle mass. Other benefits included a significant decrease in fatigue and an increase in energy. I recommend a very small dose of 25 mg per day.

• *Glutamine* is an amino acid that helps to eliminate cravings for cookies, cakes, and other simple carbohydrates and creates a sense of well-being in most people who take it. For best results take 500 to 1,000 mg an hour before meals.

• *Fiber.* You need 30 to 50 grams daily. There's no denying how important fiber-rich fruits, vegetables, and grains are to overall good health. But if you need to keep your carbohydrate levels low because of insulin resistance, you can still get your fiber from supplements. Both soluble and insoluble fiber from bran, flaxseeds, guar gum, and psyllium will help to lower insulin resistance as well as work to prevent bowel cancer, diabetes, and heart disease. Fiber also helps us process fats better. This may be why people who follow a Mediterranean diet, one that combines fiber-rich foods with fat from olive oil, tend not to gain weight.

• *L-tyrosine* is an amino acid that's important for proper thyroid functioning. It will also help to prevent adrenal exhaustion when taken in conjunction with thermogenic aids. For most people 250 mg a day are recommended.

• *DHEA (Dehydroepiandrosterone)*, sometimes called the fountain-of-youth hormone, is produced in increasingly lower quantities as we age. Small amounts of this adrenal gland hormone may help to improve immune response and to curb the appetite. As a rule, young people should avoid DHEA; it becomes more important after age forty-five, and even then should be used sparingly, in a daily dose of 10 to 25 mg. Before taking DHEA you should be tested to see if you are in fact deficient. If you are not deficient, it should not be used as a supplement.

• *Conjugated linolenic acid,* or CLA, is a new item that is reportedly good for changing the body composition through the utilization of fat. The benefit here is that you look leaner, although this is not necessarily reflected on the scale. One to two grams, or 500 mg, of CLA a day will produce an effect in most people.

A COMPLETE NUTRIENT PROTOCOL

In a recent weight-loss protocol given to study group participants, I included the following comprehensive list of nutrients and dosages, which group members then tailored to their own individual situations. Naturally, if you do not suffer from diabetes or a thyroid condition, you won't have need for the supplements that work specifically for these problems. You should use this information as a starting point only; remember, when planning your own supplementation, seek a medical doctor's okay to prevent possible contraindications. What's health-promoting for someone else may not be for you if you are taking particular medications, are pregnant, or have certain medical problems. That said, here are some general guidelines: In order to safely begin a vitamin protocol, start with a dosage that is one-fifth of the ideal. Increase one-fifth per month for five months. Then go off the nutrients for one week and begin the same process over again. Do this so the body doesn't develop tolerance.

Acetyl-L-carnitine: 500 mg
Alpha-lipoic acid: 200 mg
Ascorbyl palmitate: 200 mg
B complex: approximately 50 mg
Beta-carotene: 10,000 IU
Boron: 3 mg

Bromelain: 20 mg

C: 2,000–10,000 mg

Calcium/magnesium citrate: 1,200 mg

Cayenne: 10 mg

Chromium: 200 mcg

Coenzyme Q10: 200 mg

DMAE: 100 mg (dimethylaminoethanol)

Folic acid: 600 mcg

Garlic: 3000 mg

Ginkgo biloba: 100 mg

Ginseng: 100 mg

Glutathione: 300 mg

Hawthorn: 15 mg

Lutein: 250 mg

Lycopene: 50 mg

Manganese: 25 mg

Milk thistle: 25 mg

Molybdenum: 100 mcg

MSM: 500 mg

Mushroom complex: 100 mg (methyl-sulfonyl-methane)

NAC: 500 mg (N-actyl-cystern)

Oil of primrose: 1,500 mg

Pantothenic acid: 300 mg

Phosphatidylcholine: 500 mg

Phosphatidylserine: 500 mg

Potassium: 300 mg

Proanthrocyanidin: 200 mg

Quercitin: 200–800 mg

Selenium: 200 mcg

Trimethylglycine: 200 mg

Vitamin A: 5,000 IU

Vitamin B complex: approximately 50 mg

Vitamin E: 200–600 IU

Chapter 11

What's Your Next Move?

In the previous chapters you've been reading about eating right to normalize weight and improve health, and I hope you've been inspired to do this. If so, that's great. But if you're planning on losing weight *only* by improving your diet, forget it. You must include exercise as part of any weight-loss and health improvement plan, or your project is going to fail. No exercise, no lasting weight control or health improvement. It's as simple as that.

Of course, that's a negative way of looking at it. A positive take on the situation is that exercise has so many benefits—both short and long term—that of course you're going to develop a personal exercise program. Let's look at some of those benefits.

HOW EXERCISE HELPS YOU—RIGHT NOW

For the person looking to lose weight, exercise helps in the short term because it immediately speeds up the metabolism. One of the hallmarks of the aging process is a lowering of metabolic activity, which causes us to gain weight and feel sluggish. Exercise helps to stem those trends and, in many cases, reverse them, bringing us back levels of agility, energy, endurance, stamina, and strength that we may not have had in years. What this means is that exercise facilitates the body's ability to do even *more* exercise, resulting in a victorious—rather than vicious—cycle of increased activity and increased levels of calorie burnoff. Exercise also speeds up the cleansing process, allowing toxins that were stored in body fat to be oxidized and, hence, properly eliminated. Moreover, exercise increases thirst, making us more likely to drink the fresh water that will hydrate our cells so that proper electrical activity will occur. Exercise also stimulates chemicals that naturally improve our mood so that we feel better about ourselves and life in general. That's important to those of us trying to lose weight as we make the sometimes difficult adjustment to new eating patterns.

The Physical Facts

Going beyond weight-loss considerations, exercise is an absolutely essential factor for achieving a healthy, well-balanced life. Without it you risk a range of problems, of which obesity is just the beginning. Other things the sedentary person may have to contend with are lack of energy, weakened muscles, a fragile immune system, depression, back problems, and poor circulation. These can all add up to a less fulfilling and shorter life. Circulation problems can lead to heart attacks and strokes. Weakened muscles can cause your organs to slip and put pressure on your vertebrae, causing discomfort from back pain. A weakened immune system makes you susceptible to viral, bacterial, and other diseases, including cancer.

Exercise aids in detoxifying the body through blood oxygenation and improvement of blood flow. Cancer has been found to thrive in oxygen-deficient areas of the body, so exercise actually can be a deterrent of cancerous growth as well as an aid in the healing process. Also, improving the blood flow is vital for the elimination of toxins and waste that would otherwise overwork the liver and cause fatigue, constipation, and possibly prostate, kidney, colon, and liver diseases. Moreover, exercise can help people with mild to moderate chronic pain have fewer and less intense episodes.

Motion and the Emotions: The Psychological Benefits of Exercise

Beside the physiological benefits of exercise, the many psychological benefits cannot be overemphasized. Exercise is a terrific cure for sluggishness and lack of energy. Sluggishness tends to feed on itself, creating an unhealthy cycle as the body lowers its metabolic rate to conserve calories. This process probably evolved millions of years ago to keep our ancestors from starving when food became scarce. It seems that our bodies are still programmed to conserve calories when we are not active, to keep from starving. The difference now is that we continue to eat every day and that conserved energy quickly transforms into fat. The excess fat and lower metabolism foster the continuation of the cycle by making us feel tired and less able to exercise. When we are not active, breathing becomes shallow and blood flow slows; therefore, less of both oxygen and blood reach the brain to wake it up. Have you ever considered the fact that the brain needs oxygen to function and concentrate? It has been found that directly after exercising, our brains are particularly alert and energized, enabling us to work, study, and socialize well.

The term "runner's high" refers to the feeling of euphoria that a person achieves after thirty to sixty minutes of running. The brain produces endorphins, which are naturally occurring, soothing substances that cause mood elevation or a pleasant sense of well-being. This makes exercise a must for the highly stressed businessperson who needs to release tension and gain a positive perspective on things.

Also, the slimming effect of exercise creates a more positive self-image, and when we feel good about ourselves we just plain feel better. In fact, a review of the research literature in psychology shows regular exercise to be an effective, inexpensive way to overcome mild to moderate depression. Feelings of lethargy and depression go hand in hand, and by mobilizing ourselves—even starting with a short walk outdoors—we can brighten our mood. Both aerobic and nonaerobic forms of exercise have been found to help. Some research also suggests that exercise may be a useful treatment for other psychological problems, including schizophrenia, substance abuse, anxiety disorders, and body image problems. More studies, however, in these latter areas are needed.

HOW EXERCISE HELPS OVER THE LONG HAUL

Over the long term, exercise helps us to normalize weight; lessen our percentage of body fat; enhance enzymatic activity and hence better utilize our food; and speed up peristalsis, which is the wavelike intestinal movement that gets food waste moving out of the system as it should. Exercise also enhances energy and brings more blood to our skin, giving us a more youthful glow.

When a person takes the time and effort to be on a proper exercise program, that attention to personal needs will generally flow over into other areas of life. A person who undertakes a regular exercise program is more likely to eat in a healthful way and to be conscious of other health needs, such as stress control and the avoidance of environmental toxins. The long-term result is likely to be a more vigorous, longer life.

AEROBICS AND ANAEROBICS— HOW BOTH FIT INTO YOUR PLANS

Together, aerobic and anaerobic exercises make for a complete workout. Both aerobic and anaerobic exercises tone muscles, but only aerobics can increase lung capacity and strengthen your heart. Aerobic exercises are defined as those that utilize large muscles continuously and rhythmically and that increase your heart rate for a sustained period of time.

In addition to a healthier heart, aerobic exercises lead to stronger lungs, larger blood vessels, and more capillaries. Walking, running, swimming, Roller Blading, and bicycling are examples of exercises that give you aerobic benefit when performed within your target heart rate range.

To calculate this range, subtract your age from 220 and multiply the result by 0.6 and then 0.8. The resulting numbers refer to the minimum and maximum number of times you want your heart to beat per minute during aerobic exercise. Staying within this desired range means that you're exercising at approximately 75 percent of your optimal aerobic capacity. More than 75 percent produces too much stress on the body. Doing this correctly will, in time, bring down your resting pulse rate. If your resting heart beats 80 times per minute, for example, and by proper systematic exercise you're able to bring this rate down to 60, you will be lengthening the life of your heart and, hence, your life in general. Aerobics are not only great for the resting pulse, but they will enable you to sustain a more rapid heartbeat when necessary.

To get a reasonable amount of benefit from an aerobic exercise, you must get your heart into the target range for twenty to forty-five minutes, at least three to five days per week. Remember, this is a target to shoot for and not necessarily the starting point. Ideally, I recommend hourlong exercise periods six days a week, but not everyone can do that, and the lower level is effective. If you haven't exercised in a while, start with just five or ten minutes of aerobics and slowly work your way up. Be careful not to go over your target rate or else you will lose steam and not be able to sustain the exercise for the full twenty minutes.

Anaerobic exercises are those that focus on muscle strength, power, and skill. They require less oxygen, as opposed to aerobics, and can be performed only in very short, intense bursts of energy. Examples of this type of exercise are weight lifting, golf (minus the walking component), archery, and racquetball (unless there are lengthy volleys that rhythmically work your body and heart, in which case it can become an aerobic workout).

A well-rounded exercise program should include both types of exercise.

Make Like an Athlete: Interval Training

Athletes use interval training to improve speed and endurance, but I highly recommend this technique for anyone who wants to condition the entire body as well as lower the metabolic rate and improve his or her energy level and circulation. Because interval training is a strenuous undertaking, though, be sure to get medical clearance from your physician before embarking on a serious program.

Basically, what's involved in interval training is alternating regular-speed and high-speed periods of performing your aerobic exercise. This method can be utilized with any aerobic exercise, including biking, swimming, and jogging, by sprinting until you get close to the top of your target heart rate range (220 minus your age, times 0.8) for thirty to sixty seconds and then easing up to the middle of that range (220 minus your age, times 0.7) for another thirty seconds. Repeat this sequence three to five times.

When you are ready to intensify the workout, you can increase either the speed of the sprint or its length as well as decrease the easing-up period.

LET'S GET SPECIFIC . . .

When you choose an aerobic exercise, you may be tempted to go for the trendy choice. Resist that temptation and pick something you truly enjoy doing. That way you'll be more likely to stick with your activity month in and month out, over the years. Of course you'll probably want to engage in more than one aerobic activity; that's called cross-training, and it works to benefit both your muscles and your psyche. Still, choose one thing that will be the backbone of your exercise program, and concentrate on that. Let's look at some of your options.

Walking

Walking is perhaps the easiest way for almost anyone to get started with aerobics. In fact, for some people, such as certain pregnant women or arthritis sufferers, it's the only acceptable form of cardiovascular exercise. You can do it almost any time of year as long as you dress appropriately; you can even walk indoors if necessary. Many shopping malls open early in the morning for walkers; in some situations hallways will suffice. Although it takes one and a half hours of walking to give you the same aerobic effect as you get from running for thirty minutes, any and all walking will be beneficial.

When walking, concentrate on maintaining a steady pace with a heel-to-toe gait. Keep your arms swinging at right angles in an easy, natural manner. Don't carry anything (such as hand weights) because doing so can unbalance you and slow you down.

Always do warm-up exercises and begin walking slowly. To reach the level of a full aerobic workout, start walking twenty to thirty minutes each day and increase your time by 10 percent each week until you are walking for one hour. Finish each session by slowing down again. If you're walking outdoors, try to stay on a soft surface of grass or earth for maximum comfort. If there's a park nearby, take advantage of it. And if you're forced to walk in the street, be sure to stay on the left side, facing traffic.

In 1990 the American Council on Sports Medicine recommended that people trying to lose weight exercise six out of seven days, walking briskly for a half hour. But Dr. Daniel S. Kirschenbaum, a clinical psychologist, director of the Center for Behavioral Medicine and Sports Psychology in Chicago, and author of *Weight Loss Through Persistence*, believes seven out of seven days is better. Walking each day first thing in the morning elevates the metabolic rate for several hours, so that you burn calories throughout the day. Moreover, Kirschenbaum believes daily walking increases focus and reinforces a positive habit. "If you're walking briskly in Chicago's winter," he states, "at some level you're going to have a debate with yourself where one side of you says 'What are you doing?' and the other side says 'You must be serious about this.' That internal dialogue, even if it is at a barely conscious level, absolutely helps."

Power Walking

If you have been instructed by a physician to avoid running due to a past injury, you might want to try race or power walking, which is as beneficial as running without the stress on your joints and impact on your body.

When running, you're raising the leg up high in the air to bring it down, increasing the pressure per square inch against the joints of the knee, ankle, foot, and hip. But when you're walking, you're not stressing the joints in this way, because one foot is always on the ground. Also, because your posture is at a five-degree angle forward, and because you're vigorously moving your arms at right angles at the waist and practicing deep breathing, you're actually gaining more benefit aerobically. When power walking you're moving approximately 20 percent more muscle groups than if you were running, where the arms don't move. In power walking, your arms are the pistons, allowing the body to go. So, in the end, you get all of the benefits of running without the joint stress and actually are using more muscle groups. The more muscle groups you are able to use—such as the upper back, shoulder, arm, triceps, biceps, and chest muscles—the more fat you are going to be burning.

There are other benefits too. In inclement weather, you'll have the opportunity to power walk with others indoors at a nearby mall. Friends who are not up for jogging can still join you in power walking, so you can enjoy each other's company. Also, if you have some previous injury that you are afraid of aggravating, power walking is ideal because you can slow or increase your pace depending on your overall physical condition.

Remember to include warm-ups and cool-downs when you power walk, drink proper amounts of fluid, and wear high-quality shoes.

Running

As with walking, running is an accessible sport that requires little more than proper footwear to begin. Running is a very effective way not only to improve your cardiovascular and circulatory systems but to reduce stress and muscle tension, making it popular with businesspeople who often are overwhelmed by day-to-day activities. Believe it or not, simple muscle tension can be extremely detrimental, decreasing energy levels and, by restricting blood and oxygen flow to the brain, causing headaches.

Because running is a high-impact exercise, it is extremely important that you take the proper steps before beginning. Make certain to warm up and cool down before and after running. Hydrate yourself before you work out and afterward. Avoid saunas after a workout, as they constrict blood capillaries so the blood does not return to your heart effectively. Wear good-quality foot gear. Your running shoes do not have to be the most expensive, but they must be of high quality to avoid injury. Both *Consumer Reports* and seasoned athletes can assist you in choosing shoes.

Swimming

One of the greatest types of cardiovascular exercise is swimming. It stretches both upper- and lower-body muscles in a coordinated, rhythmic movement and helps flexibility. The water's buoyancy reduces pressure on bones and joints, so you avoid injuries common in other sports. The feeling of being suspended in water, relatively free of gravity, provides a boost for many overweight people.

If you're not a seasoned swimmer, you can start by water jogging, or simply by walking back and forth in water approximately waist deep, swinging your arms naturally as if you were walking on land. If you are a swimmer already, be sure to do warm-up exercises and determine your resting pulse before doing laps. Start with an easier stroke like the breast or sidestroke, then switch to butterfly or freestyle. If this gets too strenuous, you may break it up with periods of swimming on your back. Try to swim for a total of twenty to thirty minutes, three to four times each week, as with other aerobic programs. Don't swim on consecutive days, however, as daily swimming can cause pulled or strained muscles. You can interval train during swimming by sprinting up to thirty seconds at a time, but slow down if you start to feel winded. After taking a thirty-second rest, repeat the sprint, then the rest again, for a total of three to five times.

Be sure to follow up a swim with stretching, paying particular attention to the rear leg muscles and anterior leg muscles (the ones in front) if you use a backstroke. Select a swimsuit based on comfort, not fashion, and swim in a moderately warm pool—77 to 81 degrees. It is wise to wear goggles to protect against conjunctivitis and a bathing cap to prevent ear infections or "swimmer's ear." For days when no swimming pool is available, have an alternative sport at the ready.

Bicycling

Bicycling is a fun way to condition your cardiovascular system as well as strengthen the anterior leg muscles. This activity is a great complement to running, which builds posterior leg muscles. Runners who also bike reduce their chance of knee and rear leg injuries.

To condition your cardiovascular system properly, you should ride below 80 percent of your target heart rate. If you are constantly sprinting and riding above that rate, you are not taking full advantage of the aerobic benefits of riding.

Try riding at thirty seconds in a sprint mode and then rest for thirty seconds at a normal pace. Repeat this sequence three to five times in a row. This will help to increase your aerobic capacity as well as your stamina.

While using a three-speed or a ten-speed is optional, it is important that your bike be sturdy and comfortable for you. You might want to use foot clips to secure your feet to the pedals, but good-quality jogging shoes will suffice. For exercising you should use upright handlebars, as opposed to the tilted ones used in racing, to take pressure off your back and enable you to sit up straighter.

Using an indoor stationary bicycle is also an effective way to exercise, and the same steps should be taken when riding one. Remember, your mind should be focused on the exercise. If you can read a novel or magazine while riding, you are not riding hard enough to gain any real cardiovascular benefits.

Jumping Rope

Although most of us haven't done it since we were kids, jumping rope is an exercise that almost anyone can do without investing in a lot of equipment. All you need is a 3/8-inch nylon rope that is twice the length from the floor to your chest. This is a fun way to give yourself a great cardiovascular workout as well as burn more calories per minute than you do running, swimming, or biking. Jumping can, however, cause damage to your legs and lower back if you don't do it properly. I actually recommend that jumping rope be used with an alternate exercise, such as swimming, so that the muscle tissue can repair and rebuild without injury. I also advise you to slowly work up to a full thirty-minute jumping workout.

Keep in mind that the older and heavier you are, the less you should jump. In any case, you should not spend more than four minutes jumping on the first day. Begin by jumping for about thirty seconds and then walking until your feel your breath return. Then begin to jump for another thirty seconds.

Small trampolines are available that are lots of fun to use and will take much of the pounding effect off your legs and lower back. These are small enough to be used indoors or on a patio during inclement weather. You should use the same thirty-second formula as with jumping rope.

Other Aerobic Alternatives

Rowing, either on a machine or outdoors, is a highly effective aerobic exercise. You also might want to try Roller Blading, walking on a treadmill, or aerobic dancing. One aerobic activity that does require equipment but that gets you out into beautiful surroundings is cross-country skiing. You can get a super calorie-burning workout as you glide and climb up and down hills with this invigorating sport. However, for those who want a lower level of exertion, skiing around a flat field is an enjoyable, less strenuous option. For the snowless, machines can help you simulate cross-country movements.

Remember, if you're doing a high-impact aerobic exercise, such as jumping or running, it's a good idea to alternate with low-impact exercise, such as swimming or rowing, on a day-to-day basis to avoid injury and to allow muscle tissue to rebuild repair itself.

Different from aerobic exercise, anaerobic exercise requires short bursts of intense energy followed by periods of lower energy output or rest. This type of exercise uses concentrated energy to build strength, power, endurance, or skilled movement of certain muscle groups.

Weight Training

Perhaps the most popular form of anaerobic exercise, weight training is an excellent method to firm and strengthen specific muscles, particularly if your primary aerobic exercise focuses on the muscles of only one part of the body. For instance, runners tend to have very strong and well-developed legs while their upper muscles are lean but in need of strengthening. Keep in mind that weak body parts tend to get injured more frequently than strong ones.

Don't try to build huge muscles during weight training; muscles weigh more than fat, and massive ones will just add weight during your aerobic workout! To improve muscle tone, use light weights—two- or five-pound weights are best—but do more repetitions, approximately twelve to fifteen per set. (If you were trying to build muscle mass, you'd use heavier weights and do fewer repetitions, approximately eight to ten.) You should be able to lift the weight fiteen times with a sixty-second rest per set, for a total of three to four sets. If the weight is too heavy, you won't be able to do three or four sets of fifteen. If it's too light, you'll be able to do far more. Let your experience be your guide.

Contrary to popular belief, it is not necessary for weight trainers to consume large amounts of protein to repair muscle tissue that breaks down during training. It is better to eat more complex carbohydrates, which also contain protein, such as beans, grains, nuts, seeds, and starchy vegetables such as potatoes and squash. To avoid injury, allow a full forty-eight hours between weight-training sessions for the muscle tissue to have time to repair itself. Remember to maintain a stretching program when utilizing weight training, because working with weights can tighten up your muscles as it strengthens them.

CREATING YOUR OWN EXERCISE PROGRAM

It would be great to be able to prescribe a one-siz-fits-all exercise program for everyone, but it wouldn't be wise, because each person begins with his or her own unique level of readiness. What *can* be said that applies to everybody is that your goal is to lower your pulse rate and increase metabolic activity, so that the body becomes more efficient at burning calories.

Ideally, you should work your way up to a situation in which you're exercising aerobically six days a week for an hour a day with your heart beating at 75 percent of its optimal level. But not everyone can reach this exercise goal. You have to do what's realistic for your own physiology, and—whatever you do—you have to do it gradually. Everyone has an individual time frame for achieving fitness. The important thing is that you're involved in the process. But how do you begin?

Let's say you're middle age, overweight, new to the world of exercise, and confused. What do you do?

- First, get medical clearance from your doctor to begin an exercise program.
- Then choose your main aerobic activity. Power walking is a great one to start with. As we've discussed, if you choose something high-impact, such as jumping rope, you should alternate it with another activity.

- Next, understand that gradualism and patience are key. So on your first day of exercising, perform your aerobic activity for only five minutes, preceded by a twenty-minute loosening-up period, and followed by a ten-minute cooling-down period.
- Follow this same routine of five-minute exercise periods for the entire first week (that is, for at most six days out of seven). Try to stay within your target heart rate range during your exercise periods.
- During the second week, exercise aerobically for ten minutes each day, again trying to stay within your target heart rate range. Be sure to include loosening-up and cooling-down periods.
- Add five minutes to your routine on a weekly basis, so that by week 12 you're up to an hour a day. Note: Not everyone will be working up to this level; if you have arthritis or high blood pressure or are on certain medications, for example, or if conditions are very hot and humid, this may not be advisable. Consult your medical professional about accommodating these basic guidelines to your particular needs.
- Always pay attention to how your body feels as you work out. If you feel dizzy or weak, stop, rest the next day, and seek professional help.

Warming Up and Cooling Down

In order to avoid injuring your muscles, you always should warm up before and cool down after you exercise. This is particularly important if you are just starting an exercise program for the first time. A few minutes of light activity gets your muscles moving and your heart pumping without causing stress to your system. It also allows you to exercise longer. For a warm-up, begin by stretching to get your muscle cells full of blood, and then do anything that makes you sweat without tiring you out— push-ups or sit-ups, for example. I recommend warming up for about twenty minutes.

The cool-down is equally important, as it is very dangerous to stop vigorous exercise suddenly. Cooling down allows your heart rate to slowly return to its resting pulse and reduces lactic buildup, which causes sore muscles. A great way to cool down is to walk for five minutes and then do some simple stretches for about ten minutes after that.

Incorporating an Anaerobic Element into Your Program

Once you're established in your aerobic activity, you'll probably want to incorporate an anaerobic exercise into your routine in order to tone more muscle groups. You should perform anaerobics before, rather than after your aerobic activity.

- Weight training is an ideal way to begin. Start with weights you can handle without struggling, as light as three or five pounds.
- Do various types of curls and arm raises. For example, with a dumbbell in each hand, raise your hands to shoulder level, hold for three seconds, and then slowly, with good resistance, bring your hands back down again. That will begin developing your inner muscle tensile strength as well as burn intramuscular fat.
- Let at least two days elapse between weight-training sessions.
- Abdominal work is another basically anaerobic activity you may want to try. Start with just five sit-ups and each week add three to five more—or whatever feels comfortable. In four months to half a year, you may be able to work your way up to 100 sit-ups (done in five sets of twenty repetitions, or "reps," with two-minute rest periods in between). But, as with aerobics, each person should do his or her own realistic goal and be patient about reaching it.

You may want to go to a health club, perhaps at your local Y, and find an instructor to help you develop your exercise program. That's fine, but avoid people who want to turn you into a bodybuilder, have you take ephedra or other harmful stimulants, or act like drill sergeants. Your goal is to get fit, lose weight, and have fun—not to suffer.

Supplements That Can Help

To lessen the stress on your cardiovascular system as you exercise, consider using the following supplements. These can all be taken together daily.

- Coenzyme Q10: 100–300 mg
- L-carnitine: 500–1500 mg
- Ginkgo biloba: 100–200 mg
- Calcium and magnesium from citrate: 1,000–1,500 mg

THE BEST FROM THE EAST: YOGA, TAI CHI, QI GONG

"If we can't feel as though we're fundamentally well, I don't think we can become well." These words, spoken by Genia Pauli Hadden, co-creator of the video *Yoga for Round Bodies*, perhaps best expresses the benefits of yoga for people of size, including those who are starting on a weight-loss program.

Yoga is a no-impact exercise that can create a sense of well-being in practitioners by helping them embrace their body as it is—something that can be a real struggle for overweight people in our thinness-obsessed society. The better you feel about yourself, the easier it is to take positive steps for self-care, including weight loss. It's been shown that diabetics who practice yoga actually can become less insulin-dependent. In addition, yoga can decrease the frequency of asthma attacks and help combat depression, anxiety, and panic. It is especially helpful in reducing stress. Stretching, strengthening, breathing, and meditation are all tension-releasing techniques incorporated into this discipline. The postures can be modified for the size and shape of the practitioner to keep the person comfortable if any movement feels too strenuous. Yoga enthusiasts stress the idea of "being comfortable in the now."

Yoga is very "user friendly." While it is best to start taking classes with a certified yoga teacher, little training is required to learn the basics. You can soon practice by yourself at home with a videotape, a book, or from memory.

Another form of exercise that uses many of the techniques and ideas of yoga is qi gong. Tai chi, which is more familiar to Westerners, is one of the many forms of qi gong. The principle behind these exercises is that they cultivate one's internal energy, so that health and appearance improve. With consistent practice you'll also reap the benefits of enhanced respiration, circulation, and metabolism.

Dr. Roger Jahnke, author of *The Healer Within: The Four Essential Self-Care Methods for Creating Optimal Health,* describes qi gong as a "moving meditation." This low-impact exercise combines three processes—physical movement and posture of the body, moderating the breath, and meditation—to remove as much tension as possible. Jahnke says that the most important aspect of practicing effective qi gong is to "sustain clarity of mind, freedom from thoughts about things, and the 'listing process.'" He explains that it's natural for people to make lists and think things through, but that, while practicing qi gong, all of that is suspended as the mind is cleared. The result is a powerful internal healing resource.

B. K. Frantzis, one of the world's leading authorities on the subject of qi gong, credits the exercise with healing his back after it was broken in a car accident, enabling him to walk again and not be dependent on a wheelchair. He explains that while Western medicine focuses mainly on what has gone wrong when someone falls ill, Eastern medicine considers a person to be basically healthy and well balanced. The Eastern view holds that disease is simply something that disturbs this balance. As an example of this philosophy, Frantzis cites the case of the classic Chinese doctor who was paid on a monthly basis for his services; if one of his patients fell ill, the doctor would give the money back for the duration of the illness.

Using the balancing powers of qi gong can be an effective method of maintaining a healthy being, warding off illness by oxygenating the body, and getting the lymphatic system flowing better. As with yoga, qi gong requires no equipment and can be practiced by individuals at every level of fitness, almost anywhere. And it should be noted that all of these Eastern disciplines are holistic in that they emphasize the importance of a good diet in conjunction with exercise.

Breathing Exercises

One of the most important things we can do to improve our physical and mental well-being is to breathe properly. Breathing coach Pam Grout, author of *Jump Start Your Metabolism: How to Lose Weight by Changing the Way You Breathe,* estimates that as many as 90 percent of us do not breathe correctly, and adds that once we learn how, we can lose weight effortlessly, since breathing properly speeds up the metabolism. "I ended up losing ten pounds just by doing breathing exercises to get more energy," she states, citing the fact that a faster metabolism means calories are burned more quickly. "It's like a charcoal grill. If it's not going very well you blow on it. Then it lights up and becomes this powerful fuel." Oxygen potentiates the fuel in our bodies, and with proper breathing we digest food better and burn calories more rapidly, even when we're not exercising. And not only do we lose weight with better breathing—we are better able to keep it off.

The average person takes shallow breaths high in the chest, which does little to supply sufficient oxygen to blood vessels. What we should do, rather, is breathe slowly and deeply from the diaphragm, a dome-shape muscle between the chest and stomach cavity, as this opens up more air passages and provides instant relaxation. Additionally, breathing fully helps to normalize pH (the acid/base balance) so that we can digest foods and eliminate wastes properly. Shallow breathing, by contrast, creates an acidic environment that hinders digestive processes.

To increase breathing awareness, place on hand on your chest and the other on your abdomen. While taking normal breaths, notice which hand goes higher—usually it's the one on the chest. Then consciously focus on breathing from the diaphragm so that the stomach lifts higher instead.

Nose breathing is more beneficial than taking breaths through the mouth. One advantage is that it gets oxygen lower into the lungs, which then stimulates feel-good endorphins. Remember this when jogging, and you will be less likely to find yourself gasping for breath and more apt to find the exercise really fun. Conversely, when you breathe shallowly while exercising, your inner talk is more likely to be "When will this be over already? I don't want to do this. I'd better quit." Start using deep, slow breathing and see how much better you begin to feel instantaneously.

In yoga, there are many easy-to-learn breathing, or *pranayama*, techniques. One, the alternate breathing technique, has you inhaling using only one nostril and exhaling out the other, then inhaling with the second nostril and breathing out the original one. Several repetitions of this technique will unblock clogged nostrils (one is usually more clogged than the other), so that the air flow is evenly distributed on both sides. According to yogic philosophy, when the air flows evenly into and out of both nostrils, equilibrium is restored between the body's metabolic and catabolic processes, the mind becomes more relaxed and focused, and the body becomes purified so that illness can dissipate.

Exercise is another good way to get ourselves breathing more fully. This gets the body moving and helps to reinforce proper breathing technique. It is important, however, to exercise in environments with clean air to avoid taking in more toxins than you are expelling. It's not a good idea, for example, to walk in an area filled with car or industrial fumes.

Since breathing can be equated with being alive, the more fully we breathe the more vital we become. Effective breathing is essential to good health because our cells crave oxygen twenty-four hours a day, yet most of us breathe at only one-third of our capacity. (Imagine how you would function on one-third the amount of sleep or food you require!) Learn to breathe properly and you will increase your energy level; improve your physical, emotional, and mental states; and increase your metabolism while decreasing your appetite.

Charm School Revisited (Why Posture Matters)

When your mother insisted that you stand up straight, she was doing more than just improving your appearance. Good posture is an important aspect of maintaining a healthy, well-functioning body. Sitting and standing straight allows you to breathe properly—slowly and deeply from your diaphragm. As we've just seen, the benefits of proper breathing range from relaxation to dispelling toxins from your body to increasing your metabolism.

Good posture also can prevent many common lower back problems. These problems stem from the lack of muscle to cushion and support the spine and are compounded by the organs succumbing to gravity and moving downward from their original positions. The result can be added pressure and weight on the lower vertebrae. Maintaining a taut stomach actually keeps you from slouching, therefore maintaining a healthy and alert posture. Now that you've learned how to incorporate exercise into your weight-loss program, let's take a look at some other, alternative methods that can help you in your quest to slim down.

Chapter 12

Alternative Approaches to Weight Loss

As we've discussed, reshaping your diet to include healthful, energy-rich foods and developing a personal exercise program are at the heart of any successful weight-loss effort. But they are not the only things that will help you slim down with lasting results. Many cultures around the world use what most of us would consider alternative methods to assist the body in losing weight. To that end, this chapter presents various lesser-known modalities that can assist you in eliminating those extra pounds. Although these methods are not for everyone—and I believe that changing your diet and starting to exercise are the critical first steps—they can be beneficial if you have tried the other methods in this book and are still struggling to keep the pounds off.

COLON CLEANSING

Sometimes overeating occurs when the body sends out hunger signals because it is not receiving the nutrients it needs, a situation that can be caused by a toxic backup of waste in the intestinal tract. Accumulations here can trap the nutrients we consume and keep them from being fully absorbed by the rest of the body.

The colon, also known as the large intestine, is a large, tubelike structure at the end of the gastrointestinal tract. The small intestine feeds food particles into the colon, where the final stages of digestion and assimilation take place and wastes are eliminated from the system. After years of eating things that are difficult to digest—such as processed foods devoid of fiber, canned foods, carbonated drinks, salt, sugar, coffee, cheese, pasteurized milk—layers of mucus develop on the lining of the colon. The body develops this thick, rubbery lining to protect the sensitive colon walls, but the mucus also can act as a safe haven for parasites, yeasts, fungi, and other toxic creatures that can then grow uninhibited. Over time, the multiple poisons produced by these harmful parasites and bacteria will overload the liver and eventually weaken the body's other systems.

These layers also trap vital nutrients and can cause severe constipation. As a result, partially decomposed wastes create a sluggish colon, further limiting proper elimination and resulting in the toxic buildup of even more wastes. Further damage is done when waste matter, unable to pass through the walls of the colon, becomes reabsorbed into the body, poisoning the blood. These accumulated wastes not only add weight to the body but are a leading cause of degenerative disease, particularly cancer of the colon.

Much grief could be avoided if more people were to heed the early warning signs of colon toxemia instead of ignoring symptoms or masking them with medicines. These early indications may include—in addition to constipation—abdominal discomfort, weight gain, belching, flatulence, headaches, insomnia, and fatigue, to name only some of the physical symptoms, as well as such emotional manifestations as depression and irritability. Many of these symptoms are fairly easy to live with, and as a result, the problem can go undiagnosed for years. We get used to them, and because so many others experience the same states of suboptimal health, we come to think of them as natural. What we should wake up to is the fact that, unless addressed, these small warnings eventually may erupt into serious problems.

Colon cleansing is an effective, safe way to restore intestinal health and allow nutrients to be absorbed easily into the body. This method of detoxifying the body can be an important step toward weight loss and renewed health. Colon therapy is administered by a therapist who thoroughly washes the large intestines by irrigating the colon with water. This gentle method removes what is essentially toxic waste in a safe and comfortable manner. During the treatment, healing herbs, such as white oak bark and slippery elm bark, may be infused into the colon to lubricate and soothe irritated areas. These herbs also can be taken afterward as teas.

If you feel that this is an appropriate treatment for you, seek out a certified colon therapist who will take special precautions, using purified water and disposable equipment. For greater comfort and better results, the therapist also should be trained to massage the stomach.

Another intestinal cleansing approach relies on beverages. A great colon-cleansing tonic can be made using psyllium husk, ground flaxseed or chia seed, and liquid bentonite clay, which helps to trap and bind the toxins being released, preventing their reabsorption into the bloodstream. It acts as a laxative and should be prepared in the following proportions:

1 teaspoon psyllium husk, ground flaxseed, or ground chia seed

1 teaspoon liquid bentonite clay

1½ cups distilled water

Drink this preparation once a week for one to two months. Remember also to eat a fiber-rich diet and to drink eight to ten glasses of water a day to further help break down mucus on the colon walls.

Colon therapy will aid in achieving a regular elimination process of the bowels. Not only will this help with weight loss, but many people report alleviation of other unhealthy conditions, including breathing difficulties, irritability and stress, chronic fatigue, arthritis, and tumors. Advocates of colon therapy say that, along with the old debris, a lot of emotional baggage is unpacked as well, resulting in a feeling of lightness and a sense of joy.

SAUNAS

As we discussed in chapter seven, the skin is another important elimina-
tory organ that gets rid of a significant portion of the toxins in our bodies. Perspiration through exercise is a terrific way to eliminate harmful
chemicals through the skin as well as to lose weight. As discussed in
Chapter 7, another way to release toxins through the skin is in a steam
sauna. If you are pregnant, or suffer from high blood pressure, diabetes,
or other chronic health conditions, be sure to consult with a health professional before using this method.

Saunas, or steam rooms, are a centuries-old tradition from Finland.
Hundreds of thousands of these structures dot the Finnish landscape
and no doubt contribute to the robust health and vitality of the country's population. The standard sauna is composed of a small wooden
structure with several benches for resting. Water is thrown over hot
rocks heated in the sauna and as a result, steam fills the room. Sauna
temperatures can go up steeply, and beginners are advised to start with
moderate heat levels. After taking a sauna, people should wash themselves in warm water and relax a long while at room temperature until
their pores close and their body temperatures return to normal. Many
Americans make the mistake of cooling themselves off too rapidly with
a cold shower, which can cause undue stress on the heart and circulatory system.

The steam sauna is extremely beneficial because of its ability to induce a fever. Although Western medicine views fever as a symptom to be
suppressed and eliminated, this is actually a miconception. Fever is the
body's way of combating illness and preventing disease by inhibiting
the growth of pathogens through a rise in internal temperature; it also
eliminates toxins. Inducing a sauna-generated body temperature increase has those same effects, and sweating also helps to speed up metabolic processes.

When taking a sauna, be sure to drink plenty of water and not to eat
for at least an hour beforehand. It's a good idea to wrap your head in a
cool towel to prevent light-headedness. After the sauna (twelve to

twenty minutes is long enough), cover yourself with a large bath towel as you allow your body to cool down naturally.

If you don't have access to a sauna, you can substitute a hot steam bath. This is simply a hot tub with added mineral-rich Epsom salts that will relax your body. To create a wonderfully enjoyable and relaxing bath, add one quart Epsom salts to comfortably hot waist-high water and relax in the bath for fifteen minutes. Heat causes your pores to open, so this is a wonderful way to clean the skin and clear the head.

LYMPHATIC THERAPY

The lymphatic system acts as one of the body's waste removal systems. Cells are constantly dying and creating waste, and a healthy lymphatic system carries this waste away, detoxifying the body. Stagnant lymph (the clear fluid that circulates through this system) can trap nutrients, the same way a blocked colon can, and keep them from reaching the rest of the body. This can generate hunger signals that result in overeating. For more energy, which is vital when starting an exercise program, and for a more effective immune system, lymphatic therapy is an easy and highly recommended method of detoxifying the body and jump-starting your metabolism.

One simple way of moving lymph is by breathing deeply. To get the lymph moving, breathe through the nose until the lungs are fully inflated, hold the air in for just a second, and then push the breath out through your mouth. Repeating this three times helps the lymph to carry waste away from the cells. Qi gong, yoga (see Chapter 11), and other techniques that concentrate on breathing and movement are also good ways to restore health to a sluggish lymphatic system. Bouncing lightly on a small trampoline, also known as a rebounder, while breathing deeply can move the lymph even more.

Another way to stimulate the lymphatic system is by dry skin brushing. Taking a natural-bristle brush and stroking the skin in the direction of the heart will help to move and clear out toxins embedded in the lymph system. This also will help to exfoliate dead skin cells and reveal fresh new skin.

A professional masseur or masseuse trained in the manual lymphatic drainage technique can be of help, too. In this type of massage, a mechanical device is used to help break larger molecules in the lymph system into smaller ones, which allows for easier elimination.

HYPNOSIS AND SELF-HYPNOSIS

Many people who try unsuccessfully to lose weight think they are unable to do so because of a lack of willpower. However, the problem actually may be unacknowledged negative emotions about themselves and their bodies that hinder their motivation and prevent them from sticking with a weight-loss program. Hypnosis is a highly effective, simple method of uncovering these emotions and helping people change the behavior patterns that cause them to remain overweight. Hypnotherapy works by tapping into the subconscious mind and instilling positive, productive thoughts, which can help to quiet anxieties, boost energy levels, and overcome eating addictions.

Hypnosis works best when the person can visit a hypnotherapist twice a week so that the positive suggestions can be regularly reconfirmed until they are a part of the person's subconscious thought processes. Hypnosis aims to alter the mind's—and thus the body's—automatic responses to situations, therefore enabling the person to change negative behavior permanently. Often the sessions will be recorded so the individual can take home a tape to listen to at night or in the early morning.

Anxiety and loneliness, two problems commonly associated with chronic overeating, can be helped greatly through hypnosis. In other instances, people overeat to suppress a fear stemming from a childhood trauma, a subconscious "method of protection" that can cause obesity. Another common situation is when controlling food intake by overeating becomes a way of making up for a lack of control in other areas of life. Hypnosis can be used to change these destructive thought-behavior links and to implement more positive ones. For instance, through hypnotherapy a patient can learn to have control over his or her food intake by making eating choices rather than by overconsumption.

During hypnosis, a patient is in a very peaceful state called the theta altered state, or a trance. This is induced, in most cases, by listening to a subliminal tape while relaxing. It is in this state that changes can be suggested and implemented. Sessions generally last for thirty-five to forty-five minutes and are much like meditation, only more directed. Suggestions are intended to stay with the patient throughout the day. If the process is successful, it will result in a permanent reversal of the negative and unproductive thought patterns that keep the person from living a healthy life.

Self-hypnosis is also an effective technique, and it's one that can be easily learned and done on a daily basis. You begin by entering a deeply relaxed state and clearing your head of all feelings and situations that cause stress and a negative self-image. In this meditative state, simply imagine a favorite place, whether it's a vacation spot, a room in your house, or a mountain retreat. Once "there," visualize the details of the area, and imagine your ideal image of yourself, at the weight and level of fitness that you are striving for. Then move this ideal image of yourself into different areas of your life—your workplace, your home, a social gathering—to envision yourself as this ideal in an ordinary, everyday setting. This type of meditation is a positive way to encourage yourself to remain with your healthy lifestyle program throughout the day.

There are many other alternative therapies that, when combined with an exercise, detoxification, and nutritious eating program, can aid you in losing weight and optimizing health.

ACUPUNCTURE

Acupuncture is an ancient Asian modality that many modern people use to increase their metabolism, reduce appetite, and lower stress. It works by stimulating the nervous system with thin steel needles; however, contrary to what you might expect, this is not a painful procedure but one that produces relaxation. Acupuncture has been used for a wide variety of medical applications, ranging from surgical anesthesia to the treatment of backache, headache, and infertility. Recent physiological research ties acupuncture's results to the body's releasing of endorphins, or natural painkillers. Patients who have undergone this therapy frequently report feeling naturally refreshed and energized as a result.

Chinese medicine views overeating as related to various systemic imbalances that can be remedied through acupuncture. Problems with appetite, according to this view, may stem from the spleen or stomach, or even from the heart or lung. Usually an acupuncturist will stimulate reflex points on the ear related to these systems. For example, to reduce appetite, a small area behind the ear corresponding to the stomach can be pinpointed. Stimulating this point is said to boost metabolism and keep energy constant throughout the day. The idea is to keep the person from feeling sluggish and thus prevent overeating in an attempt to feel more energized.

Acupuncture is especially effective when it's combined with other therapies, such as herbal remedies, exercise, and juicing. When it's used as an integral part of a health and weight-loss protocol, weight management is more effective and lasts longer.

AROMATHERAPY

If our mood affects our eating behavior, then one of our weight-loss strategies should be to coax ourselves into the kind of mood in which we're less likely to turn to food. Because our sense of smell has an immediate impact upon the way we feel, we might want to consider aromatherapy. Dr. Alan Hirsh, author of *Scentsational Weight Loss, a New, Easy, Natural Way to Control Your Appetite*, explains that smells have a very strong impact on our moods and behavior, because the olfactory lobe, the part of the brain that interprets smell, is directly connected to the limbic brain, or the brain's emotional center. We are all familiar with the ability of certain smells to evoke powerful memories. If we associate certain smells with comfort and security as children—such as the scent of our mother's favorite perfume or the hickory smell of our grandfather's pipe—these smells will continue to evoke these positive feelings for the rest of our lives. Similarly, certain specific aromas, such as lavender, eucalyptus, and rose, act on our limbic system to put us in a relaxed state in which we are less likely to overeat.

Aromatherapy also can help in a more direct way, by suppressing the appetite. We may not realize it but 90 percent of what we call taste is actually smell. If you hold your nose, you will not be able to fully taste what you are eating. Try this trick and you'll soon discover that vanilla and chocolate ice cream taste just about the same and that a fresh carrot or apple tastes like chalk. The brain's olfactory lobe is closely connected to the hypothalamus, which is the part of the brain that tells us when we are sated and should stop eating. Thus, by smelling a particular food or aroma, we can fool the hypothalamus into thinking that we have already eaten; therefore, our bodies will crave less. This is one more reason we should eat slowly, paying attention to the taste and smell of our food. By hurrying through our meals, we cheat ourselves of the aromatic component of the experience and thus don't trigger this important response.

Lemon, orange, lime, tangerine, grapefruit, and onion are some of the fragrances recommended by aromatherapists to control appetite. You can buy these scents in the form of essential oils and apply them to your wrists, smelling them throughout the day. Aromatherapy practitioners also tell us that sluggish digestion may be helped by the aromas of cinnamon, bergamot, fennel, peppermint, rosemary, or sage, and a nervous digestion may be soothed with caraway, anise seed, coriander, or orange blossom. Stress-reducing aromatherapy aids include rose, lavender, chamomile, and sage.

HYDROTHERAPY

Hydrotherapy, or water therapy, first gained popularity in nineteenth-century European spas and was once considered a treatment of choice by most naturopathic physicians. Although the technique has fallen out of vogue, it is still a helpful tool practiced by some holistic physicians. Many spas offer this treatment, which generally costs about $50.

Naturopathic physician Peter Bennett, founder of the British Columbian Halios Clinic and author of *Seven Day Detox Miracle*, explains that hydrotherapy works by stimulating reflex points on the body with streams of water of alternating temperatures. (Hot and cold packs are sometimes used instead.) As these exterior reflex point are said to correspond to inner organs, activating certain parts of the skin is intended to improve the circulation to the corresponding organs. By stimulating the digestive organs through hydrotherapy, the processes of nutrient absorption and total-body detoxification are aided. Improved circulation also will improve the liver's ability to handle toxins.

PRESSURE POINT THERAPY

Pressure point therapy, also called acupressure, is a practice similar to acupuncture in that it works on the nervous system and the body's energy meridians. But instead of needles to stimulate reflex points, light pressure is applied with the fingers. This modality is easy to learn and can be applied alone or with the help of a partner to release stress that keeps us from functioning at our best.

Pressure point therapy can be an effective aid to weight loss, by working to improve the flow of energy into the digestive tract. For example, you can press lightly on one of two small indentations at the back of the neck, located behind a bump known as the mastoid near both ears. These cavities contain pressure points that are related to the digestive tract. If you press these areas and find one to be tender, your body is telling you that your digestive tract is irritated. Applying pressure to this spot for fifteen to thirty seconds will release the knot in the muscle crimped around the nerve in that irritated area. The nerve is the vagus, the longest nerve in the body, which extends from the back of the ear all the way down to the digestive tract. Once the vagus nerve is relieved of the pressure from the stressed muscle, it can again relax and receive information on digestion from the brain and convey that information to your digestive tract. As a result, you are likely to start eating less because your system will absorb nutrients more efficiently and not signal starvation.

Pressure point therapy expert and author D. Michael Pinkus recommends one therapeutic technique called the wheel. You can try this simple technique while lying in bed before getting up in the morning or before going to sleep. To begin, place your fingers over the top part of the stomach just below your breast bone—this is what is known as the 12 o'clock position. Gently push in for a few seconds and release. Moving left and slightly downward to the one o'clock position, do the same. At two o'clock, just under the left rib cage, once again push in and release. Repeat this gentle pushing all the way around the wheel two to three times. Sometimes you will hit a tender spot that relates to some aggravated area of the intestines. The wheel exercise releases toxins that have accumulated in different parts of the intestines that correspond to where you've placed your fingers. Releasing these toxins helps with elimination and appetite control, which in turn assists in weight loss. The wheel also works as a resistance exercise to firm up stomach muscles.

ZEN PRACTICE

Techniques that aid in losing weight require that you be willing to work *with* your body and not against it. Doing this means being very conscious of the foods that you eat. But Dr. Ronna Kabatznick, a weight management specialist who worked as a psychological consultant at Weight Watchers for nine years, asserts that we have to go beyond this and begin to understand our food in a different way. She calls this type of awareness the Zen of eating, and cites the example of religious fasting and how effortless it seems for people to fast when the food represents something more than just a sandwich, a cookie, or a piece of cake.

Zen is an ancient spiritual practice that encourages participants to become consciously focused on everything they do and think. Most of us go through the day with our minds jumping from topic to topic, from daydreams to anxieties, to what we're going to do on the weekend, to why we weren't invited to a friend's party. When we begin to practice Zen meditation, we learn to quiet this constant mind chatter, maintain a sense of focus, and keep our goals firmly in our mind's eye. This practice can be applied to just about anything, and it works particularly well for dietary goals. You can learn to look at a healthful food and focus on how

330 · *Gary Null's Ultimate Lifetime Diet*

important it is to your body, what it can do for your weight-loss goals, and how healing it is. When people have respect for food, they also will develop a respect for what it can do to their bodies. Similarly, when people are given an opportunity to break their diet with unhealthful foods, Zen will remind them that they do not want to do anything that will dishonor the body, mind, or spirit. Zen teaches people to exclude that which does not honor the body and to seek out foods that do. Once people achieve that kind of consciousness in their eating habits, they will begin to make better and healthier decisions.

A good exercise to try when looking to cultivate this new type of relationship with food is to ask yourself: If you are what you eat, would you rather be a Twinkie, a hot dog, or a fresh, healthy organic tomato? If you were to become what you eat, what would happen to you if you subsisted on a junk-food diet and what would happen if you subsisted on a vegetarian one? Visualize the changes that take place within your body as you ingest each different type of food.

Kabatznick considers this awareness to be one of the keys to ending emotional nourishment, which is very often the cause of overweight conditions and obesity. She stresses that we must seek true fulfillment from other sources, such as our jobs, our relationships, intellectual pursuits, or religion, and not the false kind of fulfillment we often try to gain from food. She suggests saving the money that we might otherwise spend on extra foods, desserts, or junk foods and donating it to an organization that feeds the hungry. The satisfaction we gain can help to keep us from overeating in an attempt to fill our emotional emptiness.

OTHER RESOURCES

Numerous spas and clinics offer many of the protocols described in this book and can assist you in your weight-loss program. One of the best holistic weight-loss clinics in the country is run by Dr. Ernie Baumstein in Fort Lauderdale, Florida. His clinic offers a wonderful program for losing weight, detoxifying, reducing stress, overcoming illness, and restoring body/mind happiness. For information, call 1-800-642-2012.

Part 3

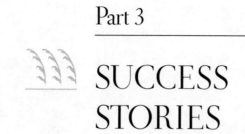

SUCCESS STORIES

Chapter 13

What We Can Learn from "Losers"

In this chapter we're going to look at the stories of people who have been in my weight-loss and detox support groups. These groups meet regularly over a period of months to be guided in the implementation of a program that is basically the same as the one outlined in this book. As you'll be reading in the accounts of these "successful losers," many have had impressive results, not just in terms of weight loss but in overall health, energy level, and outlook on life.

You'll also see that, besides following the physical steps that lead to maximal health, many of these people have integrated diet and exercise with a process of looking within and deciding what was truly important to them and what attitudes and activities they could jettison. You could call this a kind of mental and emotional detox, and it's just as vital to good health and weight loss as anything physical you can do. We'll be talking more about this later in Chapter 15.

My intent here is not to get every reader to sign up for a health support group. Yes, these groups are great for participants in that they get reinforcing feedback from others who have the same concerns. And they're great for me because I get to use them as study groups to see what works and what doesn't. But you don't have to be in any organized group to lose weight and gain energy; you can do it all on your own. I've included these group participants' stories because they're available to me and also because I know a lot of these people personally and know that what they're saying is true. I've actually seen the pounds disappear from their bodies, and I've seen the enthusiasm reflected in their faces.

So here's my hope for what you get out of this chapter, which you can read in its entirety for a big jolt of good news or peruse at your leisure:

- The knowledge that it *is* possible to lose weight and improve other aspects of your health dramatically, because many people have done so
- An insight into how people did it
- Inspiration to do it yourself

Enjoy these success stories.

Joyce ✦ *"I now share clothes with my seventeen-year-old daughter."*

At the beginning of the program, I had a multitude of physical ailments. During the spring and fall, I would experience horrible allergy symptoms, including runny, itchy eyes, running nose, head congestion, wheezing, and headaches. The headaches occurred at least once a week throughout the year. My periods were heavy and painful with premenstrual syndrome (PMS) beginning at least a week in advance. I am 5 feet 5 inches tall and I weighed 165 pounds. The extra weight made me look and feel older than I actually was. It also made me feel self-conscious and took its toll on my self-confidence. In the winter my hands would crack and split. It felt like I had paper cuts all over my hands, and it was very painful.

Almost immediately after starting the program I began to see and feel improvements in my health. My weekly headaches are completely gone. I haven't had any allergy symptoms at all! My periods are much lighter and not as painful. Now the only PMS symptom I have is sore and tender breasts. I am still working to alleviate this problem, and it is my goal to feel great on the first day of my period, as if it were any other day. Without even trying or focusing on my weight, I had lost twenty-five pounds by the fourth month in the program. I look and feel younger and I now share clothes with my seventeen-year-old daughter. Because I feel so good about the changes in my physical health and my looks, my self-confidence has grown tremendously! Everywhere I go I receive compliments and I'm told that my face and skin are radiant. For the first time in my adult life, my skin is soft, and this past winter my hands didn't crack and split. I'm still a work-in-progress, but my improvements have been phenomenal!

Donna ✦ *"For the first time in my life, my nutritional health is a priority."*

I had my doubts whether I would be able to stick to this program, but with a powerful tenacity, I have lost approximately twenty pounds. I feel absolutely wonderful. As I walk, my whole body feels lighter. It is much easier for me to bend, and I can now cross my legs! For the first time in my life, my nutritional health is a priority. I care what I put into my body. I actually crave healthy foods now.

As to physical differences and improvements, my skin is much softer, my enlarged facial pores have shrunk, and my hair is soft and shiny. I no longer experience intense mood changes, angry outbursts, or crying spells due to PMS.

My endurance has increased tremendously. I can now bike seventeen miles easily and go up hill after hill, and I power walk three to four miles. My health and the good feeling I get from exercise are too important to now put on the back burner.

The introspective questions we talk about in the groups have given me a chance to take the time to just think privately and honestly about my lifestyle, my philosophy of life, my actions and reactions toward situations, my successes and failures. I have had a lot of "aha" moments. I thank you for them.

Dorothy ✦ *"I will not allow myself to become the victim of someone else's dysfunction."*

During the program I have lost fifty pounds and many inches. Not only has the size of my clothing been reduced five sizes, my shoe size and bra size have also been reduced. My skin tone and elasticity has improved, and my energy level has increased. I have had my hair cut several times, and during the past month it has not only grown but has become thicker.

Through the program, I have increased my self-esteem and learned how to handle stress and negativity. I set aside personal time for meditation, reading, and reflection. This I find very rewarding and helpful not only at the end of the day, but any time feelings of stress or negativity try to creep into my thoughts. I have begun to set minigoals to help me focus on the things I want to do in my life.

I have [begun] focusing on solutions, not the problem, and focusing on my needs. I have created personal affirmations in the present tense, which I affirm throughout the day. I use the practice of self-acceptance to look at my thoughts, feelings, actions, and emotions without denial. I focus on what I want to have, where I want to go, and on having positive and confident expectations as to what I want to do. I have followed the steps for creative problem solving, using the superconscious mind to help me. I have learned to recognize the benefits of change—again to stay focused on what I want to do, not on the negative factors brought on by the change. I practice living purposefully. And I have begun to outline and define goals to create the mission statement of my life, setting a higher level of standards than before.

I have recognized that my personal strengths are far greater than I ever realized. I know that I am a work-in-progress, and I have felt and am dealing with the emotions of this change. I am processing them and I am able to forgive, learn the lesson, and leave the garbage behind. I will not allow myself to be the victim of someone else's dysfunction.

Lorna ✦ *"Yes you can!"*

Before I started the weight loss study group, I weighed 245 pounds and I was miserable. I felt physically handicapped, and I was an emotional wreck because I couldn't understand why I couldn't commit myself to working out, eating healthfully, and losing weight. The first very big lesson: There are no excuses! The second: Yes you can!

Eight months later I weigh around 196 pounds. Close to 50 pounds of fat is gone. My body is stronger. My heart is stronger. My blood pressure is down. I no longer suffer from heartburn. My head is clearer. I've not had the chronic bronchitis that I suffered with since 1994. I haven't had any colds, and there is a recognizable reduction of mucus in my nasal passages.

The best part of this is that I feel in control of my life. I choose to go to the gym. I choose to make my body stronger. I choose good foods. I recognize that my actions have a consequence. I had a glass of champagne on my birthday—and had a headache for the next six hours. It's no longer worth it to me to suffer with headaches; I no longer drink champagne.

I've become more aware of my old thinking patterns and how I can make decisions or simply run my life based on wrong assumptions. I now question why I have certain beliefs. This program has been about making a commitment to myself. Through this commitment and discipline I've achieved something very important—self-esteem, self-reliance, and the notion that I'm the hero in my life. I'm becoming clearer and clearer about how I live my life, and I see how the old ways don't work.

I've taken responsibility. A year ago that responsibility was cast to the wind. I've reclaimed my life, and I rest in the fact that my self-exploration will continue and my perspective on life will only continue to improve.

Terry ✦ *"I had to look deep inside myself."*

I started gaining weight during and after my first pregnancy, but I did little or no exercise. And when I wanted to lose weight I would take diet pills or not eat at all. When I did eat I ate until I couldn't breathe. It was a never-ending process of gaining and losing weight. I did lose weight on [a popular commercial weight-reduction and monitoring program], but now I know what I was putting in my body wasn't really helping at all.

When I started this [health support group] program, my blood pressure was being regulated by pills and my heart rate was too! I did not exercise on a regular basis, and I needed something almost every night to help me sleep. I drank caffeinated coffee with milk and sugar all day and night and did not take one vitamin. I didn't think that I had enough discipline to start the program, and it scared me to death when I found out that I had to look deep inside myself to resolve issues that I had kept hidden for a long time. I didn't know how to take care of myself.

After I started juicing, I experienced such a surge of energy that I wanted more. The better I felt, the more committed I became. It was a little harder to change my way of eating, but once I felt how good it was to leave a table being able to move, I've been more creative with the foods that I eat. Now I want to exercise more and more. I can sleep now without medication and wake up feeling like I slept. My doctor has decreased my blood pressure medication! This proved to me that I was in control of my life all along but was never brave enough.

I've lost ten pounds and I've lost inches; I'm no longer hiding myself in my clothes! I have more to go but now I know I can do it, and I have the confidence and the desire not to put anything in my mouth that will affect my health and well-being.

Megan ✦ *"I lost twenty-five pounds effortlessly."*

After I delivered my daughter, I nursed for a year and food never tasted better, so I ate and ate! I put on twenty-five pounds. I had very achy joints and leg pain and because of this I had extreme difficulty going up and down stairs. My feet were in such terrible shape that I had to wear orthotics. Overall I was miserable! Within four months of the program, I had lost twenty-five pounds effortlessly. I now get up and go, run up and down the stairs, and no longer wear orthotics, and my arthritis is gone. Now I am much more energized, I sleep more soundly, and my skin is very soft.

Olga ✦ *"I no longer run out of breath."*

I was always fatigued, overweight, and depressed—just not happy with myself. Often I was very cold, had headaches, stomachaches, and lower back pain. I now have energy. I have no more headaches or stomachaches, and in the process of following the program I have lost seventeen pounds. When I exercise I no longer run out of breath, and I have become more reliant on others instead of [feeling the need to do] everything myself.

Effie ✦ *"My body is lighter and tighter."*

Before I started this program I had sinus headaches periodically and exceptionally dry skin. I was always worried, uptight, and could not focus on doing one thing at a time.

With persistence I continued the program and my energy increased tremendously. I lost fifteen pounds. My body is much lighter and tighter, my skin much softer. I'm more relaxed, feel more sure of myself, and my anger has decreased tremendously.

I feel much better about myself physically, emotionally, and spiritually. I now am able to focus on one thing at a time and complete a task without worrying about the outcome.

Henry ✦ *"I started the program at about 400 pounds."*

I started the program at about 400 pounds. My knees, hands, and joints were always painful. I was unable to stand up or walk for more than a minute or two at the time. Since my blood pressure was high I was told I had to take medication. I had palpitations that would come and go. I am also a diabetic, having a blood glucose level of 150 to 200 and over.

The program has helped me lose fifty pounds. My knee pain only bothers me every now and then and isn't nearly as severe. My hands are also much better. It seems that the more water I drink, the better my joints are. I can move around much more easily even though I'm still heavy. My blood pressure is always normal even when I forget to take the medication. Now I must check my blood glucose to make sure it isn't too *low!* It's between 80 and 95 now. It's been normal despite the brown rice, legumes, veggies, and fruit as staples.

Reny ✦ *"The program has helped me take responsibility for my own life and thoughts."*

I used to drink eight cups of coffee a day, each with four teaspoons of sugar, and at least a gallon of soda a day, and eat two gallons of ice cream weekly. I could eat a whole pizza. I visited as many of the all-you-can-eat buffets as I could. I used to sleep twelve to fourteen hours a night and still felt very tired. Since following the program, I'm sleeping only four and a half to six and a half hours per night. My back pain has decreased greatly and my skin has cleared almost totally. I am now able to walk two to three miles daily.

I used to worry about everything and criticize myself for what I thought I had done wrong. I also blamed many people for my own self-righteousness. The program has helped me to stop blaming others I thought affected my life and instead take responsibility for my own life and thoughts. I am able to listen to people without forcing my opinions on them.

People smile at me more frequently than in the past. I think this is because I'm happier and it shows.

Marlene ✦ *"This is the what I used to weigh when I was nineteen years old!"*

My weight used to fluctuate up and down. I now maintain a weight of 110 pounds instead of 130. I found that I maintain the weight effortlessly by following the program. This is what I used to weigh when I was nineteen years old! It's wonderful. I require less sleep than before and wake up alert and energized for the day. I've gotten no colds or flu since I've been in the program. I had been going to a dermatologist before the study for acne and rosacea. The topical medication he prescribed for rosacea did not help. I also used to take Tylenol every four to six hours for the first forty-eight hours or more for menstrual pain.

Since following the program I no longer have acne and my rosacea has greatly improved. My hair is silkier and thicker and the number of gray hairs is becoming fewer and fewer. This is great! People often assume I am ten or more years younger than my age. I am also feeling younger. My menstrual pain has lessened very significantly, and I take no medication now whatsoever. I no longer have premenstrual puffiness and headaches like I used to. Emotionally I'm better able to deal with day-to-day stress and traumatic events. Overall, I feel more calm and positive than I did before the program.

Joan ✦ *"By the fourth month I lost twelve pounds."*

When I had the opportunity to get into [Dr. Null's] program, I made the decision to do it. By the fourth month I lost twelve pounds.

I drink five glasses of organic vegetable juices a day. My family and I eat organically now. I feel things are starting to go in the right direction. My big lesson is learning to take time for myself. Now I'm learning to get out in the sun and exercise. I am learning to have patience with myself. I do attribute the weight loss to the diet, the love I have for myself, and the pride I have in what I'm doing.

Thomas ✦ *"I was eating all I wanted and the weight was just rolling off."*

In 1994 my daughter graduated from college. During the ceremonies, she and I took a picture together. When I saw myself in the picture, I could not believe that it was me. I was fifty-two years old, 265 pounds, with puffy eyes and paunch belly. I looked terrible. . . . I resolved then that I would change. I didn't succeed. I kept procrastinating.

One day at work I received a note that was made up of words cut out of a newspaper. The note said that I should buy new suits because the ones that I had do not fit. They were too small. I bought larger suits. I lost a few pounds but I still held out for my comfort foods.

Then in early 1997 I heard about [the support groups that Gary was starting for people who did not have any particular condition but just wanted to get healthy]. It sounded good to me so I joined. I was still overweight at 255 pounds. My family has a history of heart disease and diabetes so I was afraid of that happening to me.

I started [in the group] and was surprised to find how easy it was to follow the program. The class was full, everyone was confident. Then Gary started to tell us what we had to do if we wanted to succeed in the program. Clean up the clutter in my life—use it, give it away, or throw it away.

Changing what I eat was hard enough, but to change the way I think and act was the most difficult thing of all. Everyone was supportive, but after a few weeks when some of the people dropped out of the class I became nervous.

My kids encouraged me by buying me a juice machine. My wife thought I was crazy to do all these things, but I continued. I started to get regular bowel movements once or twice a day.

I was taught how to power walk. That was great due to the low impact it had on my joints. I have had problems with my hip joints for a long time. They would click when I did exercises on my back. I also had varicose veins on my left leg due to a sports injury while in high school.

I learned to start cooking for myself. My family would look at the food and walk away. Then they started to taste it and helped themselves to it. I was glad about this. I was eating all I wanted and the weight was just rolling off.

I started to be less compliant to others and looked at my own needs. This was difficult for me to do since I wanted everyone to like me. Writing "forgiveness letters" helped a lot. I learned that to be happy I must be happy with myself. I must stay away from negative people and situations that will drain all of my positive energy. My body, mind, and spirit had to be focused on positive things in order for my life to turn around and change all those negative things in my life. I learned and listened and thought about what I wanted in my future. I had to learn to dream those dreams from my childhood all over again. I remembered and I acted. My life changed.

After the first six months of detoxing, I started the rebuilding process. I had lost twenty-five pounds in three months and felt great. I had much more energy, my skin was so much smoother, and people were asking me what I was doing. When I told them they listened with interest, but as with my own earlier efforts, giving up their comfort foods was impossible.

I continued my program. The second six months my hair looked darker and thicker. Some body moles that I had all my life started disappearing. My varicose veins shrank. I could work twelve to fourteen hours a day and still be full of energy.

I feel great and look great. I've lost forty pounds so far . . . The gift I was given is something that I pass along to whoever asks me. I feel so alive, so different. . . . positive thinking is contagious! Just remind yourself and others what you think is what you are. Think positive, be positive.

Monique ✦ *"The first four weeks of the program I lost fifteen pounds."*

During at least five years prior to joining the detox program, I had tried different types of diets, during which time I lost some weight and gained it back. It was a frustrating and at times stressful situation. I had some hesitation about joining the program for fear that the difficulties I might face would prevent me from completing it. But one day I took a look at myself in the mirror and told myself that never again do I ever want to look that fat. So I decided to join the program in January 1998 and make whatever sacrifice would be required to complete it and get positive results.

I had the pleasant surprise of discovering that the whole person was given attention in the process. Not only were nutritional aspects taken into account, but also the psychological, mental, spiritual, and social aspects of life were given attention. This program facilitated a total change in my attitude toward food. I used to have cravings for bagels and muffins. Now I don't even think about them.

One of the amazing things about the program is that I lost weight without making any effort. The first four weeks of the program I lost fifteen pounds, and I have not had any fluctuation in weight. Now I am in control of my weight. Last summer I had the great pleasure of wearing clothes that I had not been able to wear for the past three years. How can I ever go back to "business as usual" after such success?

Things have not been easy. I have been under a lot of pressure from friends and relatives, particularly when I am invited out for dinner at their home. The usual comment is "Going off the program once in a while is not going to make any difference." My best way of dealing with the pressure is just to tell them that I have invested too much into the program to go back to my past eating habits. And I mean that too.

Mudiwa ✦ *"Since beginning the program I have lost twenty pounds."*

At the beginning of the program, I had low energy level. I was beginning to top 170 pounds. I was addicted to sweets, chocolate, bread, eggs, and dairy. My eyes were blurry and I was constipated often. I also had serious outbreaks of eczema on my legs and arms. I also had a large cyst under my left arm. The eczema under my arms has healed and the discoloration is leaving. The cyst is gone.

In addition, for the first time in two years I have had my menses for a week. I am forty-nine and I thought I wouldn't have a menses ever again. The joy of it is I realize that I am detoxing at a very high rate. I am very proud of how my body is responding to the protocol. Since beginning the program I have lost twenty pounds.

I am very aware of myself now. If I begin to have fear or anger, or am self-critical, I can pull back from that behavior. I also used to gossip about people but now I am too busy to give away my energy for that kind of activity. I remind myself of my purpose and why it's important to stay with the program.

Jemma ✦ *"This has been an amazing trip, and it is still continuing."*

I was born chubby and all throughout my childhood I was teased. I remember this was a very difficult and self-conscious time for me. As a teenager, I just wanted to fit in. I explored nutrition and followed other programs, but the weight stayed with me. I went through a very rough divorce after eleven years of an abusive marriage. I put on more weight. This caused a deep sadness and depression in me. I joined one of Gary's groups but dropped out.

Six months later I joined another one of his groups. This time everything clicked. I lost seventy pounds. In the program I shared from my heart and my darkest soul. The program became easy as my energy increased. The weight just kept coming off, and I was not on a "diet." My sadness and depression has greatly diminished. I am off all medication.

I had candida, parasites, and aching knee joints. Now I am parasite-free and the candida is much better. The aching in my knee joints is pretty much gone. Overall, I am extremely healthy. I used to awaken several times a night. I needed eight to nine hours of sleep. Now I only require five and a half to six. I have made my health and my happiness a priority. I have learned not to fear being genuine with my feelings and with who I am. I am strong enough now to stand for what I believe in and still be compassionate.

This has been an amazing trip, and it is still continuing. One thing I've noticed and am amazed at is when I drive now, I do not get angry; I laugh at situations in which, before, I would have wanted to "kill" the other driver.

Louie ✦ *"I now look forward to every new day. . . ."*

Being on the program has changed every part of my life. [Initially I was] looking for help with depression and emphysema. I had been on many prescription drugs and had developed cataracts. Since I joined the program they've disappeared. An additional bonus was that I lost fifty pounds.

Through the program I learned to take full responsibility for everything that has happened to me. This awareness has helped me to make changes in my life and not think everyone and everything around me had to change. Being able to stay focused on positive thoughts, words, and actions has helped me remain happy and healthy. I also focus my attention on solutions and don't become overloaded with any problems. I now look forward to every new day. . . .

Marina ✦ *"I have more energy, so I am more active."*

I started gaining weight at forty-seven years old. When I joined I felt tired and had many medical complications. I started drinking juice and changed my way of eating. I walk three to five miles a day. I lost twenty-seven pounds in five months. I have more energy, so I am more active.

Jennifer ✦ *"Within three months . . . I lost twelve pounds and looked good in a bikini."*

Before I started the program I had no energy and I felt like I was getting old. Within three months of being on the program, I felt years younger and more energetic. I lost twelve pounds and looked good in a bikini. I exercised forty minutes three times a week and learned to power walk, which I do at least five days a week. . . I have also learned to be true to myself.

Santina ✦ *"In a short time, the positive domino effect was giving me great results. . . ."*

I never felt so focused on what I had to do yet so out of control. Exercise and eating right were never an issue until my father's death this past September 1998. As the holidays approached, I looked to food for comfort. As a result, I quickly gained ten pounds, was sick with the flu and unmotivated to exercise. Not only was my personal appearance out of control, but my professional life was in a lull. I was going down a path I didn't like. It was a negative domino effect. . . .

When I started [the detoxification program] in January of '99, I had the flu, a migraine, and fatigue. . . . Within three days of starting the program, I was better emotionally, physically, and spiritually. By the second week, I was running, walking, and doing step aerobics three to four times per week. I never thought I'd reach this level because of a sprained ankle that was healing. In a short time, the positive domino effect was giving me great results, encouraging me to continue the program. It was easy to stay committed to juicing and the dietary changes.

Thoughts and questions from Gary's talks went into my journal. This helped me shed ten pounds and the past self [and find] a new and vibrant self. To some, ten pounds may not seem like a great accomplishment. However, I am five feet tall with a petite frame, and ten pounds looks and feels like much more weight.

Presently I am in a growth, expansion, and awareness phase creatively, working on several projects in my profession. . . . I have learned to shed worry and anger. At this time, I am happy to focus my energy on deeper and more fulfilling issues.

Fred ✦ *"I buy almost all organic foods now, lots of different herbs and spices, nuts and greens."*

My problems started when I was very young. I was a twin. But my sister was stillborn because of an umbilical cord problem. I got all the nutrients and she didn't get any. My father blamed me. Later on when I was an overweight child my father would call me a glutton. "Even in the womb you were a glutton," he'd say. I believe this affected my behavior.

School was a disaster. I was just pushed through though I wasn't getting much real education. I was totally out of control by junior high school. I was asked not to come back, and just like that I was out of school.

Nobody wanted to hire me because of my size, though I did get a job in a movie with Robert DeNiro because of my size. I played JoJo the Whale. Other people called after that to offer me movie work, but I didn't want a job just because of my size and I never accepted any other offers.

I have tried any kind of diet you could name. I could never stick to it. I was six months away from death. I had congestive heart failure. I was retaining water, vomiting blood. I couldn't lie down any more at the end because of water crushing my lungs. A doctor in Manhattan wanted to cut out 75 percent of my stomach and remove part of my intestine, but I refused to do it. I wanted to try once more to lose the weight. He told me I was out of time. I had gone too far. I made a deal with him that if I came back to him showing weight gain on his scale, he could operate the very next week.

That was nine months ago. I was 175 pounds heavier then. The first fifteen days I juiced constantly. I would eat two meals a day as well. I eliminated carbonated soda and caffeine. I eventually eliminated dairy products, though occasionally I'll have a small amount of something I shouldn't. I buy almost all organic foods now, lots of different herbs and spices, nuts and greens.

Exercise is still very difficult. I have arthritis in my knees and back. I do walk one half hour to forty-five minutes each day. I try not to lose my temper anymore. I have gotten rid of a lot of friends who caused me stress.

I've lost 175 pounds . . . I've changed a lot. I feel much better. . . . I've got a much better outlook on life.

Hueston ✦ *"I have said good-bye to swollen ankles, restless nights, and poor eating habits."*

In my first three months on the program I lost 25 pounds. Since then I lost another 5 pounds. I now weigh in at a light and spry 208 pounds on my 6-foot, 5-inch frame.

I have a tremendous amount of energy and have never felt better in my life. I have said good-bye to swollen ankles, restless nights, and poor eating habits. I was a heavy meat, dairy, and sugar eater for over fifty years. I cut all of that out immediately after starting the weight-loss protocol.

Before beginning the program I had an infected big toe. My podiatrist said that even if the nail was removed, the toe would never be completely normal. Well, the infection is completely gone and the toe is perfect.

This is my first detox program. Health, happiness, and a renewed spirituality are now a way of life for me.

Karen ✦ *"Without trying I lost eleven pounds, and am still counting."*

I am a thirty-five-year-old woman. I became type 1 diabetic when I was ten. Shortly thereafter it became a constant struggle to control my weight. I would sometimes go on diets of 500 to 700 calories per day in order to lose the weight. I went through periods when I exercised six hours or more each day till I was so exhausted that I would collapse.

When I first joined the detox group I was overweight again. I then had all the major complications of diabetes, including poor circulation; nerve damage to my hands, feet, and calves; wounds and cuts that wouldn't heal; severe fungus under my nails; extremely high blood pressure, cholesterol, and blood sugar. I suffered from severe constipation, loss of some vision due to retinopathy, kidney disease, and an underactive thyroid, and I'd had a diabetic ministroke to my eye.

I found this program very easy to follow, especially since I had a fierce desire to get completely well. It's hard to find all the types of fruits and vegetables I needed for my juices where I live, so I found using green and red [nutrient supplement] powders very convenient. When I'm home I mix up my juices in a matter of minutes and I drink them throughout the day.

I've found a vegetarian diet very easy to follow. When I switched to organic food I found that everything tasted so much better, and I felt so much better after eating it too. I like to explore the health food stores to discover new things. I like that I'm putting only good things into my body, things that will help me to heal and stay healthy. I've learned better ways to exercise. I warm up first and I breathe properly. I get the proper amount of oxygen into my system and I don't get extremely fatigued.

Learning how to deal with stress was one of the most important things for me. . . . I used to feel that I had no real control over my life or my destiny. I no longer feel that way, and I'm actively planning a new life for myself. I'm planning to do things I never thought could be possible.

I've learned to look at the good and bad in life as a learning process rather than as luck and failures. I find I'm able to give more to people in a healthy way without losing myself in the process. I set up healthy boundaries. I have eliminated my anger toward other people and myself because I don't allow myself to try to give more than I really can or should.

I didn't actually enter the program to lose weight. I had much more serious issues to deal with. But without trying I lost eleven pounds, and am still counting. I'm starting to build healthy lean muscle and I feel alive again. . . . I'm even training to run in the New York City Marathon. . . .

Most of my diabetic complications have reversed themselves—just nine months after I was told by my doctors that all of my conditions would just continue to deteriorate.

Kevin ✦ *"I feel so much better about myself and have learned to trust in the whole process of life."*

I remember when I was ten years old I was not allowed to play football because I was too fat. That really devastated me because I really loved the game and all of my friends were on the team. I remember crying because I never had the self-control to stop eating long enough to lose weight.

In more recent years, I've pretty much resigned myself to the fact that I'll always be overweight. I have sometimes managed to lose some weight for short periods of time, but no matter what I did the weight always came back on.

Finally, for this year's New Year's resolution I decided to commit myself to getting rid of this large gut. So in January when I heard about Gary Null's detox protocol, I investigated to see if I could incorporate his program into my life.

I started juicing and taking the recommended supplements. I followed the dietary guidelines of eating organically and doing the breathing and meditation exercises. I became aware that good health is not only what you eat. It's also a state of mind that includes having a positive attitude, paying attention to your emotional needs, and developing an awareness of your own spirituality.

I have lost twenty pounds in the last four months. I no longer drink alcohol, smoke, or do drugs. I now have the resolve I need to stay on this path. I feel so much better about myself and have learned to trust in the whole process of life.

Ted ✦ *"It's worth it. It works. I feel really good!"*

I am sixty-six years old. I started to gain weight about twelve years ago at age fifty-four. I first began to be concerned in 1990 at age fifty-seven after three years of constant weight gain. I made some modifications in my diet and tried to control my food intake. I never made any progress in reducing the weight. I felt bad about not being in control of my own body. My clothes were too tight and I began to tire easily. I found I lacked enthusiasm for anything mildly athletic. I was not happy with myself at all! By late 1998 I was up to 210 pounds. I followed the detox program and four months later I weighed 189 pounds . . . down 21 pounds.

I made significant changes in my lifestyle. I am avoiding involvement with "toxic," negative people. I am spending more time on myself and with those who are really important to me. I am seeking a better understanding of my place in society and am deciding how I want to spend the rest of my long life. I plan to be healthy at 125 years of age.

I know I can stay with this program. It's worth it. It works. I feel really good!

Narline ✦ *"My life has not been the same since I've been on the protocol."*

I [began the detox program] in January 1999 without being sure what changes were going to occur. I was not really overweight, but I always had the majority of fat right around my waist so that when I sat down my waistline would look like it had four bicycle tires stacked one on top of the other. I didn't like the way it looked or felt. In the past I've tried losing it by exercising, doing crunches, some running, and eating the right foods. Nothing really helped.

When I began Gary's program I weighed 122 pounds. I wasn't physically sick but felt tired all the time. I was easily fatigued. I wanted to incorporate some physical activity into my life but had no energy to pursue it.

My life has not been the same since I've been on the protocol. My fatigue is gone. I'm running three to four miles five days a week and training for the New York City Marathon in November. I no longer experience menstrual cramps or the terrible accompanying mood swings.

My diet has changed radically to wholesome unrefined foods. I now cook for myself. I am implementing the behavioral aspects of the program, making my life much simpler by really focusing on me. This enables me to work on the things that are really important such as good mental health, being positive, not arguing. I'm feeling much more self-sufficient as I eliminate stress from my life or make stressful situations less significant. I've lost eight pounds since I began the program. Each day I am a more positive person. I feel optimistic about life and I believe I have more control and choices than I realized before.

Good health and happiness are priorities in my life. I feel a lot sexier, and, most important, I'm getting to know myself better and I'm falling in love with me.

Sue Ellen ✦ *"I feel better now than I did in my twenties."*

After only eleven months of following this program, I finally lost the twenty extra pounds I have been carrying around with me since giving birth seven years ago. I am now in my early forties and I feel great! I feel better than I did in my twenties, and I'm sure that it's the detox program that facilitated all the new changes in my life.

In addition to the weight loss, my skin has become clearer, my eyes sparkle, and I have a greatly increased energy level. I am generally sharper with better memory, and I am experiencing greater mental stability. I have much greater focus and discipline about my daily life and my long-term life goals. I exercise, meditate, eat right, and take supplements daily. I am enacting long-term goals with ease instead of with fear about procrastination and perfectionism. Dry skin on my feet cleared up, thinning hair improved, allergies are gone. I have not had any colds or flu since beginning the program. I need less sleep and wake up refreshed and ready for a wonderful day.

The dietary changes expanded my food choices. In place of meat, dairy, sugar, and wheat items, I found a whole new world of grains, beans, legumes, fruits, vegetables, and fish to eat. I enjoy exercising but never made time for it on a regular basis, and now I do.

I always considered meditation a waste of time but now enjoy the twenty or thirty minutes of introspection and silence. I have learned to accept both my strengths and weaknesses. My new motto is "just get the job done." Spiritually, my relationships with friends, family, and the environment have improved, and I'm reevaluating the beliefs and actions that didn't work for me. I'm taking charge of my life.

In summary, I have achieved that which I set out to do: I am healthier in body, mind, and spirit. I look forward to waking up each day with good health, happiness, and fulfillment.

Kevin ✦ *"Everything I do now seems to require much less effort."*
When I began Gary's program I had been putting on some weight. But my big problem was insomnia, insomnia that was caused in large part by medications I was taking for asthma. The medicines would not allow my body to relax enough to fall asleep. As a result I was getting two to four hours of sleep a night. Now I am cutting down on some of the medicines, which does help my sleep. However, I think the combination of less medication plus no caffeine, sugar, or wheat in my diet is making the big difference. I am now able to sleep. My other troublesome condition was that I had lost all sense of smell and taste. Now, after four and one-half months, I have both back.

Before joining Gary's program I was feeling lethargic and gaining weight. I have lost twenty-eight pounds and my energy level is much higher. There is a new lightness to my being. I feel great. I no longer have headaches. I can exercise regularly. Everything I do now seems to require much less effort.

Martin ✦ *"When I leave my office, I may take some of my work home, but I leave all of the problems there. Animosity is a waste of time."*

I'll be sixty-nine years old. I used to weigh 184. I'm down to 164. I feel much better. Over the past several years I have tried a variety of diets in order to control my weight. Sometimes they worked for a short period of time. But [in January 1999] my wife took me to see Gary and we learned a lot of new information.

Now we no longer eat any meat. I have quit coffee. I used to have four or five cups a day with at least two spoons of sugar in each one. In the afternoon every day I used to have coffee with pound cake, but I stopped all of that. Now we're on a diet of fish and vegetables. We have green juice. We have a protein drink. We walk for one hour every morning before I leave for work . . . about five miles a day. My wife does a good job of planning meals on the program. And doing all of this I've lost twenty pounds.

The only exercise I've been doing is the daily walking. I should do more to build muscle tone. It would be a good thing for me but so far I haven't done that. I don't really want to lose any more weight. I'm close to six feet. I feel much more energetic without those twenty pounds. . . . My facial skin looks much nicer. My wife says I look much more rested. . . .

We go to the meetings every two weeks. They talk about ridding your mind of all the negativity. You know, though, I do that anyhow. When I leave my office, I may take some of my work home, but I leave all of the problems there. Animosity is a waste of time.

I believe that if you're going to do a thing, you just do it. It wasn't easy giving up my cravings for sugars and coffee. I thought I was getting more energy from coffee. But since giving it up, I find I don't miss it. My wife makes sure I get enough water. She makes sure I have my juices when I leave the house. I used to think I was doing myself good by drinking these so-called natural drinks. Now I only drink the real thing. It makes quite a difference. When we go to birthday parties or weddings, it's very hard to fit in with the crowd. I restrict myself to vegetables and potatoes. If I really want one, I'll have one-half of a piece of the cake. I used to have two slices. My clothes fit me again. I like the way that feels and I want to keep it that way.

I believe you should make this commitment. Go one way or the other. This commitment is something you do for yourself. No one else is watching you when you leave your home. No one knows what you're doing. It's all up to you.

Philip ✦ *"I was getting really discouraged about my life but now I feel I'm making some progress."*

I'm forty-seven years old and I guess, like most people, I've had some health problems along the way. One consistent problem in particular has been my weight. I'm a taxi driver and of course I sit in the same position all night long and I work under stressful conditions. . . .

I'm learning to stay on the program even when I have bad feelings. Sometimes I have disappointments, and I used to tend to overeat to feel better. I still have the desire but I am learning to stay in control. I spend more time thinking about what I'll eat. I am not just grabbing a hamburger. I'm finding I can relieve the pressure by rushing to a salad bar instead of a fast-food place.

With Gary's program I've found the right mix of supplements. My body is able to eliminate toxins and fats. And with my improving diet things are beginning to change for the better. I was getting really discouraged about my life but now I feel I'm making some progress.

John ✦ *"We have the power to make life better for ourselves . . ."*

At the start of this program I was overweight. I had no motivation to make any changes. Although I could work for others, I was never able to take care of myself. In the past I had stomach disorders and suffered with diverticulosis. I have always had very dry skin. And I had fungus on my toes.

In only three months I have had some major changes happen. I have lost about fifteen pounds. My skin is clearing up. The fungus on my toes is gone. Due to changing my diet and lifestyle, my stomach is trouble-free. I have much more energy now, and with approximately six hours of sleep I am more alert to my environment and with people that I come into contact with. I'm currently working out, walking, Roller Blading.

I am happy to report that I have learned to put myself first, thinking before I speak. I still work too much but I have become much less critical of myself as well as others. I have come to understand that we are all human and I have to let some things flow in a natural way. It's up to us to make something good of our lives.

In the past . . . I was stuck in a rut. Now I am becoming more and more aware of my inner self and all of the life energies around me. Since beginning the program I feel stronger both physically and mentally. I now work on enjoying my life daily by staying in a positive state of mind. We have the power to make life better for ourselves and the people around us one step at a time, day by day.

Lawrence ✦ "I am much more comfortable in the world."

When I began the program I weighed 210 pounds. So far, I have lost 15 pounds. I feel much better about myself now. Since following the protocol I need much less sleep. When I wake up in the mornings I feel wide awake. Before the program I would wait till the very last minute to get out of bed.

I find that I am much more comfortable in the world. My attitude has changed dramatically for the better. The people around me are changing also. Through my newfound confidence I have been able to help my sister see that she too can insist on being treated with respect. We have put many of these new attitudes to the test, and I am happy to say we are experiencing great success.

Sigrid ✦ "I've lost twenty-eight pounds. I feel good about my body now."

Once I made up my mind to participate in the detox program, I found that I was able to stay firm from the beginning. Many of the people around me tried to challenge me. Friends and coworkers and others

tried to discourage me, warning me of the dangers of becoming a vegetarian. I remember that I went to a wedding and . . . I brought along my
own bottled water and ate only the salad, the salmon, and the caviar—
but nothing else. When I got through the entire affair without being
tempted by all those "goodies," I knew I was well on my way.

Mentally, the program has made a tremendous difference. I am more
organized in my mind. I can think more clearly. And I have begun a
process of eliminating unnecessary clutter from my life. I am so much
more disciplined and patient. Impatience was my biggest problem before. I have reached many new plateaus in my life. One example is my
relationship to my father. We were never friends. But we have begun to
communicate on a different level. I now see him in a different light. I am
able to just accept him the way he is and I don't try to correct him any
more. I truly operate on a different level. . . .

Several weeks into the program I started to feel real good about myself. I lost some weight without any real effort. I started to feel younger. I
began to feel like I did when I was really young. Altogether I've lost
about twenty-eight pounds. I feel good about my body now. I'm often
complimented on my skin. I am so much more joyful, more happy,
more positive today than I was a year ago when I began the program.
Life is more exciting and I feel ready to meet the day.

The program has also helped me spiritually. . . . I am just a more joyful being. My relationship to all people has improved. I have begun to
meditate. I feel much more peaceful.

Michael ✦ *"I can finally see some of that muscle I always thought
I had."*

I started the program four months ago. At the time I was carrying around
a bulging belly. I always felt bloated and sometimes had back pain because of it. When I started Gary's protocol I immediately lost 15 pounds
in less than two weeks. I have stopped eating meat and dairy. I was 170
pounds, which was much too much for my body. Now I weigh 155
pounds and my stomach is almost gone.

Juicing is easy. I started with four juices a day. Then I went to eight juices, which is where I am now. I no longer eat anything that is no good for my body. I stick strictly to the protocol. I exercise daily, practice deep breathing, and laugh whenever I can. I eat some fish daily.

Losing fifteen pounds has enabled me to live a much more active life. I can finally see some of that muscle I always thought I had.

Nancy ✦ *"It was even difficult to sit in a chair. Now I actually exercise by walking."*

In the beginning my state of health was just okay. I have had a lower back problem and numbness in my hands from neck problems. I had a lot of breathing and environmental allergy problems, lots of sinus pressure and headaches. I had trouble getting out of bed or just walking. I had problems with my knees, especially going down the stairs. My weight has made me extremely uncomfortable. It's even been difficult to sit in a chair at times. My hair has always been thin and wouldn't grow much. I tire easily and often want to sleep as much as possible. I was prone to bronchitis.

After following the protocol I find that finally I am able to breathe. I no longer have to take allergy, breathing, and headache medications. Not only am I more comfortable moving, but sometimes now I actually exercise by walking and also follow an aerobics program twice a day. At times I find I can walk down steps normally and have days without any sort of back pain. These things are very new to me. Hand numbness, which was common for me, subsides for long periods of time. I have more energy throughout the day. I've lost weight and I am considerably more comfortable.

Behaviorally, I notice that before I was very judgmental, critical, angry, defensive, and blaming. My moods were very erratic and I loved gossiping to put people down. I'd worry about everything. My temper would often flare up over nothing serious. I was mad at the world and tortured my own family and friends because of it. I was extremely regimented and inflexible.

I am happy to be able to say that now I am much calmer. I do not find the need to criticize everyone and prefer to look for the good in people.

I am a lot more understanding and do not get angry as often. I have become a more compassionate person.

Spiritually, I have changed. I was numb and in denial. Anything I did in the religious realm was external. I was totally disconnected, and I did what I was supposed to do to appear to be a good Catholic. I prayed the rote prayer and was mechanical. Now, after being involved in this program, my prayer is coming more from inside me. I get glimmers of total connectedness. Religion is personally meaningful for me. . . .

Susan ✦ *"I'm honoring myself. I'm pleased and I'm grateful."*

I've had chronic pain and fatigue for years, spending most of my energy and money seeking health. I was miserable and stumped and made a bargain. God would send help and I would follow through. If I couldn't improve my life in two years, I'd take tranquilizers and accept my fate. Enter Gary Null on PBS.

Shortly before I began Gary's protocol, I developed sharp and dull pains in my legs when I tried to rise from a low seat or kneeling position. Frightened and in tears, I'd push myself up. Soon after beginning the protocol, I realized I was standing effortlessly, naturally.

I had hypoglycemia before Gary's diet and controlled my symptoms with the wrong foods and began to gain weight. My weight would fluctuate twenty pounds. I had food cravings for sugar, carbohydrates, and animal protein, and binged often. Now there are no cravings. My protein comes from soy, nuts, fish, and legumes. I drink three to six glasses of a vegetable-based supplement drink daily. I take my drink and nuts on the road, which keeps me satisfied until mealtime. My blood sugar is elevated greatly. . . .

I still don't exercise regularly. But I can walk again and exercise is the next step for me. I plan to begin with a walking machine at home, and return to yoga or try tai chi. . . .

I've lost eighteen pounds on the program. My life is changing as I center and focus. I had a long way to go and I was running in place. I'm moving forward now. I'm honoring myself. I'm pleased and I'm grateful.

Alexandra ✦ *". . . one morning I woke up filled with energy."*

When I started the program I had a real lack of energy. I was sleeping ten to twelve hours a night and was always tired by 4:00 P.M. At the very beginning of the detox program I was more tired than ever and struggled just to complete everyday chores.

Then one morning I woke up filled with energy. No more naps at 4:00 P.M. Now my sleep is down to six to eight hours each night. I still can't believe it.

I also lost ten pounds just from the elimination of sugar, dairy, and wheat, and I maintain a regular exercise program.

Dimitrios ✦ *"I lost fifteen pounds and I have been able to keep it off for over a year."*

Weight loss was the first thing I noticed [as a result of the detox program]. I lost fifteen pounds and I have been able to keep it off for over a year. I'm also starting to build muscle from working out three times a week, which I now do. Thanks to the program my self-esteem, which was not very good, is much higher. . . . I am more confident and much less intimidated, even by doctors. Before I was in a rut, but now I am motivated to try lots of new things, such as studying a third language. I take dance lessons. I play soccer once a week. I've stopped listening to commercial radio stations and no longer watch much TV. Instead, I have gotten much more into reading. When I'm working I listen to books on tape. Just one year ago I wouldn't have considered doing any of those things. Last month I ran a five-mile race. I feel great about that.

Finally, I am happy to be able to report that I no longer seem to need toxic relationships in my life. If something is not right I move on. Since I am following the protocol I am aware that I hardly experience any sickness. If I do it never lasts long—and you can't complain about that!

Jacob ✦ *"I like loving myself a little."*

Before I began the program I had a very low energy level. I needed a sugar boost through the day. My digestion was not great and the sugar cycle confused by thinking.

I have been on the program only three months and have lost ten pounds. Overall, my energy level is greatly increased. My thinking is much clearer and I am much more conscious of my interaction with people throughout the day. My body functions have become more regulated. I am much more aware of what and when I choose to eat. Generally, my attitude is much better.

I like that I am able to listen better and hear what it is people are saying to me. I am more patient with people and have become more aware of my own needs. I am even able to express them sometimes.

Before the program I was upset with my work—feeling trapped by myself. I felt that my work controlled me and that I had no power. I felt as if I always had to get things done but was never able to feel joy in doing them.

Now, after following the program, I am beginning to take more control of my work time. And I have started to take control of my nonwork time. I am able now to step back and congratulate myself on small steps taken. I have a more positive view of the future. I like feeling better. I like loving myself a little.

Patricia ✦ *"I guess when you're ready, you're ready."*

Physically, right now I'm feeling fantastic. I started working with the protocol four months ago. Before I began I was always feeling tired. I tried to improve my lifestyle but I wasn't having much success. I was gaining weight; I wasn't really getting the nutrients I needed. I never exercised.

But once I got on the program it changed everything. Things come to me so much more easily now. I have more clarity. I have more energy. My mind feels alert, sharp. I can't believe the energy I have. It's fantastic. My skin has cleared up. It's smooth and soft now. I had varicose veins. They used to really bulge. They're lightening up.

I used to weigh about 196 pounds at 5 feet 8 inches. Last time I got on the scale I was about 184 pounds. I'm down a size and a half. . . . I used to binge on potato chips and sometimes sweets. But now I never crave these things. I don't feel the need to binge. I think I'm learning to love myself. I understand that I don't want those poisons in my body. I have a sense of calmness now. I feel peaceful now. I used to run, run, run. That disharmony was causing me to overeat. I just don't feel the need to eat. I used to love chicken. But even chicken, my favorite thing, no longer appeals to me.

I've had a card to a health club here in New Jersey for five years that I never used. I paid the fee every year even though I never went. I used to ask myself "Why am I paying for this? I never use it." But finally, now I go. I'm there three days a week for water aerobics. I feel so good doing the exercise in the pool.

Now that I have more mental clarity, I don't get all wrapped up in negative stuff. I stay more centered around with what's going on with me. I take care of me and not everybody else. Since I stopped trying to tell everyone how to get healthy, people seem to come to me more for advice. They see I'm not the one in the hospital. They see I look fifteen years younger than my age. I have no desire to go backward.

Even when the groups are finished, I'll be fine now. Now I know that everybody's watching me. I'm inspiring people to do the right thing. Even my own children are starting to follow some of the protocol. I guess when you're ready, you're ready.

Donna ✦ *"I dove right into the protocol. I have lost about twenty-five pounds."*

Being overweight only became a problem for me in my adult life. In my thirties I went through a difficult divorce. I was emotionally devastated. I had been smoking and drinking to numb the pain. I decided that I would stop smoking and cut back on the wine. But this became more of a hurdle than I had envisioned. I guess I turned to food to fill the void I felt in my gut. I gained weight steadily and kept it on for over ten years. I was unhappy with the way I looked, but I didn't have the will to do anything about it.

I tried a couple of techniques to lose the weight. I tried food combining and met with some success. Shortly after that I joined the health support group. My general health was not bad but I was terribly uncomfortable with the extra weight.

I dove right into the protocol. I juice every morning. I have eliminated meat, dairy, and wheat. I take all of the supplements and meditate every morning. I also have read books and listened to several tapes recommended by Gary. The one aspect of the protocol that I have been less than consistent with is exercise. Focusing on being positive, setting boundaries, and detaching from toxic relationships has been very liberating.

I have been in the program for nine months and I have lost about twenty-five pounds. I am a new energized person. I have taken control of a situation where I felt dissatisfied and helpless. The protocol has become a way of life.

Donna ✦ *"The last time I can remember feeling this vital was when I was a child."*

When I started Gary's program I had just left work on a medical disability from my hospital laboratory job of twenty-one years. Due to improper use of toxic chemicals and insufficient and improper cleaning of the ventilation system, my health was deteriorating daily. My hair began falling out in clumps, I suffered from intense mood swings, chest pain, headaches every day, continuous coughing, difficulty breathing, exhaustion, and lower abdominal pain. My menses completely arrested and I gained fourteen pounds. . . . I was diagnosed with chemically induced asthma and put on three different kinds of inhalers in order to breathe.

The gynecologist said I was now in menopause and some people go through it earlier than others.

Since beginning the program I no longer use inhalers, my menses are regulated, as are my hormone levels and mood swings. My pulmonary function tests have returned to normal. I have a tremendous amount of energy. My hair is no longer falling out and is growing faster and thicker. I have lost the fourteen pounds that I had gained. I'm building muscle and have decreased my body fat from 30 percent to 20 percent.

The last time I can remember feeling this vital was when I was a child.

Bernard ✦ *"Since following the protocol I only require a maximum of six hours sleep."*

Before I began Gary's protocol I was experiencing a very low energy level. I was napping during the day. I experienced indigestion at least once or twice during the week at dinnertime. My joints and my lower back were starting to ache.

Since following the protocol I only require a maximum of six hours sleep, and sometimes less than that. I wake up refreshed and remain that way throughout the day. I haven't had a bout of indigestion since beginning the program. My sense of smell has increased greatly. The pain in my joints has just about disappeared.

Since being involved in the program I have made other behavioral changes as well. I have stopped blaming others for things that I refused to take responsibility for. I have become less defensive and acknowledge my fears and anger. I look inside for what is really going on when the self-critical, righteous, and defensive part of my emotions surface.

In the past I felt unconnected to religion. I have started to see my place in this universe. I have always loved nature, and my sense of the spiritual continues to grow.

Bernie ✦ *"I somehow feel that I have more control over my life."*

I joined the detox support group nine months ago, and because of that there have been major changes occurring in my life. I used to spend long periods of time brooding and holding on to anger. Now there are times when I still get angry, but I have learned to let it go. I am very much more appreciative and understanding of the people around me. I also have a much greater enjoyment of life. I make sure to spend more quality time with my three children and with my wife. Each weekend includes at least one fun thing to do. My wife and I now talk about more meaningful things. We discuss spiritual concepts. We discuss things like diet, interpersonal issues, and psychology. I am less concerned about what would happen if I lost my job. I somehow feel that I have more control over my life.

Another very big change is that I have become more involved in the community. I never used to get involved at all. Now I am on the board of one local group and on the leadership committee of another. Both of these groups want me to take on even more responsibility, which I look forward to doing.

While following the program I have lost fifteen pounds. My total cholesterol dropped from 272 to 232. LDL cholesterol dropped from 183 to 145. My triglycerides have dropped 20 points from 255 to 235. I have become a vegetarian and no longer eat out of boredom.

Sharon ✦ *"After one year on the program I have lost twenty pounds and reduced my cholesterol level by over thirty points."*

Upon hearing Gary was having an orientation for weight management, I finally said to myself, "That's it, no more excuses." The major issue I was faced with was being "slightly overweight" most of my life. But "slightly overweight" turned into "very overweight" after the birth of my three children. I was very lazy, not exercising, and eating everything. Hips and backside became wider, arms were heavier, and my nickname was "thunder thighs."

I wondered if I could really follow Gary's healthy protocol. Could I go through the detox and change to a completely different lifestyle? I needed the support of the group. But I also needed the support of my family. Our meals would be taking a whole different turn. I took a deep breath and decided to take it one day at a time. I made a six-month commitment. It is now one year later and I am thrilled to say that I made it.

After one year on the program I no longer suffer with the excruciating pain from heel spurs. The protocol has helped me immeasurably. After losing twenty pounds the spurs are almost completely cleared up. I have also reduced my cholesterol level by over 30 points. I started at 190, and at the six-month blood workup it read 157.

Angelo ✦ *"I am ecstatically happy now. And so is my family!"*

It is my wife who discovered the Gary Null detox program. She is the inspiration for the success we are both experiencing. I was ready for a major change, whatever it was. I'm glad it was this protocol. I had always believed that I was eating properly in the past. However, I was blind to reality. I was getting fatter and fatter and my health was declining quickly....

Since beginning the program five months ago I have lost approximately 105 pounds. My blood pressure is 120/80 and my cholesterol level has dropped to 158. I feel superb. As I walk I feel like I am on air and that I could walk for as long as the day is long. I have much more flexibility. I can perform many physical tasks that I could not do before. Before I could not cross my legs or even tie my shoe laces. Now I can bike, jog, or power walk for long periods of time....

I have learned to laugh every chance I get. I still get the job done but now I am able to enjoy myself at the same time. I will not tolerate any negativity at all. If I am wrong I have learned to apologize.

When I meditate at church or in the quiet of my own home I think about how my life is changed and I break down. I am ecstatically happy now. And so is my family!

Barbara ✦ *"As a result of my new way of living I lost twenty pounds and have abundant energy."*

I began Gary's detox program after learning about it on his radio program "Natural Living." My goal was to enjoy optimum health and vitality, which I believed was a physically oriented goal.

I was ready to make the commitment. I kept to the dietary guidelines outlined in the protocol. I juiced every day and visited the gym more than I ever had before. As a result of my new way of living I lost twenty pounds and have abundant energy.

The result that I hadn't expected was my new attitude concerning life, happiness, and my future. When the workshop began I had been working in a middle-management position. Although I was unhappy with my twenty years of working experiences, I did not have the courage or confidence to make a change. I sometimes felt angry and depressed.

Somewhere during the six-month workshop I internalized Gary's voice whispering in my ear, "Are you enough to be enough?" Somehow

I knew that I needed to become . . . "enough" in my own eyes. Being physically fit is a major part of health. But with Gary's instruction I learned to take responsibility for my mental as well as my physical health.

Linda ✦ *"I found out that you cannot diet. You must change your whole attitude about what food is about and what's good for you."*

. . . I came to the program overweight, short of breath, and diabetic. I had tried several diets and weight-loss programs over the years to no avail. The programs were either too restrictive or did not teach me how to change my relationship with food. Gary's program did.

I found out that you cannot diet. You must change your whole attitude about what food is about and what's good for you. I learned to replace unhealthy foods loaded with chemicals, sugars, or fats with nutritious natural foods that taste great. My old way of eating was monotonous and boring. My new way of eating affords me a large variety of foods, and finding new recipes to try has become an adventure. I have a new appreciation for food and how to eat it for life. I eat all I want without being concerned about calories.

As of this date, I have lost twenty-nine pounds. I walk two miles a day without being short of breath, and my diabetes is under control.

Joseph ✦ *"I have improved strength and staimina."*

Since beginning the detox program I have improved strength and stamina. For example, I used to run ten-minute miles prior to my participation and presently I run eight- to nine-minute miles. I could only do 50 sit-ups. After just four months I can do 360 sit-ups. Also I notice when getting up in the morning my joints, particularly my ankles, don't ache any more. My blood pressure is now 110/70. My hiatal hernia doesn't bother me as it did before the study.

If you want to know how my behavior has changed you may want to ask my wife and daughters. I always blamed someone in the past. Now if I start to blame, I stop myself. I am more aware. In the past I always acted defensively. This behavior is occurring less and less. I used to worry constantly. This is the area of greatest improvement for me. Most of the time I refuse to worry. I used to suffer with lots of anxiety. Most of the time I would not have been able to explain why. Now I have little or no anxiety. I used to experience a bout of anger at least once a day. Now—maybe one time a week.

I used to look at animals as a source of protein. Now I look at these creatures from a perspective that they also have a spirit.

Part 4

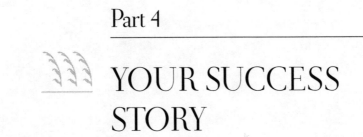

YOUR SUCCESS STORY

Chapter 14

Looking Within

Many people sense that part of the reason they are over-weight is that they don't have the power to run their lives the way they want to. They feel stressed out at their jobs, where information comes in faster than ever and our responses must be equally quick. The number of hours we work is on the rise, and many employees worry about job security. But even after we leave the office, our problems may continue at home. Many of us feel lonely and stay stuck in unrewarding friendships and relationships for fear of being isolated. If we're married and have children, we may live in households where no one communicates or shares feelings with one another. Quality time with our friends and family is difficult to find in an era when parents must work two or three jobs to keep up with the bills and children rush through dinner in order to get to the next activity, watch television, or play video games.

Our lives also are filled with short-term crises—an exam at school, a heated argument, or getting stuck in traffic on the way to an important meeting. These minor stresses have no lasting effect on our bodies and immune systems, notes Dr. Joan Borysenko, one of the pioneering scientists of psychoneuroimmunology, the study of how emotions act as a link between the body, mind, and immune system. Rather what does us in is the chronic stress we feel from a negative outlook that can develop as a result of these minor irritations and setbacks.

If we begin to view life as stressful rather than challenging, our body behaves as if it's in a constant state of emergency, stimulating the adrenal glands to produce cortisone, epinephrine, and norepinephrine, hormones that give us more energy to surmount these everyday obstacles. "That's great if you have to leap out of the way of a speeding train," says Borysenko, "but if you see life as a speeding train, you're going to increase your blood pressure and become prone to cardiovascular disease." In addition, various facets of the immune system suffer, creating a condition of immunosuppression that makes us more receptive to illness. We also may attempt to relieve our stress through eating, which can result in weight gain and poor overall health.

Some of us handle stress better than others, a concept known as stress hardiness by researchers in this field. Superior adaptation to stress depends on three factors: challenge, control, and commitment. Instead of letting ourselves become unhinged by troublesome events, we need to view each difficult situation as a challenge, take control, and commit ourselves to resolving it. Borysenko, who considers herself a poor adapter, uses a personal example to illustrate how stress hardiness makes a difference in how two people cope with the same situation.

She and her three children were riding in their motor boat down a river. Being inexperienced, she did not heed the warning of the red and green barrels floating in their path telling them to remain within their boundaries. As a result, they ran the boat into a low-tide area and became stuck on a sandbar. The sun was going down, and the crew was wet and getting colder by the minute. Panicked, Borysenko started imagining the worst possible scenario: They were going to get sick and develop hypothermia. She had been a terrible mother to let this happen.

Meanwhile, her fifteen-year-old son was glowing. This was his opportunity to rescue the family and become a hero! Viewing the stressful event as a challenge, instead of a threat, gave him a sense of control and commitment to resolving the situation. Drawing on his creative resources, it took him just thirty seconds to figure out a plan. He asked the family to get out of the boat as he cast the anchor into deeper waters. The weight of the sinking anchor dislodged the boat, and once everyone had climbed back in, they motored away.

Borysenko, who teaches people how to deal with stress, explains that optimists seek creative solutions to difficult situations while pessimists tend to blame themselves and see no way out. But rather than fall apart and engage in destructive patterns of behavior, people with a negative outlook can learn to alter their perceptions by asking such questions as "What is the challenge here?" and "How can I grow from it?" We can't control the external realities, she says, but we can control our response to them.

This chapter looks at ways for you to become more stress hardy. It will help you to pinpoint the areas of stress in your life that may be contributing to overeating and work to resolve them in a positive way. As you become clearer and more centered, you will gain a better sense of command and commitment, and the loss of control around food and other avenues of escape will naturally disappear.

JOURNAL WRITING

Keeping a journal is an excellent way to work through stress-related issues. Although some people find it difficult to get started—in the information age, writing has become something of a lost art—the journaling habit can be easily developed just by taking the time each day to do it. And the results are well worth the effort. If some vague stress or feeling of dissatisfaction is haunting you, reflecting on your life through writing can help you determine what actually is bothering you and then figure out what to do about it. Once you have determined the cause of your stress, it will be that much easier to determine solutions, and you'll increase the likelihood of accomplishing your goals.

One way that we can relieve stress is to pinpoint and then dismiss irrational beliefs that keep us from being happy, healthy, and productive individuals. These thoughts can manifest themselves as either exaggerated or absolute statements. Words such as "should," "ought," "must," "have to," "need to," "never," and "always" can help us to identify such thoughts, which are often the root of negative emotions, such as anxiety, depression, rage, frustration, shame, and embarrassment, and can lead to self-defeating behaviors. When starting a diet, we may find ourselves saying "I *have to* lose twenty pounds by my birthday." If our parents are pressuring us to follow in their footsteps career-wise, we may think "I really *should* go to medical school." Repeating these absolute statements over and over can lead us to place counterproductive pressure on ourselves and to feel discouraged and powerless if we don't live up to these goals.

When these types of stress-producing, irrational thoughts arise, we can use a journal to vigorously and persistently dispute these beliefs—and encourage ourselves in other ways. For instance, you can ask yourself such questions as:

- Where is the evidence to support the existence of this belief?
- Is my belief logical? Or is it a result of peer pressure or invalid interpretation?
- Where is this belief getting me? Is it helpful or self-defeating?

We also can use a journal specifically to help us achieve our weight-loss goals. With it, we can systematically monitor what we are doing diet- and exercise-wise. Although we will be more pleased with ourselves some days than others, the main point of a diet journal is to ensure that we're staying in the struggle, persisting, and staying focused. The most important thing is to focus on not giving up and to be proud of making that kind of effort. You should feel free to use your journal as a space to boast about your accomplishments and pat yourself on the back for your success.

Dream journals are another vehicle that we can use to work on our life's issues. Dreams open up another world when our senses shut down during sleep, and although they sometimes seem silly or illogical, dreams can be a window into the subconscious mind. If we pay attention to our dreams, we can get to the source of many personal issues and possibly begin the process of healing. Try this: Before going to sleep, write down a question and instruct your dreams to answer it. In the morning, record your dream and see whether it answers the question. You may be surprised at the results.

OTHER SELF-ACTUALIZATION TECHNIQUES

Beyond journal writing, there are a variety of ways of smoothing out the bumpy aspects of life so you'll have an easier time reaching your weight-loss goals. One that I recommend to every group I work with is to simplify your home environment. Many therapists have seen the value of this approach in helping their clients lead more relaxed, fulfilling lives.

Unclutter Your Life

When patients wishing to lose weight talk to therapist Dr. Peter Reznik, one of his first questions is "How's your closet?" Trained in mind/body medicine, Reznik works on the premise that a disorder on one level is always reflected on other levels. He also asserts, and I agree, that you can successfully start a process of change on any of these levels and it will have direct repercussions on the others. People who want to let go of excess weight but can't often are unable to let go in every aspect of their life. As a result, their closets and homes are clogged with old clothes, papers, books, furniture, and dust-collecting trinkets. An initial step to change, then, is to start cleaning your house or apartment, getting rid of everything that you no longer have use for. You'll find that this can contribute greatly to an enhanced sense of well-being.

The emotional makeup of an overweight individual often reflects this pattern as well, with the person hanging on to memories, perhaps painful ones, that no longer serve a purpose. The regrets and resentments we hold on to from the past keep us from living fully in the present. Instead of being in the now, we think about how our parents didn't treat us right, or about the poor choices we made or about the opportunities we passed up. We carry around old hurts and grudges, and it's almost as if they're stored in the tissues of the body.

These types of negative thoughts keep us chronically stressed and have a negative impact on our immune system. When a traumatic or stressful event occurs, our limbic system—the part of the brain related to emotions—secretes neuropeptides, or information molecules, that pass through the blood/brain barrier and bind to cell receptors throughout the body. These neuropeptides affect all our body systems, inhibiting the immune system, increasing blood pressure, and adding stress. From that point on, whenever something happens that reminds us of that particular stress, our immune response drops.

To begin the healing process, Reznik has his patients clean out their inner closets by remembering past stressors and releasing them. Unlike more traditional models of therapy, where people talk about a hurtful situation and then store it in their mind so that it continues to rule their life, Reznik's approach teaches patients how to resolve the painful memory differently. For example, if a patient has suffered abuse, he would ask him or her to return to the experience, feel the pain, and then transform it by creating a better ending. Instead of remembering feelings of being trapped and powerless, the patient is encouraged to use his or her imagination to fight back. In rewriting the memory, the new ending is stored in the mind along with the old one, and the experience of "I am a victim; I can do nothing" will change to "I can fight back." While it's true the actual experience will never change, the way that memory is now processed *has* changed, and that's what's important for healthy functioning.

Another method is to look squarely at the traumatic event and seek the meaning in what happened. If you are still upset over a past divorce, for example, realize how it helped you to stand on your own two feet, gain self-respect, and so on. Suddenly your past challenges become empowering, and your brain will begin to secrete different chemicals, ones that enhance your immune system. By confronting hurtful personal issues and memories and reframing them in a more positive light, we open the path for positive thinking on all fronts and can achieve our weight-loss goals more easily.

Get in Touch with Your Demons

Eating for emotional reasons happens more when we are unsure about what's bothering us. Once we get a clear picture of what's really going on, the urge to take solace in food is likely to diminish and eventually disappear. Clinical psychologist Dr. Edward Abramson therefore encourages his patients to pay close attention to events that precipitate eating episodes: "I frequently ask people, 'What were you thinking about before you started eating?' Not just 'Where did I leave the peanut butter?' but 'What was I thinking about before I asked where I left the peanut butter?'" This method helps people identify what was going on in their head at the time and enables them to connect a particular feeling to the urge to eat. It may be an upcoming job interview or other work-related situations that cause anxiety, for example, or the memory of someone who is absent that precipitates loneliness.

It's important to realize that most of us have been conditioned to cover our feelings, and if we're not turning to chocolate cake for comfort, we're turning to Prozac or other antidepressants that mask an uncomfortable state of mind. Instead of shutting down our mind's internal message, we need to become more aware of what our inner voice is saying and learn to live in accordance with that voice. Ask yourself honestly what it is that makes you feel anxious about your job, or why a particular person's absence makes you feel lonely. Don't be embarrassed and don't shut out the answers that come to you. Once you acknowledge these feelings, you can begin to work through and overcome them.

One method for tuning in to yourself is to get involved in something creative. Using art is a simple way to open the door to better self-understanding and self-expression. You don't have to be Picasso; just the act of generating images that are meaningful to you through sketching, painting, or doing collage can help. The expression-through-art technique is especially good for people who have difficulty talking about their problems, and the process actually can start a flow of dialogue as you begin to open up. It's inexpensive, without side effects, and can be extremely beneficial. For example, you might use art to explore the circumstances in your life that compelled you to gain weight in the first place.

Note that, in addition to visual art, music, drama, dance, and creative writing are other avenues of artistic expression that can lead to better self-understanding.

Seek Social Support

When something is bothering you, it's important to get it off your chest. Hiding your feelings and pretending they are not there does absolutely no good. This goes for all negative emotions as well as insecurities about your weight and body image. Try sharing what's on your mind with someone who cares. A good friend, a therapist, or a support group can help you to see your situation in a larger frame of reference and realize that you are not alone. Scientific studies reveal there to be considerable health benefits from social support; people who express their feelings have better immune systems and less illness than people with similar life stressors who keep their problems to themselves.

Use Imagery

Human beings are different from other creatures in one very important respect—we have the ability to shape ourselves and our world through our own thought processes. Stephen Twigg, one of Britain's leading holistic health practitioners, stresses that we can be lots of different things, depending on who we think we are. Although our original perception of ourselves is based largely on who we learned we are while growing up, as adults, our health and well-being are largely our own responsibility.

To leave behind your old image and perceived self and start taking responsibility for a new you, it's important to ask yourself some important questions. Ask yourself, "Do I want to be who I am right now?" If you sense that the image you have of yourself is destructive and is preventing you from leading a full and happy life, you can work to change it through affirmation and visualization. "Without changing this inner model," Twigg says, "you're not going to change the model's effect, such as weight gain, on your mind/body process." If you have a weight problem, once you make changes to your inner model you can support the new model with changes in your eating patterns. In fact, as you start to change who you think you are, then what you want to eat and what you enjoy will begin to change automatically.

To Dr. Peter Reznik, imagery encompasses the use of our entire sensory system to stimulate the imagination. Rather than focus on outside realities, as we usually do, imagery allows us to reshape our reality from within and bring about positive physical and emotional changes. Imagination is constantly at work in our lives, but we can purposefully direct it for specific outcomes. For instance, as in the following exercise, it can be used to help you speed up your metabolism.

Close your eyes and breathe gently and evenly with long, slow inhalations—nice and easy inhalations—breathing out twice as slowly as you breathe in. Envision yourself lying lazily in your bed in the morning. Now envision yourself jumping up and quickly putting on a red jogging suit. Bolt out of the house, and quickly run to the football field—very quickly—faster, faster, faster. Get to the football field. Run one circle and then a second circle. Go faster—third circle—faster—fourth circle—faster—fifth circle, sixth circle, seventh circle, eighth circle, ninth circle.

Very quickly run back home. Take off the jogging suit, and put it in the laundry. Go into the shower. Turn on the hot water. Now as hot water is pouring down, envision yourself squeezing your body just as you would a sponge, and squeezing out all the excess fat. See the fat coming out and the hot water washing it off. Now put cold water on. Now hot water again. See yourself squeezing your body, making it perfect. The hot water is washing the fat off; the cold water is solidifying your new body. Turn off the water, dry your body. And open your eyes.

Reznik says the key to impacting the body is to keep the exercise short, generally no longer than ten to fifteen seconds, and filled with unexpected images. Changing the images gives little shocks to the cells, just enough to get the energy unstuck and moving again. This is somewhat akin to the idea behind Chinese medicine, where disorders are seen as stagnant qi, or energy. By stimulating the cells, you can redirect your thought patterns, and soon these new patterns will impact your physical body as well.

Engage in Positive Self-Talk

Very few of us have been fortunate enough to grow up in unconditionally supportive households. Generally, we've been controlled and corrected and made to feel that we were not okay the way we were. Friends and family members can be especially harsh if we fail to fit into the standards of acceptable appearance, which can make us feel self-conscious and even lead to self-loathing. As a result, all sorts of negative thoughts pop up in our minds, often without our even realizing it. We frequently find ourselves saying unkind words to ourselves, such as "You're so fat," or "You're lazy," or "You have no willpower."

You may not be able to control what others feel and say, but you certainly can control what thoughts you allow to remain in your own head. The next time negativity strikes and you catch yourself engaging in self-criticism, try responding in a new way. For instance:

- *Have a debate with yourself.* Expressing your negative thoughts aloud and arguing against them can be therapeutic and help you to feel better about yourself.
- *Make criticism work for you.* If someone is suggesting that you are fat and unhealthy, take the attitude that the person is telling you this because he or she cares about you. Treat it as constructive criticism and consider taking the person up on their challenge.
- *Be patient with your process of change.* If you ate too much over the holidays, rather than admonishing yourself with criticisms like "I was

bad; I have no control," have compassion for yourself, and recognize that change is a process. Don't engage in self-sabotage because of one small setback. Realize that getting to where you want to go sometimes means that you will take three steps forward and one step back; this is only natural and a part of the process. Try to realize *why* you took that backward step, and use it as a learning experience.

- *Use affirmations.* Affirmations are positive words that help us break from negative thought patterns so that we may move in the direction of our goals. For instance, instead of saying "I don't exercise enough," words that keep us stuck in the same lazy cycle, we should say "I am exercising more frequently." Rather than cry "I can't stop eating chocolate!" state "I do want to eat foods that are good for me." Even if you are stressed out because you don't have a defined weight-loss goal, your affirmation can be "I am evaluating possible goals."

- *Start the day right.* Instead of just getting up and adjusting to whatever the day brings, use the early morning to get into the type of mind-set that assures a more purposeful, satisfying day. Start by asking yourself "What is going to be good about today?" and determining how you will be productive and what you have to look forward to. Next, focus on how good that is going to make you feel. This will cause a shift in your body chemistry that adds greater health and happiness to your life. In the evening, when you assess the day, you will feel as if you have accomplished something.

- *Acknowledge your successes.* While most of us are quick to focus on our failures, few of us commend ourselves for the little successes we have. For instance, if you're at a party and successful at passing up the high-fat hors d'oeuvres, tell yourself, "I did something good; I'm moving forward." That will keep you thinking positive and on track.

Cultivate a Low-Stress Lifestyle

The ways in which people deal with stress often can lead to more stress, which only exacerbates the problem. Overeating is one counterproductive coping mechanism as it results in your feeling bad about your body, so you have another thing to be stressed about. Other counterproductive responses to stress include smoking, drug or alcohol abuse, and compulsive gambling or shopping. These solutions are all short term, don't resolve the situation, and lead to further problems.

One of the reasons we're so stressed today is that people tend to be overscheduled and overcommitted. So a long-term approach to de-stressing your life is to go through your date book or calendar, determine what activities or commitments are no longer serving you well, and then, whenever possible, cut them out of your schedule. One way to begin reprioritizing is to stop everything for an hour or so, sit quietly, and ask yourself where you are in your daily schedule. If you're like most of us, you've probably been concentrating on doing things for others rather than for yourself. Take the time to rewrite your to-do list, this time focusing on *your* needs. Try to pinpoint the people and events in your life who waste your time, rob you of energy, and create stress. Then figure out a way to eliminate these negative forces. If you need to exercise first thing in the morning, pencil it in, and let those who might try to distract you know that this is your personal time and not negotiable. Realize that it's okay to let the answering machine pick up your calls or delegate responsibility to others who are capable. Try to prepare larger meals that you can then freeze and serve as leftovers throughout the week. You're not expected to be superman or superwoman—you need time for rest and relaxation, and the schedule you create for yourself should reflect that.

Relax

In order to free ourselves from stress and worry, we need to step outside of our busy minds. Deep diaphragmatic breathing is an ancient technique that can help us to escape the mind and feel more relaxed. When people are anxious, they tend to breathe shallowly and rapidly. By taking a moment to breathe deeply, we oxygenate our entire body and immediately feel more at ease. In just seconds you will notice a dramatic improvement in how you feel.

Deep breathing has been found to have a profound impact on our overall health. Holistic physician Dr. Magid Ali reports: "We did studies with blood gases, chemistries, pH, and lactic acid, and we found that by breathing deeply you can profoundly alter your body chemistry so that it slides back into the spontaneous healing mode rather than into the stressful disease-causing mode." Dr. Roger Jahnke, of Santa Barbara, California, agrees, saying that worry, fear, and frustration are powerful defeaters of the medicine within: "The good news is that when you straighten your posture and take a deep breath you are turning this medicine on." Other simple methods for relaxation include imagining birds flying across the sky or the sounds of waves crashing against the shore, rubbing your ears vigorously, or using your thumb to apply pressure to the palms.

Practicing relaxation on a regular basis also helps us sleep better at night. To overcome insomnia, Jahnke asks his patients to do some breathing exercises; massage their hands, ears, and feet; and then guide themselves through a session of deep muscle relaxation. This alleviates tension in the muscles that is associated with anxiety. To do this, focus first on tensing each muscle group and then relaxing it completely by saying "Now my feet are relaxed; now my legs are relaxed; now my hands are relaxed," and so on. If you are relaxed, you will be less likely to indulge in unhealthy foods on account of stress and anxiety.

Cognitive Behavior Therapy

Unlike old-school psychoanalysis with its focus on the past, cognitive behavior therapy centers on the present to help us resolve current issues. Rather than try to unravel subconscious conflicts generated in early childhood, it works with people's present attitudes, thoughts, and feelings about who they are. For example, if a person has an eating disorder, a therapist trained in cognitive behavior therapy will help him to overcome his dysfunctional dietary patterns by developing healthy ones instead that he can put into practice on a daily basis. *Why* the eating disorder actually developed is not of particular concern.

Cognitive therapy also can help us develop coping mechanisms for dealing with high-risk situations that trigger eating episodes. Binge eating is often emotionally triggered, and the job of the cognitive behavior therapist is to help a client identify emotionally charged situations—such as a fight with a spouse or difficulties at school—that are likely to precipitate an eating episode and then learn how to deal with those situations in a more constructive way. Once we recognize the situations that impede our weight-loss attempts, we experience "cognition," or awareness, that helps us overcome the problem.

You don't need to work with a therapist to do this—I recommend using your journal to try to pinpoint emotion-laden situations and then making a list that you carry with you. When you feel one of the situations coming on, look at your list and remember your resolve to not let circumstance get the better of you. Ask yourself, "Do I need this tiramisu? Do I need to have a beer with dinner? Can I really afford to skip exercising today?" This type of self-discipline can be extremely challenging, so don't get discouraged if you can't always talk yourself away from certain temptations. You will get better the more practice you have, and as we said earlier, awareness is the first step.

Integrative Body Therapy

Developed by Sigmund Freud's student Wilhelm Reich, integrative body therapy is based on the belief that psychological traumas have physical counterparts, so that when we become psychologically wounded, our physical bodies become wounded as well. Integrative body therapy is a process that aims to uncover the wounds that are at the root of our problems and holds that eating disorder behaviors are associated with feelings of abandonment and loneliness. To escape our painful feelings of inner emptiness, we attempt to develop a comforting relationship with something outside of ourselves, be it food, money, or certain people. But since the object in focus can never satisfy our longing and doesn't address the basis of the problem, we never feel satisfied. And we're never at peace.

Integrative body therapy works to heal the problem at its essence, and, once this is done, behaviors such as eating disorders begin to disappear. Integrative body therapist Jane Latimer cautions that this is not a quick process, as most people with emotional eating issues are so disconnected from their bodies that they cannot access that deeper, inner wounding at the beginning. The major part of the therapist's job is to help patients reconnect with what they are feeling underneath. "They need to start connecting the trigger, the thing that started them feeling out of control," Latimer says. "If they can connect the trigger with some of the older wounding, then they can begin the healing and actually start putting the pieces back in place."

Clarify Your Values

The people who live long and happy lives are those who are able to express who they really are. Unfortunately, many of us do not live according to our beliefs, and even worse, we may not even be sure what we do believe in. Being out of touch with our spiritual ideals, values, and emotional needs contributes to an unhealthy psyche, and it is bound to take its toll on our appearance and our health.

This connection has been recognized by many holistic practitioners, including naturopathic physicians Charles and Maxine Cropley, authors of the now-famous book, *The Mind Body Connection*. In their own practice, the Cropleys noticed that their patients wanted to improve their health and appearance but, despite good intentions, found themselves unable to change to patterns of eating and exercise that would produce desired results. So the Cropleys started looking more closely at what was going on inside their clients' minds that prevented them from attaining their weight-loss goals. What they ultimately discovered was that people had trouble losing weight because there was a spiritual void in their lives. Charles Cropley says, "What we find is there's an inner quality missing in people, and the quality is that of motivation. So the question becomes, how can we raise a person's level of motivation?" Most people, they realized, need to believe in something greater than just the idea of losing weight.

To help their patients get in touch with their spiritual needs, the Cropleys give their patients an "emotional exam." It begins with questions that help people tune in to different areas of their life that may be unsettling. For instance, people are asked how they feel about their primary relationship—be it with a spouse, sibling, or child—their work, and other areas of their lives, and then are asked to rate those areas on a scale of one to ten that ranges from ease to dis-ease. The uneasy areas of life are usually the ones that trigger hormonal responses that adversely affect health and eating patterns. Once these stressful areas have been identified, patients can begin to work through their issues and understand how they impact their eating habits.

Then there are questions to help people clarify their values and what it is they want out of life. Patients ask themselves: If you had all the time in the world, what would you do? If you had all the money that you wanted, what would you want to do, or have, or be? If you knew you couldn't fail, what would you attempt? If you were witnessing your own funeral, what would people say about the kind of person you were and about your accomplishments? What would you want to hear at the end of your life that would be so fulfilling that you would say "It's time for me to go because I've done all I wanted"?

By getting in touch with our hearts, we have a much better chance of gaining power over our health and weight. When you become clear about what it is you really want, your health becomes more valuable and you feel inspired to change. The next chapter offers some specific questions to help you get started on this process.

Chapter 15

Starting Over

Who are you? You might answer that question with such responses as "I'm an American," or "I'm a forty-seven-year-old woman," or "I work for XYZ Company," or "I'm a 200-pound man who wants to weigh 170." But these are all superficial answers to the question. "Who are you?" in a deeper sense refers to the characteristics that most define the way you think, work, and interact; the combination of talents that is uniquely yours; and the values that guide your life. Some people never ask themselves who they are on this more meaningful level, and they end up adopting a lifestyle that isn't really suited to their true selves. Whether they know it or not, there's a disparity between who they are and how they're living, so they carry around a constant sense of unease. In an attempt to dull that feeling, they indulge in escapist habits, such as drug or alcohol addiction, overwork, oversocializing, overcommitment, compulsive gambling, or excessive TV watching. Or they overeat. In fact, when you see someone whose life is ruled by one of these addictive behaviors, there's a good chance that the "Who are you?" question hasn't been dealt with satisfactorily.

I base this assertion on years of counseling individuals and working with groups. One of the reasons I wrote the book *Who Are You, Really?* a few years ago was to help people answer the question for themselves and see if there was a mismatch between their true identities and the paths they were following. In that book I described seven natural life energies. It's been my observation that people tend to fall into one of seven ways of being and interacting in the world, and I described these. I explained that by seeing where you fit into this picture and working with your natural life energy rather than against it, you could have a more fulfilling life. Obviously, everyone's unique, and so it's inaccurate to pigeonhole people. And obviously, many people are going to exhibit characteristics of more than one life energy group. The point is, if certain patterns are there and you're cognizant of them, you'll be better off than someone who hasn't thought about these issues. You'll be in a position to say, for example, "Hey, I think I'm basically an Adaptive Supportive. But I've been trying to live my life as a Dynamic Aggressive, because that's what my parents expected me to do. Maybe that's why I'm anxious all the time. Maybe that's why I overeat all the time. Maybe it's time to reevaluate my life."

This example describes a particularly uncomfortable mismatch of life energy and lifestyle, because a true Dynamic Aggressive is someone who's a natural "mover and shaker," someone with a CEO-type overview of situations and an innate drive to organize and direct large endeavors. A true Dynamic Aggressive actually thrives on stress and the challenges of creating new systems. An Adaptive Supportive, by contrast, is a person most comfortable following directions rather than thinking them up. The vast majority of the population are Adaptive Supportives, but since it's more prestigious to have a Dynamic-Aggressive kind of job, sometimes an Adaptive Supportive will be pushed, or push him- or herself, into living a false life. This is a tremendous strain, and healthwise, the results are not good.

Placing this example in the context of the seven life energies paradigm, I see most of the energies falling into one of two major groups, the Dynamics and the Adaptives. The former are the charismatic change-initiators of society; the latter, those who follow along the paths laid out by Dynamics. To tell you something about the five life energies I haven't yet described, Dynamic Assertives are not looking for control of systems the way Dynamic Aggressives are, but they are very involved in the world of ideas and beliefs and in molding or changing these. Dynamic Supportives are the compassionate people naturally suited to the healing, teaching, and communicating professions. They try to effect change by helping others directly. Adaptive Aggressives are those who operate well in tandem with Dynamic Aggressives; they're the master manipulators who serve as the facilitators of the Dynamics' plans. Adaptive Assertives use practical organizational and work skills to help keep things humming. Creative Assertives constitute the one group that are not necessarily Dynamic or Adaptive; they're our artists, musicians, and writers, who live with their own rhythm of high and low activity and interaction levels.

This is just a whirlwind run-through of the life energies, and you may want to read *Who Are You, Really?* for a deeper understanding of how they affect our lives. At my lectures and in talking with people individually, I've noticed that a tremendous number of people can relate to the idea of trying to live out the wrong life energy. Since the lifestyles of certain energies—particularly Dynamic Aggressives and Adaptive Aggressives—tend to be more financially rewarding than those of others—particularly Adaptive Supportives and Creative Assertives—many of us end up in the wrong occupations. Some also end up forging the wrong relationships, living in the wrong places, and adopting the wrong kinds of daily schedules.

But as many people have discovered, it's never too late to realize that you're on the wrong course and to start life over in a sense by making new choices. In my health support groups we often discuss who-are-you? type issues. Sometimes we use a natural-life-energy framework and sometimes we don't. But what we always do is ask and answer questions that go to the heart of the choices people make in their lives. I offer my own ideas on answering the questions, with the understanding that these are just my own thoughts, not necessarily *the* answers. We talk about some of the issues in the group meetings, and I also give people lists of unanswered questions to take home and think about or use as jumping-off points in the kind of journal writing that we discussed earlier.

Members of my groups have told me that the question-and-answer process has helped them immensely, not just in terms of destressing their lives and achieving a feeling of personal peace but in terms of improving their physical health. Note that the support groups I'm discussing always focused on physical health goals, with weight control being a primary issue. But as I've explained before, the only way people seem to achieve these goals and—most important—to maintain them for any length of time is if they integrate a thorough examination of life values into their protocols. Now I always include such examinations with whatever group I'm working with.

Of course, you don't need a group to examine your life—you can do it totally on your own. To get you started, I've provided two sections of sample questions that I've given to people to think about. These questions cover a wide variety of issues, from materialism, to relationships, to the ways we label ourselves. Some of the questions will be more relevant to you than others. Use the ones that strike a chord of recognition within you. There may only be a few, but if you give those few your honest evaluation, the experience can open your eyes, change your life, and help you reach both your weight-loss and lifelong goals.

As you go, pause and reflect on each question. Jot down your responses on a sheet of paper if it helps you to organize your thoughts. The first section, with twenty questions, includes my answers and comments. The second section, of one hundred questions, includes no answers. But for all of these, *your* answers are the ones that are important.

1. Do your comforts limit you?

We work toward making our lives comfortable. Comforts provide a sense of security. But they also prevent us from trying anything new. We become afraid to quit our jobs and find new work, change relationships, or even change the way we eat, dress, or comb our hair. New situations create discomfort. We have no way of predicting how we are going to feel and what is going to happen to us. Comfort also creates complacency. Complacency stops the growth process. It prevents us from asking questions that are critical to growth and improvement.

Look at what happens to so many of us in the urban environment. People tend to find comfort in their apartments and in the things they buy, but not with other people. They forget how to communicate with each other. I gave a lecture on making new friends during which I asked people to turn to the person next to them and say hello to someone new. Until I made that request, no one had asked anyone else around them a single question. Imagine that—a lecture on friendship and they were afraid to say hello to someone next to them! They needed my permission and encouragement; their established comfort level wouldn't allow them to risk talking to someone new on their own.

It is important to challenge yourself by pushing through discomfort. This helps you to expand and grow. Then what was once uncomfortable becomes completely comfortable. Suddenly you will find that you can make decisions, make changes, and let go of old notions that no longer serve you. As you get rid of the old you can allow in the new. You can meet new people and do things you never thought you could do. You are able to say things you wouldn't have said before and eat foods you wouldn't have eaten. These are just a few of the wonderful things that can happen when you step outside of your comfort zone.

2. Can separating from our possessions set us free?

How much of your life is spent maintaining and guarding possessions? What do they mean to you? Can you see yourself without them? Picture yourself without one-third of your possessions. Without half of them. Without three-quarters of them. Mentally choose which ones you might jettison. How do these images make you feel?

When you were a young child, possessions weren't viewed as permanent but were used to explore, experience, and let go of. Your joy was in using and sharing more than in owning. Once we become adults, though, we don't want anyone else to touch our things. One floor in our office building is only for the president, the executive vice president, and the executive secretary. Everyone else is kept out. But the president, the executive vice president, and the executive secretary may not be as well off as you might imagine. They may get their identities from their titles and from the fact that they have their own floor—but they may not be any happier for it, or know who they really are.

What happens when you cease to base your identity on what you have? You find other things more meaningful, things you can't possess to give you happiness—like a sunset, a meaningful conversation with a friend. Without so many permanent possessions to keep you locked in to your old identity, you're freer to experiment with new jobs, new activities, new environments for living, new people. I truly believe that unless you are able to separate yourself from unnecessary possessions, you will never find true pleasure or see the beauty in this world.

3. Do you know the difference between having new experiences and acquiring new things?

Having a new experience can enliven you for a long while afterward and even provide you with a new perspective that lasts a lifetime. Simply getting something new, on the other hand, frequently ceases to be exciting after about a week. Then you realize that this new possession isn't doing all that much for you and that you'll now have to clean and maintain it perpetually. What's more, if you have been in the habit of getting new things, you may not even have a place to put it.

A lot of people have a dirty little secret—a dirty *big* secret, actually. While at first glance their houses may look uncluttered, if you go into their basements or garages, you see the material overflow of their lives, and it's astounding. There's a floor-to-ceiling collection of toys, appliances, clothing, kitchen equipment, knickknacks, games, and gadgets that makes Macy's basement look understocked by comparison. How much of this stuff was bought because the people, who were dissatisfied with their lives, really needed new experiences but went out and got new possessions instead?

4. *What are you willing to get rid of?*

Having too many things is not only a substitute for having new experiences, it actually can get in the way of having new experiences. You have to spend time and money acquiring, taking care of, and storing all your things. Then you don't want to leave them to go somewhere else on an adventure.

This is one of the reasons I advocated not having too many possessions and why I think it's a good idea to ask yourself periodically, What can I get rid of? Do I really need five TV sets in the house? Do I really need that fondue pot from a 1970s bridal shower? I haven't fondued anything in decades. Do I really need all these clothes? These shoes? These knickknacks that make my living room look like a gift shop about to have a fire sale? Am I dusting them all for a reason?

Do you know those bumper stickers that say "I'd rather be golfing" or "I'd rather be dancing"? When you're dusting your knickknacks, ask yourself what you'd rather be doing.

5. *Make a list of the new experiences you've tried as an adult.*

Childhood is cram-packed with new experiences, but they're not necessarily ones that you've chosen. As an adult, your new experiences are probably fewer and farther apart, but they're more likely to be ones that you've opted for—ones that are tailored to your interests and aptitudes. Doing new things can be harder for an adult than for a child, but the experiences are just as rewarding.

A list of the new things you've undertaken as an adult might include your first trip to Africa, to Europe, or to a neighboring state. It might include learning to sky-dive or learning to swim or to drive, going rock-climbing, enrolling in a continuing education course, or getting your first dog. Your list might contain three items, or it might be so long as to be impossible to complete. The last thing on it might have occurred yesterday or two decades ago.

The point is not how long your list is or how adventurous you've been. Rather, it's to get you thinking about the experience of trying something new. Remember how you felt, for instance, learning to swim. It was a little scary, but it was exciting too, because suddenly there was a whole new element you could get around in, a whole new way you could exercise and have fun. The experience probably energized you and made all of life livelier for a while.

Perhaps it's time to try something new again.

6. *What are you willing to do that's different?*

How many times have you had an opportunity to do something but decided not to do it because you prejudged that you wouldn't like it, that something would be wrong about it for you, or that you wouldn't fit in with the others there? Later someone said, "You should have come. It was fun." And you made an excuse.

What are you willing to do that's different? Are you willing to spend a Saturday doing something totally different from what you usually do on Saturdays? Are you willing to wear your hair differently? To wear different types of clothes? How many things in your life are you willing to change? Or is your life just a routine, predictable pattern?

I have friends who have never done one single thing differently for years. I can tell you what they're going to say, what they'll eat, how they will treat people, what their apartment looks like, what they will do when they go on vacation. To me, that's boring. When people are that boring, they get old real fast. And when they get old, they stop taking risks.

When people stop taking risks, they stagnate. Joy is no longer there, and they don't see the happy side of life. They are only bitter and cynical. Why? Because the only perspective they have is one of the fermentation that is occurring around them. Who creates that fermentation? They do. But whom are they going to blame? Everybody else. They blame circumstances.

When you are willing to act differently and take some risks, before long you will begin to feel comfortable doing something else differently. Soon you will start looking forward to experiencing life and not being afraid. Suddenly your tiny view of life expands and you are all the richer for it.

7. Do you fully engage in life?

Either we give of ourselves completely or we do not. Don't try something halfheartedly. You won't get as much in return as you could if you gave yourself over to the experience completely.

Many people build escape mechanisms into what they try. Ted invites Bob to go camping, for example. "Bob, would you like to go camping?"

"Sure," Bob replies, "I'd love to."

"Let's go next month."

Next month arrives, and as they are preparing to leave, Ted asks, "Bob, what have you got here? You've got a cellular telephone, a tent with a CD player in it, a security system for insects, and a heater with a thermostat. This isn't camping. This is merely trying to create a suburban environment in the woods."

Bob isn't engaging in life fully—in fact, he's going out of his way to create artificial circumstances in an artificial setting. He is avoiding the reality of the camping experience as much as possible. Why bother going camping at all?

The next time you catch yourself avoiding an opportunity to grow and change—or even just to experience something different from your norm—make a conscious effort to open up and embrace the situation. Instead of dragging your television and cell phone along on your camping trip, for example, take the bare minimum with you and enjoy the experience of being without modern conveniences and creature comforts. Allow yourself to become a minimalist like Thoreau or Audubon—even if it is only for a few days. You'll be surprised at how wonderful and inspiring the world can be when you stop running from what it has to offer.

8. Is your thinking "on automatic"?

Despite what you may believe, our thoughts are not truly our own. They have been passed on to us, not genetically, but through our conditioning. We have thousands of preset associations in our mind by the time we're ten years old. When we think of something, an image comes up to identify it. We think of the word "pretty" and up comes an image to tell us what pretty is. We don't create that image. We are given different formulations that stay in the mind and that can pop up automatically without our ever questioning them.

What if how we are taught to respond is flawed? Then we can form negative emotions around concepts that aren't necessarily negative. If we are conditioned to believe that being poor is terrible, and we don't have much money, then every day we will wake up thinking that we are rotten and miserable because we lack wealth. The whole day we will perpetuate those images as we compare ourselves to others. We'll see someone in a car that we don't have. We'll see someone in a dress or suit that we can't afford. We'll see someone who has a fancier apartment than we do. Our thoughts probably will be negative if we're on automatic, and they in turn will create other negative thoughts and emotions.

At some point we need to ask ourselves: Where do these thoughts come from? Whose perceptions are they? What can I put in their place? Until we learn to replace them, we'll continue to live by them. We need to be a little more choosy about our thoughts and to honor only those that create the most positive reactions. Those are the ones we need to focus on.

9. Do you need a label?

We have an identity problem in this society, and we think we need labels to solve it. What's more, we all want to have the "right" label.

School starts the process. In school there is one right answer, and we base our sense of self-worth on what other people identify as right. Then too, it's in school that we first learn whether we are "high achievers" or in "the slow group." And this labeling process is repeated ad nauseam every day of our life. Are we working class or middle class? Lower-middle class or upper-middle class? Are we black or white? Jewish or Christian? Catholic or Protestant? Perhaps we're Hispanic or Pacific Islander. We're supposed to know what boxes to check off in the questionnaire of life.

A friend of mine tells me of an experience she had looking for an apartment in a New York suburb. A prospective landlady seemed ready to rent her a place, but she had a question first.

"What are you?" she said.

Hoping that her status as a human and a female were obvious, my friend said, "I'm an American." But of course the landlady still looked puzzled, because what the woman really wanted to know was what religious or ethnic label she could attach to this person. To attach "person" to her just wasn't enough. My friend thought it was, and she didn't take the apartment.

"Person" isn't enough for a lot of people. Did you ever go to a Mets or Yankees game and see how some of the fans have to grasp at an identity that isn't really theirs? Some of them are fanatics who dress up like the athletes and live through them. It's one thing to enjoy a sport or participate in one. But when we begin to identify with something that is totally outside of ourselves, we can lose part of our real selves in the process. We are a culture that's learned that copying styles, copying language, copying slogans, and copying rituals can give us our identity.

Brand names are big deals in our society. People use these to identify themselves as having good taste or as having money. They actually wear brand names emblazoned on their clothes in a way that would have been considered crass until a few years ago. Instead of wearing a name tag that says "Hi! My name is John," people wear a company name or logo on their clothes that says "Hey! I've got the sense and the bucks to buy such-and-such a brand. In fact, it's part of who I am. Admire me."

But is that shirt company really part of who you are? Once you've paid your money to the department store, the shirt *company* cares about you about as much as that athletic team whose hat you're wearing does once you've paid for game tickets. They don't identify with *you;* why identify with them? Instead, let your own unique assets and characteristics define who you are. We're looking for identity in all the wrong places.

10. *What defines your sense of self?*

Wealth? Some people get their sense of self from the money they have. Others may look at them and assume they have got to be intelligent and deserving people to be wealthy. But it's not necessarily so. For example, there are many families with old wealth and no one living today has worked for any of that money. Their bank accounts are not a reflection of their drive or integrity—they're a reflection of the efforts of those who came before them.

Popularity? The popular person gets his or her sense of self from being charismatic and charming. But that doesn't mean such people are entitled to good self-esteem. Think of all the charismatic salespeople who have charmed people out of their life savings. Charm and charisma may come in handy, but they aren't the basis for self-worth. Think of the charismatic politicians who have no integrity.

Others' fear? I know a lot of people who get their sense of self from the fear they generate in others. They call it respect, but there's often an element of fear there. It's not just organized groups like the Mafia that I'm referring to but many of today's military generals, CEOs and politicians. And almost everyone remembers the neighborhood bully who pushed the smaller kids around when they were growing up. Instilling fear in others isn't something to be proud of—and using it as a basis for self-esteem is more damaging to you than to those who are afraid.

Winning? We consider winners to be people who are successful and have a good sense of self. But being a winner is not essential to anything. There are a lot of winners who are bad people. We've all heard of those winners in sports who are ungracious with their fans, abusive to their families, or megalomaniacs who think they deserve the world on a silver platter.

Winning doesn't mean much if you don't treat those around you with honor and respect—it's a fleeting accomplishment that doesn't count for much in the larger picture.

What have you done that was meaningful, and what do you hope to do in the future? These things make more sense as ways of defining who you are. Think back to something you've done that has affected who you are today. Also, ask yourself: What was the best year of my life? What was the worst? How did I react to the wonderful times and to the negative experiences, and how did all of this mold me?

Ask yourself what accomplishments you're proudest of. Sometimes the things a person is proudest of are not the stereotypical ones, such as getting a college degree or being promoted at work. They're more private acts or accomplishments that others don't necessarily know about. They could be something like seeing an opportunity and seizing it when the temptation was to stay comfortable and let it slide by. They could be something like befriending a person and then finding out many years later that that person always remembered the kindness. It pays to pinpoint your greatest accomplishments, especially if they include "little" ones like these, because doing so will help you define who you are in ways that go beyond that line on your résumé that reads "Ph.D. in chemistry."

Ask yourself what you want to accomplish in the future too. Do you want to get a second Ph.D.? Do you want to become a skier? Scaling down, do you want to be able to dine alone in a good restaurant and actually enjoy the solitude? Will these plans encourage you to grow as a person and allow you to contribute to society? Again, small plans as well as large ones are what really define who you are.

11. *Do you focus on your weaknesses or your strengths?*

If you are like most people, you focus on your weaknesses. One of the best ways to learn to focus on your strengths is to challenge yourself. Only through challenge are people forced to use those strengths that they may forget about from time to time. If you train for a marathon, for example, and push yourself to go out in bad weather as well as good because you know you have to run each and every day if you're going to be able to do twenty-six miles, you are not only enhancing your physical strength but honing your mental discipline and endurance. By challenging yourself in this way, you are building strengths you didn't know you had.

The next time someone asks you what your strengths are, rather than drawing a blank, call to mind your response to your most recent challenge. Don't be shy about your accomplishments—be proud of them, embrace them as a part of who you are, and incorporate them into your everyday life.

12. *Are you looking for someone else to change the circumstances of your life?*

People are naturally drawn to gurus and other charismatic leaders because we are looking for someone to guide us, solve our problems, or protect us. Similarly, when people look for love, often they're really looking for social acceptance, because being part of a couple is society's ideal. Half the single people in America hate being single because of how others perceive them. "You're thirty-five and single?" others ask, implying that there's something wrong with you. When I grew up in West Virginia, if you were over twenty-five and single, you were pronounced either dysfunctional, incorrigible, or too ugly for anyone to want to be with. No one ever considered that you might not want to be married. We, as a society, have very strict standards about what we will and will not accept.

Sometimes we are terrified of being alone because we equate being alone with loneliness. We assume there's a void and that the void can be filled by a warm body. We embark on a relationship looking for the other person to absolve us of our loneliness and insecurity. And most of the time, these relationships fail, because only you can change your set of circumstances.

Instead of looking to someone else to improve your self-esteem or infuse your life with purpose, try looking to yourself first. After all, no one knows better than you what *you* need. Only when you are a whole and satisfied person will you be able to have healthy, fulfilling relationships with those around you.

13. Is what we gain or what we give up more essential?

When we give something up, we are then free to have something take its place. If we gain something but still hold onto everything else from the past, in reality we have gained very little. When you start giving things up, you automatically gain the ability to have a whole new reality. And, of course, I'm referring not just to possessions but to attitudes, notions, and emotions.

You cannot have a whole new reality if you are not willing to give up the notions that framed your old reality in the first place. Then you are still looking at the world with the same mind. You are using the same old biases, fears, and limitations to interpret events and solve problems. If these same notions couldn't create a solution in the past, how are they going to create one now?

When you give up your old way of thinking, the new mind takes over and everything is possible. You look at your problem from a new perspective, with new feelings, new awareness, and new ways of integrating thoughts and emotions. That's why when someone has a problem and says, "I think I'll sleep on it," it makes sense. In a dream state the mind is unfettered, fluid, able to take new perspectives and make new connections. In a dream, your mind can let go of what's not essential and hold on to what's really meaningful to you. Thus dreams can provide a new way of looking at problems and even real inspiration.

14. Is being good always a good thing?

A lot of people assume that by doing good things they will feel better about themselves. Problems can arise, though, if in the process, they deny their own needs. Think of the people in your life who are good to others but not to themselves. These are the people who have no real sense of self-esteem—they get self-esteem from being good, but not because they feel good about themselves.

If you are "trying" hard to be good and you have a hidden agenda, then you aren't being truly good. There is a conflict between what you want to be and who you actually are. Being authentic is essential, as whatever you do becomes who you are.

15. How do you know that your beliefs and feelings are authentic?

When you know what is right, it resonates as being right. You feel inner peace and balance. When something does not feel right, but you want to make it so, you force yourself into believing it. You argue with yourself, try to convince yourself, talk to yourself, and sell yourself ideas.

If after all your arguments and mind games, another idea still resonates, pay attention to it—that other idea is your truth. And that's what should be followed. Your intuition, your inner voice that comes from your authentic self, is talking to you. Listen to it.

16. Do you acknowledge others?

How often in a day do you compliment people? How often do you acknowledge them? We often forget that what's important is the bond between people and that acknowledgment of others is the basis of communication. It makes relationships intimate and personal.

If you've got a dog, did you ever notice how when you come home, it immediately runs over and starts licking you? Ten minutes later, if you come in again, it's the same thing. What if you had someone in your life who gave you the same kind of love and attention? What if every time when that person saw you he or she said warmly, "Gee, it's good to see you."

Learn to acknowledge others. Always look for something good that you can say. Genuine compliments are important because they're a form of acknowledgment—they let us love and be loved by others.

17. When you want to release tension, what do you do?

There are many positive ways to release tension. You can go for a walk, listen to music, laugh, take deep breaths, dance, have sex, exercise, meditate, or party. There are negative ways as well. You can drink, take drugs, overeat, oversleep, shop compulsively, hold feelings in, let out destructive anger, project your negative thoughts on others, or break things. These are all outlets for dealing with the same feelings.

The moment you start feeling tense, a process occurs. By paying attention to the process, you are in control of your behavior. Tension happens slowly. It starts with the idea that it is what you should feel. You start to visualize tension. You have something in your mind that shows you what tension looks like. What you see in your mind causes your emotions to react.

You can't stop the feeling, but you can control the way that it manifests itself. For example, you can change your outlet from alcohol to music, from bursts of negative energy to meditation, from hurting something to deep breathing. These types of things will change your whole energy flow. You have a choice about the energy that you feel and internalize and whether it is going to manifest itself constructively or destructively.

18. Are you active or supportive?

Believe it or not, both of these traits are important. Many of us tend to think we should all be dynamic. But this is wrong. We should be our true natures. Some people are best at supporting the energies of others. They have a natural caring nature. Others have a natural leadership nature.

Honoring the energy inherent in your character will make all the difference in the way you feel about yourself. There's nothing more frustrating than feeling that you should be leading when you're always following. Or being forced into being the leader when it doesn't come naturally to you and doesn't feel comfortable. You're suppressing your natural energy and pretending to be someone you aren't. Of course, there always are opportunities to expand on your nature and change in the way you relate to people. Growth and change are things we should all strive for, but being in touch with who you are creates a sense of internal balance.

19. If a society is not vital or healthy, why participate?

I don't do anything just because I'm supposed to do it. I go out and create my own social context, my own friends, my own life, my own career, my own day. Last night I worked all through the night. I didn't say "Uh-oh, it's ten o'clock. Time to go to bed to get my eight hours of sleep." I felt there were other, more essential things to do. The bottom line is that society and your day-to-day experience in it is what you make of it.

You've got to understand that what you embrace you become. Be very careful about the routines, activities, and people you have embraced. Be honest about what they mean to you. If they are important, if they honor you, if they're healthy, that's fine. If not, then ask yourself whether you can disengage and and rebuild your life and your society in a better fashion. If you are honest with yourself, you can.

Take a look at everything that you are a part of. Ask: Is this essential to what I want to be? I had friends who were essential to me at one point in my life but who aren't now. I had things that I needed, but I don't need those same things now. It's not a matter of good and bad. It's a matter of what's essential to you and your happiness at this stage of your life.

20. *Can you reaffirm your life?*

Every morning I wake up knowing that everything I am going to do that day will be life-affirming. Each day has meaning to me. Life is not about fame or fortune but rather about the quality of the energy that is shared. You can make the world a better place if you choose to do so because you are an essential ingredient in society. It doesn't matter whether you are rich or poor. You have something special to share.

No matter what your situation, if you are working on improving it, you will be happy with yourself. For instance, when you look in the mirror you can't lie about what you see. If you are overweight, you'll see it. Yet if you are overweight but working on a better body, you will be happy with what you see. You will appreciate yourself for working on the process of change.

Affirmations are an important ritual for helping you to focus on the purpose of your life. They help you to keep focused on your vision. Affirm health and you will eat only foods that enhance health. Affirm love and you will approach everything you do and everyone you meet lovingly. Affirm beauty and you will see it everywhere. This is a daily process.

Further Questions

1. About what parts of your life are you in denial?
2. Do you tend to take appropriate or inappropriate risks?
3. How much time and effort do you spend trying to control your emotions?
4. Do you tend to react from fear of abandonment?
5. Are you an accuser?
6. Are you realistic about what others should do or be in your life?
7. Do you develop stress-related illnesses?
8. Do you trust your own values, perceptions, and needs?
9. In what ways are you consistent?
10. What choices do you make out of fear?
11. Are you self-centered?
12. Do you respect others' boundaries?
13. Do you honor the trust placed in you by others?
14. What parts of your being do you identify as weak?
15. Do you feel a need for perfection on all levels, and, if so, how does this affect you?
16. What are you doing that is vital, engaging, life-affirming?
17. Do you try first to meet your own or others' needs, and do you feel you've made the correct choice?
18. Are you a caretaker? How does it affect you?
19. Do you try to manipulate the feelings or attitudes of others?
20. What changes do you fear?
21. What would you do differently if there were no punishments or rewards?
22. Do you honor your promises to yourself? To others?
23. What have you achieved through discipline, determination, and attention?
24. What excuses do you commonly use?
25. How strong is your willpower? Do you actually use it?
26. Do you tend to think and not feel, or vice versa?
27. What do you really need that is tangible? Intangible?

28. What drives you?
29. What do you find effortless and spontaneous?
30. How do you use intuition, and when do you not trust it?
31. Do you fear failure?
32. What is divine within and outside of ourselves?
33. When you work hard at something, what do you really want?
34. Where does your life need organizing? Discipline? Focus? Attention?
35. Do you judge yourself by what's in your heart and mind, or by your accomplishments?
36. Do you avoid anger?
37. As a child, teenager, young adult, and mature adult, how have you processed anger?
38. How do you perceive power?
39. Do you allow or actively seek new beginnings?
40. What part of your life—professionally, personally, or socially—is a testament to your greatest efforts?
41. Do you find insecurity and self-doubt occur when you feel your place at work, in the community, or in relationships is challenged?
42. How can you use self-doubt as a vehicle for change?
43. What do you fear losing?
44. Are you a complainer?
45. What life circumstances are you willing to change in order to achieve a goal?
46. How can you make change exciting rather than intimidating?
47. How predictable are you, and, specifically, do you ever surprise people with changes you've made?
48. If you knew you had only three more years to live, what would you change?
49. Do you act on impulse or, at the other extreme, think things through indefinitely?
50. What have you allowed yourself to experience that lies outside conscious control?
51. Where do you obtain meaning?
52. Are you focused too much, or not enough, on your physical self?

53. When and how did you make a major life adjustment?

54. When all is said and done, who are you?

55. What would change if you truly freed your mind, body, and spirit?

56. What do you alter that makes you appear as something other than what you really are?

57. Where are you inflexible, and where are you open?

58. Why do you choose wrong actions?

59. As a child you learned important lessons. Which ones do you actualize now?

60. In a typical day, do you do too little or too much?

61. What is your inspiration, and do you reaffirm it daily?

62. Do you say yes when you want to say no?

63. Do you use guilt to try to control people, or are you yourself controlled by it?

64. If you told the truth about your real self and needs, what type of confrontations would occur? What would change?

65. What first step are you willing to take to begin change?

66. Are you willing to undertake change alone?

67. How do you share love, intimacy, vulnerability, anger, pain, despair, and hope, and with whom do you share?

68. What have you ignored that is essential?

69. How have you allowed yourself to be used by others?

70. Do you accept your imperfections?

71. Do you allow passion to be a part of your communication and shared experience?

72. What effects—positive or negative—do you have on those in your life?

73. How is your life affected by your need for love?

74. Do you alter your communications so as to be more appreciated, needed, connected?

75. Can you experience the giving and receiving of love if you are invulnerable?

76. Do you feel hopeful or hopeless about the important issues in your life?

77. What characteristics of your parents have you incorporated into your own behavior?
78. Whom or what do you turn to when you've reached your limits?
79. How do you deal with reality when it doesn't match your expectations?
80. Do you distort your perceptions to match your conditioning?
81. In what areas and to what extent are you willing to share your life with others?
82. Do you allow temporary situations to become permanent?
83. What does children's unconditional love of people, places, and things teach us?
84. How strongly do you affirm what you will and won't do?
85. When are you completely yourself?
86. When are you least yourself?
87. Who grants you your choices?
88. Do you take more than you give, or vice versa?
89. What's the most constructive attitude you share?
90. Where is your passion and excitement?
91. What parts of your behavior are addictive?
92. What type of behavior do you exhibit when you are afraid?
93. What in your life represents gender compliance?
94. What aspects of life have you yet to explore?
95. In what ways do you feel empowered?
96. Does opinion, rather than knowledge, play too large a part in your life?
97. Do you feel whole or fragmented?
98. In what types of activities do you lose your sense of the passage of time?
99. What freedoms do you have that you're not taking advantage of?
100. Are you stronger than you pretend to be?

As you continue on your weight-loss program, come back to these questions every day. How you respond to a particular question may vary dramatically depending on your mood or frame of mind; this is a normal part of the process. In addition, probably there will be a few questions that you never feel like you have full closure on. This is nothing to be concerned about. By continuing to ponder these questions, we continue to evolve as individuals, and as we change, our responses will too. By looking deep within ourselves to find the answers, we open the door to new ways of thinking, of eating, of viewing our bodies, and of living healthier, happier lives.

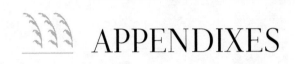

APPENDIXES

Appendix A

Phytochemical Activities

(+)–CATECHIN: Anticoagulant; Anticomplementary; Antimutagenic; Antioxidant; Antiperoxidant; Antiradicular; Cancer Preventive; Cardiotonic; Dermatitigenic; Hemostat; Hepatoprotective; Immunostimulant; Phagocytotic; Vasoconstrictor; cAMP-Phosphdiesterase Inhibitor.

(–)–EPICATECHIN: Allelochemic; Antianaphylactic; Antidiabetic; Anti-EBV; Antihpatitic; Antileukemic; Antimutagenic; Antioxidant; Antiperoxidant; Antiviral; Bactericide; Cancer Preventive; Cardiotonic; Choline Sparing; Hypocholesterolemic; Hypoglycemic; Insulinogenic; Lipoxygenase Inhibitor; Pancreatogenic; Pesticide; Xanthine-Oxidase Inhibitor.

1,4–DICAFFEOYLQUINIC-ACID: Choleretic.

1,8–CINEOLE: AchE Inhibitor; Allelopathic; Allergenic; Anesthetic; Anthelmintic; Antiallergic; Antialzheimeran; Antibronchitic; Anticatarrh; Anticholinesterase; Antihalitosic; Antilaryngitic; Antipharyngitic; Antirhinitic; Antiseptic; Antitussive; Bactericide; Choleretic; CNS Stimulant; Counterirritant; Dentifrice; Expectorant; Fungicide; Hepatotonic; Herbicide; Hypotensive; Insectifuge; Nematicide; Pesticide; Rubefacient; Sedative.

2–VINYL-4H-1,3–DITHIN: Antiaggregant; Antithrombotic; Pesticide.

3–N-BUTYKPHTHALIDE: Antitumor 60 mg/mus/6 days.

3',4',5,6,7,8–HEXAMETHOXYFLAVONE: Cancer Preventive.

4–HYDROXYCINNAMIC-ACID: Cancer Preventive.

5–HEXYL-CYCLOPENTA-1,3–DIONE: Antiseptic; Pesticide.

5–HYDROXYTRYPTAMINE: Antidepressant; Antidote (Manganese) to 3/g/man/day; Antimutilation; Antiparkinsonian; Antitourette 400 mg/4xday/or1/man; Cancer Preventive; Cerebrophilic; Hypertensive; Insecticide; Pesticide; Secretogogue; Spasmogenic; Ulcerogenic; Vasoconstrictor.

413

5–METHOXYPSORALEN: Antipsoriac; Cancer Preventive; Carcinogenic.

5–OCTYL-CYCLOPENTA-1,3–DIONE: Antiseptic; Pesticide.

5,7–DIHYDROXYCHROMONE: Antifeedant; Bactericide; Herbicide; Pesticide.

8–METHOXYPSORALEN: Antialopecic; Antilymphomic; Antimycotic 20–50 mg/man/day; Antipsoriac 20–50 mg/man/day; Antitumor; Antiviral; Bactericide; Fungicide; Lymphocytogenic; Mitogenic; Mutagenic; Pesticide; Phototoxic; Viricide.

24–METHYLENE-CYCLOARTANOL: Cancer Preventive.

ABCISSIC-ACID: Juvabional; Pesticide; Phytohormonal.

ACETIC-ACID: Acidulant; Antiotitic; Antivaginitic 1–2%; Bactericide 5,000 ppm; Expectorant; Fungicide; Keratitigenic; Mucolytic; Osteolytic; Pesticide; Protisticide; Spermicide; Ulcerogenic; Verrucolytic.

ACETYLCHOLINE: Allergenic; Antiamblyopic; Antidiuretic; Anti-ileus; Antitachycardic; Cardiodepressant; Cerebrostimulant; Histaminic; Hypotensive; Miotic; Myocontractant; Myopic; Myotonic; Neurotransmitter; Parasympathomimetic; Peristaltic; Sialogogue; Spasmogenic; Vasodilator.

ACETYLDEHYDE: Fungicide; Pesticide; Respiraparalytic.

ACTINIDIN: Proteolytic.

ADENINE: Antianemic 1.5 g/day; Antigranulocytopenic; Antiviral; CNS Stimulant; Diuretic; Hyperuricemic; Insectifuge; Lithogenic; Myocardiotonic; Pesticide; Vasodilator; Viricide.

ADENOSINE: Antiaggregant; Antiarrhythmic; Antiendotoxic 500 mg/kg ipr mus; Antilipolytic; Antitachycardic 50–250 ug/kg/ivn; Arteriodilator; Hypoglycemic; Insulinic; Respirastimulant; Secretomotor; Vasodilator.

ADENOSINE-TRIPHOSPHATE: Antienzymatic; Antirheumatic; Antitachycardic; Myotonic.

AESCULETIN: Analgesic; Antiarrhythmic; Antiasthmatic; Anti-Capillary Fragility; Antidysentric; Anti-inflammatory.

AESCULIN: Antiarthritic; Anti-Capillary Fragility; Antihistaminic; Cardiotonic; Diuretic; Hypertensive; Lipoxygenase Inhibitor; Sunscreen.

AJOENE: Antiaggregant; Antimalarial 50 mg/kg; Antimutagenic; Antithrombotic; Fungicide; Hypocholesterolemic; Lipoxygenase Inhibitor; Pesticide; Prostaglandin Inhibitor.

ALANINE: Antioxidant; Cancer Preventive; Oxidant.

ALFALFONE: Plant.

ALLANTOIN: Antidandruff; Anti-inflammatory; Antipeptic 30–130 mg/man/day; Antipsoriac 2%; Antiulcer; Immunostimulant; Keratolytic; Sunscreen; Suppurative; Vulnerary.

ALLICIN: Amebidice 30 ug/ml; Antiaggregant; Antibiotic; Antidiabetic; Antihypertensive; Antimutagenic; Antiprostaglandin; Antitumor; Bactericide; Candidicide; Fungicide; Hypocholesterolemic; Hypoglycemic; Insecticide; Insulin Sparing 100 mg/kg/man; Larvicide; Lipoxygenase Inhibitor; Mucokinetic; Pesticide; Trichomonicide; Vibriocide.

ALLIIN: Antiaggregant; Antibiotic; Antihepatoxic; Antioxidant; Antiradicular; Antithrombotic; Bactericide; Hypocholosterolemic; Pesticide.

ALLISTATIN-I: Bactericide; Pesticide.

ALLISTATIN-II: Bactericide; Pesticide.

ALLYL-ISOTHIOCYANATE: Allergenic; Antiasthmic; Antifeedant; Antimutagenic; Antiseptic; Cancer Preventive; Counterirritant; Decongestant; Embryotoxic; Herbicide; Insectiphile; Mutagenic; Nematiovistat 50 ug/ml; Pesticide.

ALLYL-MERCAPTAN: Acantholytic; Pemphigenic; Spice.

ALLYL-SULFIDE: Acantholytic; Allergenic; Bactericide; Pemphigenic; Pesticide; Respiradepressant.

ALPHA-AMYRIN: Antitumor; Cytotoxic.

ALPHA-BISABOLOL: Antiarthritic; Antiburn; Anti-inflammatory; Antipyretic; Antiseptic; Antispasmodic; Antitubercular; Anti-ulcer; Bactericide; Candidicide; Cosmetic; Fungicide; Musculotropic; Pesticide; Protisticide; Spasmolytic; Vulnerary.

ALPHA-CHACONINE: Antialzheimeran; Antifeedant; Cholinesterase Inhibitor; Fungicide; Memranolytic; Nematistat; Pesticide; Teratogenic.

ALPHA-CURCUMENE: Anti-inflammatory; Antitumor.

ALPHA-HUMULENE: Antitumor.

ALPHA-LINOLENIC ACID: Antimenorrhagic; Antiprostatitic; Cancer Preventive.

ALPHA-PHELLANDRENE: Dermal; Insectiphile; Irritant; Pesticide.

ALPHA-PINENE: Allelochemic; Allergenic; Antiflu; Anti-inflammatory; Antiviral; Bactericide; Cancer Preventive; Colcoptiphile; Expectorant; Herbicide; Insectifuge; Pesticide; Sedative; Tranquilizer.

ALPHA-SOLANINE: Antifeedant; Fungicide; Pesticide.

ALPHA-TERPINEOL: Anticariogenic; Antiseptic; Bactericide; Motor Depressant; Nematicide; Pesticide; Sedative; Termiticide.

ALPHA-TOCOPHEROL: Antimutagenic.

ALUMINUM: Antisilicotic; Antivaginitic; Candidicide; Encephalopathic; Pesticide.

AMYGDALIN: Anti-inflammatory; Antitussive; Cancer Preventive; Cyanogenic; Expectorant.

ANETHOLE: Allergenic; Antihepatotic; Antiseptic; Bactericide; Cancer Preventive; Carminative; Dermatitogenic; Digestive; Estrogenic; Expectorant; Fungicide; Gastrostimulant; Immunostimulant; Insecticide; Lactagogue; Leucocytogenic; Pesticide; Spasmolytic.

ANISALDEHYDE: Antimutagenic; Insecticide; Pesticide.

ANNONACIN: Antimalarial; Artemicide; Cytotoxic; Larvicide; Nematicide; Pesticide.

ANONAINE: Antiseptic; Bactericide; Candidicide; Cytotoxic; Dopamine-Adenylate-Cyclase Inhibitor; Fungicide; Hypotensive; Insecticide; Mycoplasmicide; Pesticide.

ANTHOCYANINS: Antimyopic 600 mg/man/orl; Antinyctalopic 600 mg/man/orl; Goitrogenic; Pesticide; Viricide.

ANTHRANILIC ACID: Antiarthritic; Antifeedant; Anti-inflammatory; Insulinase Inhibitor; Insulinotonic.

APIGENIN: Antiaggregant; Antiallergic; Antiarrhythmic; Antidermatitic; Antiestrogenic; Antiherpetic; Antihistamine; Anti-inflammatory; Antimutagenic; Antioxidant; Antispasmodic; Antithyroid; Antiviral; Bactericide; Calcium Blocker; Cancer Preventive; Choleretic; Cytotoxic; Deiodinase Inhibitor; Diuretic; Hypotensive; Musculotropic; Myorelexant; Nodulation Signal; Pesticide; Sedative; Spasmolytic; Vasodilator.

APIIN: Aldose-Reductase Inhibitor; Antiarrhythmic; Antibradykinic; Spasmolytic.

APIOLE: Abortifacient; Antipyretic; Diuretic; Emmenagogue; Hepatotoxic; Insecticide; Intoxicant; Pesticide; Secretolytic; Spasmolytic; Synergist; Uterotonic.

ARABINOGALACTAN: Anticomplementary; Antileishmanic 250 ug/ml; Immunostimulant 3.7–500 ug/ml; Interferonogenic 3.7–500; Mitogenic; Phagocylotic.

ARACHIDONIC-ACID: Antidermatitic; Antieczemic; Antipsoriatic; Cancer Preventive; Hepatoprotective; Insulinogenic; Insulin Sparing; Pesticide; Urinary Antiseptic.

ARBUTIN: Allelochemic; Antiseptic 60–200 mg/man; Antitussive; Artemicide; Bactericide; Candidicide; Diuretic 60–200 mg.

ARGININE: Antidiabetic; Antiencephalopathic; Antihepatic; Anti-infertility 4 g/day; Antioxidant; Diuretic; Hypoammonemic; Spermigenic 4 g/day.

ASARONE: Anticonvulsant; Antielleptic; Cardiodepressant; CNS Depressant; Emetic; Febrifuge; Fungicide; Hypothalmic Depressant; Myorelaxant; Pesticide; Psychoactive; Sedative; Tranquilizer.

ASCORBIC ACID: Acidulant; Analgesic 5–10 g per day; Antiarthritic 1 g per day; Antiasthmatic 2g per day; Antiatherosclerotic; Anticataract 350 mg/day; Anticold 1–2 g/man/day; Anti-Crohn's 50–100 mg/day/or/man; Antidecubtic 500 mg/man/2x/day; Antidepressant 2g/day; Antidote (Aluminum); Antidote (Cadmium); Antidote (Lead); Antidote (Paraquat); Antieczemic 3.5–5 g/day; Antiedemic 1 g/man/day; Antiencephalitic; Antigingivitic; Antiglaucomic 2 g/day; Antihemorrhagic 1 g/man/day; Antihepatic 2–6 g/man/day; Antihepatoxic; Antiherpetic; 1–5 g/day; Antihistaminic; Anti-infertility 1 g/day; Anti-inflammatory; Antilepric 1.5 g/man/day; Antimeasles; Antimigraine; Antimutagenic; Antinitrosic 1 g/man/day; Antiobesity; 1 g/3xday; Antiorchitic; Antiosteoarthritic 1 g/2xday; Antiosteoporotic 500 mg day; Antioxidant 100 ppm; Antiparkinsonian 1 g/2xday; Antiparotitic; Antiperiodontitic 1 g/2xday; Antipneumonic; Antipodriac; Antipoliomyelitic; Antiscorbutic 10 mg/man/day; Antiseptic; Antishingles; Antiulcer; Antiviral 1–5 g/day; Asthma Preventive 1 g/day/orl; Bactericide; Cancer Preventive; Cold Preventive; 1–2 g/day; Detoxicant; Diuretic 700 mg/man/orl; Febrifuge; Fistula Preventive; Hypocholesterolemic 300–1,000 mg/day; Hypotensive; 1 mg/man/day; Interferonogenic; Lithogenic; Mucolytic 1 g/wmn/day; Pesticide; Uricosuric 4 g/man/day; Urinary Acidulant; Viricide; Vulnerary.

ASIATIC ACID: Collagenic.

ASIMICIN: Antifeedant; Antimalarial; Aphicide; Artemicide; Cytotoxic; Larvicide; Nematicide; Pesticide.

ASPARAGINE: Antisickling; Diuretic.

ASPARAGUSIC ACID: Allelopathic; Nematicide 50 ug/ml; Nativoistat 50 ug/ml; Pesticide.

ASPARTIC ACID: Antimorphinic; Neuroexcitant; Roborant.

ASTRAGALIN: Aldose-Reductase Inhibitor; Antileukemic; Expectorant; Hypotensive; Immunostimulant.

AUBERGENONE: Phytoalexin.

AURAPTEN: Antiaggregant; Spasmolytic.

AUREUSIDIN: Iodothyronine-Deiodinase Inhibitor.

AVENIN: Neuromyostimulant.

AVICULARIN: Aldose-Reductase Inhibitor; Antibiotic; Diuretic; Pesticide.

AZULENE: Antiallergic; Anti-inflammatory; Antiseptic; Antiulcer; Bactericide 500 ppm; Febrifuge; Pesticide.

BENZALDEHYDE: Allergenic; Anesthetic; Antipeptic; Antiseptic; Antispasmodic; Antitumor; Insectifuge 50 ppm; Motor Depressant; Narcotic; Nematicide; Pesticide; Sedative.

BENZOIC ACID: Allergenic; Anesthetic; Antiotitic; Antiseptic; Bactericide; Choleretic; Expectorant; Febrifuge; Fungicide; Insectifuge; Pesticide; Phytoalexin; Uricosuric; Vulnerary.

BENZYL-ALCOHOL: Allergenic; Anesthetic; Antiodontalgic; Antipruritic; Antiseptic; Pesticide; Sedative.

BENZYL-BENZOATE: Acaricide; Allergenic; Antiasthmatic; Antidysmenorrheic; Antispasmodic; Antitumor; Artemicide; CNS Stimulant; Hypotensive; Myorelaxant; Pediculicide; Pesticide; Scabicide.

BENZYL-ISOTHIOCYANATE: Allergenic; Antiasthmatic; Antimutagenic; Antineoplastic; Antitumor; Bactericide; Fungicide; Herbicide; Laxative; Pesticide.

BERGAPTEN: Antiapertif; Anticonvulsant; Antihistamine; Anti-inflammatory; Anti-jet-lag; Antileukodermic; Antimitotic; Antipsoriatic; Antitumor; Calcium Antagonist; Cancer Preventive 5–25 ug/ml; Clastogenic; DME Inhibitor; Hypotensive; Insecticide; Molluscicide; Mutagenic; Pesticide; Phototoxic; Piscicide; Spasmolytic.

BETA-BISABOLENE: Abortifacient; Antirhonoviral; Antiulcer; Antiviral.

BETA-CAROTENE: Allergenic; Androgenic; Anticarcinomic; Anticoronary 50 mg/man/2 days; Antihyperkeratotic; Anti-ichysthoyotic; Antileukoplakic; Antilupus 150 mg/man/day/2 mos; Antimastitic; Antimutagenic; Antioxidant; Antiozenic; Antiphotophobic 30–300 mg man/day; Anti-PMS; Antipsoriac; Antiradicular; Antistress; Antitumor; Antiulcer 12 mg/3xday/man/orl; Antixerophthalmic; Cancer Preventive 22 ppm; Immunostimulant 180 mg/man/day/orl; Mucogenic; Phagocytotic; Thymoprotective; Ubiquiot.

BETA-ELEMENE: Anticancer (Cervix).

BETA-EUDESMOL: Antianoxic; Antipeptic; CNS Inhibitor; Hepatoprotective.

BETA-IONONE: Anticariogenic; Antitumor; Bactericide; Cancer Preventive; Fungicide; Hypocholesterolemic; Nematicide.

BETA-MYRCENE: Cancer Preventive.

BETA-PHELLANDRENE: Expectorant.

BETA-PINENE: Allergenic; Flavor; Herbicide; Insectifuge; Pesticide.

BETA-SANTALENE: Anti-inflammatory.

BETA-SESQUIPHELLANDRENE: Antirhinoviral; Antiulcer; Pesticide.

BETA-SITOSTEROL: Androgenic; Anorexic; Antiadenomic; Antiandrogenic; Antiestrogenic; Antifeedant; Antifertility; Antigonadotrophic; Antihyperlipoproteinaemic; Anti-inflammatory; Antileukemic; Antimutagenic 250 ug/ml; Antiophidic 2.3 mg mus; Antiprogestational; Antiprostatadenomic; Antiprostatitic; Antitumor; Antiviral; Artemicide; Bactericide; Cancer Preventive; Candidicide; Estrogenic; Gonadotrophic; Hepatoprotective; Hypoglycemic; Hypolipidemic; Pesticide; Spermicide; Ubiquiot; Viricide.

BETA-SITOSTEROL-D-GLUCOSIDE: Antitumor; CNS Depressant; CNS Stimulant; Convulsant; Hypoglycemic; Spasmolytic.

BETA-SOLAMARINE: Antisarcomic; Antitumor.

BETAINE: Abortifacient; Antigastric; Antihomocystinuric; Antimyoatrophic; Bruchiphobe; Emmenagogue; Hepatoprotective; Lipotropic.

BETULINIC-ACID: Anticarcinomic; Anti-HIV; Anti-inflammatory; Antimelanomic; Antitumor; Antiviral; Cytotoxic.

BIOCHANIN-A: Antimutagenic; Antiprostatedenomic; Cancer Preventive; Estrogenic; Fungicide; Fungistat; Herbicide Safener; Hypocholesterolemic; Hypolipidemic; Pesticide; VAM Simulant.

BIOTIN: Antialopecic; Antidermatitic 3 mg/2x/day; Antiseborrheic 3 mg/2x/day.

BORNEOL: Analgesic; Antibronchitic; Anti-inflammatory; CNS Toxic; Febrifuge; Hepatoprotectant; Herbicide; Insectifuge; Nematicide; Pesticide; Spasmolytic.

BORNYL-ACETATE: Antifeedant; Bactericide; Expectorant; Insectifuge; Pesticide; Sedative; Spasmolytic; Viricide.

BORON: Androgenic 3 mg/man/day; Antiosteoarthritic; Antiosteoporotic 3 mg/man/day; Estrogenic 3 mg/man/day.

BOWMAN-BIRK INHIBITOR: Antinutrient; Antitrypsic; Antitumor; Cancer Preventive.

BROMELAIN: Antiaggregant; Antianginal 1,500 mg/day; Antiappetant; Antiarthritic; Antibronchitic; Anticellulitic; Antidysmenorrheic; Antidyseptic; Antiecchymotic; Antiedemic; Antiepisiotomic; Anti-infective; Anti-inflammatory; Antileukemic; Antimetastatic; Antiplaque; Antipneumonic; Antiprostaglandin; Antiradiation; Antisclerodermic; Antisinusitic; Antithrombophlebitic; Antithrombotic 60–800 mg; Antitumor; Antitussive; Antiulcer; Bactericide; Chemopreventive; Digestive; Emetic; Fibrinolytic; Hypotensive; Laxative; Lipolytic; Mucolytic; Myorelaxant; Nematicide; Pesticide; Proteolytic 400–600 mg/3xdaily/; Spasmolytic; Vermifuge; Vulnerary.

BULLATACINE: Antileukemic; Aphicide; Artemicide; Cytotoxic; Larvicide.

BULLATACINONE: Artemicide; Cytotoxic; Pesticide.

BUTYLIDENE-PHTHALIDE: Abortifacient; Anti-inflammatory; Antispasmodic; Emmenagogue; Spasmolytic.

BUTYRIC ACID: Anticancer; Bruchifuge; Nematistat 880 ug/ml; Pesticide.

BYAKANGELICIN: Antiestrogenic; Antigonadotropic.

CADAVERINE: Phytohormonal.

CADMIUM: Hypertensive; Lithogenic; Nephrotoxic.

CAFFEIC-ACID: Allergenic; Analgesic; Antiadenoviral; Antiaggregant; Anticarcinogenic; Antidedemic; Antiflu; Antigonadotropic; Antihemolytic 25 uM; Antihepatotoxic; Antiherpectic 50 ug/ml; Anti-HIV; Antihypercholesterolemic; Anti-inflammatory; Antimutagenic; Antinitrosaminic; Antioxidant; Antiperoxidant; Antiradicular 10 uM; Antiseptic; Antispasmodic; Antistomatitic; Antithiamin; Antithyroid; Antitumor; Anti-Tumor Promoter; Antiulcerogenic; Antivaccinia; Antiviral; Bactericide; Cancer Preventive; Cholagogue; Choleretic; Clastogenic; CNS Active; DNA Active; Diuretic; Fungicide; Hepatoprotective; Hepatotropic; Histamine Inhibitor; Insectifuge; Leukotriene Inhibitor; Lipoxygenase Inhibitor; Metal Chelatory; Ornithine-Decarboxylase Inhibitor; Pesticide; Prostaglandigenic; Sedative 500 mg; Spasmolytic; Sunscreen; Tumorigenic; Viricide; Vulnerary.

CAFFEINE: Analeptic 200 scu mus; Antiapneic; Antiasthmatic 5–10 mg/kg/orl/man; Anticarcinogenic; Antidermatic; Antiemetic; Antifeedant; Antiflu; Antiherpetic; Antihypotensive 250 mg/day/orl/man; Antinarcotic; Antiobesity; Antioxidant; Antirhinitic 140 mg/day/orl/man; Antiserotonergic; Antitumor; Antivaccinia; Antiviral; Cancer Preventive; Cardiotonic; Catabolic; Choleretic; CNS Stimulant; Diuretic; Ergotamine Enhancer; Herbicide; Hypertensive; Hypoglycemic; Insecticide; Neurotoxic; Pesticide; Respirastimulant; Stimulant; Teratogenic; Vasodilator; Viricide; Phosphodeiesterase Inhibitor.

CALCIUM: AntiPMS 1 g/day; Antiallergenic 500 mg/day; Antianxiety; Antiatherosclerotic 500 mg/day; Antidepressant; Antidote (Aluminum); Antidote (Lead); Antihyperkinetic; Anti-insomniac; Antiosteoporotic 500 mg/day; Antiperiodontitic 750 mg/day; Antitic; Hypocholesterolemic 500 mg/day; Hypotensive 1 g/day.

CAMPHENE: Antilithic; Antioxidant; Hypocholesterolemic; Insectifuge; Pesticide; Spasmogenic.

CAMPHOR: Abortifacient; Allelopathic; Analgesic; Anesthetic; Antiacne; Antiemetic 100–200 mg/man/orl; Antifeedant; Antifibrositic; Antineuralgic; Antipruritic; Antiseptic; Cancer Preventive; Carminative; CNS Stimulant; Convulsant; Counterirritant; Decongestant; Deliriant; Ecbolic; Emetic; Expectorant; Fungicide; Herbicide; Insectifuge; Irritant; Nematicide; Occuloirritant; Pesticide; Respirainhibitor; Respirastimulant; Rubefacient; Spasmolytic; Stimulant; Verrucolytic.

CANAVANINE: Allelochemic; Antifeedant; Antiflu; Antimetabolic; Antitumor; Antiviral; Bactericide; Cytotoxic; Fungicide; Herbicide; Juvabional; Lupus Generating; Mitogenic; Pesticide.

CAPRYLIC ACID: Candidicide 300 mg/man/12xday; Fungicide; Irritant; Pesticide.

CAPSAICIN: 5-Lipoxygenase Inhibitor; Analgesic; Anaphylactic; Anesthetic; Antiaggregant; Anticolonospasmic.

CAPSIDOL: Fungicide; Pesticide; Phytoalexin.

CARPAINE: Amebicide; Antitubercular; Antitumor; Bactericide; Cardiodepressant; Cardiotonic; CNS Depressant; Diuretic; Hypotensive; Paralytic; Pesticide; Respiradepressant; Trichuridiede; Vasoconstrictor; Vermicide.

CARPOSIDE: Anthelminthic; Antienteritic; Cardiac; Pesticide.

CARVACROL: AchE Inhibitor; Allergenic; Anesthetic; Anthelminithic; Antialzheimeran; Anticholinesterase; Antidiuretic; Anti-inflammatory; Antimelanomic; Antioxidant; Antiplaque; Antiradicular; Antiseptic; Bactericide; Carminative; Enterorelxant; Expectorant; Fungicide; Nematicide; Pesticide; Prostaglandin Inhibitor; Spasmolytic; Tracheorelaxant; Vermifuge.

CARVEOL: SNS Stimulant.

CARVONE: Allergenic; Antiseptic; Cancer Preventive; Carminative; CNS Stimulant; Insecticide; Insectifuge; Motor Depressant; Nematicide; Pesticide; Sedative; Vermicide.

CARYOPHYLLENE: Anticariogenic; Antiedemic; Antifeedant 500 ppm; Anti-inflammatory; Antitumor; Bactericide; Insectifuge; Pesticide; Spasmolytic; Termitifuge.

CARYOPHYLLEN OXIDE: Antiedemic; Antifeedant; Anti-inflammatory; Antitumor; Insecticide; Pesticide.

CASUARIN: Antiperoxidant; Lipoxygenase Inhibitor; Xanthine-Oxidase Inhibitor.

CATALASE: Antioxidant.

CATECHIN: Allelochemic; Antialcoholic; 2g/man/day; Antiarthritic; Anticariogenic; Antiedemic; Antiendotoxic; Antifeedant.

CATECHOL: 5-Lipoxygenase Inhibitor; Allelochemic; Allergenic; Antigonadotropic; Antioxidant; Antiseptic; Antistomatitic; Antithiamin; Antithyreotropic; Antiviral; Cancer Preventive; Convulsant; Dermatitigenic; Pesticide.

CELLULOSE: Hemostat.

CEPHALIN: Hemostat.

CHARANTIN: Abortifacient; Antidiabetic; Antitesticular; Hypoglycemic 50 mg/kg/orl/rbt.

CHAVICOL: Fungicide; Nematicide; Pesticide.

CHELIDONIC ACID: Antiwart; Irritant.

CHLORINE: Antiherpetic; Antiseptic; Bactericide; Candidicide; Fungicide; Pesticide; Viricide.

CHLOROGENIC ACID: Allergenic; Analgesic; Anti-EBV; Antifeedant; Antigonadotropic; Antihemolytic; Antihepatotoxic; Antiherpetic; Anti-HIV; Antihypercholesterolemic; Anti-inflammatory; Antimutagenic; Antinitrosaminic; Antioxidant; Antiperoxidant; Antipolio; Antiradicular; Antiseptic; Antithyroid; Anti-Tumor Promoter; Antiulcer; Antiviral; Bactericide; Cancer preventive; Cholagogue; Choleretic; Clastogenic; CNS Active; CNS Stimulant; Diuretic; Fungicide; Hepatoprotective; Histamine Inhibitor; Immunostimulant; Insectifuge;

Interferon Inducer; Juvabional; Larvistat; Leukotriene Inhibitor; Lipoxygenase Inhibitor; Metal Chelator; Ornithine-Decarboxylase Inhibitor; Oviposition Stimulant; Pesticide.

CHLOROPHYLL: Antidecubitic; Antihalitosic; Antimenorrhagic 25 mg/day/wmn/orl; Antimutagenic; Antioxidant.

CHOLINE: Antialzheimeran 5–16 g/man/day: Antichorcic; Anticirrhotic 6,000 mg/man/day; Anticystinuric; Antidiabetic; Antidyskinetic 150–200 mg.

CHROMIUM: Amphiglycemic; Antiatherosclerotic 20 ug/day; Anticorneotic; Antidiabetic; Antidote (Lead); Antiglycosuric; Antitriglyceride 20 ug/day; Hypocholesterolemic 20 ug/day; Insulinogenic.

CHRYSIN: Antiaggregant; Antiallergic; Antimutagenic; Antispasmodic; Antithrombic; Anxiolytic; Cancer Preventive; Cyclooxygenase Inhibitor; Fungicide; Myorelaxant; Pesticide; Termitifuge.

CHRYSOERIOL: Aldose-Reductase Inhibitor; Antimutagenic; Antirhinoviral; Antiviral; Cancer Preventive.

CICHORIC ACID: Antiflu; Antistomatitic; Antiviral; Immunostimulant 10–100 ug/ml; Pesticide; Phagocytotic 10–100 ug/ml; Viricide.

CICHORIIN: Antiaggregant; Antifeedant.

CINCHONINE: Antimalarial; Pesticide.

CINNAMALDEHYDE: Allelochemic; Allergenic; Antiaggregant; Antiherpetic; Antimutagenic; Antiulcer 500 mg/kg/orl; Antiviral; Cancer Preventive; Choleretic 500 mg/kg/orl; Chronotropic; Circulostimulant; CNS Depressant; CNS Stimulant; Cytotoxic; 5–60 ug/ml; Febrifuge; Fungicide; Herbicide; Histaminic; Hypoglycemic; Hypotensive; Hypothermic; Inotropic; Insecticide; Mutagenic; Nematicide; Pesticide; Sedative; Spasmolytic; Sprout Inhibitor; Teratogenic; Tranquilizer.

CINNAMIC ACID: Allergenic; Anesthetic; Anti-inflammatory; Antimutagenic; Bactericide; Cancer Preventive; Choleretic; Dermatitigenic; Fungicide; Herbicide; Laxative; Lipoxygenase Inhibitor; Pesticide; Spasmolytic; Vermifuge.

CINNAMIC-ACID-ETHYL-ESTER: Cancer Preventive.

CINNAMYL ALCOHOL: Allelochemic; Antimutagenic; Herbicide; Nematicide; Pesticide.

CIS-3,5,4'-TRIHYDROXY-4–ISOPENTENYLSTILBENE: Fungicide; Pesticide.

CITRAL: Allergenic; Antiallergic; Antihistamine; Antiseptic; Antishock; Bactericide; Bronchorelaxant; Cancer Preventive; Expectorant; Fungicide; Herbicide; Nematicide; Pesticide; Sedative; Teratogenic.

CITRANTIN: Antifertility; Contraceptive.

CITRIC ACID: Allergenic; Antiaphthic 20,000 ppm; Anticalculic; Anticoagulant; Antimutagenic; Antioxidant Synergist; Antiseborrheic; Antitumor; Disinfectant; Hemostat; Laxative; Litholytic; Refrigerant.

CINTRONELLAL: Allergenic; Antiseptic; Bactericide; Embryotoxic; Insectifuge; Motor Depressant; Mutagenic; Nematicide; Pesticide; Sedative; Teratogenic.

CITRONELLOL: Allergenic; Bactericide; Candidicide; Fungicide; Herbicide; Nematicide; Pesticide; Sedative.

CITRULLINE: Antiasthenic 180 mg/kg/day; Antihepatotic; Antiosteoporotic; Diuretic.

CNIDILIDE: Abortifacient; Anti-inflammatory; Emmenagogue; Fungicide; Pesticide; Spasmolytic.

COBALT: Cardiomyopathogenic; Erythrocytogenic.

COPPER: Antiarthritic; Antidiabetic 2–4 mg/day; Anti-inflammatory; Antinociceptive; Contraceptive; Hypocholesterolemic; Schizophrenic.

COREXIMINE: Antihypertensive; Respirastimulant.

CORILAGEN: ACE Inhibitor; Antiallergic; Antiasthmatic; Xanthine-Oxidase Inhibitor.

CORYDINE: Antitumor; Cardiodepressant; CNS Depressant; Hypnotic; Respirodepressant; Sedative.

COSMOSIIN: Aldose-Reductase Inhibitor; Bactericide; Candidicide.

COUMARIN: Allelochemic; Antiaggregant; Antiandrogenic; Antibrucellosic; Antiedemic; Anti-inflammatory; Antimelanomic; Antimitotic; Antimutagenic; Antisporiac; Antitumor; Bruchiphobe; Cancer Preventive; Cardiodepressant; DME Inhibitor; Emetic; Fungicide; Hemorrhagic; Hepatotoxic; Hypnotic; Hypoglycemic; Immunostimulant; Juvabional; Lymphocytogenic 100 mg/day; Ovicide; Pesticide; Phagocytogenic; Piscicide; Rodenticide; Sedative.

COUMESTROL: Antimicrobial; Estrogenic; Fungicide; Nematicide; Nemistat 5–25 ug/ml; Peroxidase Inhibitor; Pesticide; Phytoalexin.

CROCETIN: Antihypoxic; Antimutagenic; Choleretic 100 mg/kg; Hypocholesterolemic; Lipolytic.

CUCURBITACIN-B: Antihepatotoxic; Anti-inflammatory; Cancer Preventive; Cytotoxic.

CUCURBITACIN-E: Antigibberellin; Antihepatotoxic; Antitumor; Cytotoxic.

CUCURBITACIN-I: Anticarcinomic; Antileukemic.

CUCURBITAN: Antihelminthic; Pesticide; Schistosomicide.

CUMINALDEHYDE: Bactericide. Fungicide; Larvicide; Pesticide.

CYANIDIN: Allelochemic; Antioxidant; Pesticide; Pigment.

CYANIN: Antipolio; Antiviral; Emetic; Pesticide.

CYNARIN: Cholagogue; Choleretic 200–250 mg/3xday; Cholesterolytic; Diuretic; Hepatoprotective 100 mg/kg; Hyperemic; Hypocholesterolemic 500 mg/man; Hypolipidemic.

CYCLOALLIIN: Lachrymatory.

CYCLOARTENOL: Anti-inflammatory; Ubiquet.

CYSTEINE: Antiaddisonian; Anticataract; Anticytotoxic; Antiophthalmic; Antioxidant; Antitumor; Antiulcer; Cancer Preventive; Detoxicant; Ophthalmic Antialkalin; Pesticide.

CYSTINE: Adjuvant; Antihomocystinuric; Anticoagulant; Cancer Preventive; Cardiotonic; Vasoconstrictor.

D-AFZELECHIN: Allelopathic.

D-CATECHIN: Anticoagulant; Cancer Preventive; Cardiotonic; Vasoconstrictor.

D-LIMONENE: Anticancer (Breast); Antimelanomic; Anti-Tumor Promoter; Cancer Preventive; Hypochlosterolemic; Litholytic; Pesticide.

DAIDZEIN: Antialcoholic; Antiarrhythmic; Antidipsomanic 150 mg/kg/day; Antihemolytic; Anti-inflammatory; Antileukemic; Antimicrobial; Antimutagenic; Antioxidant; Antispasmodic; Coronary Dilator; Estrogenic; Fungicide; Hypotensive; Lipase Inhibitor; Spasmolytic.

DAIDZIN: Antialcoholic; Antidipsomanic 150 mg/kg/day; Antioxidant; Antispasmodic; Cancer Preventive; Estrogenic; Fungicide; Hypotensive; Lipase Inhibitor; Pesticide; Spasmolytic.

DAPHNORETIN: Anticarcinomic; Antitumor.

DAUCOSTEROL: Antileukemic; Antitumor; Hypoglycemic; Spasmolytic.

DECAN-1-AL: Cancer Preventive.

DELPHINIDIN: Allelochemic; Allergenic; Antioxidant; Cancer Preventive; Pesticide.

DELTA-3–CARENE: Allergenic; Anti-inflammatory; Bactericide; Dermatitigenic; Insectifuge.

DELTA-CADINENE: Anticariogenic; Bactericide; Pesticide.

DIALLYL-SULFIDE: Antimutagenic; Antitumor; Cancer Preventive (Esophagus) 200 mg/kg; Hypocholesterolemic; Occuloirritant; Pesticide.

DIALLYL-TRISULFIDE: Antiseptic; Hypocholesterolemic; Hypoglycemic; Insecticide; Larvicide; Pesticide.

DIAZEPAM: Amnesigenic; Anesthetic 1–40 mg/man; Antialcoholic; Anticonvulsant; Antiepileptic; Antimyocarditic; Antischizophrenic.

DIHYDROCAPSAICIN: Hypocholesterolemic.

DIMETHYL-DISULFIDE: Antithyroid.

DIOSGENIN: Antifatigue; Anti-inflammatory; Antistress; Estrogenic; Hypocholesterolemic.

DIOSMETIN: Aldose-Reductase Inhibitor; Antimutagenic; Antirhinoviral; Cancer Preventive.

DIOSMIN: Anti-Capillary Fragility 300 mg/2x/day/woman; Antihemorrhoidal; Anti-inflammatory; Antimetrorrhagic.

DIPENTENE: Antiviral; Bactericide; Expectorant; Pesticide; Sedative; Viricide.

DOPA: Antiparkinsonian.

DOPAMINE: Adreneric; Antilactagogue; Antimyocontractant; Antineurogenic; Antiparkinsonian; Antishock; Antithyreotropic; Cardiotonic; Hypertensive; Inotropic; Myocontractant; Neurotransmitter; Sympathomimetic; Teratogenic; Vasoconstrictor; Vasodilator.

ELEMICIN: Antiaggregant; Antidepressant; Antifeedant; Antihistamine; Antiserotonic; Antistress; DNA Binding; Hallucinogenic; Hypotensive; Insecticide; Insectifuge; Neurotoxic; Pesticide; Schistosomicide.

ELLAGIC ACID: ACE Inhibitor; Aldose-Reductase Inhibitor; Anti-HIV; Anticataract; Antimutagenic.

ELLAGITANNIN: Antiallergic; Anti-HIV; Antioxidant; Antitumor; Cardiotoxic; Immunostimulant; Interferon Stimulant; Rt Inhibitor.

EPICATECHIN: Allelochemic; Anticomplementary; Antidiabetic; Anti-EBV; Anti-inflammatory; Antileukemic; Bactericide; Hepatotropic; Pesticide.

EPSILON VINIFERIN: Fungicide; Pesticide.

ERIODICTYOL: Antifeedant; Cancer Preventive; Expectorant; Pesticide.

ERUCIC ACID: Antitumor.

ESCULIN: Antiarthritic; Anti-Capillary Fragility; Antidermatotic; Antifeedant; Antihistaminic; Anti-inflammatory; Antioxidant; Bactericide; Cancer Preventive; Cardiotonic; Choleretic; Diuretic; Expectorant; Hypertensive; Juvabional; Lipoxygenase Inhibitor; Pesticide; Sunscreen.

ESTRAGOLE: Antiaggregant; Cancer Preventive; DNA Binder; Hepatocarcinogenic; Hypothermic; Insecticide; Insectifuge.

ESTRONE: Aphrodisiac; Anti-impotency; Antimenopausal 0.7–2.8 mg/day/orl/wmn; Antiprostatadenomic; Antivaginitic; Estrogenic.

ETHANOL: Anesthetic; Antihydrotic; Antipruritic; Antiseptic; Bactericide; CNS Depressant; Hepatotoxic; Hypnotic; Hypocalcemic; Neurolytic; Pesticide; Rubefacient; Sclerosant; Teratogenic; Tremorilytic; Ulcerogenic.

ETHYL ACETATE: Antispasmotic; Carminative; CNS Depressant; Spasmolytic; Stimulant.

ETHYLENE: Anesthetic.

EUGENOL: Analgesic; Anesthetic; Antiaggregant; Anticonvulsant; Antiedemic; Antifeedant; Anti-inflammatory; Antimitotic; Antimutagenic; Antinitrosating; Antioxidant; Antiprostaglandin; Antiradicular; Antiseptic 3 ml/man/day; Antithromboxane; Antitumor; Antiulcer; Apifuge; Bactericide; Cancer Preventive; Candidicide; Carcinogenic; Carminative; Choleretic; CNS Depressant; Cytotoxic 25 ug/ml; Dermatitigenic; Enterorelaxant; Febrifuge 3 ml/man/day; Fungicide; Herbicide; Insecticide; Insectifuge; Irritant; Juvabional; Larvicide; Motor Depressant; Nematicide; Neurotoxic; Pesticide; Sedative; Spasmolytic; Trichomonistat; Trypsin Enhancer; Ulcerogenic; Vermifuge.

EUGENOL-METHYL-ETHER: Cancer Preventive; CNS Depressant; DNA Binding; Hypothermic; Myorelaxant.

EUPHOL: Abortifacient.

FALCARINDIOL: Analgesic; Bactericide; Fungicide; Pesticide; Phytoalexin.

FARNESOL: Antimelanomic; Nematicide; Juvabional; Pesticide.

FENCHONE: AchE Inhibitor; Antialzheimeran; Anticholinesterase; Counterirritant; Secretolytic.

FERULIC ACID: Allelopathic; Analgesic; Antiaggregant; Antidysmenorrheic; Antiestrogenic; Anti-inflammatory; Antimitotic; Antimutagenic; Antinitrosamine; Antioxidant 3,000 uM; Antioxidant; Antiserotonin; Antitumor; Anti-Tumor Promoter; Antiviral; Arteriodilator; Bactericide; Cancer Preventive; Candidicide; Cardiac; Cholagogue; Choleretic; Fungicide; Hepatotrophic; Herbicide; Hydrocholerectic; Immunostimulant; Insectifuge; Metal Chelator; Ornithine-Decarboxylase Inhibitor; Pesticide; Phagocytotic; Preservative; Prostaglandigenic; Spasmolytic; Sunscreen; Uterosedative.

FIBER: Antidiabetic; Antiobesity; Antitumor; Antiulcer; Cardioprotective; Cancer Preventive; Hypocholesterolemic; Hypotensive 10 g/man/day; Laxative.

FICIN: Anti-inflammatory; Dermatitigenic; Irritant; Pesticide; Proteolytic; Pruritogenic; Trichuricide; Vermifuge.

FISETIN: Antihistamine; Antimutagenic; Antioxidant; Antiviral; Cyclooxygenase Inhibitor; Iodothyronine-Deiodinase Inhibitor; Lipoxygenase Inhibitor; Oxidase Inhibitor; Pesticide.

FLUORIDE: Anticariogenic; Antiosteoporotic; Antiosteosclerotic.

FOLACIN: Antianemic 5–20 mg/man/day; Anticervicaldysplasic 8–30 mg/wmn/day/orl; Anticheilitic; Antidepressant; Antigingivititic 2–5 mg/day/man; Antiglossitic; Antimyelotoxic 5 mg/day/orl/man; Antineuropathic; Antiperiodontitic; Antiplaque; Antipsychotic; Anti-Spina Bifida; Hematopoietic; Uricosuric; Xanthine-Oxidase Inhibitor.

FORMALDEHYDE: Anesthetic; Anticystitic; Antiplantar; Antiseptic; Antiviral; Fungicide; Irritant; Neoplastic; Pesticide; Scolicide; Viricide.

FORMIC ACID: Antiseptic; Antisyncopic; Astringent; Counterirritant; Fungitoxic; Pesticide.

FORMONONETIN: Abortifacient; Antifeedant; Antiulcer; Cancer Preventive; Estrogenic; Fungicide; Herbicide Safener; Hypocholesterolemic; Hypolipidemic; Pesticide; VAM Stimulant.

FRIEDELIN: Anti-inflammatory 30 mg/kg; Diuretic.

FRUCTOSE: Antialcoholic; Antidiabetic; Antihangover; Antiketotic; Antinauseant; Neoplastic.

FUMARIC ACID: Acidulant; Antidermatatic; Antipsoriatic; Antihepatocarcinogenic; Antioxidant; Antitumor.

FURFURAL: Antiseptic; Fungicide; Insecticide; Pesticide.

GABA: Analeptic; Anticephalgic; Antichoreic 1–32 g/man/day; Anti-insomniac; Antitinnitic; Diuretic; Hypotensive 1–4 g/day; Neuroinhibitor; Neurotransmitter; Tranquilizer.

GALACTOSE: Sweetener.

GALLIC ACID: ACE Inhibitor; Antiadenovirus; Antiallergenic; Antianaphylactic; Antiasthmatic; Antibacterial; Antibronchitic; Anticarcinomic; Antifibrinolytic; Antiflu; Antihepatotoxic; Antiherpetic; Anti-HIV; Anti-inflammatory; Antimutagenic; Antinitrosaminic; Antioxidant; Antiperoxidant; Antipolio; Antiseptic; Antitumor; Antiviral; Astringent; Bacteristatic; Bronchodilator; Cancer Preventive; Carcinogenic; Choleretic; Cycloosygenase

Inhibitor; Floral Inhibitor; Hemostat; Immunosuppressant; Insulin Sparing; Myorelaxant; Nephrotoxic; Pesticide; Styptic; Viricide; Xanthine-Oxidase Inhibitor.

GAMMA-DECALACTONE: Cancer Preventive.

GAMMA-LINOLENIC ACID: Antiacne; Antiaggregant; Antialcoholic; Antiarthritic 540 mg/day; Antiatherosclerotic; Antieczemic; Antimenorrhagic; Anti-MS; Antiobesity; Anti-PMS; Antiprostatic; Antitumor; Hypotensive.

GAMMA-TERPINENE: Antioxidant; Insectifuge; Pesticide.

GENTISIC ACID: Analgesic; Antifeedant; Anti-inflammatory; Antirheumatic; Bactericide; Pesticide; Viricide.

GERANIAL: Bactericide; Pesticide.

GERANIIN: ACE Inhibitor; Adrenocorticotrophic; Antiallergenic; Antiasthmatic; Antiherpetic; Anti-HIV; Antihypertensive; Antilipolytic; Antiradicular; Antimutagenic; Antioxidant; Antiperoxidant; Antiradicular; Antiviral; Juvabional; Larvistat; Pesticide; Vasodilator; Viricide; Xanthine-Oxidase Inhibitor.

GERANIOL: Anticariogenic; Antimelanomic; Antiseptic; Antitumor; Bactericide; Cancer Preventive; Candidicide; Emetic; Fungicide; Insectifuge; Nematicide; Pesticide; Sedative; Spasmolytic.

GERMACRENE-D: Pesticide; Pheromone.

GLAUCINE: Adrenalytic; Antisuperoxidgogenic; Antitussive; Hypoglycemic; Hypotensive; Respiradepressant; Spasmolytic.

GLUCOSE: Acetylcholinergic; Antiedemic; Antihepatoxic; Antiketotic; Antivaricose; Hyperglycemic; Memory Enhancer.

GLUCURONIC ACID: Detoxicant.

GLUTAMIC ACID: Antalkaline 500–1,000 mg/day/orl/man; Antiepileptic Antihyperammonenic; Antilithic; Antiretardation; Anxiolytic; Neurotoxic.

GLUTAMINE: Antialcoholic 1,000 mg/man/day/orl; Antidepressant; Antisickling; Antiulcer 1,600 mg/man/day/orl.

GLUTATHIONE: Anticytoxic; Antidote (Heavy Metals); Antieczemic; Antihepatitic; Antioxidant; Cancer Preventive.

GLYCERIC ACID: Antalkaline 500–1,000 mg/day/orl/man; Antiepileptic; Antihyperammonenic; Antilithic; Antiretardation; Anxiolytic; Cholesterolytic; Diuretic; Hepatotoxic.

GLYCINE: Antiacid; Antialdosteronic; Antidote (Hypoglycin-A); Antiencephalopathic; Antigastric; Antiprostatic; Antipruritic; Antisickling; Antiulcer; Cancer Preventive; Neuroinhibitor; Uricosuric.

GLYCITEIN: Antioxidant; Cancer Preventive; Estrogenic; Fungicide; Pesticide.

GLYCOLIC ACID: Cholesterolytic; Diuretic; Hepatotonic; Irritant.

GOITRIN: Antithyroid; Goitrogenic.

GOLD: Antiarthritic; Antiulcer; Nephrotoxic.

GOSSYPETIN: Antimutagenic; Antioxidant; Bactericide; Lipoxygenase Inhibitor; Pesticide.

GOSSYPOL: Amebicide; Anaphrodisiac; Antibiotic; Antibiotic; Anticancer; Anti-Corpus Luteum; Antiencephalitic; Antiestrogenic; Antifeedant; Antifertility 30 mg/kg; Antiflu; Antiherpetic; Anti-HIV; Antimplantation; Antikeratitic; Antimalarial; Antioxidant; Antiprogesterone; Antiproliferant; Antirabies; Antispermatogenic; Antistomatitic; Antitestosterone; Antitumor; Antiviral; Avicide; Bactericide; Contraceptive (Male) 10 mg/man/day; Cytotoxic 25 uM; Fungicide; Hepatotoxic; Hypokalemic; Immunostimulant; Insectifuge; Interferon Inducer; Larvicide; Libidolytic; Mutagenic; Nematistant 125 ug/ml; Paralytic; Pesticide; Plasmodicide; Prostaglandigenic; Spermicide 0.2–100 uM; Trypanocide; Trypanosomicide; Tumorigenic; Viricide.

GUAIACOL: Anesthetic; Antidermatitic; Antieczemic; Antiesophagitic; Antiseptic; Antitubercular; Bactericide; Expectorant 0.3–0.6 ml/man; Insectifuge; Pesticide.

GUAIAZULENE: Antiallergic; Anti-inflammatory; Antileprotic; Antipeptic; Antipyretic; Antiulcer.

HCN: Antiasthmatic; Antidote (Amyl Nitrate); Antitussive; Bronchosedative; Insecticide; Pesticide; Respirastimulant; Rodenticide; Vasomotor Stimulant.

HARDWICKIC ACID: Antiseptic; Bactericide; Fungicide; Pesticide.

HERACLENIN: Anticoagulant; Anti-inflammatory.

HESPERIDIN: Antiallergenic; Antibradykinic; Anti-DNA; Antiflu; Anti-inflammatory 100 mg/kg; Antioxidant; Anti-RNA; Antistomatitic; Antivaccinia; Antiviral; Capillariprotective; Catabolic; Chlorectic; Pesticide; Vasopressor.

HESPERETIN: Antifeedant; Antilipidolytic; Bactericide; Cancer Preventive; Fungistatic; Hepatoprotective; Pesticide; Viricide.

HETEROSIDE-B: Choleretic; Hepatotonic.

HEXANAL: Pesticide.

HIGENAMINE: Antiarrhythmic; Antithrombic; Antitussive; Cardiotonic.

HISTAMINE: Antichilblain; Anti-Menière's; Antimigraine; Bronchostimulant; Cardiovascular; Gastrostimulant; Histaminic; Hypotensive; Myostimulan; Radioprotective; Secretogogue; Spasmogenic; Tachycardic; Vasodilator.

HISTIDINE: Antiarteriosclerotic; Antinephritic; Antioxidant; Antiulcer; Antiuremic.

HORDENINE: Antiasthmatic; Antidiarrheic; Antifeedant; Bronchorelaxant; Cardiotonic; Hepatoprotective; Pesticide; Vasoconstrictor.

HYDROQUINONE: Allelochemic; Allergenic; Antilithic; Antimalarial; Antimelanomic; Antimelasmic; Antimenorrhagic; Antinephritic; Antioxidant; Antipertussic; Antiseptic; Antithyreotropic; Antitumor; Astringent; Bactericide; Carcinogenic; Co-carcinogenic; Convulsant; Cytotoxic; Depigmentor; Emetic 1 g/orl; Herbicide; Hypertensive; Pesticide; Trypanosomicide.

HYDROXYPHASEOLIN: Fungicide; Pesticide.

HYDROXYPROLINE: Vulnerary.

HYOSCYAMINE: Analgesic; Anticholinergic 150–300 ug/4xday/man; Antidote (Anticholinesterase); Antiemetic; Antiherpetic; Antimeasles; Antimuscarinic; Antineuralgic; Antiparkinsonian; Antipolio; Antisialogogue; Antispasmodic; Antiulcer; Antivertigo; Antivinous; Bronchodilator; Bronchorelaxant; Cardiotonic; CNS Depressant; CNS Stimulant; Mydriatic; Pesticide; Photophobigenic; Psychoactive; Sedative; Spasmolytic; Viricide.

HYPERIN: Aldose-Reductase Inhibitor; Antihepatotoxic; Anti-inflammatory; Antioxidant; Antitussive; Antiviral; Capillarifortificant; Capillarigenic; Diuretic; Hepatoprotective; Hypotensive; Pesticide; Viricide.

HYPEROSIDE: Anti-Capillary Fragility; Antidermatitic; Antiflu; Anti-inflammatory; Antiviral; Bactericide 250–500 ug/ml; Cancer Preventive; Capillarifortificant; Capillarigenic; Diuretic; Hypotensive; Pesticide; Viricide; cAMP Inhibitor.

IMPERATORIN: Anti-Tumor Promoter; Antialopecic; Anticonvulsant; Anti-inflammatory; Antileukodermic; Antimutagenic; Antivitiligic; Calcium Antagonist; DME Inhibitor; Hepatotoxic; Molluscicide.

INDOLE: Anticariogenic; Bactericide; Cancer Preventive; Insectiphile; Nematicide.

INDOLE-3–ACETIC ACID: Allelochemic; Cancer Preventive; Herbicide; Hypoglycemic; Insulinase Inhibitor; Insulinotonic.

INDOLE-3–CARBINOL: Antitumor; Cancer Preventive.

INOSITOL: Antialopeic; Anticirrhotic; Antidiabetic; Cholesteroelytic 200 mg/man/day; Lipotropic.

INULIN: Antidiabetic; Immunostimulant.

IODINE: Acnegenic; Antigoiter; Antithyrotoxic; Dermatitigenic; Goitrogenic; Thyrotropic.

IRON: Antiakathisic; Antianemic; Anticheilitic; Antimenorrhagic 100 mg/day/wmn/orl.

ISOCHLOROGENIC ACID: Antioxidant; Antiseptic; Cancer Preventive; Pesticide.

ISOFERULIC ACID: Hypothermic.

ISOFRAXIDIN: Antileukemic; Antimalarial; Cancer Preventive; Choleretic.

ISOIMPERATORIN: Anti-Tumor Promoter; Artemicide; DME Inhibitor; Pesticide.

ISOLEUCINE: Antiencephalopathic; Antipellagric.

ISOLIQUIRITIGENIN: Aldose-Reductase Inhibitor; Antiaggregant; Antidepressant; Antidiabetic; Antiulcer; Cancer Preventive; MAO Inhibitor; Spasmolytic.

ISOORIENTIN: Larvistat; Pesticide.

ISOPIMPINELLIN: Antiappetant; Antifeedant; Anti-inflammatory 100 ppm; Antitubercular; Calcium Antagonist; Diuretic 125 mg/kg; Insecticide; Molluscicide; Mutagenic; Pesticide.

ISOQUERCITRIN: Aldose-Reductase Inhibitor; Antifeedant; Antioxidant; Bactericide; Cancer Preventive; Capillarigenic; Diuretic 10 ppm; Hypotensive; Insectiphile; Pesticide.

ISORHAMNETIN: Antihistaminic; Anti-inflammatory; Antioxidant; Bactericide; Cancer Preventive; Hepatoprotective; Pesticide; Spasmolytic.

ISORHAMNETIN-3-GLUCOSIDE: Hepatoprotective.

ISOVALERIC-ACID—ETHYL-ESTER: Cancer Preventive.

ISOVITEXIN: Antioxidant; Cancer Preventive.

JASMONE: Anticariogenic 800–1,600 ug/ml; Bactericide 800–1,600 ug/ml; Cancer Preventive; Insectiphile; Nematicide; Pesticide.

JUGLONE: Allelochemic; Antidermatophytic; Antifeedant; Antimenorrhagic 100 mg/day/wmn/orl; Antiparasitic; Antiseptic; Antitumor; Antiviral; Bactericide; Fungicide 500 ug/ml; Keratolytic; Pesticide; Sedative; Sternutatory.

KAEMPFERITRIN: Anti-inflammatory.

KAEMPFEROL: 5-Lipoxygenase Inhibitor; Antiallergic; Antifertility 250 mg/kg/60 days/orl; Antihistaminic; Anti-implantation; Anti-inflammatory 20 mg/kg; Antileukemic 3.1 ug/ml; Antilymphocytic; Antimutagenic; Antioxidant; Antiradicular; Antispasmodic; Anti-tumor Promoter; Antiulcer; Antiviral; Bactericide; cAMP-Phosphodiesterase Inhibitor; Cancer Preventive; Choleretic; Cyclooxygenase Inhibitor; Diaphoretic; Diuretic; HIV-RT Inhibitor; Hypotensive; Iodothyronine-Deiodinase Inhibitor; Lipoxygenase Inhibitor; Mutagenic; Natriuretic; Spasmolytic; Teratologic; Viricide.

KAEMPFEROL-3-GLUCOSIDE: Choleretic.

KAEMPFEROL-3-RHAMNOSIDE: Aldose-Reductase Inhibitor.

LACTIC ACID: Antileukorrheic; Antivaginitic; Antixerotic; Keratolytic.

LANOSTEROL: Cancer Preventive.

LECITHIN: Antialzheimeran 40–100 g/man/day/orl; Antiataxic; Anticirrhotic; Antidementic; Antidyskinetic 40–80 g/man/day/orl; Antieczemic; Antilithic; Antimanic; Antimorphinistic; Antioxidant Synergist; Antipsoriac; Antisclergermic; Antiseborrheic; Antisprue; Antitourette's 20–50 g/man/day/orl; Cholinogenic; Hepatoprotective; Hypocholesterolemic 20–30 g/man/day; Lipotropic.

LEPTINE: Antifeedant; Insecticide; Pesticide.

LEUCINE: Antiencephalopathic.

LEUCOANTHOCYANIN: Antioxidant.

LEVULOSE: Sweetener.

LIGNIN: Anticancer; Anticoronary; Antidiarrheic; Anti-HIV; Antinitrosamine; Antioxidant; Antiviral; Bactericide; Chelator; Hypocholesterolemic; Laxative; Pesticide; Viricide.

LIGNOCERIC ACID: Antihepatotoxic.

LIGUSTILIDE: Antiasthmatic; Spasmolytic.

LIMONENE: AchE Inhibitor; Allergenic; Antialzheimeran; Anticancer; Antiflu; Antilithic; Antimutagenic; Antitumor; Antiviral; Bactericide; Cancer Preventive; Candistat; Enterocontractant; Expectorant; Fungiphilic; Fungistat; Herbicide; Insecticide; Insectifuge; Irritant; Nematicide; Pesticide; Sedative; Spasmolytic; Viricide.

LIMONIN: Anticataleptic; Antifeedant; Antimalarial; Antileukemic; Pesticide.

LINALOOL: Allergenic; Antiallergenic; Anticariogenic; Antihistamine; Antiseptic; Anti-shock; Antiviral; Bactericide; Bronchorelaxant; Cancer Preventive; Candistat; Expectorant; Fungicide; Insectifuge; Motor Depressant; Nematicide; Pesticide; Sedative; Spasmolytic; Termitifuge; Anti-Tumor Promoter; Viricide.

LINALYL-ACETATE: Sedative; Spasmolytic.

LINARIN: Aldose-Reductase Inhibitor.

LINOLEIC ACID: Antianaphylactic; Antiarteriosclerotic; Antiarthritic; Anticoronary; Antieczemic; Antifibrinolytic; Antigranular; Antihistaminic; Anti-inflammatory; Antimenorrhagic; Anti-MS; Antiprostatic; Cancer Preventive; Carcinogenic; Hepatoprotective; Immunomodulator; Insectifuge; Metastatic; Nematicide.

LIRIODENINE: Analgesic; Antidermatophytic; Antitumor; Bactericide; Candidicide; Cytotoxic; Fungicide; Sedative.

LITHIUM: Antidepressant; Antihyperthyroid; Antimanic; Anti-PMS; Antipsychotic; Antischizophrenic; Deliriant; Nephrotoxic.

LUPEOL: Antirheumatic; Antitumor; Antiurethrotic; Cytotoxic 50–500 ppm.

LUTEOLIN: Aldose-Reductase Inhibitor; Anticataract; Antidermatic; Antifeedant; Antiherpetic; Antihistaminic; Anti-inflammatory; Antimutagenic; Antioxidant; Antipolio; Antispasmodic; Antitussive; Antiviral; Bactericide; Cancer Preventive; Choleretic; Deiodinase Inhibitor; Diuretic; Iodothyronine-Deiodinase Inhibitor; Spasmolytic; Xanthine-Oxidase Inhibitor.

LUTEOLIN-7–O-BETA-GLUCOSIDE: Cancer Preventive; Cholagogue.

LYCOPENE: Antioxidant; Antiradicular; Antitumor; Cancer Preventive.

LYSINE: Antialkalotic; Antiherpetic 1g/man/day; Hypoarginanemic; 250 mg/kg.

MAGNESIUM: Antiaggregant; Antianorectic; Antianxiety 400 mg/day; Antianginal 400 mg/day; Antiarrhythmic; Antiarthritic; Antiasthmatic; Antiatherosclerotic 400 mg/day; Anticonvulsant; Antidepressant; Antidiabetic 400 mg/day; Antidysmenorrheic 100 mg/4xday; Antiepileptic 450 mg/day; Antihyperkinetic; Antihypoglycemic; Anti-inflammatory 100 mg/4xday; Anti-insomniac; Antilithic; Antimastalgic; Antimigraine 200 mg/day; Antineurotic; Antiosteoporotic 500–1,000 mg/day/wmn/oral; Anti-PMS 400–800 mg/day/wmn/orl; Antispasmophilic 500 mg/day; Calcium-Antagonist; CNS Depressant; Hypocholesterolemic 400 mg/day; Hypotensive 260–500 mg/day; Myorelaxant 100 mg/4xday; Uterorelaxant 100 mg/4xday; Vasodilator.

MALIC ACID: Bacteristat; Bruciphobe; Hemopoietic; Laxative; Pesticide; Sialogogue.

MALTOSE: Sweetener.

MANGANESE: Antialcoholic; Antianemic; Antidiabetic; Antidiscotic; Antidyskinetic; Antiepileptic 450 mg/day; Antiotic.

MANNITOL: Allergenic; Anthelminthic; Antiglaucomic; Anti-inflammatory; Antimutagenic; Antinephritic; Antioxidant; Antiradicular; Anti-Reye's; Diuretic; Emetic; Laxative; Nephrotoxic; Pesticide; Spasmolytic.

MASLINIC ACID: Antihistaminic; Anti-inflammatory.

MAYSIN: Juvabional; Larvistat; Pesticide.

MEDICAGENIC ACID: Aphicide; Candidicide; Fungicide 7.5–25 ppm; Molluscicide 7.5–25 ppm; Pesticide.

MEDICAGOL: Fungicide; Pesticide.

MENTHOL: Analgesic; Anesthetic; Antiaggregant; Antiallergic; Antibronchitic; Antidandruff; Antihalitosic; Antihistaminic; Anti-inflammatory; Antineuralgic; Antiodontalgic; Antipruritic; Antirheumatic; Antiseptic; Antisinusitic; Bactericide; Bradycardiac 65 mg/3xday/woman; Bronchomucolytic; Bronchomucotropic; Bronchorrheic; Calcium Antagonist; Carminative; Ciliotoxic; CNS Depressant; CNS Stimulant; Congestant; Convulsant; Counterirritant; Decongestant; Dermatitigenic; Diaphoretic; Enterorelaxant; Expectorant; Gastrosedative; Myorelaxant; Nematicide; Neurodepressant; Neuropathogenic; Nociceptive; Pesticide; Refrigerant; Rubefacient; Spasmolytic; Vibriocide.

MENTHONE: Analgesic; Antiseptic; Cancer Preventive; Sedative; Spasmolytic.

METHIONINE: Anticataract; Antidote (Acetominaphen) 10 g/6hr/man/orl; Antidote (Paracetamol) 10 g/16 hr/man/orl; Antieczemic; Antihepatotic; Antioxidant; Antiparkinsonian 1–5 g/day; Cancer Preventive; Emetic; Essential; Glutathionigenic; Hepatoprotective; Lipotropic; Urine Acidifier 200 mg/3xday/man/orl; Urine Deodorant.

METHYL-GALLATE: Antileukemic; Antiseptic; Antitumor; Bactericide; Pesticide; Reverse-Transcriptase Inhibitor; Xanthine-Oxidase Inhibitor.

METHYL-SALICYLATE: Allergenic; Analgesic; Anti-inflammatory; Antipyretic; Antiradicular; Antirheumatalgic; Cancer Preventive; Carminative; Counterirritant; Dentifrice; Insectifuge.

MOLYBDENUM: Anticancer.

MUCILAGE: Cancer Preventive; Demulcent.

MYRCENE: Allergenic; Analgesic; Antimutagenic; Antinociceptive 10–20 mg/kg ipr mus; Antinociceptive 20–40 mg/kg scu mus; Antioxidant; Bactericide; Fungicide; Insectifuge; Pesticide; Spasmolytic.

MYRICETIN: Allelochemic; Antiallergenic; Antifeedant; Antigastric; Antigonadotrophic; Antihistamine; Anti-inflammatory; Antimutagenic; Antioxidant; Bactericide; Cancer Preventive; Candidicide; Diuretic; Hypoglycemic; Larvistat; Lipoxygenase Inhibitor; Mutagenic; Oxidase Inhibitor; Pesticide; Tyrosine-Kinase Inhibitor.

MYRISTIC ACID: Cancer Preventive; Nematicide.

MYRISTICIN: Amphetaminagenic; Anesthetic; Antiaggregant; Antidepressant; Anti-inflammatory; Antioxidant 25–100 mg/kg/orl; Antistress; Cancer Preventive 10 mg/mus/orl/day; Hypnotic; Hypotensive; Insecticide; Insecticide Synergist; MAO Inhibitor; Neurotoxic; Oxytoxic; Paralytic; Pesticide; Psychoactive; Sedative; Serotinergic; Spasmolytic; Tachycardiac; Uterotonic.

N-BUTYLPHTHALIDE: Anticonvulsant.

N-HENTRIACONTANE; Anti-inflammatory; Diuretic.

N-HEXACOSANE: Bacteristat; Pesticide.

N-METHYL-TYRAMINE: Cancer Preventive.

NARCOTINE: Analgesic; Antitussive; Sedative.

NARINGENIN: Aldose-Reductase Inhibitor; Antiaggregant; Antihepatotoxic; Antiherpetic; Anti-inflammatory 20 ppm; Antileukemic 10 ug/ml; Antimutagenic; Antioxidant; Antiperoxidant; Antispasmodic; Antiulcer; Antiviral; Bactericide 500 ug/ml; cAMP-Phosphodiesterase Inhibitor; Cancer Preventive; Choleretic; Decarboxylase Inhibitor; Fungicide; Fungistatic; Pesticide; Serotonin Inhibitor.

NARINGIN: Antidermatitic; Anti-inflammatory; Antioxidant; Antiviral; Cancer Preventive; Pesticide.

NEOANNONIN: Larvicide 72–70 ppm diet; Ovicide 62–70 ppm diet.

NERAL: Bactericide; Pesticide.

NEROL: Bactericide, Pesticide.

NIACIN: Antiacrodynic; Antiallergenic 50 mg/2xday; Antiamblyopic; Antianginal; Antichilblain; Anticonvulsant 3 g/day; Antidermatic; Antidysphagic; Anticleptic 3 g/day; Antihistaminic 50 mg/2x/day; Antihyperactivity 1.5–6 g/day; Anti-insomniac; Anti-Menière's; Antineuralgic; Antiparkinsonian 100 mg day; Antipellagric; Antiscotomic; Antispasmodic 100 mg/2xday; Antivertigo; Cancer Preventive; Hepatoprotective; Hypoglycemic; Hypolipidemic; Sedative; Serotenergic; Vasodilator.

NICKEL: Antiadrenaline; Anticirrhotic; Insulin Sparing.

NICOTINE: ANS Paralytic; ANS Stimulant; Antifeedant; Cholinergic; Dopaminigenic; Ectoparasitiede; Herbicide; Insecticide; Pesticide.

NICOTINAMIDE: Cancer Preventive; Depressant.

NOBILETIN: Antiallergic; Antihistamine; Antiproliferative; Cancer Preventive; Chloinergic; Fungicide; Fungistatic; Pesticide.

NODAKENIN: Antiaggregant.

NONACOSANE: Antimutagenic 250 ug/ml; Antiviral.

NOOTKATONE: Antiulcer.

NORADRENALIN: Adrenergic; Antishock; Hypertensive; Inotropic; Neurotransmitter; Sympathomimetic; Vasoconstrictor.

NORHARMAN: Tremorogenic.

O-CRESOL: Allelochemic; Antimutagenic; Antiseptic; Cancer Preventive; Pesticide; Rodenticide.

OBACUNONE: Anticataleptic; Antifeedant; Pesticide.

OCTACOSANOL: Antiviral; Hypolipidemic.

ODORIN: Bactericide; Pesticide.

OLEANOLIC ACID: Abortifacient; Anticariogenic; Antifertility; Antihepatotoxic; Anti-inflammatory; Antioxidant; Antisarcomic; Cancer Preventive; Cardiotonic; Diuretic; Hepatoprotective; Uterotonic.

OLEANIC-ACID-METHYL-ESTER: Hemolytic.

OLEIC ACID: Anemiagenic; Cancer Preventive; Choleretic 5 ml/man; Dermatigenic; Insectifuge; Percutaneostimulant.

OLEUROPEIN: Antiarrhythmic; Antihypertensive; Bacteristat; Coronary Dilator; Hypotensive; Spasmolytic; Vasodilator.

ORIENTIN: Anti-inflammatory; cAMP-Phosphodiesterase Inhibitor; Cancer Preventive.

ORNITHINE: Anticholesteremic; Antiencephalopathic; Hypoammonemic; Hyparginanemic.

OSTHOLE: Antimalarial; Juvabional; Pesticide.

OXYPEUCEDANIN: Antitumor Promoter; Calcium Antagonist; DME Inhibitor.

OXYPEUCEDANIN-HYDRATE: Calcium Antagonist.

P-AMINOBENZOIC ACID: Antineoplastic; Antirickettsial; Bactericide; Cancer Preventive; Choleretic; Lipoxygenase Inhibitor; Pesticide; Sunscreen.

P-COUMARIC ACID: Allelopathic; Antifertility; Antihepatotoxic; Antineoplastic; Antioxidant; Antiperoxidant; Antitumor; Bactericide; Cancer Preventive; Choloretic; Lipoxygenase Inhibitor; Pesticide; Prostaglandin-Synthesis Inhibitor.

P-CRESOL: Allelochemic; Antimutagenic; Antiseptic; Cancer Preventive; Parasiticide; Pesticide; Rodenticide.

P-CYMENE: Analgesic; Antiflu; Antirheumatalgic; Antiviral; Bactericide; Fungicide; Herbicide; Insectifuge; Pesticide; Viricide.

P-HYDROXYCINNAMIC ACID: Antioxidant.

P-HYDROXYBENZALDEHYDE: Antifeedant.

P-HYDROXYBENZOIC ACID: Antimutagenic; Antioxidant; Antisickling; Bactericide; Cancer Preventive; Fungistat; Immunosuppressant; Pesticide; Phytoalexin; Prostaglandigenic; Ubiquiot.

PALMITIC ACID: Antifibrinolytic; Hemolytic; Nematicide; Pesticide.

PANGAMIC ACID: Antifibrinolytic; Hepatoprotective.

PANTOTHENIC ACID: Antiallergenic; Antiarthritic; Anticephalagic; Anticlaudificant; Antidermatic; Antihypercholestorlemic; Antifatigue; Anti-ielus; Anti-insomniac; Antirheumatic; Cancer Preventive.

PARAFFIN: Antihemorrhoidal; Antiproctalgic; Emollient; Laxative 45 ml/day/orl/man.

PATULETIN: Cholagogue; Spasmolytic.

PECTIN: Antiatheromic 15 g/man/day; Antidiabetic 10 g/man/day/orl; Antidiarrheic; Antitumor; Antitussive; Antiulcer; Bactericide; Cancer Preventive; Demulcent; Hemostat; Hypocholesterolemic; Pesticide.

PECTINASE: Pectinolytic.

PELARGONIDIN: Antiherpetic; Antiviral; Cancer Preventive.

PELLETIERINE: Antithelminic; Cestodicine; Emetic; Hypertensive; Mydriatic; Oxyuricide; Pesticide; Taenicide.

PHASEOL: Fungicide; Pesticide.

PHASEOLLIN: Antiseptic 25 ug/ml; Fungicide; Pesticide.

PHELLANDRENE: Hyperthermic; Spasmogenic.

PHELLOPTERIN: Calcium Antagonist.

PHENETHYLAMINE: Insectifuge; Irritant; Pesticide.

PHENOL: Anesthetic; Anodyne; Antihemorrhoidal; Antihydrocoele; Anti-incontinence; Anti-MS; Antionychogryphotic; Antiotitic; Antioxidant; Antiprostatitic; Antipyruvetic; Antiseptic; Antisinustic; Antispastic; Antiviral; Antiwrinkle; Bactericide; Cancer Preventive; Carcinogenic; CNS Depressant; Emetic; Fungicide; Hemolytic; Pesticide; Rodenticide; Vasodilator; Viricide.

PHENYLALANINE: Anti-Attention Deficit Disorder 587 mg/day/orl; Antidepressant 50–500 mg/day/man; Antiparkinsonian 200–500 mg/day/man; Antisickling; Antivitiligic 100 mg/kg/day/orl/man; Monoamine Precursor; Tremorigenic 1,600–12,600 mg/man/day.

PHLORETIN: Antiallergic; Antifeedant; Bactericide 30 ppm; Lipoxygenase Inhibitor.

PHLORIZIN: Anticonvulsant; Antifeedant; Antimalarial; Glucosuric 100 ppm; Neuroparalytic; Pesticide; Sedative.

PHOROGLUCINOL: Antiseptic; Antitumor Promoter; Cancer Preventive; Decalcifier; Fungicide; Pesticide.

PHOSPHATIDYL-CHOLINE: Antialzheimeran 25 g/day/orl; Antimanic 15–30 g/man/day/orl.

PHOSPHORUS: Antiosteoporotic; Immunostimulant; Osteogenic.

PHYTIC ACID: Cancer Preventive.

PHYTOHAEMAGGLUTININ: Anticancer; Lectin.

PINENE: Antiseptic; Bactericide; Expectorant; Fungicide; Herbicide; Pesticide; Spasmogenic; Spasmolytic.

PIPERIDINE: CNS Depressant; Insectifuge; Pesticide; Spinoconvulsant.

PINITOL: Antidiabetic; Antifeedant; Expectorant; Insectifuge; Pesticide.

PIPERITONE: Antiasthmatic; Herbicide; Insectifuge; Pesticide.

PISATIN: Bactericide 50 ug/ml; Fungicide; Pesticide.

POTASSIUM: Antiarrhythmic; Antidepressant; Antifatigue; Antihypertensive; Cardiotoxic 18,000 mg/man/day; Spasmolytic.

PROPIONIC ACID: Fungicide; Pesticide.

PROTOCATECHUIC ACID: Antiarrhythmic; Antiasthmatic; Antihepatotoxic; Antiherpetic; Anti-inflammatory; Anti-ischemic; Antiophide; Antioxidant; Antiperoxidant; Antitussive; Antiviral; Bactericide; Fungicide; Immunostimulant; Pesticide; Phagocytotic; Prostaglandigenic; Ubiquiot; Viricide.

PRUNASIN: Cyanogenic.

PSORALEN: Antileukemic; Antileukodermic; Antimitotic; Antimutagenic; Antipsoriac; Antitubercular; Antitumor; AntiTumor Promoter; Antiviral; Artemicide; Bacteriophagicide; Calcium Antagonist; Cancer Preventive; Contraceptive; Cytotoxic; Fungicide; Genotoxic; Hypotensive; Mutagenic; Pesticide; Photocarcinogenic; Phototoxic; Phytoalexin; Viricide.

PTEROSTILBENE: Antidiabetic; Bactericide; Hyperglycemic; Hypoglycemic 10-50 mg/kg; Insecticide; Pesticide; Phytoalexin.

PUCHIIN: Bactericide; Pesticide.

PUFA: Antiacne; Antieczemic; Anti-MS; Antipolyneuritic.

PULEGONE: AchE Inhibitor; Antialzheimeran; Antihistaminic; Antipyretic; Avifuge; Bactericide; Cancer Preventive; Candidicide; Cerebrotoxic; Encephalopathic; Fungicide; Glutathionalytic; Hepatotoxic; Herbicide; Insecticide; Insectifuge; Nephrotoxic; Neurotoxic; Perfumery; Pesticide; Pulifuge; Pulmonotoxic; Sedative.

PUNICALAGIN: Anti-HIV; Pesticide.

PUNICALIN: Anti-AIDS; HIV-RT Inhibitor; Pesticide.

PYRIDOXINE: Antiacne; Antiaggregant; Antianemic 50–400 mg/man/day; Antiautistic; Anti-Carpal Tunnel 100–150 mg/day 12; Anticheilitic; Antidepressant; Antidermatitic; Antidiabetic; Antidote (Hydrazine) 10 g; Antidyskinetic 250–300 mg/man/4x/day; Antiemetic 20–200 mg/man/day; Antiepileptic; Antiglossitic; Antihyperkinetic; Anti-Morning Sickness; Antinephritic; Antineurotic 150 mg/man/day; Antioxaluric; Antiparkinsonian; Anti-PMS 100 mg/day/orl/wmn; Antiprolactin; Antiradiation; Antischizophrenic 50 mg/man/3x day; Antiseborrheic; Antisickling; Antiulcer; Antivertigo; Dopaminergic; Neurotoxic 2–6 g/day for 2–24 months.

PYROGLUTAMIC ACID: Antilipolytic; Insulinic.

QUERCETIN: 5–Lipoxygenase Inhibitor; Aldose-Reductase Inhibitor; Allelochemic; Allergenic; Antiaggregant; Antiallergic; Antianaphylactic; Antiasthmatic; Anticarcinomic (Breast); Anticataract; Anti-Crohn's 400 mg/man/3xday; Anticolitic 400 mg/man/3x/day; Antidermatic 400 mg/man/3x day; Antidiabetic; Antiencephalitic; Antiestrogenic; Antifeedant; Antiflu; Antigastric; Antigonadotropic; Antihepatotoxic; Antiherpetic; Antihistaminic; Antihydrophopbic; Antihypertensive; Anti-inflammatory; Antileukotrienic; Anti-Lipo-Peroxidant; Antimalarial; Antimutagenic; Antimyocarditic; Antioxidant; Antiperiodontal; Antipermeability; Antiperoxidant; Antipharyngitic; Antiplaque; Anti-PMS 500 mg/2xday/wmn; Antipodriac; Antipolio; Antiprostanoid; Antipsoriac; Antiradicular; Antispasmodic; Antithiamin; Anti-Tumor Promoter; Antiviral; ATPase Inhibitor; Bactericide; Bradycardiac; Calmodulin Antagonist; cAMP-Phosphodiesterase Inhibitor; Cancer Preventive; Capillariaprotective; Carcinogenic; Catabolic; Cyclooxygenase Inhibitor; Diaphoretic; Hepatomagenic; HIV-RT Inhibitor; Hypoglycemic; Insulinogenic; Juvabiol; Larvistat; Lipoxygenase Inhibitor; Mast-Cell Stabilizer; Mutagenic; Ornithine-Decarboxylase Inhibitor; Pesticide; Protein-Kinase-C Inhibitor; Spasmolytic; Teratologic; Tumorigenic; Tyrosine-Kinase Inhibitor; Vasodilator; Xanthine-Oxidase Inhibitor.

QUERCETIN-3–GALACTOSIDE: Anti-inflammatory.

QUERCETIN-3–O-BETA-D-GLUCOSIDE: Anti-inflammatory; Cancer Preventive.

QUERCETIN-3–RIIAMNOGLUCOSIDE: Anti-inflammatory; Choleretic; Diuretic; Spasmolytic.

QUERCITRIN: Aldose-Reductase Inhibitor; Antiarrhythmnic; Anticataract; Antiedemic; Antifeedant; Antiflu; Antihemorrhagic; Antihepatotoxic; Antiherpetic; Anti-inflammatory; Antimutagenic; Antioxidant; Antipurpuric; Antispasmodic; Antithombogenic; Antitumor; Antiulcer; Antiviral; Bactericide; Cancer Preventive; Cardiotonic; Choleretic; CNS Depressant; Detoxicant; Diuretic; Hemostat; Hepatotonic; Hypoglycemia; Hypotensive; Insectiphile; Paralytic; Pesticide; Spasmolytic; Vasopressor; Viricide.

QUINIC ACID: Choleretic.

RAPHANIN: Bactericide; Fungicide; Pesticide.

RESVERATROL: Artemicide; Bactericide; Fungicide; Hypocholesterolemic; Pesticide; Phytoalexin.

RETICULINE: Analgesic; Antidopaminergic; Bactericide; CNS Stimulant; Convulsant; Hyperthermic; Spasmolytic.

REYNOUTRIN: Aldose-Reductase Inhibitor.

RHOIFOLIN: Aldose-Reductase Inhibitor; Antiarrhythmic.

RIBOFLAVIN: Antiarabiflavinotic 2–10 mg/oral/day; Anti-Carpal Tunnel 50 mg/day; Anticataract 15 mg/day; Anticheilitic; Anticheilotic; Antidecubitic; Antiglossitic; Antikeratitic; Antimigraine; Antipellagric; Antiphotophobic; Cancer Preventive.

RIBONUCLEASE: Analgesic; Antiarthritic.

RIBONUCLEIC ACID: Antiasthenic; Antidementic; Memorigenic.

RICINOLEIC ACID: Carcinogenic; Spermicide.

RISHITIN: Pesticide; Phytoalexin.

ROSMARINIC ACID: AchE Inhibitor; Antianaphylactic 1–100 mg/kg orl; Anticomplementary; Antiedemic 0.316–3.16 mg; Antigonadotropic; Antihemolytic; Antihepatotoxic; Antiherpetic 50 ug/ml; Anti-inflammatory; Antileukotrienic; Antilipoperoxidant; Antioxidant; Antipulmonotic; Antiradicular; Antishock; Antithyreotropic; Antithyroid; Antiviral; Bactericide; Cancer Preventive; Deiodinase Inhibitor; Pesticide; Viricide.

RUTIN: Aldose-Reductase Inhibitor; Antiapoplectic; Antiatherogenic; Anti-Capillary Fragility 20–200 mg orl/man; Anticataract; Anticonvulsant; Antidermatitic; Antidiabetic; Antiedemic; Antierythemic; Antifeedant; Antiglaucomic 60 mg/day; Antihepatotoxic; Antiherpectic; Antihistaminic; Antihmaturic; Antihypertensive; Anti-inflammatory 20 mg/kg; Antimalarial; Antimutagenic; Antinephritic; Antioxidant; Antipurpuric; Antiradicular; Antithrombogenic; Antitrypanosomic 100 mg/kg; Anti-Tumor Promoter; Antivaricosity; Antiviral; Bactericide; Cancer Preventive; Capillariprotective; Catabolic; Estrogenic; Hemostat; Hypotensive; Insecticide; Insectiphile; Juvabional; Larvistat; Lipoxygenase Inhibitor; Mutagenic; Myorelaxant; Oviposition Stimulant; Pesticide; Phosphodiesterase Inhibitor; Spasmolytic; Vasopressor; Viricide.

S-ALLYL-CYSTEINE-SULFOXIDE: Antiatherogenic; Antioxidant; Antiperoxidant; Hypocholesterolemic; Lipolytic.

SAFROLE: Anesthetic; Antiaggregant; Anticonvulsant; Antiseptic; Bactericide; Cancer Preventive; Carcinogenic; Carminative; CNS Depressant; DNA Binder; Hepatoregenerative; Hypothermic; Nematicide; Neurotoxic; Pediculide; Pesticide; Psychoactive; Tremorigenic.

SAKURANETIN: Antiseptic; Bactericide; Fungicide; Pesticide.

SALICYLIC ACID: Analgesic; Antidermatotic; Anticirrhotic; Anticoronary; Antidandruff; Antidote (Mercury); Antieczemic; Anti-ichthyosic; Anti-inflammatory; Antikeshan; Antineuralgic; Antionychomycotic; Antioxidant; Antiperiodic; Antipodagric; Antipsoriac; Antipyretic; Antirheumatic; Antiseborrheic; Antiseptic; Antitumor; Antitympanitic; Bactericide; Cancer Preventive; Comedolytic; Cyclo-Oxygenase Inhibitor; Dermatitigenic; Febrifuge; Fungicide; Hypoglycemic; Insectifuge; Keratolytic; Pesticide; Tineacide; Ulcerogenic.

SCOLYMOSIDE: Choleretic.

SCOPOLETIN: Allelochemic; Analgesic; Antiasthmatic; Antiedemic; Antifeedant; Anti-inflammatory; Antileukotriengoenic; Antiseptic; Antitumor; Cancer Preventive; CNS Stimulant; Hypoglycemic; Hypotensive; Myorelaxant; Pesticide; Phytoalexin; Spasmolytic; Uterosedative.

SCUTELLAREN: Aldose-Reductase Inhibitor; Antihemolytic; Cancer Preventive; Phospholipase A1-Inhibitor.

SELENIUM: Analgesic 200 ug/day; Anorexic; Antiacne 200 ug/day; Antiaggregant; Anticirrhotic; Anticoronary 200 ug/day; Antidandruff; Antidote (Mercury); Antikeshan; Antileukotrienic; Antimyalgic 200 ug/day; Antiosteoarthritic; Antioxidant; Antiulcerogenic; Cancer Preventive; Depressant; Fungicide; Pesticide; Prostaglandin Sparer.

SELINENE: Expectorant.

SERINE: Cancer Preventive.

SEROTONIN: Abortifacient; Antiaggregant; Antialzheimeran; Antigastric; Antigastrisecretogogic; Bronchoconstrictor.

SESELIN: Fungicide; Pesticide.

SHIKIMIC ACID: Bruchifuge; Carcinogenic; Ileorelaxant; Mutagenic; Pesticide; Spasmolytic.

SILICON: Antiarteriosclerotic.

SILVER: Astringent; Bactericide.

SINAPIC ACID: Antihepatotoxic; Antioxidant; Bactericide; Cancer Preventive; Fungicide; Pesticide.

SINIGRIN: Cancer Preventive; Larvicide; Pesticide; Phagostimulant.

SOLAMARGINE: Antitumor; Cytotoxic; Erythrocytolytic; Fungicide; Hepatoprotective; Membranolytic; Pesticide.

SOLANIDINE: Antifeedant; Pesticide.

SOLANINE: Antiasthmatic; Antibronchitic; Antiepileptic; Antiparkinsonian; Cardiodepressant; Cardiotonic; Hemolytic; Memranolytic; Myostimulant; Narcotic; Sedative; Teratogenic.

SOLASODINE: Antiandrogenic 200 mg/kg; Anti-inflammatory; Antispermatogenic; Antitumor; Contraceptive; Cytotoxic; Fungicide; Hepatoprotective; Pesticide; Teratogenic.

SOLASONINE: Antitumor; Cardiodepressant; Cardiotonic; Erythroyctolytic; Hemolytic; Hepatoprotective; Insecticide; Memranolytic; Molluscicide; Myostimulant; Pesticide.

SORBITOL: Antidiabetic (Insuling Sparing) 30 g/man/day; Antiketotic; Cathartic; Diuretic; Laxative 5–15 g/man/day; Purgative.

SPIRAEOSIDE: Aldose-Reductase Inhibitor.

SQUALENE: Antitumor; Bactericide; Cancer Preventive; Immunostimulant; Lipoxygenase Inhibitor; Pesticide.

SQUAMOCIN: Cytotoxic; Larvicide; Ovicide.

STACHYDRINE: Cardiotonic; Emmenagogue; Insectifuge; Lactagogue; Oxytocic; Systolic Depressant.

STARCH: Absorbent; Antidote (Iodine); Antinesidioblastosic; Emollient; Poultice.

STIGMASTEROL: Antihepatotoxic; Anti-inflammatory; Antiophidic; Antiviral; Artemicide; Cancer Preventive; Estrogenic; Hypocholesterolemic; Ovulant; Sedative; Viricide.

SUCCINIC ACID: Antifeedant; Bruchiphobe; Cancer Preventive; Pesticide.

SUCROSE: Aggregant; Antihiccup 1 tsp; Antiopthalmic; Antioxidant; Atherogenic; Flatugenic; Hypercholesterolemic.

SULFUR: Acarifuge; Antiacne; Antidandruff; Antigrey; Antiseborrheic; Antiseptic; Comedogenic; Keratolytic; Laxative; Triglycerolytic; Uricogenic; Vulnerary.

SYNEPHRINE: Cancer Preventive.

SYRINGALDEHYDE: Antidemic; Anti-inflammatory; Cancer Preventive.

SYRINGIN: Adaptogenic; Antistress; Immunostimulant; Neurotropic; Tonic.

TANGERETIN: Antiallergic; Antihistaminic; Antiproliferative; Cancer Preventive.

TANNIN: Antidiarrheic; Antidysenteric; Antimutagenic; Antinephritic; Antiophidic; Antioxidant; Antiradicular 500 mg/kg/da/orl; Antirenitic; Antiviral; Bactericide; Cancer Preventive; Hepatoprotective; Immunosuppressant; Pesticide; Psychotropic; Viricide.

TARTARIC ACID: Acidifier; Antioxidant; Synergist.

TERPINEN-4–OL: Antiallergic; Antiasthmatic; Antiseptic; Antitussive; Bacteriostatic; Diuretic; Fungicide; Herbicide; Insectifuge; Nematicide; Pesticide; Spermicide; Vulnerary.

TERPINOLENE: Deodorant; Fungicide; Pesticide.

TETRAMETHYLPYRAZINE: Antiaggregant; Antianginal; Anticholinergic; Antidecubitic; Antideliriant; Antidysmenorrheic; Antiembolic; Antiencephalopathic; Antifatigue; Antigastritic; Antiheartburn; Antiherpetic; Antihistaminic 1 mg/kg; Antihypertensive; Antimigraine; Antimyocarditic; Antineuropathic 50 mg; Antipolio; Arteriodilator; Bactericide;

Cardiotonic; Diuretic; Hypotensive; Insectifuge 75–150 mg/man/day; Pesticide; Schisto-somidice; Spasmolytic; Uterosedative.

THIAMIN: Analgesic 1–4 g/day; Antialcoholic; Antialzheimeran 100–3,000 mg/day; An-tianorectic; Antibackache 1–4 g/day; Antiberiberi; Anticardiospasmic; Anticolitic; Antide-cubitic; Antideliriant; Antiencephalopathic; Antiheartburn; Antiherpetic; Antimigraine; Antimyocarditic; Antineurasthenic; Antineuritic; Antipoliomyelitic; Insectifuge 75–150 mg/man/day; Pesticide.

THYMOL: AchE Inhibitor; Anesthetic; Anthelminthic; Antiacne; Antiaggregant; An-tialzheimeran; Antibronchitic; Antihalitosic; Antiherpetic; Anti-inflammatory; Antimela-nomic; Antineuritic; Antioxidant; Antiplaque; Antiradicular; Antirheumatic; Antiseptic; Antispasmodic; Antitussive; Bactericide; Carminative; Counterirritant; Dentifrice; Deodor-ant; Dermatitigenic; Enterorelaxant; Expectorant; Fungicide; Gastroirritant; Larvicide; My-orelaxant; Pesticide; Spasmolytic; Sprout Inhibitor; Tracheorelaxant; Urinary Antiseptic; Vermicide.

THREONINE: Antioxidant; Antiulcer.

TIN: Antiacne; Bactericide; Pesticide; Taenicide.

TOLUENE: Encephalopathic.

TOMATIDINE: Antifeedant; Pesticide.

TOMATINE: Anti-inflammatory; Bactericide; Fungicide; Molluscicide; Pesticide.

TRANS-BETA-FARNESENE: Insectifuge; Pesticide; Pheromone.

TRANS-FERULIC ACID: Antioxidant; Cancer Preventive.

TRANS-ISOASARONE: Bactericide; Bronchospasmolytic; Pesticide; Secretolyic.

TRIACONTANAL: Antihepatotoxic; Hormone; Hypolipidemic.

TRICIN: Antileukemic 6–12 mg/kg; Antioxidant; Antitumor; Estrogenic.

TRIGONELLINE: Anticancer; Antihyperglycemic; Antimigraine; Antiseptic; Hypocholes-terolemic; Hypoglycemic 500–3,000 mg/man/day; Pesticide.

TRIFOLIN: Aldose-Reductase Inhibitor.

TRYPTAMINE: Hypertensive; Vasopressor.

TRYPTOPHAN: Analgesic 750 mg/4xday/orl/man; Antianxiety 500-1,000 mg/meal; Anti-depressant 1–3 g/3xday/orl/man; Antidyskinetic 2–8 g/orl/wmn/day; Antihypertensive; Anti-insomniac 1–3 g/day; Antimanic 12 g/man/day/orl; Antimenopausal 6 g/day; An-timigraine 500 mg/man/4xday; Antioxidant; Antiparkinsonian 2 g/3xday; Antiphenylke-tonuric; Antipsychotic 12 g/man/day; Antirheumatic; Carcinogenic; Hypnotic; Hypoglycemic; Hypotensive 3 g/day; Insulinase Inhibitor; Insulinotonic; Monoamine Pre-cursor; Prolactinogenic; Sedative 3–10 g/man/day; Serotonigenic 6–12 g/day/orl/man.

TUBEROSIN: Antistaphylococcic; Antitubercular; Bactericide; Fungicide; Pesticide.

TULIPOSIDE-A: Antiallergic.

TYRAMINE: Adrenergic; Antiaggregant; Insectifuge; Pesticide; Vasopressor.

TYROSINASE: Antihypertensive.

TYROSINE: Antidepressant; Antiencephalopathic; Antiparkinsonian 100 mg/kg/day; Antipheylketonuric; Antiulcer; Cancer Preventive; Monoamine Precursor.

UBIQUINONE-10: Anticardotic; Cardioprotective.

UMBELLIFERONE: Allelochemic; Antihistaminic; Anti-inflammatory; Antimitotic; Antimutagenic; Antiprostaglandin; Antiseptic; Antispasmodic; Bactericide; Cancer Preventive; Choleretic; Fungicide; Lipoxygenase Inhibitor; Pesticide.

URSOLIC ACID: Antiarthritic; Anticholestatic 28–100 mg/kg orl; Antidiabetic; Antiedemic; Antihepatotoxic 5–20 mg/kg; Antihistaminic; Anti-inflammatory; Antileukemic; Antimutagenic; Antiobesity; Antioxidant; Antitumor; Anti-Tumor Promoter; Antiulcer; Cancer Preventive; Choleretic 5–20 mg/kg orl; CNS Depressant; Cytotoxic; Diuretic; Hepatoprotective; Hypoglycemic; Pesticide; Piscicide; Potassium Sparing; Prostisticide; Sodium Sparing.

UVAOL: Antitumor; Cytotoxic 100–200 ppm.

VALERIANIC ACID: Spasmolytic.

VALINE: Antiencephalopathic.

VANADIUM: Antiatherosclerotic; Anti-infertility; Antimanic; ATPase Inhibitor; Cancer Preventive; Cardioprotective; Hypocholesterolemic.

VANILLIC ACID: Anthelminthic; Antifatigue; Antioxidant; Antisickling; Ascaricide; Bactericide; Cancer Preventive; Choleretic; Immunosuppressant; Laxative; Pesticide; Ubiquiot.

VANILLIN: Allelochemic; Antimutagenic; Antipolio; Antiviral; Cancer Preventive; Fungicide; Immunosuppressant; Insectifuge; Irritant; Pesticide.

VERBASCOSIDE: Antiseptic; Antitumor; Bactericide; Immunosuppressant; Pesticide.

VICENIN-2: Anti-inflammatory.

VITEXIN: Aldose-Reductase Inhibitor; Antiarrhythmic; Antibradinquinic; Antidermatic; Antihistaminic; Anti-inflammatory; Antiserotoninic; Antithyroid; cAMP-Phosphodiesterase Inhibitor; Cancer Preventive; Goitrogenic; Hypotensive; Thyroid-Peroxidase Inhibitor.

XANTHOPHYLL: Bruchifuge; Insectifuge; Pesticide.

XANTHOTOXIN: Antidermatitic; Antifeedant; Antihistaminic; Anti-inflammatory 20 mg/man/day; Antikerato, Antileucodermic; Antilymphomic 600 ug/kg; Antimitotic 5–25 ug/ml; Antimutagenic; Antimycotic; Antipityriasic; Antipruritic; Antipsoriac; Antiscleromyxoedemic; Antispasmodic; Anti-Tumor Promoter; Antivitligic 20 mg/man/day; Artemicide; Bactericide; Bufocide; Calcium Antagonist; Cancer Preventive; Cytotoxic; Dermatitigenic; Emetic; Fungistat; Herbicide; Hypertrichotic; Insectiside; Pesticide; Phytoalexin; Spasmolytic.

XANTHOTOXOL. Antihistaminic; Antinicotinic; Cancer Preventive.

XANTHOXYYLETIN: Anticonvulsant.

XANTHYLETIN: DME Inhibitor.

XYLITOL: Anticarcinogenic; Antiplaque; Diuretic; Hepatoprotective; Hyperuricemic; Laxative; Sweetener.

XYLOSE: Antidiabetic; Diagnostic.

Z-LIGUSTILIDE: Antiasthmatic; Spasmolytic.

ZEATIN: Mitotic.

ZINC: Antiacne; Antiacrodermatitic 8–34 mg/day/orl/chd; Antialopecie; Antianorexic; Antiarthritic 50 mg/3x/day/orl/man; Anticanker 100 mg/day; Anticataract 30 mg/day; Anticoeliac; Anticold 50 mg; Anticolitic; Anti-Crohn's; Antidandruff; Antidote (Cadmium); Antieczemic; Antiencephalopathic; Antiepileptic 100 mg/day; Antifuruncular 45 mg/3x/day; Antiherpetic 25 mg/day; Anti-impotency; Anti-infective 50 mg/day; Anti-infertility 60 mg/day; Anti-insomniac; Antilepric; Antiplaque; Antiprolactin; Antiprostatic 50 mg/man/day/orl; Antirheumatic; Antistomatic 50 mg/man/3x/day; Antitinnitic 60–120 mg/day; Antiulcer 50 mg/3x/day/man; Antiviral; Astringent; Deodorant; Immunostimulant; Immunosuppressant 300 mg/day/6 weeks/orl/man; Mucogenic; Pesticide; Spermigenic 60 mg/day; Testosteronigenic 60 mg/day; Trichomonicide; Vulnerary.

Fruit Phytochemicals

Phytochemicals are as important if not more important, than vitamins, minerals, and enzymes. Each fruit and vegetable has from several dozen to nearly 200 different phytochemicals. Each of these phytochemicals has the capacity to prevent cancer, kill viruses and bacteria, stimulate the immune system, and cleanse and rebuild our bodies. Some plants, such as broccoli, soy beans, cabbage, cauliflower, kale, and mustard greens have multiple anticancer phytochemicals. You can construct a meal plan or juice therapy that would contain the most beneficial anticancer phytochemicals in dosages that have therapeutic benefit.

APPLE

Chemicals in *Malus domestica BORKH.* (*Rosaceae*)—Apple

D-GLUCITOL Plant
1,3,3-TRIMETHYL-DIOXA-2,7-
  BICYCLO(2,2,1)HEPTANE Fruit
1-BUTANOL Plant
1-DECYL-ACETATE Plant
1-MONO-LINOLEIN Seed
1-NONYL-ACETATE Plant
1-OCTYL-ACETATE Plant
19-HYDROXYURSOLIC-ACID Plant
19-HYDROXYURSONIC-ACID Plant

2,4-METHYLENE-CHOLESTEROL Pollen or
  Spore
2-BUTANOL Plant
2-HEPTANOL Plant
2-HEXENAL Plant
2-METHYL-2,3-EPOXY-PENTANE Fruit
2-METHYL-BUT-2-EN-1-AL Fruit
2-METHYL-BUT-3-EN-1-OL Fruit
2-METHYL-BUTAN-2-OL Plant
2-METHYL-PENTAN-2-OL Plant
2-METHYL-PROPEN-1-AL Fruit
2-PENTANOL Plant
2-PHENETHYLACETATE Plant
2-PROPANOL Plant

ppm = parts per million

tr = trace

20-HYDROXYURSOLIC-ACID Plant

3,4-BENZOPYRENE Fruit

3-BETA-19-ALPHA-DIHYDROXY-2-OXO-URS-12-EN-28-OIC-ACID Wood 1,000 ppm

3-HYDROXY-OCTYL-BETA-D-GLUCOSIDE Fruit

3-PENTANOL Plant

4-HYDROXYMETHYLPROLINE Plant

5,6-EPOXY-10'-APO-5,6-DIHYDRO-BETA-CAROTENE-3,10'-DIOL Plant 20,000 ppm

6-METHYL-HEPTEN-5-EN-2-ONE Fruit

7-HEXANOIC-ACID Plant

ABSCISIC-ACID Fruit

ACETALDEHYDE Plant

ACETIC-ACID Plant

ACETIC-ACID-AMYL-ESTER Plant

ACETONE Plant

ADENINE Root

ALANINE Fruit 70–435 ppm

ALPHA-ALANINE Fruit

ALPHA-AMINO-BUTYRIC-ACID Plant

ALPHA-LINOLENIC-ACID Fruit 180–1,120 ppm

ALPHA-OXOGLUTARIC-ACID Plant

ALPHA-TOCOPHEROL Fruit 2–37 ppm

ALUMINUM Fruit 0.4–129 ppm

AMMONIA(NH3) Fruit Epidermis 235–1,029 ppm

AMYGDALIN Seed 6,000–13,800 ppm

AMYL-ACETATE Plant

AMYL-BUTYRATE Plant

AMYL-PROPIONATE Plant

ANILINE Fruit 1.5 ppm Fruit Epidermis 1.7 ppm

ARABINOSE Plant

ARGININE Fruit 60–373 ppm

ARSENIC Fruit 0.001–0.43 ppm

ASCORBIC-ACID Fruit 20–402 ppm

ASCORBIDASE Plant

ASH Fruit 2,300–43,000 ppm

ASPARAGINE Fruit 171 ppm

ASPARTIC-ACID Fruit 210–2,115 ppm

AVICULARIN Fruit

BARIUM Fruit 0.22–8.6 ppm

BENZOIC-ACID Plant

BENZYL-ACETATE Plant

BENZYL-AMINE Fruit 0.3–3 ppm Fruit Epidermis 0.6 ppm

BETA-ALANINE Fruit

BETA-CAROTENE Fruit 76 ppm

BIOTIN Plant

BORON Fruit 1–110 ppm

BROMINE Fruit

BUTANOL Plant

BUTYL-ACETATE Plant

BUTYL-BUTYRATE Plant

BUTYL-CAPROATE Plant

BUTYL-PROPIONATE Plant

BUTYL-VALERIANATE Plant

CADMIUM Fruit 0.002–0.026 ppm

CAFFEETANNIN Plant

CAFFEIC-ACID Fruit 85–1,270 ppm

CALCIUM Fruit 43–570 ppm

CALCIUM-OXALATE Plant

CAPROALDEHYDE Plant

CAPROIC-ACID-AMYL-ESTER Plant

CAPRYLIC-ESTER Plant

CARBOHYDRATES Fruit 152,250–948,550 ppm

CAROTENOIDS Plant 126 ppm

CATALASE Plant

CHLOROGENIC-ACID Fruit

CHLOROPHYLL Fruit 1 ppm

CHROMIUM Fruit 0.005–0.3 ppm

CIS-2,TRANS-4-ABSCISIC-ACID Bark

CIS-N-HEX-3-EN-1-OL Plant

CITRAMALIC-ACID Plant

CITRIC-ACID Plant

COBALT Fruit 0.005–0.043 ppm

COPPER Fruit 0.24–4 ppm

COUMARIC-ACID Plant

CREATINE Shoot

CUTIN Fruit Epidermis

CYANIDIN Leaf

CYANIDIN-3,5-DIGLUCOSIDE Cotyledon

CYANIDIN-3-ARABINOSIDE Plant

CYANIDIN-3-GALACTOSIDE Plant

CYANIDIN-7-ARABINOSIDE Plant

CYSTINE Plant 30–187 ppm

D-2-METHYLBUTAN-1-OL Plant

D-CATECHIN Fruit

D-GALACTURONIC-ACID Plant 13–54 ppm

D-GLUCONIC-ACID Plant

D-L-NONACOSANOL Plant

DECENOIC-ACID Plant

DEHYDROASCORBIC-ACID Plant

DIASTASE Plant

DIETHYL-AMINE Fruit 3 ppm

DIGALACTOSYL-DIGLYCERIDE Fruit 49–107 ppm

DIHYDROXYTRICARBALLYLIC-ACID Fruit 1 ppm

DIPHOSPHATIDYL-GLYCEROL Fruit 4–6 ppm

EO Fruit 25–35 ppm

ESTRAGOLE Essential Oil

ESTRONE Seed 0.1–0.13 ppm

ETHANOL Plant

ETHYL-ACETATE Plant

ETHYL-AMINE Fruit 3 ppm

ETHYL-BUTYRATE Plant

ETHYL-CAPROATE Plant

ETHYL-CROTONATE Plant

ETHYL-DECENOATE Plant

ETHYL-DODECANOATE Plant

ETHYL-HEXANOATE Plant

ETHYL-ISOBUTYRATE Plant

ETHYL-METHYLBUTYRATE Plant

ETHYL-NONANOATE Plant

ETHYL-OCTANOATE Plant

ETHYL-PENTANOATE Plant

ETHYL-PHENACETATE Plant

ETHYL-PROPIONATE Plant

ETHYL-VALERIANATE Plant

FARNESENE Fruit Epidermis

FAT Fruit 3,210–34,200 ppm Seed 180,000–230,000 ppm

FERULIC-ACID Fruit 4–95 ppm

FIBER Fruit 5,200–131,000 ppm

FLUORINE Fruit 0.1–2.1 ppm

FOLACIN Fruit 0.02–0.2 ppm

FORMIC-ACID Plant

FR Plant

FRUCTOSE Fruit 50,100–60,800 ppm

FUMARIC-ACID Plant

GALACTANASE Plant

GALACTARIC-ACID Plant

GAMMA-GUANIDINOBUTRAMIDE Shoot

GAMMA-GUANIDINOBUTYRIC-ACID Shoot

GAMMA-GUANIDINOPROPIONIC-ACID Shoot

GAMMA-METHYL-PROLINE Plant

GERANIOL Plant

GLUCOCEREBROSIDE Plant 34–49 ppm

GLUCOSE Fruit 17,200–18,200 ppm

GLUTAMIC-ACID Fruit 156–1,244 ppm

GLUTAMINE Plant 20 ppm

GLYCERIC-ACID Plant

GLYCINE Plant 80–497 ppm

GLYCOLIC-ACID Plant

GLYOXYLIC-ACID Plant

GUANIDINE Shoot

GUANIDINOACETIC-ACID Shoot

GUANIDINOSUCCINIC-ACID Shoot

HEMICELLULOSE Plant

HEPTACOSANE Plant

HEPTENOIC-ACID Plant

HEXACOSANOL Plant

HEXANOL Plant

HEXYL-ACETATE Plant

HEXYL-BUTYRATE Plant

HEXYL-FORMATE Plant

HISTIDINE Fruit 30–187 ppm

HYDROXYCINNAMIC-ACID Fruit 1,340 ppm

HYPERIN Plant

HYPEROSIDE Fruit

I-BUTYL-OCTANOATE Plant

I-BUTYL-PROPIOANTE Plant

I-DECANOIC-ACID Plant

I-HEXANOIC-ACID Plant

I-PENTANOIC-ACID Plant

I-PENTANOL Plant

I-PENTYL-FORMATE Plant

I-PENTYL-I-PENTANOATE Plant

I-PROPANOL Plant

IDAEIN Plant

INDOLE-3-ACETIC-ACID Plant

INOSITOL Plant

IODINE Plant

IRON Fruit 1.1–123 ppm

ISOAMYL-BUTYRATE Plant

ISOAMYL-PROPIONATE Plant

ISOBUTYL-ACETATE Plant

ISOBUTYL-BUTYRATE Plant

ISOBUTYL-FORMATE Plant

ISOCHLOROGENIC-ACID Plant

ISOCITRIC-ACID Plant

ISOLEUCINE Fruit 50–497 ppm

ISOPROPYL-BUTYRATE Plant

ISOQUERCITRIN Fruit

JASMONIC-ACID Fruit

KILOCALORIES Fruit 3,419 /kg

L-EPICATECHIN Fruit

L-MALIC-ACID Plant

L-QUINIC-ACID Plant

LACTIC-ACID Plant
LAURIC-ACID Fruit 10–63 ppm
LEAD Fruit 0.002–64 ppm
LECITHIN Plant
LEUCINE Fruit 120–746 ppm
LINOLENIC-ACID Fruit 870–5,411 ppm
LITHIUM Fruit 0.044–0.172 ppm
LUTEIN Fruit 0.4–5 ppm
LUTEOXANTHIN Fruit
LYSINE Fruit 20–746 ppm
MAGNESIUM Fruit 48–478 ppm
MALVIDIN-MONOGLYCOSIDE Plant
MANGANESE Fruit 29 ppm
MANNOSE Plant
MERCURY Fruit 0.02 ppm
METHANOL Plant
METHIONINE Plant 20–124 ppm
METHYL-2-METHYL-BUTYRATE Plant
METHYL-2-XI-ACETOXY-20–BETA-HYDROXY-
    URSONATE Fruit Epidermis
METHYL-ACETATE Plant
METHYL-AMINE Fruit Epidermis 4.5 ppm
METHYL-BUTYRATE Plant
METHYL-CAPROATE Plant
METHYL-FORMATE Plant
METHYL-GUANIDINE Shoot
METHYL-HEXANOATE Plant
METHYL-I-PENTANOATE Plant
METHYL-N-PENTANOATE Plant
METHYL-PROPIONATE Plant
METHYL-VINYL-KETONE Fruit
MEVALONIC-ACID Fruit 30–36 ppm
MOLYBDENUM Fruit 0.077–0.43 ppm
MONOGALACTOSYL-DIGLYCERIDE Plant
    12–42 ppm
MUFA Fruit 150–935 ppm
MYO-INOSITOL Pollen Or Spore 4,500 ppm
MYRISTIC-ACID Fruit 20–124 ppm
N-ALPHA-ACETYL-AGGININE Shoot
N-BUTANOL Plant
N-BUTYL-DECANOATE Plant
N-BUTYL-FORMATE Plant
N-BUTYL-N-HEXANOATE Plant
N-BUTYL-OCTANOATE Plant
N-BUTYL-PROPIONATE Plant
N-COUMARYL-QUINIC-ACID Plant
N-DECANOL Plant
N-HEHYL-N-HEXANOATE Plant

N-HEPTANOIC-ACID Plant
N-HEPTANOL Plant
N-HEX-1-EN-3-OL Plant
N-HEXANOL Plant
N-HEXYL-OCTANOATE Plant
N-HEXYL-PROPIONATE Plant
N-METHYL-BETA-PHENETHYLAMINE Fruit 1.2
    ppm
N-METHYL-PHENETHYLAMINE Exocarp 1.3
    ppm Fruit 1.2 ppm
N-NONANOIC-ACID Plant
N-NONANOL-2-NONANOL Plant
N-OCTANOL-2-OCTANOL Plant
N-OCTANONE Plant
N-PENTANOIC-ACID Plant
N-PENTENOIC-ACID Plant
N-PENTYL-2-METHYLBUTYRATE Plant
N-PENTYL-AMINE Fruit 0.3 ppm
N-PENTYL-DECANOATE Plant
N-PENTYL-FORMATE Plant
N-PENTYL-OCTANOATE Plant
N-PROPANOL Plant
N-PROPIONIC-ACID Plant
NEO-CHLOROGENIC-ACID Plant
NEOXANTHIN Fruit Epidermis
NIACIN Fruit 1–7 ppm
NICKEL Fruit 0.004–0.645 ppm
NITROGEN Fruit 280–4,000 ppm
NONACOSANE Plant
NONENOIC-ACID Plant
OCTA-CIS-3-CIS-5-DIEN-1-OL Essential Oil
OCTA-CIS-3-CIS-5-DIEN-1-OL-ACETATE Essen-
    tial Oil
OCTA-TRANS-3-CIS-5-DIEN-1-OL Essential Oil
OCTA-TRANS-3-CIS-5-DIEN-1-OL-ACETATE Es-
    sential Oil
OCTACOSANOL Plant
OCTENOIC-ACID Plant
OLEIC-ACID Fruit 140–871 ppm
OXALIC-ACID Plant
OXALOACETIC-ACID Plant
P-COUMARIC-ACID Fruit 15–460 ppm
P-COUMARYL-QUINIC-ACID Fruit
P-HYDROXY-BENZOIC-ACID Fruit
PALMITIC-ACID Fruit 480–2,986 ppm
PALMITOLEIC-ACID Fruit 10–62 ppm
PANTOTHENIC-ACID Fruit 1–4 ppm
PECTASE Plant

PECTIN Fruit 1,400–66,585 ppm
PECTIN-DEMETHOXYXYLASE Plant
PENTANOL Plant
PENTYL-BUTYRATE Plant
PENTYL-HEXANOATE Plant
PEROXIDASE Plant
PHENOLICS Plant 1,100–3,400 ppm
PHENYLALANINE Fruit 50–311 ppm
PHLORETAMIDE Fruit
PHLORETIN Leaf
PHLORETIN-4'-O-BETA-D-GLUCOPYRA-
  NOSIDE Fruit 6,486 ppm
PHLORETIN-XYLOGLUCOSIDE Fruit
PHLORIZIN Plant
PHOSPHATIDYL-CHOLINE Fruit 189–214 ppm
PHOSPHATIDYL-ETHANOLAMINE Fruit
  101–124 ppm
PHOSPHATIDYL-GLYCEROL Fruit 8–27 ppm
PHOSPHATIDYL-INOSITOL Fruit 53–59 ppm
PHOSPHATIDYL-SERINE Fruit 4 ppm
PHOSPHATIDYLIC-ACID Fruit 3–6 ppm
PHOSPHORUS Fruit 68–925 ppm
PHYTOSTEROLS Fruit 120–745 ppm
PIPECOLINIC-ACID Plant
POLYGALACTOSYL-DIGLYCERIDE Plant
POLYGALACTURONASE Plant
POLYPHENOLASE Plant
POMOLIC-ACID Plant
POMONIC-ACID Plant
POTASSIUM Fruit 1,110–12,140 ppm
PROCYANIDINS Leaf
PROLINE Plant 20–435 ppm
PROPANOL Plant
PROPYL-2-METHYLBUTYRATE Plant
PROPYL-ACETATE Plant
PROPYL-BUTYRATE Plant
PROPYL-FORMATE Plant
PROPYL-N-PENTANOATE Plant
PROPYL-PROPIONATE Plant
PROTEIN Fruit 1,870–12,800 ppm
PROTOCATECHUIC-ACID Fruit
PUFA Fruit 1,050–6,535 ppm
PYROXIDINE Plant
PYRROLIDINE Fruit Epidermis 1.5 ppm
PYRUVIC-ACID Plant
QUERCETIN Pericarp 58–263 ppm
QUERCETIN-3-0–RUTINOSIDE Plant

QUERCETIN-3-O-ALPHA-
  ARABINOFURANOSIDE Plant
QUERCETIN-3-O-ALPHA-
  GALACTOSIDE Fruit Epidermis
QUERCETIN-3-O-BETA-D-GLUCOSIDE Plant
QUERCETIN-3-O-RHAMNOSIDE Plant
QUERCETIN-3-O-XYLOSIDE Fruit Epidermis
QUERCETIN-3-RHAMNOGLUCOSIDE Plant
QUERCETIN-ARABINOSIDE Plant
QUERCITRIN Fruit
REYNOUTRIN Fruit
RIBOFLAVIN Fruit 1 ppm
RUBIDIUM Fruit 0.27–10 ppm
RUTIN Fruit Epidermis
SELENIUM Fruit
SERINE Fruit 80–497 ppm
SFA Fruit 580–3,610 ppm
SHIKIMIC-ACID Plant
SILICON Fruit 1–70 ppm
SILVER Fruit 0.011–0.086 ppm
SINAPIC-ACID Fruit
SODIUM Fruit 133 ppm
SORBITOL Leaf
STEARIC-ACID Fruit 70–435 ppm
STRONTIUM Fruit 0.165–8.6 ppm
SUCCINIC-ACID Plant
SUCROSE Fruit 24,000–36,200 ppm
SUGAR Fruit 60,100–166,000 ppm
SULFUR Fruit 1.65–23 ppm
TETRADECENYL-ACETATE Leaf
TETRADECYL-ACETATE Leaf
THIAMIN Fruit 1–2 ppm
THREONINE Fruit 30–435 ppm
TITANIUM Fruit 0.055–3 ppm
TRANS-2-HEXENOIC-ACID Plant
TRANS-ABSCISIC-ACID Fruit
TRANS-N-HEX-2-EN-1-OL Plant
TRANS-N-HEX-3-EN-1-OL Plant
TRIACONTANOL Plant
TRIGLYCERIDE Plant 45–50 ppm
TRYPTOPHAN Fruit 20–124 ppm
TYROSINE Fruit 40–249 ppm
URONIC-ACID Fruit 7–1,440 ppm
URSOLIC-ACID Fruit Epidermis
VALINE Fruit 40–560 ppm
VIT-B-6 Fruit 1–3 ppm
VOMIFOLIOL-1-O-BETA-D-XYLOPYRANOSYL-
  6-O-BETA-D-GLUCOPYRANOSIDE Plant

WATER Fruit 809,000–896,000 ppm

XYLOSE Plant

ZINC Fruit 35 ppm

ZIRCONIUM Fruit 0.22–0.86 ppm

APRICOT

Chemicals in *Prunus armeniaca L.*
(*Rosaceae*)—Apricot

2-METHYL-BUTYRIC-ACID Plant

ACETIC-ACID Essential Oil

ALANINE Fruit 680–4,980 ppm

ALPHA-ESTRADIOL Seed

ALPHA-TERPINEOL Essential Oil

AMYGDALIN Seed 80,000 ppm

AMYLASE Fruit

ARGININE Fruit 450–3,300 ppm

ASCORBIC-ACID Fruit 100–745 ppm

ASH Fruit 7,000–105,000 ppm Seed
     10,000–30,000 ppm

ASPARTIC-ACID Fruit 3,140–23,000 ppm

BENZYL-ALCOHOL Fruit

BETA-CAROTENE Fruit 13–189 ppm Seed

BETA-SITOSTEROL Seed

BORON Fruit 1–70 ppm

CAFFEIC-ACID Plant

CALCIUM Fruit 134–1,899 ppm Seed
     930–1,522 ppm

CALCIUM-PECTATE Fruit 10,000 ppm

CAMPESTEROL Seed

CAPRONIC-ACID Fruit

CARBOHYDRATES Fruit 111,200–873,000 ppm
     Seed 140,000 ppm

CHLOROGENIC-ACID Fruit

CIS-EPOXYDIHYDROLINALOL Plant

CITRIC-ACID Fruit

COPPER Seed 1–16 ppm

CYANIDIN Plant

CYSTINE Fruit 30–220 ppm

DELTA-24-CHOLESTEROL Seed

DELTA-OCTALACTONE Fruit

DEXTROSE Seed 81,000–116,000 ppm

EMULSIN Fruit

EO Seed 8,000–16,000 ppm

ESTRONE Seed

FAT Fruit 2,200–41,000 ppm Seed
     400,000–514,000 ppm

FIBER Fruit 6,000–132,000 ppm Seed 33,000
     ppm

FOLACIN Fruit 0.07–0.7 ppm

FRUCTOSE Fruit 14,000–42,000 ppm

GAMMA-CAPRALACTONE Fruit

GAMMA-CAPROLACTONE Fruit

GAMMA-CAROTENE Fruit

GAMMA-DECALACTONE Plant

GERANIAL Essential Oil

GERANIOL Essential Oil

GLUCOSE Fruit 32,000–48,000 ppm

GLUTAMIC-ACID Fruit 1,570–11,500 ppm

GLYCINE Fruit 400–2,930 ppm

GLYCOSIDES Leaf 29,000–36,000 ppm

HCN Seed

HISTIDINE Fruit 270–1,980 ppm

INVERTASE Fruit

IODINE Fruit 0.05 ppm

IRON Fruit 5–79 ppm Seed 42–48 ppm

ISOBUTYRIC-ACID Fruit

ISOLEUCINE Fruit 410–3,000 ppm

ISOQUERCITRIN Fruit

KAEMPFEROL Leaf

KAEMPFEROL-3-0-GALACTOSIDE Plant

KAEMPFEROL-3-0-GLUCOSIDE Plant

KAEMPFEROL-3-0-RUTINOSIDE Leaf

KILOCALORIES Fruit 480–3,515 /kg

LEUCINE Fruit 770–5,640 ppm

LIMONENE Essential Oil

LINALOL Fruit

LINOLEIC-ACID Fruit 770–5,640 ppm Seed
     56,000–411,200 ppm

LYCOPENE Fruit

LYSINE Fruit 970–7,105 ppm

M-INOSITOL Plant

MAGNESIUM Fruit 76–615 ppm Seed 1,750 ppm

MALIC-ACID Fruit 7,000–22,000 ppm

MANGANESE Seed 1–11 ppm

METHIONINE Fruit 60–440 ppm

MUFA Fruit 170–1,245 ppm

MYRCENE Essential Oil

NEO-CHLOROGENIC-ACID Fruit

NIACIN Fruit 6–61 ppm Seed 17 ppm

OLEIC-ACID Fruit 170–1,245 ppm Seed
     248,000–411,200 ppm

P-COUMARIC-ACID Plant

P-CYMENE Leaf

PALMITIC-ACID Fruit 240–1,760 ppm

PANGAMIC-ACID Seed

PANTOTHENIC-ACID Fruit 2.4–17.6 ppm

PHENYLALANINE Fruit 520–3,810 ppm

PHOSPHORUS Fruit 180–2,982 ppm Seed 3,000 ppm

PHYTOSTEROLS Fruit 180–1,320 ppm

POTASSIUM Fruit 2,824–22,565 ppm Seed 4,180–7,783 ppm

PROLINE Fruit 1,010–7,400 ppm

PROTEIN Fruit 10,000–127,000 ppm Seed 315,000 ppm

PUFA Fruit 770–5,640 ppm

QUERCETIN Plant

QUERCITIN Fruit

QUERCITIN-3-DIGLUCOSIDE Fruit

QUERCITIN-3-GALACTOSIDE Plant

QUERCITIN-3-GLUCOSIDE Plant

QUERCITIN-3-RHAMNOSIDE Plant

QUERCITIN-3-RUTINOSIDE Plant

QUINIC-ACID Fruit

RIBOFLAVIN Fruit 0.4–4.4 ppm Seed 5.3 ppm

RUTIN Leaf 17,700 ppm

SERINE Fruit 830–6,080 ppm

SFA Fruit 270–1,980 ppm

SODIUM Fruit 10–88 ppm Seed 18–19 ppm

SORBITOL Plant

SQUALENE Seed 200 ppm

STEARIC-ACID Fruit 30–220 ppm

SUCCINIC-ACID Fruit

SUCROSE Fruit 14,000–54,000 ppm

TANNIN Fruit 600–1,000 ppm

TARTARIC-ACID Fruit

TERPINOLENE Essential Oil

THIAMIN Fruit 0.3–2.5 ppm Seed 1.5 ppm

THREONINE Fruit 470–3,445 ppm

TRANS-2-HEXENAL Essential Oil

TRANS-EPOXYDIHYDROLINALOL Fruit

TRYPTOPHAN Fruit 150–1,100 ppm

TYROSINE Fruit 290–2,125 ppm

VALINE Fruit 470–3,445 ppm

VIT-B-6 Fruit 0.5–4 ppm

WATER Fruit 963,500 ppm

XYLOSE Plant

ZINC Seed 2–38 ppm

AVOCADO

Chemicals in *Persea americana MILLER* (*Lauraceae*)—Avocado

1,2,4-TRIHYDROXYHEPTADECA-16-ENE Plant

24-METHYLENE-CYCLOARTENOL Plant

ALANINE Fruit 960–4,625 ppm

ALPHA-CAROTENE Fruit 0.19–1 ppm

ALPHA-TOCOPHEROL Fruit 13–49 ppm

ANETHOLE Bark

ARGININE Fruit 470–2,293 ppm

ASCORBIC-ACID Fruit 65–994 ppm

ASH Fruit 6,000–56,000 ppm

ASPARTIC-ACID Fruit 2,270–11,000 ppm

BETA-CAROTENE Fruit 0.3–27 ppm

BETA-SITOSTEROL Leaf

BIOTIN Fruit 0.1–0.4 ppm

BORON Fruit 5–13 ppm

CAFFEIC-ACID Fruit

CALCIUM Fruit 60–964 ppm

CAMPESTEROL Plant

CARBOHYDRATES Fruit 8,000–629,000 ppm

CHLOROGENIC-ACID Fruit

CHOLESTEROL Plant

COPPER Fruit 2–11 ppm

CRYPTOXANTHIN Fruit 0.38–2 ppm

CYCLOARTENOL Plant

CYSTINE Fruit 170–816 ppm

D-ARABINITOL Seed

D-ERYTHRO-D-GALACTO-OCITTOL Fruit

D-ERYTHRO-L-GLUCO-NONULOSE Fruit

D-GLYCERO-D-GALACTO-HEPITTOL Fruit

D-GLYCERO-D-GALACTO-HEPTOSE Fruit

D-GLYCERO-D-GALACTO-OCTULOSE Fruit

D-GLYCERO-D-MANNO-OCTULOSE Fruit

D-MANNOHEPTULOSE Fruit

D-MANNOKETOHEPTOSE Fruit

D-TALOHEPTULOSE Fruit

DOPAMINE Fruit

EO Leaf 5,000 ppm

EPSILON-CAROTENE Plant

FAT Fruit 61,000–864,000 ppm

FIBER Fruit 10,000–106,000 ppm

FOLACIN Fruit 0.3–2.8 ppm

GALACTITOL Seed

GLUTAMIC-ACID Fruit 1,660–8,045 ppm

GLYCEROL Fruit

GLYCINE Fruit 660–3,226 ppm

HENTRIACOSANE Fruit

HEPTACOSANE Fruit

HISTIDINE Fruit 230–1,127 ppm

IRON Fruit 6–71 ppm

ISOLEUCINE Fruit 570–2,759 ppm

ISOLUTEIN Fruit

KILOCALORIES Fruit 940–6,700 /kg

LECITHIN Fruit

LEUCINE Fruit 990–4,780 ppm

LINOLEIC-ACID Fruit 24,340–505,440 ppm

LINOLENIC-ACID Fruit 245–28,510 ppm

LUTEIN Fruit 3.2–16 ppm

LYSINE Fruit 750–3,653 ppm

MAGNESIUM Fruit 370–1,740 ppm

MANGANESE Fruit 2–10 ppm

METHIONINE Fruit 290–1,438 ppm

METHYL-CHAVICOL Leaf

MUFA Fruit 96,080–373,400 ppm

MYO-INOSITOL Fruit

NIACIN Fruit 14–101 ppm

NONACOSANE Fruit

OLEIC-ACID Fruit 27,450–691,200 ppm

P-COUMARIC-ACID Fruit

P-COUMARYL-QUINIC-ACID Fruit

PALMITIC-ACID Fruit 4,270–266,000 ppm

PALMITOLEIC-ACID Fruit 6,430–25,000 ppm

PANTOTHENIC-ACID Fruit 8–37.7 ppm

PARAFFIN Leaf

PENTACOSANE Fruit

PERSEITOL Seed 89,000 ppm

PHENYLALANINE Fruit 540–2,643 ppm

PHOSPHORUS Cr 260–3,030 ppm

PHYTOSTEROLS Fruit

PINENE Leaf

POTASSIUM Fruit 2,780–27,470 ppm

PROLINE Fruit 620–2,993 ppm

PROTEIN Fruit 11,000–81,000 ppm

PUFA Fruit 19,550–76,000 ppm

PYRIDOXINE Fruit 6–23 ppm

QUERCETIN Leaf

RIBOFLAVIN Fruit 1–7.7 ppm

SERINE Fruit 810–3,148 ppm

SEROTONIN Fruit

SFA Fruit 24,370–94,700 ppm

SODIUM Fruit 20–520 ppm

STEARIC-ACID Fruit 120–4,320 ppm

TANNIN Leaf 47,000 ppm

TARTARIC-ACID Fruit 200 ppm

THIAMIN Fruit 0.5–4.2 ppm

THREONINE Fruit 530–2,565 ppm

TRIACOSANE Fruit

TRYPTOPHAN Fruit 170–816 ppm

TYRAMINE Fruit

TYROSINE Fruit 390–1,904 ppm

VALINE Fruit 970–3,770 ppm

VIOLAXANTHIN Fruit

VIT-B-6 Fruit 10.9 ppm

VIT-D Fruit

VOLEMITOL Seed

WATER Fruit 716,000–830,000 ppm

ZINC Fruit 4–16 ppm

BANANA

Chemicals in *Musa x paradisiaca L.*
(*Musaceae*)—Banana, Plantain

(24R)-4ALPHA,14ALPHA,24-TRIMETHYL-
5ALPHA-CHOLESTA-8,25(27)-3BETA-OL
Plant

(24S)-24-METHYL-25-DEHYDROCHOLES-
TEROL Fruit

2,4-METHYLENE-CHOLESTEROL Fruit

24-METHYL-CHOLESTEROL Fruit

24-METHYLENE-31-NOR-5ALPHA-CYCLOAR-
TAN-3-ONE Fruit

24-METHYLENE-31-NOR-5ALPHA-LANOST-
9(11)-3BETA-OL Fruit

24-METHYLENE-CYCLOARTENOL Fruit Plant

24-METHYLENE-CYCLOARTENOL-PALMITATE
Fruit

24-METHYLENEPOLLINASTANOL Fruit

31-NOR-24BETA-METHYL-9,19-CY-
CLOLANOST-25-EN-3ALPHA-OL Flower

31-NORCYCLOLAUDENOL Fruit

31-NORCYCLOLAUDENONE Fruit

5-HYDROXYTRYPTAMINE Plant

6G-BETA-D-FRUCTOFURANOSYLSUCROSE
Fruit

ACETIC-ACID Fruit

ALANINE Fruit 390–1,515 ppm

ALPHA-CAROTENE Fruit 0.12–0.36 ppm

ALPHA-KETO-GLUTARIC-ACID Leaf

ALPHA-LINOLENIC-ACID Fruit 330–1,282
ppm

ALPHA-TOCOPHEROL Hull Husk 30 ppm

ALUMINUM Fruit 1–35 ppm

AMYLASE Fruit

AMYLOSE Fruit 205,000 ppm

ANHYDROGALACTURONIC-ACID Fruit

ARABINOSE Fruit

ARGININE Fruit 470–1,826 ppm
ARSENIC Fruit 0.04–0.35 ppm
ASCORBIC-ACID Fruit 88–367 ppm Hull Husk 1,380 ppm
ASCORBIC-ACID-OXIDASE Fruit
ASH Flower 12,000 ppm Fruit 7,100–31,900 ppm Hull Husk 121,000 ppm Leaf 88,000 ppm Pith 6,000 ppm Shoot 11,710–158,300 ppm Sprout Seedling 143,000 ppm
ASPARTIC-ACID Fruit 1,130–4,390 ppm
BETA-CAROTENE Fruit 0.4–2.1 ppm Hull Husk 0.6–16.6 ppm
BETA-SITOSTEROL Fruit Leaf
BIOTIN Fruit
BORIC-ACID Fruit
BORON Fruit 1–17.7 ppm
BROMINE Fruit 0.3–27 ppm
BUTYRIC-ACID Fruit Plant
CADMIUM Fruit
CALCIUM Flower 300 ppm Fruit 40–460 ppm Leaf 7,500 ppm Pith 100 ppm Sprout Seedling 11,600 ppm
CALCIUM-PECTATE Fruit 42,000 ppm
CAMPESTEROL Fruit
CAPRIC-ACID Fruit 10–39 ppm
CAPROLIC-ACID Plant
CAPRYLIC-ACID Plant
CARBOHYDRATES Flower 50,000 ppm Fruit 234,300–910,256 ppm Hull Husk 631,000 ppm Leaf 695,000 ppm Pith 97,000 ppm Shoot 39,000–527,000 ppm Sprout Seedling 810,000 ppm
CATALASE Fruit
CELLULOSE Fruit
CHLORINE Fruit 1,250 ppm
CHLOROPHYLL Hull Husk 52–103 ppm
CHOLESTEROL Fruit
CHROMIUM Fruit 0.02–0.15 ppm
CITRIC-ACID Fruit
COBALT Fruit
COPPER Fruit 1–7 ppm
CYANIDIN Inflorescence
CYCLOARTENOL Fruit
CYCLOEUCALENOL Fruit
CYCLOEUCALENONE Fruit
CYCLOLAUDENOL Fruit
CYSTINE Fruit 170–660 ppm
DEHYDROASCORBIC-ACID Fruit 10–51 ppm

DELPHINIDIN Inflorescence Plant
DOPA Fruit
DOPAMINE Fruit Hull Husk 700 ppm
ERUCIC-ACID Plant
FAT Flower 2,000 ppm Fruit 3,450–23,693 ppm Hull Husk 87,000 ppm Leaf 118,000 ppm Pith 1,000 ppm Shoot 8,480–115,000 ppm Sprout Seedling 23,000 ppm
FIBER Flower 19,000 ppm Fruit 5,000–19,425 ppm Hull Husk 100,000 ppm Leaf 240,000 ppm Pith 8,000 ppm Shoot 13,210–178,600 ppm Sprout Seedling 205,000 ppm
FLUORINE Fruit 0.1–0.4 ppm
FOLACIN Fruit 0.2–0.9 ppm
FORMIC-ACID Fruit
FRUCTOSE Fruit 35,000 ppm
GABA Fruit
GADOLEIC-ACID Plant
GALACTOSE Fruit
GAMMA-GUANIDINO-N-BUTYRIC-ACID Fruit
GAMMA-GUANIDINOBUTYRIC-ACID Fruit
GLUCOSE Fruit 45,000 ppm
GLUTAMIC-ACID Fruit 1,110–4,312 ppm
GLUTARIC-ACID Leaf
GLYCERIC-ACID Leaf
GLYCINE Fruit 370–1,437 ppm
GLYCOLIC-ACID Leaf
GLYOXALIC-ACID Leaf
HEMICELLULOSE Fruit
HISTIDINE Fruit 810–3,147 ppm
INDOLE-3-ACETIC-ACID Fruit
INOSITOL Fruit 340 ppm
INVERTASE Fruit
IRON Flower 1 ppm Fruit 3–25 ppm Pith 11 ppm
ISOFUCISTEROL Fruit
ISOLEUCINE Fruit 330–1,282 ppm
ISOVALERIANIC-ACID Plant
KAEMPFEROL Fruit Plant
KILOCALORIES Fruit 920–3,574 /kg
L-OCTACOSANOL Plant
L-TRIACONTAOL Plant
LATEX Hull Husk 20,000 ppm
LAURIC-ACID Fruit 20–78 ppm
LEAD Fruit 0.02–0.2 ppm
LEUCINE Fruit 710–2,758 ppm
LEUCOCYANIDIN Fruit
LEUCODELPHINIDIN Fruit

LIGNIN Fruit
LINOLEIC-ACID Fruit 560–2,176 ppm
LIPASE Fruit
LUTEIN Fruit 0.033–0.1 ppm
LYSINE Fruit 480–1,865 ppm
MAGNESIUM Fruit 277–1,465 ppm
MALIC-ACID Fruit 530–3,730 ppm
MALONIC-ACID Leaf
MALTOSE Fruit
MALVIDIN Inflorescence
MANGANESE Fruit 1.4–18 ppm
MERCURY Fruit 0.001–0.007 ppm
METHIONINE Fruit 110–427 ppm
MFA Fruit 410–1,593 ppm
MOLYBDENUM Fruit
MUFA Fruit 410–1,593 ppm
MYRISTIC-ACID Fruit 30–117 ppm
NEO-BETA-CAROTENE-U Hull Husk 0.1–0.3 ppm
NIACIN Flower 6 ppm Fruit 5–23 ppm Hull Husk 50 ppm Pith 2 ppm
NICKEL Fruit 0.01–0.1 ppm
NITROGEN Fruit 1,600–15,000 ppm
NONACOSANE Plant
NOREPINEPHRINE Fruit Hull Husk 122 ppm
OBTUSIFOLIOL Fruit
OLEIC-ACID Fruit 270–1,049 ppm
OXALIC-ACID Fruit 22–5,240 ppm Leaf
OXYGENASE Fruit
PALMITIC-ACID Fruit 1,250–4,856 ppm
PALMITOLEIC-ACID Fruit 120–466 ppm
PANTOTHENIC-ACID Fruit 2.6–10.1 ppm
PECTIN Fruit 7,000–40,000 ppm Hull Husk 3,800–12,800 ppm
PELARGONIDIN Inflorescence
PEONIDIN Inflorescence
PEROXIDASE Fruit
PETUNIDIN Inflorescence
PHENYLALANINE Fruit 380–1,476 ppm
PHOSPHATASE Fruit
PHOSPHORIC-ACID Fruit
PHOSPHORUS Flower 500 ppm Fruit 200–1,190 ppm Leaf 2,400 ppm Pith 100 ppm
PHYTOSTEROLS Fruit 160–622 ppm
PIPECOLIC-ACID Fruit
POTASSIUM Fruit 3,100–16,150 ppm
PROLINE Fruit 400–1,554 ppm

PROTEASE Fruit
PROTEIN Flower 61,000 ppm Fruit 10,040–41,026 ppm Leaf 99,000 ppm Pith 5,000 ppm Shoot 18,930–255,900 ppm Sprout Seedling 24,000 ppm
PUFA Fruit 890–3,458 ppm
PYRUVIC-ACID Leaf
QUERCETIN Fruit Plant
QUINIC-ACID Fruit
RHAMNOSE Fruit
RIBOFLAVIN Fruit 1–3.9 ppm
RUBIDIUM Fruit 2.5–20 ppm
RUTIN Fruit
SELENIUM Fruit 0.001–0.04 ppm
SERINE Fruit 470–1,826 ppm
SEROTONIN Fruit Hull Husk 47–93 ppm
SFA Fruit 1,850–7,187 ppm
SHIKIMIC-ACID Leaf
SILICA Fruit 238 ppm
SILICON Fruit 70–350 ppm
SITOINDOSIDE Fruit
SITOSATEROL Fruit
SODIUM Fruit 6–44 ppm
STARCH Fruit 7,000–17,500 ppm Stem 50,000 ppm
STEARIC-ACID Fruit 60–233 ppm
STIGMASTEROL Fruit
SUCCINIC-ACID Fruit Leaf
SUCROSE Fruit 119,000 ppm
SULFUR Fruit 78–500 ppm
TARTARIC-ACID Fruit
THIAMIN Fruit 0.45–1.7 ppm
THREONINE Fruit 340–1,321 ppm
TOCOPHEROL Fruit 2–11 ppm
TRYPTOPHAN Fruit 120–466 ppm
TYROSINE Fruit 240–932 ppm
VALINE Fruit 470–1,826 ppm
VANILLIC-ACID Plant
VIT-B-6 Fruit 6–22.5 ppm
WATER Bulb 902,000 ppm Flower 902,000 ppm Fruit 738,790–746,410 ppm Latex Exudate 114,600 ppm Pith 883,000 ppm Shoot 926,000 ppm
XANTHOPHYLLS Hull Husk 1–7.3 ppm
XYLOSE Fruit
ZINC Fruit 1.5–10 ppm

BLACKBERRY

Chemicals in *Rubus fruticosus* (*Rosaceae*)—Blackberry

2-HYDROXYURSOLIC-ACID Plant
ARBUTIN Leaf
ASCORBIC-ACID Leaf
BETA-AMYRIN Leaf Plant
BORON Fruit 0.1–21 ppm
CHLOROGENIC-ACID Fruit
FERULIC-ACID Fruit
HYDROQUINONE Leaf
INOSITOL Leaf
LACTIC-ACID Leaf
MALIC-ACID Leaf
NEO-CHLOROGENIC-ACID Fruit
OXALIC-ACID Leaf
RUBINIC-ACID Plant
RUBITIC-ACID Plant
SITOSTEROL Plant
STIGMASTEROL Plant
SUCCINIC-ACID Leaf
TANNIN Leaf
URSOLIC-ACID Plant

BLACK CHERRY

Chemicals in *Prunus serotina subsp. serotina* (*Rosaceae*)—Black Cherry, Wild Cherry

2-ALPHA-3-ALPHA-DIHYDROXYURS-12-EN-28-OIC-ACID Leaf
3,4,5-TRIMETHOXYBENZOIC-ACID Bark
ACETYL-CHOLINE Plant
ALUMINUM Leaf 14–1,440 ppm Stem 540 ppm
ASH Leaf 29,000–96,000 ppm Stem 1,900–54,000 ppm
BARIUM Leaf 1–960 ppm Stem 6–810 ppm
BENZALDEHYDE Bark
BETA-GLYCOSIDASE Seed
BORON Leaf 2–48 ppm Stem 54 ppm
CAFFEIC-ACID Plant
CALCIUM Leaf 4,060–32,640 ppm Stem 323–18,360 ppm
CHROMIUM Leaf 2.88 ppm Stem 0.81 ppm
COBALT Stem 5.4 ppm
COPPER Leaf 0.8–29 ppm Stem 1.3–378 ppm
CYANIDIN Plant
EMULSIN Bark
EUDESMIC-ACID Bark

HCN Bark 500–1,500 ppm Leaf 2,500 ppm
IRON Leaf 20–1,440 ppm Stem 0.19–810 ppm
KAEMPFEROL Plant
LANTHANUM Leaf 0.8–19 ppm Stem 0.06–16 ppm
LEAD Leaf 0.3–67 ppm Stem 0.2–108 ppm
MAGNESIUM Leaf 435–9,600 ppm Stem 28–5,400 ppm
MOLYBDENUM Leaf 1.9 ppm Stem 0.19 ppm
NEODYMIUM Leaf 2–19 ppm
NICKEL Leaf 6.7 ppm Stem 2.7 ppm
P-COUMARIC-ACID Bark
PHOSPHORUS Leaf 261–4,608 ppm Stem 114–2,592 ppm
POTASSIUM Leaf 1,624–26,880 ppm Stem 80–15,120 ppm
PRUNASIN Bark
QUERCETIN Plant
SCOPOLETIN Bark
SILVER Leaf 0.48 ppm Stem 0.1 ppm
STRONTIUM Stem 0.5–480 ppm
TANNIN Bark
TITANIUM Leaf 0.6–144 ppm Stem 0.02–38 ppm
URS-12-EN-28-AL-3-BETA-OL Flower
URSOLIC-ACID Leaf
VANADIUM Leaf 0.14–4.8 ppm Stem 1.6 ppm
YTTERBIUM Leaf 0.05–0.67 ppm Stem 0.27 ppm
YTTRIUM Leaf 0.14–14.4 ppm Stem 0.001–3.78 ppm
ZINC Leaf 3–192 ppm Stem 0.5–216 ppm
ZIRCONIUM Leaf 0.6–6.7 ppm Stem 0.04–1.6 ppm

BLUEBERRY

Chemicals in *Vaccinium corymbosum L.* (*Ericaceae*)—Blueberry

(+)-CATECHIN Plant
1,8-CINEOLE Fruit
2-METHOXY-5-VINYL-PHENOL Fruit
2-METHYL-BUTANOIC-ACID Fruit Juice 0.05 ppm
2-PHENYLETHANOL Fruit 0.02–0.3 ppm
3-PHENYL-PROPAN-1-OL Fruit
4-HYDROXYCINNAMIC-ACID Plant
4-VINYL-PHENOL Fruit Juice 0.07 ppm

ACETIC-ACID Fruit Juice 0.7 ppm
ACETIC-ACID-HEXYL-ESTER Fruit Juice
ALANINE Fruit 280–1,820 ppm
ALPHA-CAROTENE Fruit
ALPHA-CEDRENE Plant
ALPHA-PINENE Fruit
ALPHA-TERPINEOL Fruit 0.01–0.03 ppm
ALPHA-TOCOPHEROL Fruit 18–116 ppm
ARGININE Fruit 340–2,210 ppm
ASCORBIC-ACID Fruit 125–878 ppm
ASH Fruit 2,070–13,845 ppm
ASPARTIC-ACID Fruit 520–3,379 ppm
BENZALDEHYDE Fruit Juice
BENZYL-ALCOHOL Fruit Juice 0.01–0.08 ppm
BETA-CAROTENE Fruit 0.6–3.9 ppm
BETA-CRYPTOXANTHIN Fruit
BETA-IONONE Plant
BETA-SITOSTEROL Plant
BORON Fruit 0.1–13 ppm
BUTAN-1-OL Fruit Juice 0.016 ppm
BUTAN-2-OL Fruit Juice 0.013 ppm
BUTANOIC-ACID Fruit Juice 0.01 ppm
BUTYRIC-ACID-HEX-TRANS-2-ENYL-ESTER
  Fruit Juice
CAFFEIC-ACID Plant
CAFFEIC-ACID-4-O-BETA-D-GLUCOSIDE Fruit
CALCIUM Fruit 58–400 ppm
CAPROIC-ACID Fruit Juice 0.05 ppm
CARBOHYDRATES Fruit 141,300–918,130 ppm
CARYOPHYLLENE Fruit
CHLOROGENIC-ACID Fruit 3,000 ppm
CHRYSANTHEMIN Leaf
CITRONELLOL Fruit 0.01–0.03 ppm
COPPER Fruit 0.5–4 ppm
CYANIDIN Fruit
CYANIDIN-3-O-ALPHA-L-ARABINOSIDE Fruit
CYANIDIN-3-O-ALPHA-L-GALACTOSIDE Fruit
CYANIN Fruit
CYSTINE Fruit 70–455 ppm
DELPHINIDIN Fruit
DELPHINIDIN-3-O-ALPHA-L-ARABINOSIDE
  Fruit
DELPHINIDIN-3-O-ALPHA-L-GALACTOSIDE
  Fruit
DELPHINIDIN-3-O-BETA-D-GLUCOSIDE Fruit
DELPHININ Fruit
ELLAGIC-ACID Plant
ESCULETIN Plant

EUGENOL Fruit 0.02 ppm
FARNESOL Fruit 0.04 ppm
FARNESOL-ACETATE Fruit 0.01–0.07 ppm
FAT Fruit 3,740–25,090 ppm
FERULIC-ACID Plant
FERULIC-ACID-O-BETA-D-GLUCOSIDE Fruit
FIBER Fruit 12,770–86,000 ppm
FOLACIN Fruit 0.05–0.5 ppm
FRUCTOSE Fruit
GALLIC-ACID Plant
GALLIC-ACID-4-O-BETA-D-GLUCOSIDE Fruit
GAMMA-DECALACTONE Plant
GERANIOL Fruit 0.01–0.03 ppm
GLUCOSE Fruit
GLUTAMIC-ACID Fruit 830–5,393 ppm
GLYCINE Fruit 280–1,819 ppm
HEX-CIS-3-EN-1-AL Fruit Juice 0.01–0.06 ppm
HEX-TRANS-2-1-AL Fruit Juice 0.02–0.5 ppm
HEX-TRANS-2-1-OL Fruit Juice 0.08 ppm
HEX-TRANS-2-EN-1-OL Fruit Juice 0.02–0.5
  ppm
HEXAN-1-OL Fruit Juice 0.04–0.4 ppm
HEXAN-1-AL Fruit Juice
HISTIDINE Fruit 100–715 ppm
HYDROXY-CITRONELLOL Fruit 0.02–0.07 ppm
HYDROXY-ISOCARVOMENTHOL Fruit
HYPEROSIDE Plant
IRON Fruit 2–11 ppm
ISOEUGENOL Fruit
ISOLEUCINE Fruit 210–1,365 ppm
ISOQUERCITRIN Leaf
ISOVALERIC-ACID-ETHYL-ESTER Plant
KILOCALORIES Fruit 560–3,638 /kg
LEUCINE Fruit 400–2,600 ppm
LIMONENE Fruit
LINALOL Fruit 0.01–0.05 ppm
LYSINE Fruit 120–780 ppm
MAGNESIUM Fruit 48–332 ppm
MALVADIN-3-O-ALPHA-L-GALACTOSIDE Fruit
MALVIDIN Fruit
MALVIDIN-3-O-ALPHA-L-ARABINOSIDE Fruit
MALVIDIN-3-O-BETA-D-GLUCOSIDE Fruit
MALVIN Fruit
MANGANESE Fruit 3–20 ppm
METHIONINE Fruit 110–715 ppm
MYRCENE Fruit
MYRICETIN Plant
MYRICETIN-3-O-BETA-D-GLUCOSIDE Fruit

MYRISTICIN Fruit

NEOMYRTILLIN Leaf

NEROL Fruit 0.02–0.08 ppm

NIACIN Fruit 3.4–24 ppm

NONAN-1-OL Fruit Juice

OCTAN-1-OL Fruit Juice

OLEANOLIC-ACID Plant

ORIENTIN Plant

P-COUMARIC-ACID Plant

P-COUMARIC-ACID-O-BETA-D-GLUCOSIDE
   Fruit

P-CRESOL Plant

P-DIMETHYL-ALPHA-STYRENE Fruit

P-HYDROXY-BENZOIC-ACID Plant

PANTOTHENIC-ACID Fruit 0.9–6 ppm

PENT-1-EN-3-OL Fruit Juice

PENTAN-1-OIC-ACID Fruit Juice

PENTAN-1-OL Fruit Juice 0.02 ppm

PENTYL-FURAN Fruit

PEONIDIN Fruit

PEONIDIN-3-O-ALPHA-L-ARABINOSIDE Fruit

PEONIDIN-3-O-ALPHA-L-GALACTOSIDE Fruit

PEONIDIN-3-O-BETA-D-GLUCOSIDE Fruit

PETUNIDIN Fruit

PETUNIDIN-3-O-ALPHA-L-ARABINOSIDE Fruit

PETUNIDIN-3-O-ALPHA-L-GALACTOSIDE
   Fruit

PETUNIDIN-3-O-BETA-D-GLUCOSIDE Fruit

PHENOL Fruit 0.01–0.06 ppm

PHENYLALANINE Fruit 240–1,560 ppm

PHLOROGLUCINOL Plant

PHOSPHORUS Fruit 96–675 ppm

PHYLLOQUINONE Fruit 300 ppm

PIPERONAL Plant

POTASSIUM Fruit 879–5,859 ppm

PROANTHOCYANIN Fruit

PROLINE Fruit 250–1,624 ppm

PROTEIN Fruit 6,520–44,720 ppm

PROTOCATECHUIC-ACID-4-O-BETA-D-GLU-
   COSIDE Fruit

PULEGONE Plant

QUERCETIN Plant

QUERCETIN-3-O-BETA-D-GLUCOSIDE Plant

QUERCITRIN Plant

RIBOFLAVIN Fruit 0.5–3.4 ppm

ROSMARINIC-ACID Plant

RUTIN Plant

SCOPOLETIN Plant

SERINE Fruit 200–1,300 ppm

SODIUM Fruit 56–414 ppm

THIAMIN Fruit 0.5–3.1 ppm

THREONINE Fruit 180–1,170 ppm

THYMOL Fruit

TRANS-CINNAMALDEHYDE Fruit

TRANS-CINNAMYL-ALCOHOL Fruit 0.01 ppm

TRYPTOPHAN Fruit 30–195 ppm

TYROSINE Fruit 80–520 ppm

URSOLIC-ACID Plant

VALINE Fruit 280–1,820 ppm

VANILLIC-ACID Plant

VANILLIN Fruit 0.01–0.05 ppm

VIT-B-6 Fruit 0.3–2.5 ppm

WATER Fruit 843,000–849,000 ppm

ZINC Fruit 1–7 ppm

BREADFRUIT

Chemicals in *Artocarpus altilis* (*PARKINS.*)
FOSBERG (*Moraceae*)—Breadfruit

ALANINE Seed 3,360–7,685 ppm

ALPHA-AMYRIN Fruit

ARGININE Seed 4,940–11,300 ppm

ARTOCARPIN Fruit

ARTOCARPINE Fruit

ASCORBIC-ACID Fruit 150–985 ppm Seed
   65–275 ppm

ASH Fruit 5,600–33,400 ppm Seed
   15,000–85,850 ppm

ASPARTIC-ACID Seed 8,170–18,685 ppm

BETA-CAROTENE Fruit 0.04–0.1 ppm Seed 3–6
   ppm

BORON Fruit 5.2–23 ppm

CALCIUM Fruit 170–1,950 ppm Seed 110–825
   ppm

CAMPHOROL Leaf

CARBOHYDRATES Fruit 179,200–922,450 ppm
   Seed 159,000–677,000 ppm

CEROTIC-ACID Latex Exudate

COPPER Fruit 0.8–7.5 ppm

CYCLOART-24-EN-BETA,25-DIOL Fruit

CYCLOART-25-ENE-BETA,25-DIOL Fruit

CYCLOARTENOL Fruit

CYCLOARTENONE Bark

CYCLOARTENYL-ACETATE Bark

CYSTINE Fruit 90–305 ppm Seed 1,160–2,655
   ppm

FAT Fruit 1,000–34,400 ppm Seed
25,900–128,000 ppm

FIBER Fruit 10,600–64,725 ppm Seed
13,400–38,700 ppm

GLUTAMIC-ACID Seed 10,360–23,690 ppm

GLYCINE Seed 4,650–10,635 ppm

HCN Leaf

HISTIDINE Seed 2,070–4,735 ppm

IRON Fruit 3–62 ppm Seed 37–58 ppm

ISOLEUCINE Fruit 640–2,175 ppm

KILOCALORIES Fruit 1,030–3,500 /kg Seed
1,910–4,370 /kg

LEUCINE Fruit 650–2,210 ppm Seed
5,630–12,875 ppm

LINOLEIC-ACID Seed 22,900–52,365 ppm

LINOLENIC-ACID Seed 6,870–15,710 ppm

LYSINE Fruit 370–1,258 ppm Seed
5,700–13,035 ppm

MAGNESIUM Fruit 220–975 ppm

MANGANESE Fruit 0.6–3.5 ppm

METHIONINE Fruit 100–340 ppm Seed
960–2,195 ppm

MUFA Seed 7,120–18,280 ppm

NIACIN Fruit 9–30 ppm

PANTOTHENIC-ACID Fruit 4–15.5 ppm Seed
8–20 ppm

PAPAYOTIN Fruit

PHENYLALANINE Fruit 260–885 ppm Seed
7,970–18,225 ppm

PHOSPHORUS Fruit 240–1,460 ppm Seed
1,750–5,385 ppm

POTASSIUM Fruit 2,930–16,700 ppm

PROLINE Seed 3,690–8,440 ppm

PROTEIN Fruit 9,000–58,240 ppm Seed
52,500–199,600 ppm

PUFA Seed 29,770–68,075 ppm

QUERCETIN Leaf

RIBOFLAVIN Fruit 0.3–1 ppm Seed 1–7 ppm

SERINE Seed 4,960–11,340 ppm

SFA Seed 15,090–34,505 ppm

SODIUM Fruit 11–98 ppm

STEARIC-ACID Seed 5,100–11,660 ppm

SULFUR Fruit 120–530 ppm

THIAMIN Fruit 1–4 ppm Seed 2–10 ppm

THREONINE Fruit 520–1,770 ppm Seed
3,850–8,800 ppm

TRYPTOPHAN Seed 1,230–2,815 ppm

TYROSINE Fruit 190–645 ppm

VALINE Fruit 470–1,600 ppm Seed
5,350–12,235 ppm

WATER Fruit 706,000–891,600 ppm Seed
562,700 ppm

ZINC Fruit 1.2–8 ppm

CANTALOUPE

Chemicals in *Cucumis melo subsp. ssp melo
var.cantalupensis NAUDIN* (*Cucurbitaceae*)—Cantaloupe, Melon,
Muskmelon, Netted Melon, Nutmeg
Melon, Persian Melon

2,4-METHYLENE-CHOLESTEROL Seed

22-DIHYDRO-SPINASTEROL Seed

22-DIHYDROBRASSICASTEROL Seed

24-BETA-ETHYL-25(27)-DEHYDROLATHOS-
TEROL Seed

24-METHYL-25(27)-DEHYDROCYCLOAR-
TANOL Seed

24-METHYL-LATHOSTEROL Seed

24-METHYLENE-24-DIHYDROPARKEOL Seed

24-METHYLENE-24-DIHYDROLANASETOL
Seed

24-METHYLENE-CYCLOARTANOL Seed

25(27)-DEHYDROCHONDRILLASTEROL Seed

25(27)-DEHYDRO-FUNGISTEROL Seed

25(27)-DEHYDROPORIFERASTEROL Seed

3,4-DIMETHOXY-ACETOPHENONE-ISOMER
Petiole

3-PHENYL-PROPYL-ACETATE Petiole

ACETALDEHYDE Petiole

ADENOSINE Fruit

ALPHA-AMYRIN Seed

ALPHA-CAROTENE Fruit

ALPHA-SPINASTEROL Stem

ALPHA-TOCOPHEROL Fruit 1.4–14 ppm

ALUMINUM Fruit 26–77 ppm

ARACHIDIC-ACID Cotyledon 10,200–55,300
ppm Seed 2,700–4,014 ppm

ARSENIC Fruit 0.004–0.006 ppm

ASCORBIC-ACID Fruit 397–4,370 ppm

ASH Fruit 6,950–110,000 ppm

AVENASTEROL Seed

BARIUM Fruit 1.3–7.7 ppm

BEHENIC-ACID Leaf

BENZALDEHYDE Petiole

BENZYL-ACETATE Petiole

BENZYL-PROPIONATE Petiole

BETA-AMYRIN Seed

BETA-CAROTENE Fruit 0.2–201 ppm

BETA-CRYPTOXANTHIN Fruit

BETA-IONONE Petiole

BETA-PYRAZOL-1-YL-ALANINE Fruit

BORON Fruit 1–16.5 ppm

BUTYL-ACETATE Petiole

CADMIUM Fruit 0.017–0.044 ppm

CAFFEIC-ACID Plant

CALCIUM Fruit 96–3,080 ppm

CAMPESTEROL Seed

CAPRIC-ACID Seed 2,400–3,570 ppm

CAPROIC-ACID Seed 3,000–5,350 ppm

CAPRYLIC-ACID Seed 6,000–8,920 ppm

CARBOHYDRATES Fruit 83,600–818,026 ppm

CERYL-ALCOHOL Seed

CHROMIUM Fruit 0.13–0.165 ppm

CINNAMIC-ACETATE Petiole

CIS,CIS-3,6-NONADIEN-1-OL Fruit

CIS-3-NONEN-1-OL Fruit

CIS-6-NONEN-1-OL Fruit

CIS-6-NONENAL Fruit

CIS-CIS-NONA-3,6-DIENYL-ACETATE Petiole

CITRIC-ACID Leaf

CITRULLINE Fruit 142–241 ppm

CLEROSTEROL Seed

COBALT Fruit 0.087–0.11 ppm

CODISTEROL Seed

COPPER Fruit 0.4–7.7 ppm

CUCURBITACIN-B Fruit

CUCURBITACIN-E Fruit

CUCURBITIN Seed

CYCLOARTENOL Seed

EPSILON-CAROTENE Fruit

ETHANOL Petiole

ETHYL-(METHYLTHIO)-ACETATE Petiole

ETHYL-2-METHYL-BUTYRATER Petiole

ETHYL-ACETATE Petiole

ETHYL-DECANOATE Petiole

EUGENOL-METHYL-ETHER Plant

EUPHOL Seed

FAT Fruit 2,600–29,355 ppm Seed 300,000–446,000 ppm

FERULIC-ACID Plant

FIBER Fruit 3,180–39,357 ppm

FOLACIN Fruit 0.1–1.9 ppm

GAMMA-GLUTAMYL-BETA-PYRAZOL-1-YL-ALA-NINE Fruit

GLOBULIN Fruit 26,000 ppm

HEPTYL-ACETATE Petiole

HEXADECENOIC-ACID Seed 2,190–3,255 ppm

HEXYL-ACETATE Petiole

HISTAMINE Juice

IRON Fruit 2–55 ppm

ISOBUTYL-ACETATE Petiole

ISOFRAXIDIN Plant

KILOCALORIES Fruit 350–3,425 /kg

LAURIC-ACID Seed 360–8,920 ppm

LEAD Fruit 1.74–2.2 ppm

LINOLEIC-ACID Cotyledon 56,100–726,700 ppm Seed 99,600–246,192 ppm

LINOLENIC-ACID Cotyledon 200,500–219,000 ppm

LITHIUM Fruit 0.348–0.44 ppm

LUPEOL Seed

MAGNESIUM Fruit 92–3,300 ppm

MALONIC-ACID Leaf

MANGANESE Fruit 0.4–7.7 ppm

MARGARIC-ACID Stem

MELONIN Seed

MELOSIDE Leaf

MELOSIDE-A-CAFFEOYL-ESTER Leaf

MERCURY Fruit 0.001–0.001 ppm

MOLYBDENUM Fruit 0.609–0.77 ppm

MULTIFLORENOL Seed

MYRISTIC-ACID Fruit 1,500–8,920 ppm

NIACIN Fruit 4.6–68 ppm

NICKEL Fruit 0.87–1.1 ppm

NONAN-1-OL Fruit

NONANAL Fruit

NONYL-ACETATE Petiole

OCTYL-ACETATE Petiole

OLEIC-ACID Cotyledon 40,500–195,300 ppm Seed 81,000–200,700 ppm

P-HYDROXY-BENZOIC-ACID Plant

PALMITIC-ACID Cotyledon 122,000–532,300 ppm Seed 9,600–58,400 ppm

PANTOTHENIC-ACID Fruit 1.2–14 ppm

PENTADECANOIC-ACID Leaf

PHOSPHORUS Fruit 121–2,640 ppm

PHYSETOLIC-ACID Cotyledon

PHYTOSTEROLS Fruit 100–978 ppm

POTASSIUM Fruit 3,018–44,000 ppm

PROPYL-ACETATE Petiole

PROTEIN Fruit 8,410–89,924 ppm Seed
   358,000 ppm
RIBOFLAVIN Fruit 0.2–2.4 ppm
RUTIN Plant
SELENIUM Fruit 0.003–0.004 ppm
SILVER Fruit 0.087–0.11 ppm
SITOSTEROL Seed
SODIUM Fruit 66–1,115 ppm
STEARIC-ACID Cotyledon 10,100–61,400 ppm
   Seed 10,080–35,145 ppm
STIGMAST-7-EN-3-BETA-OL Stem
STIGMASTEROL Seed
STRONTIUM Fruit 2.6–16.5 ppm
SUGAR Fruit 20,000–30,000 ppm
SULFUR Fruit 139–198 ppm
TARAXEROL Seed
THIAMIN Fruit 0.3–4.4 ppm
TIRUCALLOL Seed
TITANIUM Fruit 0.435–2.2 ppm
TRANS,CIS-2,6-NONADIEN-1-OL Fruit
TRANS,CIS-2,6-NONADIENAL Fruit
TRANS-2-NONEN-1-OL Fruit
TRANS-2-NONENAL Fruit
TRIDECANOIC-ACID Root
TRIGONELLINE Seed 2–6 ppm
VIT-B-6 Fruit 1–13 ppm
WATER Fruit 896,000–938,000 ppm
ZINC Fruit 1.5–31 ppm
ZIRCONIUM Fruit 1.7–2.2 ppm

COCONUT

Chemicals in *Cocos nucifera L.* (*Arecaceae*)—Coconut

1,3-DIPHENYLUREA? Seed
ACETOSYRINGONE Leaf
ACETOVANILLONE Leaf
ALPHA-TOCOPHEROL Oil 18 ppm
ALUMINUM Seed 7.2 ppm
ANTIMONY Seed 0.1 ppm
ARSENIC Seed 0.02 ppm
ASCORBIC-ACID Seed 20–88 ppm
ASH Seed 9,000–22,000 ppm
BARIUM Seed 0.1 ppm
BORON Seed 3–5.2 ppm
BROMINE Seed 4 ppm
CADMIUM Seed 0.03 ppm
CALCIUM Seed 71–476 ppm

CALCIUM-OXIDE Leaf 2,700 ppm
CAPRIC-ACID Seed 2,628–69,743 ppm
CAPROIC-ACID Seed 117–3,595 ppm
CAPRYLIC-ACID Seed 3,154–68,305 ppm
CARBOHYDRATES Seed 94,000–331,000 ppm
CELLULOSE Hull Husk 266,000 ppm
CESIUM Seed 0.1 ppm
CHLORINE Seed 1,007 ppm
CHROMIUM Seed 0.2 ppm
CITRIC-ACID Seed
COBALT Seed 0.2 ppm
COPPER Seed 3.2–33 ppm
D-GALACTOSE Seed
D-GALACTURONIC-ACID Seed
EUROPIUM Seed 0.1 ppm
FAT Seed 58,400–719,000 ppm
FERULIC-ACID Leaf
FIBER Seed 30,000–115,000 ppm
FLUORINE Seed 2.7 ppm
FRUCTOSE Resin, Exudate, Sap 2,100 ppm
GABA Seed
GALACTOMANNAN Seed 16,000 ppm
GAMMA-TOCOPHEROL Oil
GLUCOSE Resin, Exudate, Sap 2,400 ppm
GOLD Plant
INOSITOL Resin, Exudate, Sap 690 ppm
IODINE Seed 0.3 ppm
IRON Seed 23–33 ppm
KILOCALORIES Seed 2,960–7,050 /kg
L-RHAMNOSE Seed
LANTHANUM Seed 0.03 ppm
LAURIC-ACID Seed 25,754–368,847 ppm
LEAD Seed 0.7 ppm
LIGNIN Hull Husk 294,000 ppm
LINOLEIC-ACID Seed 584–18,694 ppm
LUTETIUM Seed 0.01 ppm
MAGNESIUM Seed 770 ppm
MAGNESIUM-OXIDE Leaf 5,700 ppm
MALIC-ACID Seed
MANGANESE Seed 9–21 ppm
MANNAN Seed
MERCURY Seed 0.1 ppm
MESO-INOSITOL Endosperm 100 ppm
METHOXYL Hull Husk 56,000 ppm
MOLYBDENUM Seed 0.03 ppm
MYRISTIC-ACID Seed 7,650–133,015 ppm
NIACIN Seed 5–10 ppm
NICKEL Seed 2.1 ppm

NITROGEN Hull Husk 1,100 ppm

OLEIC-ACID Seed 2,920–58,958 ppm

P-COUMARIC-ACID Leaf

P-HYDROXY-BENZOIC-ACID Leaf

PALMITIC-ACID Seed 4,380–75,495 ppm

PECTIN Seed

PENTOSANS Hull Husk 277,000 ppm

PHOSPHORUS Seed 830–2,400 ppm

PHOSPHORUS-OXIDE-(P2O5) Leaf 1,700 ppm

PHYTOSTEROLS Seed

POTASSIUM Seed 2,560–11,491 ppm

POTASSIUM-OXIDE-(K20) Leaf 52,300 ppm

PROTEIN Seed 32,000–77,000 ppm

QUINIC-ACID Seed

RAFFINOSE Resin, Exudate, Sap 900 ppm

RIBOFLAVIN Seed 0.2–0.7 ppm

RUBIDIUM Seed 16 ppm

SAMARIUM Seed 0.04 ppm

SCANDIUM Seed 0.002 ppm

SCYLLITOL Endosperm 500 ppm Leaf 3,200 ppm

SELENIUM Seed 0.02 ppm

SHIKIMIC-ACID Seed

SILICON Seed 370 ppm

SODIUM Seed 145–626 ppm

SORBITOL Endosperm 15,000 ppm

SQUALENE Seed

STEARIC-ACID Seed 584–23,008 ppm

STRONTIUM Seed 2.8 ppm

SUCCINIC-ACID Seed

SUCROSE Resin, Exudate, Sap 134,000 ppm

SULFUR Seed 440–1,370 ppm

SYRINGALDEHYDE Leaf

SYRINGIC-ACID Leaf

TANTALUM Plant

THIAMIN Seed 0.3–1 ppm

THORIUM Plant

TIN Seed 1.5 ppm

TITANIUM Seed 5.6 ppm

TRIDECANOIC-ACID Seed

TUNGSTEN Seed 0.3 ppm

UNDECANOIC-ACID Seed

URONIC-ANHYDRIDES Hull Husk 35,000 ppm

VANADIUM Seed 0.004 ppm

VANILLIC-ACID Leaf

VANILLIN Leaf

VIT-E Seed 2 ppm

WATER Hull Husk 80,000 ppm Leaf 84,500 ppm Seed 363,000–546,000 ppm

YTTERBIUM Seed 0.1 ppm

ZINC Seed 13–17 ppm

CRANBERRY

Chemicals in *Vaccinium macrocarpon AITON* (*Ericaceae*)—American Cranberry, Cranberry, Large Cranberry

2-METHYL-BUTYRIC-ACID Fruit

ALPHA-TERPINEOL Fruit

ALPHA-TOCOPHEROL Fruit 9–81 ppm

ALUMINUM Fruit 2–15 ppm

ANISALDEHYDE Fruit

ANTHOCYANOSIDES Fruit

ASCORBIC-ACID Fruit 75–1,003 ppm

ASH Fruit 1,800–17,000 ppm

BENZALDEHYDE Fruit

BENZOIC-ACID Fruit

BENZYL-ALCOHOL Fruit

BENZYL-BENZOATE Fruit

BETA-CAROTENE Fruit 0.2–2.6 ppm

BORON Fruit 1–8 ppm

CADMIUM Fruit 0.03–0.23 ppm

CALCIUM Fruit 70–1,157 ppm

CARBOHYDRATES Fruit 108,000–942,050 ppm

CATECHINS Fruit

CHLOROGENIC-ACID Fruit

CHROMIUM Fruit 0.01–0.08 ppm

COBALT Fruit

COPPER Fruit 0.5–4.7 ppm

CYANIDIN-3-ARABINOSIDE Fruit

CYANIDIN-3-GALACTOSIDE Fruit

CYANIDIN-3-GLUCOSIDE Fruit

EUGENOL Fruit

FAT Fruit 2,000–58,000 ppm

FIBER Fruit 12,000–116,000 ppm

FOLACIN Fruit 0.1–0.2 ppm

IRON Fruit 2–41 ppm

KILOCALORIES Fruit 490–3,800 /kg

LEAD Fruit 0.2–2 ppm

LUTEIN Fruit 0.28–2 ppm

MAGNESIUM Fruit 50–690 ppm

MALIC-ACID Fruit

MANGANESE Fruit 1.4–200 ppm

MERCURY Fruit 0.001–0.007 ppm

MOLYBDENUM Fruit 0.1–0.7 ppm

NIACIN Fruit 1–8.3 ppm
NICKEL Fruit 0.05–0.38 ppm
NITROGEN Fruit 650–5,000 ppm
OXALIC-ACID Fruit
OXYCOCCRIYANINE Fruit
PANTOTHENIC-ACID Fruit 2.2–16 ppm
PEONIDIN-3-ARABINOSIDE Fruit
PEONIDIN-3-GALACTOSIDE Fruit
PEONIDIN-3-GLUCOSIDE Fruit
PHOSPHORUS Fruit 90–1,075 ppm
POTASSIUM Fruit 250–6,777 ppm
PROTEIN Fruit 3,900–33,000 ppm
QUERCETIN Fruit 100–250 ppm
QUINIC-ACID Fruit
RIBOFLAVIN Fruit 0.2–1.7 ppm
RUBIDIUM Fruit 0.5–3.5 ppm
SELENIUM Fruit
SODIUM Fruit 10–165 ppm
SULFUR Fruit 65–500 ppm
THIAMIN Fruit 0.3–2.5 ppm
VIT-B-6 Fruit 0.6–5.4 ppm
WATER Fruit 865,400–879,000 ppm
ZINC Fruit 1–19 ppm

CUSTARD APPLE

Chemicals in *Annona reticulata L.* (*Annonaceae*)—Custard Apple

1,2-DISEHYDRONORCOCLAURINE Plant
14-HYDROXY-25-DESOXYROLLINICIN Bark
ANONAINE Bark 1,200 ppm
ASCORBIC-ACID Fruit 150–1,400 ppm
ASH Fruit 5,000–11,100 ppm
BETA-CAROTENE Fruit 0.2 ppm
CALCIUM Fruit 176–1,270 ppm
CARBOHYDRATES Plant 185,000–884,000 ppm
COCLAURINE Plant
COUMARINS Plant
DOPAMINE Plant
FAT Fruit 2,000–21,000 ppm Seed 400,000 ppm
FIBER Fruit 8,000–119,000 ppm
HCN Plant
HEXADECANOIC-ACID Plant
IRON Fruit 4–47 ppm
KILOCALORIES Fruit 800–3,540 /kg
LEUCOANTHOCYANINS Plant

LINOLEIC-ACID Plant
LIRODENINE Root
LYSINE Fruit 370–1,300 ppm
MAGNESIUM Fruit 180–630 ppm
METHIONINE Fruit 40–140 ppm
MICHELALBINE Plant
MURICININE Root
MYRISTIC-ACID Plant
NIACIN Fruit 5–38 ppm
NICOTINIC-ACID Fruit 0.5–2.5 ppm
NORCOCLAURINE Plant
NORCOCLAURINE-CARBOXYLIC-ACID Plant
OLEIC-ACID Plant
PALMITIC-ACID Plant
PANTOTHENIC-ACID Fruit 5–17 ppm
PHOSPHORUS Fruit 147–1,475 ppm
POTASSIUM Fruit 3,300–22,810 ppm
PROTEIN Fruit 11,700–89,000 ppm
RETICULINE Root
RIBOFLAVIN Fruit 0.7–5.5 ppm
SALSOLINOL Plant
SODIUM Fruit 25–275 ppm
STEARIC-ACID Plant
TANNIC-ACID Plant
TANNIN Bark
THIAMIN Fruit 0.7–5 ppm
TRYPTOPHAN Fruit 70–245 ppm
VIT-B-6 Fruit 2–8 ppm
WATER Fruit 683,000–801,000 ppm

DATE PALM

Chemicals in *Phoenix dactylifera L.* (*Arecaceae*)—Date Palm

2,3,4-TRI-O-METHYLXYLOSE Fruit
2,3-DI-O-METHYLXYLOSE Fruit
2-O-METHYLXYLOSE Fruit
3,5,4'-TRIHYDROXYSTILBENE Stem
3,5-DIHYDROXY-4-METHOXY-BENZOIC-ACID
  Stem
3,5-DIHYDROXY-4-METHOXYBENZALDEHYDE
  Stem
3-CAFFEOYLSHIKIMIC-ACID Fruit
4-HYDROXY-3-METHOXY-CINNAMIC-ACID
  Stem
4-HYDROXY-3-METHOXYBENZALDEHYDE
  Stem
5-ALPHA-STIGMAST-22-ENE-3,6-DIONE Stem

5-ALPHA-STIGMASTAN-3,6-DIONE Stem

5-OXYPIPECOLIC-ACID Fruit

5ALPHA-CAMPESTERAN-3,6-DIONE Stem

6-BETA-HYDROXY-STIGMAST-4-EN-3-ONE
Stem

6BETA-HYDROXYCAMPEST-4-ENE-3-ONE Stem

6BETA-HYDROXYSTIGMASTA-4,22-DIEN-3-
ONE Stem

7BETA-GLUCOSYL-CHRYSOERIOL Stem

ACETALDEHYDE Fruit

ALANINE Fruit 80–1,290 ppm

ALUMINUM Fruit 51 ppm Seed 3–13 ppm

APIGENIN Stem

ARABINOSE Fruit

ARACHIDIC-ACID Seed

ARGININE Fruit 620–2,090 ppm

ASCORBIC-ACID Fruit 750 ppm

ASH Fruit 15,600–44,800 ppm Seed
9,000–18,000 ppm

ASPARAGINE Fruit 2,300–4,500 ppm

ASPARTIC-ACID Fruit 20–3,150 ppm

BAIKIAIN Fruit

BEHENIC-ACID Seed

BENZOIC-ACID Stem

BETA-AMYRIN Pollen Or Spore

BETA-CAROTENE Fruit 1–3.6 ppm

BETA-SITOSTEROL Pollen Or Spore

BORON Fruit 7 ppm

BRASSICASTEROL Seed

CADMIUM Seed 9 ppm

CALCIUM Fruit 140–2,000 ppm Seed 18–436
ppm

CAMPEST-4-EN-3,6-DIONE Stem

CAMPEST-4-EN-3-ONE Stem

CAMPESTAN-4-EN-3-ONE Stem

CAMPESTEROL Stem

CAPRIC-ACID Seed

CAPRYLIC-ACID Seed

CARBOHYDRATES Fruit 735,100–948,500 ppm
Seed 655,000–853,000 ppm

CHLORIDE Seed 1,610 ppm

CHLORINE Fruit 270–310 ppm

CHLOROGENIC-ACID Fruit

CHLOROPHYLL Fruit 410 ppm

CHOLESTEROL Fruit

CIS-3,5,3',5'-TETRAHYDROXY-4-METHYLSTIL-
BENE Stem

COPPER Fruit 2–4 ppm Seed 0.6–2 ppm

COUMARIN Leaf

CYSTEINE Fruit 110–1,140 ppm

CYSTINE Fruit 7–580 ppm

D-MANNOSE Seed

DACTYLIFRIC-ACID Fruit

DEHYDRO-BETA-CAROTENE Fruit

ELLAGITANNIN Plant 9,900 ppm

ERGOSTEROL Seed

ESTROGEN Seed

ESTRONE Seed

FAT Fruit 1,000–25,000 ppm Seed
68,000–100,000 ppm

FIBER Fruit 22,000–83,000 ppm Seed
136,000–300,000 ppm

FLAVOXANTHIN Fruit

FOLACIN Fruit 0.08–0.17 ppm

FRUCTOSE Fruit 308,000 ppm Seed 15,300
ppm

GABA Fruit 2,660–3,370 ppm

GALACTOSE Fruit

GALACTURONIC-ACID Fruit

GALLO-TANNIN Plant 4,300–27,800 ppm

GLUCOSE Fruit 357,000 ppm Seed 16,800
ppm

GLUTAMIC-ACID Fruit 400–6,160 ppm

GLUTAMINE Fruit 650–870 ppm

GLYCINE Fruit 40–3,010 ppm

GLYCOSYLAPIGENIN Leaf

HENEICOSANOIC-ACID Seed

HISTIDINE Fruit 10–390 ppm

INVERTASE Fruit

IODINE Fruit 0.06 ppm

IRON Fruit 10–151 ppm Seed 5–17 ppm

ISOCHLOROGENIC-ACID Fruit

ISOFUCOSTEROL Fruit

ISOLEUCINE Fruit 20–4,650 ppm

KILOCALORIES Fruit 2,750–3,550 /kg

LACTOSE Seed

LAURIC-ACID Seed 5,600–54,000 ppm

LEAD Seed 0.1–4 ppm

LEUCINE Fruit 5–1,140 ppm

LEUCOANTHOCYANIN Fruit

LINOLEIC-ACID Seed 7,000–8,000 ppm

LINONELIC-ACID Seed

LUPEOL Stem

LUPYL-ACETATE Stem

LUTEIN Fruit

LUTEOLIN-7-GLYCOSIDE Leaf

LUTEOLIN-7-RUTINOSIDE Leaf
LYCOPENE Fruit
LYSINE Fruit 30–2,450 ppm
MAGNESIUM Fruit 325–790 ppm
MALTOSE Seed
MANGANESE Fruit 3–45 ppm Seed 16 ppm
MARGARIC-ACID Seed
METHIONINE Fruit 5–2,190 ppm
MYRISTIC-ACID Seed 2,800–23,000 ppm
NIACIN Fruit 10–135 ppm
OLEIC-ACID Seed 31,500–51,000 ppm
OXALIC-ACID Seed
P-HYDROXY-BENZOIC-ACID Stem
P-HYDROXYBENZALDEHYDE Stem
PALMITIC-ACID Seed 17,000–17,500 ppm
PALMITOLEIC-ACID Seed
PANTOTHENIC-ACID Fruit 8–10 ppm
PECTINS Fruit 7,200–39,000 ppm
PENTOSANS Fruit 38,800 ppm Seed 43,600 ppm
PEROXIDASE Fruit
PHENYLALANINE Fruit 8–740 ppm
PHOSPHORUS Fruit 370–8,795 ppm Seed 1,120 ppm
PIPECOLIC-ACID Fruit
POLYPHENOLS Fruit 30,000 ppm
POTASSIUM Fruit 6,250–8,780 ppm Seed 28–2,440 ppm
PROLINE Fruit 120–1,590 ppm
PROTEIN Fruit 19,000–43,000 ppm Seed 52,000–58,000 ppm
QUERCETIN Pollen Or Spore
RAFFINOSE Seed 3,000 ppm
RHAMNOSE Fruit
RIBOFLAVIN Fruit 0.2–1.3 ppm
RIBOSE Fruit
RUTIN Pollen Or Spore
SERINE Fruit 60–1,960 ppm
SEROTONIN Fruit 8–9 ppm
SILICON Fruit 660 ppm
SODIUM Fruit 10–380 ppm Seed 15–820 ppm
SORBITOL Fruit
STACHYOSE Seed 2,200 ppm
STARCH Fruit 206,000 ppm
STEARIC-ACID Seed 3,000–7,000 ppm
STIGMAST-4,22–DIENE-3,6-DIONE Stem
STIGMAST-4-ENE-3,6-DIONE Stem
STIGMAST-4-ENE-3-ONE Stem

STIGMASTEROL Fruit
SUCROSE Fruit 400,000 ppm Seed 38,200 ppm
SUGARS Fruit 380,000–850,000 ppm
SULFUR Fruit 510–590 ppm
TANNIN Fruit 200–18,000 ppm
TANNINS Plant 7,500–44,800 ppm
THIAMIN Fruit 0.1–1.7 ppm
THREONINE Fruit 10–980 ppm
TRANS-3,5,3',5'-TETRAHYDROXY-4-METHYL-STILBENE Stem
TRICOSANOIC-ACID Seed
TRYPTOPHAN Fruit 500–645 ppm
TYROSINE Fruit 10–1,730 ppm
URONIC-ACID Pollen Or Spore
VALINE Fruit 5–2,710 ppm
VIOLAXANTHIN Fruit
VIT-B-6 Fruit 2–3 ppm
WATER Fruit 153,000–225,000 ppm Seed 79,000 ppm
WAX Fruit
XYLOSE Fruit
ZINC Fruit 3–4 ppm Seed 0.6–29 ppm

ELDERBERRY

Chemicals in *Sambucus canadensis L.* (*Caprifoliaceae*)—American Elder, Elderberry

ALANINE Fruit 300–1,485 ppm
ALPHA-AMYRIN-PALMITATE Plant
ARACHIDIC-ACID Seed 1,206–1,920 ppm
ARGININE Fruit 470–2,326 ppm
ASCORBIC-ACID Fruit 360–1,782 ppm
ASH Fruit 6,150–32,918 ppm
ASPARTIC-ACID Fruit 580–2,871 ppm
BALDRIANIC-ACID Bark
BETA-AMYRIN-PALMITATE Plant
BETA-CAROTENE Fruit 4–18 ppm
BETA-SITOSTEROL Plant
CALCIUM Fruit 380–1,881 ppm
CAMPESTEROL Plant
CARBOHYDRATES Fruit 184,000–910,800 ppm
CYSTINE Fruit 150–742 ppm
FAT Fruit 5,000–24,750 ppm Seed 201,000–320,000 ppm
FIBER Fruit 70,000–346,000 ppm
GLUTAMIC-ACID Fruit 960–4,752 ppm
GLYCINE Fruit 360–1,782 ppm

HISTIDINE Fruit 150–742 ppm
IRON Plant 16–79 ppm
ISOLEUCINE Fruit 270–1,336 ppm
LEUCINE Fruit 600–2,970 ppm
LINOLEIC-ACID Seed 106,530–169,600 ppm
LINOLENIC-ACID Seed 68,340–108,800 ppm
LYSINE Plant 260–1,287 ppm
METHIONINE Fruit 140–693 ppm
MORRONISIDE Shoot 500–1,000 ppm
MUCILAGE Seed
NIACIN Fruit 5–25 ppm
OLEIC-ACID Seed 8,040–12,800 ppm
PALMITIC-ACID Seed 11,658–18,560 ppm
PANTOTHENIC-ACID Fruit 1–7 ppm
PHENYLALANINE Fruit 400–1,980 ppm
PHOSPHORUS Fruit 369–2,036 ppm
POTASSIUM Fruit 2,699–14,356 ppm
PROLINE Fruit 250–1,238 ppm
PROTEIN Fruit 6,180–24,750 ppm Seed
    106,000 ppm
RESIN Seed
RIBOFLAVIN Fruit 1–3 ppm
RUTIN Flower Leaf 35,000 ppm
STEARIC-ACID Seed 5,628–8,960 ppm
STIGMASTEROL Plant
TANNIN Seed
THIAMIN Fruit 1–3 ppm
THREONINE Fruit 270–1,336 ppm
TRYPTOPHAN Fruit 130–559 ppm
TYROSINE Fruit 510–2,524 ppm
VALINE Fruit 330–1,634 ppm

FIG

Chemicals in *Ficus carica L.* (*Moraceae*)—
Fig

ACIDS Fruit 1,000–4,400 ppm
ALANINE Fruit 450–2,154 ppm
ALKALOIDS Fruit 500 ppm Leaf 1,700 ppm
APIGENIN-GLYCOSIDES Fruit
ARABINOSE Fruit
ARACHIDIC-ACID Seed 2,520–3,150 ppm
ARGININE Fruit 170–814 ppm
ASCORBIC-ACID Fruit 20–2,013 ppm Leaf
    1,050 ppm
ASH Fruit 5,000–57,000 ppm Leaf
    53,000–167,000 ppm
ASPARTIC-ACID Fruit 1,760–3,447 ppm

BERGAPTEN Leaf 3,900 ppm
BETA-AMYRIN Leaf
BETA-CAROTENE Fruit 0.3–16 ppm
BETA-SITOSTEROL Leaf
BORIC-ACID Fruit
BORON Fruit 1–100 ppm
CADALENE Leaf
CAFFEIC-ACID Plant
CALCIUM Fruit 350–4,228 ppm Leaf 31,600
    ppm
CAOUTCHOUC Latex Exudate 24,000 ppm
CARBOHYDRATES Fruit 98,000–918,143 ppm
    Leaf 164,000–632,000 ppm
CAROTENE Leaf 20 ppm
CEROTINIC-ACID Latex Exudate
CHLOROPHYLL-A Fruit
CHLOROPHYLL-B Fruit
CITRIC-ACID Fruit 1,000–4,400 ppm
COPPER Fruit 0.6–3.6 ppm
COUMARINS Leaf 8,000 ppm
CYSTINE Fruit 120–574 ppm
DIASTASE Latex Exudate
ESTERASE Latex Exudate
FAT Fruit 2,000–24,000 ppm Leaf
    17,000–59,000 ppm Seed 240,000–
    300,000 ppm
FERULIC-ACID Plant
FIBER Fruit 12,000–154,000 ppm Leaf
    47,000–171,000 ppm
FICIN Latex Exudate
FICUSIN Leaf
FLAVONOIDS Leaf 5,300 ppm
FRUCTOSE Fruit 22,950 ppm
FUCOSOGENIN Leaf
FUMARIC-ACID Fruit
FURANOCOUMARIN Leaf 600 ppm
GALACTOSE Leaf
GALACTURONIC-ACID Leaf
GLUCOSE Fruit 31,050 ppm
GLUTAMIC-ACID Fruit 720–3,447 ppm
GLYCINE Fruit 250–1,197 ppm
GLYCOSIDES Fruit 500 ppm
GUAIACOL Leaf
GUAIAZULENE Root
HEMICELLULOSE Fruit 11,200 ppm
HISTIDINE Fruit 110–527 ppm
INVERT-SUGAR Fruit 500,000–700,000 ppm
IRON Fruit 3–57 ppm

ISOLEUCINE Fruit 230–1,101 ppm
ISOSCHAFTOSIDE Fruit
KAEMPFEROL Plant
KILOCALORIES Fruit 420–3,600 /kg
LEUCINE Fruit 330–1,580 ppm
LINOLEIC-ACID Fruit 1,440–6,893 ppm Seed
 84,000–105,000 ppm
LINOLENIC-ACID Seed 115,200–144,000 ppm
LIPASE Latex Exudate
LUPEOL Leaf
LUTEIN Fruit
LYSINE Fruit 300–1,436 ppm
MAGNESIUM Fruit 158–872 ppm
MALIC-ACID Fruit 30,200 ppm Leaf 23,400
 ppm
MALONIC-ACID Fruit
MANGANESE Fruit 1–7 ppm
METHIONINE Fruit 60–287 ppm
MUCILAGE Fruit 8,000 ppm
MUFA Fruit 660–3,159 ppm
MYRISTIC-ACID Fruit 20–96 ppm
NEOXANTHIN Leaf
NIACIN Fruit 3–32 ppm
OLEIC-ACID Fruit 660–3,159 ppm Seed
 47,520–59,400 ppm
OXALIC-ACID Fruit
P-CYMENE Leaf
PALMITIC-ACID Fruit 460–2,202 ppm Seed
 12,552–15,690 ppm
PANTOTHENIC-ACID Fruit 3–14 ppm
PECTIN Fruit 18,000–50,000 ppm Leaf 48,400
 ppm
PENTOSAN Leaf 36,000 ppm
PENTOSANS Fruit 8,300 ppm
PHENYLALANINE Fruit 180–862 ppm
PHOSPHORUS Fruit 129–2,764 ppm
PHYTOSTEROLS Fruit 310–1,484 ppm
POTASSIUM Fruit 1,770–11,662 ppm
PROLINE Fruit 490–2,346 ppm
PROTEASE Latex Exudate
PROTEIN Fruit 7,220–130,000 ppm Leaf
 43,000–142,000 ppm
PSORALEN Leaf 4,100 ppm
PUFA Fruit 1,440–6,893 ppm
PYRROLIDINE-CARBOXYLIC-ACID Fruit
QUERCETIN Plant
QUINIC-ACID Fruit
RHAMNOSE Leaf

RIBOFLAVIN Fruit 5.7 ppm
RUTIN Leaf 500–1,000 ppm
SCHAFTOSIDE Fruit
SERINE Fruit 370–1,771 ppm
SFA Fruit 600–2,872 ppm
SODIUM Fruit 10–366 ppm
STEARIC-ACID Fruit 120–574 ppm Seed
 5,232–6,540 ppm
STIGMASTEROL Leaf
SUCCINIC-ACID Fruit
SUCROSE Fruit 2,250 ppm
THIAMIN Fruit 3.3 ppm
THREONINE Fruit 240–1,149 ppm
TRYPTOPHAN Fruit 60–287 ppm
TYROSINE Fruit 320–1,532 ppm
UMBELLIFERONE Leaf
VALINE Fruit 280–1,340 ppm
VIOLAXANTHIN Fruit
VIT-B-6 Fruit 1–5.4 ppm
WATER Fruit 775,000–877,000 ppm Leaf
 676,000 ppm
XANTHOTOXIN Leaf
XANTHOTOXOL Leaf
XYLOSE Leaf
ZINC Fruit 1–7 ppm

GRAPE

Chemicals in *Vitis vinifera L. (Vitaceae)*—
European Grape, Grape, Wine Grape

(DL)-GALLOCATECHIN Leaf
2,2,6-TRIMETHYL-8-(1-HYDRFOXY-ETHYL)-7-
 OXA-BICYCLO-(4,3,0)-NONA-4,9-DIEN Fruit
2,6-DIMETHYL-TRANS,TRANS-OCTA-2,6-DIEN-
 1,8-DIOL Fruit
2,6-DIMETHYL-TRANS-OCTA-2,7-DIEN-1,6-
 DIOL-6-O-ALPHA-D-ARABINOFURANOSYL-B
ETA-D-BETA-D-GLUCOPYRANOSIDE Fruit
2,6-DIMETHYL-TRANS-OCTA-2,7-DIEN-1,6-
 DIOL-BETA-D-GLUCOPYRANOSIDE Plant
2-METHOXY-3-ISOBUTYL-PYRAZINE Stem
2-PHENYLETHAN-1-OL Leaf
2-PHENYLETHAN-2-OL-6-BETA-D-APIOFURA-
 NOSYL-BETA-D-GLUCOSIDE Fruit
2-PHENYLETHYL-AMINE Fruit Juice
24-METHYL-CYCLOARTENOL Stem
3,7-DIMETHYL-OCT-1-ENE-3,6,7-TRIOL Fruit
3,7-DIMETHYL-OCT-1-ENE-3,7-DIOL Fruit

3,7-DIMETHYL-OCTA-1,5,7-TRIEN-3-OL Fruit

3,7-DIMETHYL-OCTA-1,5-DIEN-3,7-DIOL Fruit

3,7-DIMETHYL-OCTA-1,6-DIEN-3,5-DIOL Fruit

3,7-DIMETHYL-OCTA-1,7-DIEN-3,6-DIOL Fruit

3-HYDROXY-BETA-DAMASCONE Fruit Juice

30-NOR-LUPAN-3-BETA-OL-20-ONE Root

9-HYDROXY-MEGASTIGM-4,6,7-TRIEN-3-ONE Fruit Juice

A-HEMICELLULOSE Fruit

ABSCISSIC-ACID Fruit

ACETIC-ACID Fruit 1,500–2,000 ppm Leaf

ACUMINOSIDE Fruit Juice

ALANINE Fruit 280–1,440 ppm

ALPHA-3-OXO-DAMASCONE Fruit Juice

ALPHA-3-OXO-IONONE Fruit Juice

ALPHA-AMYL-AMINE Fruit Juice

ALPHA-AMYRIN Stem

ALPHA-CAROTENE Fruit

ALPHA-HYDROXY-CAROTENE Fruit

ALPHA-LINOLENIC-ACID Fruit 390–2,006 ppm

ALPHA-TERPINEOL Leaf Essent. Oil 108,000 ppm

ALPHA-TOCOPHEROL Fruit 6–31 ppm

ALPHA-VINIFERIN Leaf 23,400 ppm

ALUMINUM Fruit 1–154 ppm Stem 1,030 ppm

ANTHERAXANTHIN Fruit

ANTHOCYANINS Fruit

ARGININE Fruit 490–2,520 ppm

ARSENIC Fruit 0.001–0.889 ppm

ASCORBIC-ACID Fruit 99–600 ppm Leaf 3,490–3,870 ppm Stem 310 ppm

ASCORBIC-ACID-OXIDASE Fruit

ASH Fruit 4,290–77,000 ppm Stem 88,000 ppm

ASPARTIC-ACID Fruit 810–4,167 ppm

ASRAGALIN Flower

B-HEMICELLULOSE Fruit

BARIUM Fruit 0.66–15.4 ppm

BENZOIC-ACID Fruit

BENZYL-6-O-BETA-D-APIOFURANOSYL-BETA-D-GLUCOSIDE Fruit Juice

BENZYL-ALCOHOL Leaf

BENZYL-ALCOHOL-6-O-L-ARABINOFURA-NOSYL-BETA-D-GLUCOPYRANOSIDE Leaf

BENZYL-ALCOHOL-BETA-D-GLUCOSIDE Leaf

BENZYL-ALCOHOL-BETA-D-RUTINOSIDE Leaf

BETA-3-OXO-DAMASCONE Fruit Juice

BETA-AMYRIN Stem

BETA-CAROTENE Fruit 0.5–2.1 ppm Stem 43 ppm

BETA-IONONE Fruit

BETA-PHENYLETHANOL-6-BETA-D-ARABINO-FURANOSYL-BETA-D-GLUCOPYRANOSIDE Fruit Juice

BETA-PHENYLETHANOL-BETA-D-GLUCOSIDE Fruit Juice

BETA-PHENYLETHANOL-BETA-D-RUTINOSIDE Fruit Juice

BETA-SITOSTEROL Fruit

BETAINE Fruit Juice

BETULINIC-ACID Root

BIOTIN Fruit

BORON Fruit 1–50 ppm

BREVILAGIN-I Leaf 533 ppm

BROMINE Fruit

CADMIUM Fruit 0.001–0.231 ppm

CAFFEIC-ACID Fruit

CAFFEOYL-TARTRATE Fruit

CAFFEYLTARTARIC-ACID Fruit

CALCIUM Fruit 92–4,774 ppm Stem 17,700 ppm

CALCIUM-PECTATE Leaf 69,000 ppm

CARBOHYDRATES Fruit 177,700–914,095 ppm

CATALASE Fruit

CATECHOL-OXIDASE Fruit

CHLOROGENIC-ACID Fruit

CHOLESTEROL Fruit

CHROMIUM Fruit 0.005–0.385 ppm Stem 9 ppm

CINNAMIC-ACID Fruit

CIS-CAFFEIC-ACID Fruit

CITRIC-ACID Fruit Leaf

CITRONELLOL Leaf

CITROSTADIENOL Stem

COBALT Fruit 0.005–0.22 ppm Stem 33 ppm

COPPER Fruit 0.7–11.6 ppm

COUMARIN Fruit

CRYPTOCHLOROGENIC-ACID Fruit

CRYPTOXANTHIN Fruit

CYANIDIN Fruit

CYANIDIN-3-GALACTOSIDE Fruit

CYANIDIN-3-GLUCOSIDE Fruit

CYCLOARTENOL Stem

CYSTINE Fruit 110–566 ppm

D-CATECHIN Fruit Leaf

DAMASCENONE Fruit Juice 0.013–0.085 ppm

DELPHINIDIN Plant
DELPHINIDIN-3,5-DIGLUCOSIDE Fruit
DELPHINIDIN-3-(6-P-COUMAROYLGLUCO-
   SIDE) Fruit
DELPHINIDIN-3-(P-COUMAROYLGLUCO-
   SIDE)-5-GLUCOSIDE Fruit
DELPHINIDIN-3-0–BETA-D-GLUCOSIDE Fruit
DELPHINIDIN-3-CAFFEOYLGLUCOSIDE Fruit
DIETHYL-AMINE Fruit Juice
DIHYDROFURAN-I Fruit Juice
DIHYDROPHASEIC-ACID-4′-BETA-D-GLUCO-
   SIDE Fruit
DIMETHYL-AMINE Fruit Juice
ELEMOL-ACETATE Leaf Essent. Oil 130.2 ppm
ELLAGIC-ACID Fruit
ENOMELANIN Fruit
ENOTANNIN Seed
EPICATECHIN Fruit
EPICATECHIN-3-GALLATE Fruit Seed
EPSILON-VINIFERIN Leaf 30,900 ppm
ERGOSTEROL Fruit
ETHYL-AMINE Fruit Juice
FAT Fruit 5,010–33,898 ppm Seed
   60,000–200,000 ppm
FERULIC-ACID Fruit
FIBER Fruit 4,210–24,640 ppm
FLAVONOIDS Leaf 40,000–50,000 ppm
FLUORINE Fruit 0.1–0.6 ppm
FOLACIN Fruit 0.03–0.23 ppm
FORMIC-ACID Fruit
FR Plant
FRUCTOSE Fruit
FUMARIC-ACID Leaf
GABA Fruit
GALACTOSE Fruit
GALACTURONIC-ACID Fruit
GALLIC-ACID Fruit
GALLOCATECHIN Hr Leaf
GAMMA-CAROTENE Fruit
GENTISIC-ACID Hull Husk
GERANIOL Fruit Leaf Essent. Oil 145,200 ppm
GERANIOL-6-O-ALPHA-L-ARABINOFURA-
   NOSYL-BETA-D-GLUCOPYRANOSIDE Fruit
GERANIOL-6-O-ALPHA-L-RHAMNOPYRA-
   NOSYL-BETA-D-GLUCOPYRANOSIDE Fruit
GERANIOL-BETA-D-GLUCOSIDE Fruit Juice
GERMANICOL Stem
GLUCOSE Fruit

GLUCOSE-6-PHOSPHATE-DEHYDROGENASE
   Fruit
GLUTAMIC-ACID Fruit 1,380–7,099 ppm
GLYCERIC-ACID Leaf
GLYCINE Fruit 200–1,029 ppm
HENTRIACONTANE Fruit
HEPTACOSAN-1-OL Root
HEXOKINASE Fruit
HIRSUTRIN Leaf
HISTIDINE Fruit 240–1,235 ppm
HYDROXY-CITRONELLOL Essential Oil
INOSITOL Leaf
IRON Fruit 1.5–154 ppm Stem 900 ppm
ISOAMYL-AMINE Fruit Juice
ISOBUTYL-AMINE Fruit Juice
ISOCHLOROGENIC-ACID Fruit
ISOLEUCINE Fruit 50–257 ppm
ISOQUERCITRIN Leaf
ISOVITILAGIN Leaf 163 ppm
JU Plant
KAEMPFEROL Leaf
KAEMPFEROL-3-MONOGLUCOSIDE Fruit
LACTIC-ACID Fruit
LEAD Fruit 0.02–9 ppm
LEUCINE Fruit 140–720 ppm
LEUCOANTHOCYANIDOLE Fruit
LEUCOCYANIDIN Plant
LIMONENE Plant
LINALOL Fruit Leaf Essent. Oil 273,000 ppm
LINALOL-6-0–ALPHA-L-ARABINOFURANOSYL-
   BETA-D-GLUCOPYRANOSIDE Fruit
LINALOL-6-0–ALPHA-L-RHAMNOPYRANOSYL-
   BETA-D-GLUCOPYRANOSIDE Fruit
LINALOL-6-0–BETA-D-APIOFURANOSYL-BETA-
   D-GLUCOSIDE Fruit Juice
LINALOL-BETA-D-GLUCOSIDE Fruit Juice
LINOLEIC-ACID Fruit 1,300–6,687 ppm Seed
   33,000–110,000 ppm
LITHIUM Fruit 0.088–0.308 ppm
LUPEOL Leaf
LUTEIN Fruit 0.7–7 ppm
LUTEIN-5,6-EPOXIDE Fruit
LUTEIN-5-8-EPOXIDE Fruit
LUTEOLIN Leaf
LUTEOXANTHIN Fruit
LYCOPENE Fruit
LYSINE Fruit 150–772 ppm

MAGNESIUM Fruit 58–2,310 ppm Stem 4,360 ppm

MALIC-ACID Fruit 1,500–2,000 ppm Plant

MALVIDIN Fruit

MALVIDIN-3-(6-P-COUMAROYLGLUCOSIDE)-5-GLUCOSIDE Fruit

MALVIDIN-3-(P-COUMAROYLGLUCOSIDE) Fruit

MALVIDIN-3-CAFFEOYLGLUCOSIDE Fruit

MALVIDIN-3-CHLOROGENIC-ACID-GLUCO-SIDE Fruit

MALVIDIN-3-GLUCOSIDE Fruit

MALVIDIN-3-O-BETA-D-GLUCOSIDE Fruit

MANGANESE Fruit 0.5–54 ppm Stem 986 ppm

MEGASTIGM-5-EN-7-YNE-3,9-DIOL Fruit Juice

MELIBIOSE Fruit

MERCURY Fruit 0.011 ppm

METHIONINE Fruit 220–1,132 ppm

MOLYBDENUM Fruit 0.1–0.539 ppm

MONO-P-COUMARYL-ACID Fruit Leaf

MONOCAFFEIC-ACID Fruit Leaf

MONOFERULYLSUCCINIC-ACID Leaf

MUFA Fruit 230–1,183 ppm

MUTATOXANTHIN Fruit

MYRICETIN Fruit

MYRICETIN-3-MONOGLUCOSIDE Fruit

MYRISTIC-ACID Fruit 50–257 ppm

N-PROPYL-AMINE Fruit Juice

NEO-CHLOROGENIC-ACID Fruit

NEOXANTHIN Fruit

NEROL Leaf

NEROL-6-0–ALPHA-L-ARABINOFURANOSYL-BETA-D-GLUCOPYRANOSIDE Fruit

NEROL-6-0–ALPHA-L-RHAMNOPYRANOSYL-BETA-D-GLUCOPYRANOSIDE Fruit

NEROL-6-0–BETA-D-APIOFURANOSYL-BETA-D-GLUCOSIDE Fruit Juice

NEROL-BETA-D-GLUCOSIDE Fruit Juice

NIACIN Fruit 3–15.4 ppm Stem

NICKEL Fruit 0.01–0.77 ppm

NITROGEN Fruit 1,100–7,220 ppm

NONACOSANE Fruit

O-HYDROXY-BENZOIC-ACID Hull Husk

OBTUSIFOLIOL Stem

OCTAN-1-OL Stem

OENIN Petiole

OLEANOLIC-ACID Leaf Wax

OLEANOLIC-ACID-METHYL-ESTER Leaf

OLEANOLIC-ALDEHYDE Stem

OLEIC-ACID Plant 230–1,183 ppm Seed 22,200–74,000 ppm

OXALIC-ACID Fruit 34 ppm

P-COUMARIC-ACID Fruit

P-COUMAROYL-CIS-TARTRATE Fruit

P-COUMAROYL-TRANS-TARTRATE Fruit

P-HYDROXY-BENZOIC-ACID Hull Husk

PAEONIDIN Fruit

PAEONIDIN-3-(6-P-COUMAROYLGLUCO-SIDE) Fruit

PAEONIDIN-3-5,-DIGLUCOSIDE Fruit

PAEONIDIN-3-CAFFEOYLGLUCOSIDE Fruit

PAEONIDIN-3-O-BETA-D-GLUCOSIDE Fruit

PALMITIC-ACID Fruit 1,620–8,333 ppm Seed 3,300–11,000 ppm

PANTOTHENIC-ACID Fruit 0.2–1.3 ppm

PECTIN Fruit 300–3,900 ppm

PECTIN-METHYL-ESTERASE Fruit

PELARGONIDIN Fruit

PEROXIDASE Fruit

PETUNIDIN-3,5-DIGLUCOSIDE Fruit

PETUNIDIN-3-(6-P-COUMAROYLGLUCOSIDE) Fruit

PETUNIDIN-3-CAFFEOYLGLUCOSIDE Plant

PETUNIDIN-3-GLUCOSIDE Fruit

PETUNIDIN-3-O-BETA-D-GLUCOSIDE Fruit

PHENYLALANINE Fruit 140–720 ppm

PHOSPHODIESTERASE Root

PHOSPHORUS Fruit 117–1,848 ppm Stem 1,710 ppm

PHYTOENE Fruit

PHYTOFLUENE Fruit

PHYTOSTEROLS Fruit 40–206 ppm

POLYPHENOL-OXIDASE Fruit

POTASSIUM Fruit 1,784–24,640 ppm Stem 20,100 ppm

PROCYANIDIN-B-2-3'-O-GALLATE Fruit

PROCYANIDINS Fruit

PROLINE Fruit 220–1,132 ppm

PROTEIN Fruit 6,350–35,236 ppm Seed 70,000–100,000 ppm Stem 89,000 ppm

PROTOPECTINASE Fruit

PTEROSTILBENE Leaf

PUFA Fruit 1,690–8,693 ppm

PYROPHOSPHATASE-NUCLOETIDE Root

PYRROLIDINE Fruit Juice

QUERCETIN Fruit

QUERCETIN-GLUCURONOSIDE Fruit
QUERCITRIN Leaf
QUINIC-ACID Fruit Leaf
RAFFINOSE Fruit
RESVERATROL Leaf 90,400 ppm
RIBOFLAVIN Plant 0.5–3.2 ppm Stem 6.9 ppm
ROSEOSIDE Fruit
RUBIDIUM Fruit 0.4–5.5 ppm
RUTIN Leaf
SALICYLIC-ACID Root
SELENIUM Fruit 0.012 ppm Stem
SERINE Fruit 320–1,646 ppm
SFA Fruit 1,890–9,722 ppm
SHIKIMIC-ACID Leaf
SILICON Fruit 1–28 ppm Stem 365 ppm
SILVER Fruit 0.022–0.077 ppm
SINAPIC-ACID Root
SODIUM Fruit 2–454 ppm Stem 156 ppm
SQUALENE Seed
STACHYOSE Fruit
STEARIC-ACID Seed 1,440–4,800 ppm
STIGMASTEROL Plant
STRONTIUM Fruit 1.54–38.5 ppm
SUCCINDEHYDROGENASE Fruit
SUCCINIC-ACID Fruit
SUGAR Fruit 30,000–189,000 ppm
SULFUR Fruit 7–888 ppm
SYRINGIC-ACID Hull Husk
TANNIN Seed
TARAXASTEROL Leaf
TARAXEROL Leaf
TARTARIC-ACID Fruit 15–20 ppm
TARTARIC-ACID-CAFFEOYL-ESTER Fruit 15–20 ppm
THIAMIN Fruit 0.8–4.9 ppm Stem 11 ppm
THREONINE Fruit 180–926 ppm
TIN Stem 12 ppm
TITANIUM Fruit 0.11–7.7 ppm
TRANS-CAFFEIC-ACID Fruit
TRIACONTAN-1-OL Root
TRIACONTAN-1-OL-TRIDECANOATE Root
TRYPTOPHAN Fruit 30–154 ppm
TYROSINE Fruit 120–617 ppm
URSOLIC-ALDEHYDE Stem
VALINE Fruit 180–926 ppm
VANILLIC-ACID Hull Husk
VIOLAXANTHIN Fruit
VIT-B-6 Fruit 1–6 ppm

VITILAGIN Leaf 89 ppm
VITISPIRANE Plant
VOMIFOLIOL Fruit
WATER Fruit 761,000–897,000 ppm Stem 792,000 ppm
XYLOSE Fruit
ZEAXANTHIN Fruit
ZINC Fruit 0.4–27 ppm Stem 75 ppm
ZIRCONIUM Fruit 0.44–1.54 ppm

GRAPEFRUIT

Chemicals in *Citrus paradisi MacFAD.* (*Rutaceae*)—Grapefruit

(+)-6-ISO-PROPENYL-4,8-ALPHA-DIMETHYL-4-ALPHA-®-5,6-®-7,8,8-ALPHA® HEXAHYDRO-2-(1H)NAPTHALENONE Fruit
(+)-8,9-DIDEHYDRO-ALPHA-VETIVONE Fruit
(+)-8,9-DIDEHYDRO-NOOTKATONE Fruit
(+)-ALPHA-CYPERONE Fruit
(+)-ALPHA-VETIVONE Fruit
(+)-NOOTKATONE Plant
1,10-DIHYDRO-ALPHA-VETIVONE Fruit
10-EPI-ALPHA-CYPERONE Fruit
2-H-18(3-BETA-D-GLUCOPYRANOSYL-OXY-2-HYDROXY-3-METHYL-BUTYL)-7-METHOXY-BENZOPYRAN-2-ONE Plant
24-METHYLENE-CYCLOARTENOL Pericarp
24-METHYLENE-LOPHENOL Pericarp
3',4',5,6,7,8-HEXAMETHOXYFLAVONE Pericarp
3,7(11)-EUDESMADIEN-2-ONE Plant
3-HYDROXY-ETHYL-HEXANOATE Fruit
4',5,6,7,8-PENTAMETHOXY-FLAVONE Pericarp
4',5,6,7-TETRAHYDROXY-FLAVONE-8-O-BETA-D-GLUCOSIDE Fruit
4',5,7-TRIHYDROXY-FLAVONE-6-C-GLUCO-SIDE Fruit
4',5-DIHYDROXY-FLAVONONE-7-O-BETA-D-RHAMNOSYL-GLUCOSIDE Fruit
5,6-DIHYDROERGOSTEROL Plant
5-(3,7-DIMETHYL-6-EPOXY-2-OCTENYL)-OXYPSORALEN Pericarp
5-(6,7-DIHYDROXY-3,7-DIMETHYL-2-OCTENYL)-OXYPSORALEN Pericarp
5-HYDROXY-4'-METHOXY-FLAVANONE-7-O-BETA-D-RHAMNOSYL-GLUCOSIDE Fruit
7-(3,7-DIMETHYL-6-EPOXY-OCT-TRANS-2-ENYL)-OXYCOUMARIN Pericarp

7-GERANYL-OXYCOUMARIN Pericarp

7-METHOXY-8(2,3-DIHYDROXY-ISOPENTYL)-
  COUMARIN Pericarp

7-METHOXY-8(2,3-EPOXY-ISOPENTENYL)-
  COUMARIN Pericarp

7-OBACUNOL Seed 8–9 ppm

ACETIC-ACID Fruit

ALANINE Fruit 90 ppm

ALPHA-AMINO-BUTYRIC-ACID Fruit 190 ppm

ALPHA-CAROTENE Fruit

ALPHA-CRYTOXANTHIN Fruit

ALPHA-LINOLENIC-ACID Fruit 50–550 ppm

ALPHA-PINENE Fruit

ALPHA-TOCOPHEROL Fruit 3–29 ppm

ALUMINUM Fruit 1–330 ppm

APIGENIN-7-O-BETA-D-RUTINOSIDE Leaf 5 ppm

ARABAN Fruit

ARGININE Fruit 470–760 ppm

ARSENIC Fruit 0.001–4.4 ppm

ASCORBIC-ACID Fruit 337–3,862 ppm

ASH Fruit 3,050–53,000 ppm

ASPARAGINE Fruit 420 ppm

ASPARTIC-ACID Fruit 810–4,700 ppm

BARIUM Fruit 0.44–22 ppm

BERGAMOTTIN Pericarp

BERGAPTOL Fruit

BETA-CAROTENE Fruit 5 ppm

BETA-SITOSTEROL Fruit

BORON Fruit 1–33 ppm

BRAYLIN Root

BROMINE Fruit

CADMIUM Fruit 0.002–0.066 ppm

CAFFEIC-ACID Fruit 40–51 ppm

CAFFEINE Flower 29 ppm

CALCIUM Fruit 117–4,270 ppm

CAMPESTEROL Fruit

CARBOHYDRATES Fruit 80,800–948,000 ppm

CARYOPHYLLENE Fruit

CATECHOL Plant

CHALCONASE Fruit

CHLORINE Plant 6 ppm

CHOLESTEROL Fruit

CHROMIUM Fruit 0.002–0.55 ppm

CIS-LINALOL-OXIDE Fruit

CITRAL Fruit

CITRIC-ACID Fruit 11,900–21,000 ppm

CITROSTADIENOL Pericarp

COBALT Fruit 0.005–0.22 ppm

CONIFERIN Pericarp

COPPER Fruit 7.7 ppm

CRYPTOXANTHIN Fruit 0.03–0.3 ppm

CYCLOARTENOL Pericarp

CYCLOEUCALENOL Pericarp

CYSTINE Fruit 2 ppm

D-CADINENE Plant

D-LIMONENE Plant 9,000 ppm

DEACETYL-NOMILIN Seed

DEACETYL-NOMILINIC-ACID-17-O-BETA-D-
  GLUCOSIDE Seed

DECYL-ALDEHYDE Fruit

DECYLIC-ACID Fruit

DEOXY-LIMONOL Seed 8 ppm

DIHYDROKAEMPFEROL Fruit

EO Fruit 6,000–10,000 ppm

EPI-ISO-OBACUNOIC-ACID-17-O-BETA-D-
  GLUCOSIDE Seed

ERIODICTYOL Fruit

ESCULETIN Fruit

FAT Fruit 1,000–19,000 ppm

FERULIC-ACID Fruit 30–34 ppm

FERULOYL-PUTRESINE Plant 15–41 ppm

FIBER Fruit 2,000–44,000 ppm

FLUORINE Fruit 0.03–0.9 ppm

FRIEDELIN Pericarp

FRUCTOSE Plant 12,400 ppm

GALACTAN Plant

GALACTURONIC-ACID Fruit

GAMMA-CAROTENE Fruit

GERANIAL Fruit 420–700 ppm

GERANIOL Plant

GERANYL-ACETATE Fruit

GERANYL-OXY-PYRANOCOUMARIN Root

GLUCOSAN Plant

GLUCOSE Fruit 19,500 ppm

GLUTAMIC-ACID Fruit 220–2,800 ppm

GLYCINE Fruit

HEPTULOSE Pericarp

HESPERETIN Fruit

HESPERIDIN Fruit

HISTIDINE Fruit 140 ppm

HORDENENE Fruit

HUMULENE Fruit

IRON Fruit 1–88 ppm

ISO-OBACUNOIC-ACID-17-O-BETA-D-GLUCO-
  SIDE Seed

ISOMERANZIN Pericarp

ISORHAMNETIN Fruit

ISORHOIFOLIN Leaf

ISOSAKURANETIN Fruit

KAEMPFEROL Fruit

KILOCALORIES Fruit 1,724 /kg

LEAD Fruit 0.02–7.7 ppm

LEUCINES Fruit 240 ppm

LIMONIN Fruit Plant 9–140 ppm

LIMONOATE-A-RING-LACTONE Fruit

LIMONOL Seed 23 ppm

LINALOL Fruit

LINALYL-ACETATE Fruit

LINOLEIC-ACID Fruit 190–2,090 ppm

LITHIUM Fruit 0.088–2.31 ppm

LUTEIN Fruit 0.095–0.95 ppm

LYCOPENE Fruit

LYSINE Fruit 160–1,760 ppm

MAGNESIUM Fruit 15–1,360 ppm

MALIC-ACID Fruit 400–600 ppm

MALONIC-ACID Fruit

MANGANESE Fruit 5 ppm

MANNOSE Fruit

MERANZIN Pericarp

MERANZIN-HYDRATE Pericarp

MERCURY Fruit 0.001 ppm

METHIONINE Fruit 3–222 ppm

METHYL-ANTHRALINATE Fruit

MOLYBDENUM Fruit 0.1–0.77 ppm

MYRCENE Fruit 72–190 ppm

N-DODECASANE Fruit

N-DORIACONTANE Fruit

N-EICOSANE Fruit

N-HENEICOSANE Fruit

N-HENTRIACONTANE Fruit

N-HEPTACOSANE Fruit

N-HEXACOSANE Fruit

N-METHYL-TYRAMINE Fruit

N-NONACOSANE Fruit

N-NONYL-ALCOHOL Fruit

N-OCTACOSANE Fruit

N-OCTYL-ACETATE Fruit

N-OCTYL-ALCOHOL Fruit

N-PENTACOSANE Fruit

N-PENTATRIACONTANE Pericarp

N-TETRACOSANE Fruit

N-TETRATRIACONTANE Pericarp

N-TRIACONTANE Fruit

NARINGENIN Fruit

NARINGENIN-7-BETA-(4-BETA-D-GLUCOSYL)-
    NEOHESPERIDOSIDE Fruit

NARINGENIN-7-BETA-(4-BETA-D-GLUCOSYL)-
    RUTINOSIDE Fruit

NARINGENIN-7-O-BETA-D-RUTINOSIDE Fruit

NARINGENIN-RUTINOSIDE Fruit

NARINGIN Fruit 245 ppm Pericarp
    4,500–14,000 ppm Seed 200 ppm

NARINGIN-4-BETA-D-GLUCOSIDE Plant

NARIRUTIN Fruit

NEOHESPERIDIN Fruit

NERAL Fruit 136–210 ppm

NEUROSPORENE Fruit

NIACIN Fruit 2–44 ppm

NICKEL Fruit 0.04–7.7 ppm

NITROGEN Fruit 990–16,360 ppm

NOMILIN Seed

NOMILINIC-ACID Plant

NOMILINIC-ACID-17-O-BETA-D-GLUCOSIDE
    Seed

OBACUNONE Seed

OCTOPAMINE Hull Husk

OCTYL-ALDEHYDE Fruit

OCTYLIC-ACID Fruit

OLEIC-ACID Fruit 120–1,320 ppm

OSTHOLE Root

OXALIC-ACID Plant

P-COUMARIC-ACID Fruit 53 ppm

P-MENTH-1-ENE-8-THIOL Fruit

PALMITIC-ACID Fruit 120–1,320 ppm

PALMITOLEIC-ACID Fruit 10–110 ppm

PANTOTHENIC-ACID Plant 3–31 ppm

PARADISIOL Fruit

PECTIN Fruit

PENTAN-1-OL Fruit

PHENYLALANINE Fruit

PHLORIN Plant

PHLOROGLUCINOL Fruit

PHOSPHORUS Fruit 76–2,545 ppm

PHYTOENE Fruit

PHYTOFLUENE Fruit

POLYGALACTURONIC-ACID Fruit

PONCIRIN Fruit

PONCITRIN Root

POTASSIUM Fruit 1,300–16,360 ppm

PROLINE Fruit 590 ppm

PROTEIN Fruit 6,000–70,290 ppm

PSI-CAROTENE Plant

QUERCETIN Fruit

QUINIC-ACID Fruit

RHOIFOLIN Leaf

RIBOFLAVIN Fruit 5 ppm

RUBIDIUM Fruit 0.26–22 ppm

SALICYLATES Fruit 70 ppm

SCOPOLETIN Fruit

SELENIUM Fruit 0.027 ppm

SERINE Fruit 150–3,100 ppm

SESELIN Root

SESLIN Root

SILICON Fruit

SILVER Fruit 0.022–0.11 ppm

SINAPIC-ACID Fruit 4–5 ppm

SODIUM Fruit 175 ppm

STEARIC-ACID Fruit 10–110 ppm

STIGMASTEROL Fruit

STRONTIUM Fruit 3.3–220 ppm

SUBAPHYLLIN Fruit Leaf

SUBEROSIN Root

SUCROSE Fruit 21,400 ppm

SUGARS Fruit 33,000–99,600 ppm

SULFUR Fruit 7–2,090 ppm

SYNEPHERINE Fruit

THIAMIN Fruit 6 ppm

THREONINE Fruit 100 ppm

TIN Fruit 0.66–3.3 ppm

TITANIUM Fruit 0.11–7.7 ppm

TRANS-OBACUNOIC-ACID-17-O-
BETA-D-GLUCOSIDE Seed

TRYPTOPHAN Fruit 20–220 ppm

TYRAMINE Fruit

TYROSINE Fruit 61 ppm

UMBELLIFERONE Fruit

URONIC-ACID Fruit

VALINE Fruit 240 ppm

WATER Fruit 847,000–930,000 ppm

XANTHOXYLETIN Root

XANTHYLETIN Fruit

XYLAN Fruit

XYLOSE Fruit

ZETA-CAROTENE Fruit

ZINC Fruit 9 ppm

ZIRCONIUM Fruit 0.44–2.2 ppm

GUAVA

Chemicals in *Psidium guajava L.*
(*Myrtaceae*)—Guava

2-ALPHA-HYDROXYURSOLIC-ACID Plant

ACETONE Fruit

ALANINE Fruit 410–2,952 ppm

ALPHA-HUMULENE Fruit

ALPHA-LINOLENIC-ACID Fruit 710–5,112 ppm

ALPHA-SELINENE Fruit

AMRITOSIDE Leaf

ARABAN Fruit

ARABINOSE Fruit

ARABINOSE-HEXAHYDROXYDIPHENYL-ACID-
ESTER Fruit 1,000 ppm

ARGININE Fruit 210–1,512 ppm

ARJUNOLIC-ACID Root

AROMADENDRENE Leaf

ASCORBIC-ACID Fruit 200–14,300 ppm

ASCORBIGEN Fruit 253–2,145 ppm

ASH Fruit 6,000–43,200 ppm Seed 30,000 ppm

ASPARTIC-ACID Fruit 520–3,744 ppm

AVICULARIN Leaf

BENZALDEHYDE Fruit

BENZENE Fruit

BETA-BISABOLENE Fruit

BETA-CAROTENE Fruit 3–46 ppm

BETA-CARYOPHYLLENE Fruit

BETA-COPAENE Fruit

BETA-FARNESENE Fruit

BETA-HUMULENE Fruit

BETA-IONONE Fruit

BETA-PINENE Fruit

BETA-SELINENE Fruit

BETA-SITOSTEROL Leaf

BUTANAL Fruit

CALCIUM Fruit 180–1,582 ppm

CALCIUM-OXALATE Leaf

CARBOHYDRATES Fruit 118,800–855,360 ppm

CARYOPHYLLENE-OXIDE Leaf

CATECHOL-TANNINS Leaf 40,000–75,000 ppm

CHLORINE Fruit 40 ppm

CINNAMYL-ACETATE Fruit

CITRAL Fruit

CITRIC-ACID Fruit

COPPER Fruit 1–9 ppm

CRATAEGOLIC-ACID Leaf

D-GALACTOSE Fruit

D-GALACTURONIC-ACID Fruit

DELTA-CADINENE Fruit

ELLAGIC-ACID Bark 8,000 ppm Fruit

EO Leaf 2,600–3,600 ppm

FAT Fruit 6,000–43,200 ppm Leaf 60,000 ppm
  Seed 100,000–143,000 ppm
FIBER Fruit 56,000–403,200 ppm Seed 424,000
  ppm
FRUCTOSE Fruit
GALLIC-ACID Fruit
GALLOYL-TANNIN Root
GLUCOSE Seed 1,000 ppm
GLUTAMIC-ACID Fruit 1,070–7,704 ppm
GLYCINE Fruit 410–2,952 ppm
GUAFINE Bark 20,000 ppm
GUAJIVERINE Leaf
GUAJIVOLIC-ACID Leaf
HISTIDINE Fruit 70–504 ppm
IRON Fruit 3–24 ppm
ISOLEUCINE Fruit 300–2,160 ppm
KILOCALORIES Fruit 510–3,670 /kg
L-MALIC-ACID Fruit
LACTIC-ACID Fruit
LEUCINE Fruit 550–3,960 ppm
LEUCOANTHOCYANIN Bark
LEUCOCYANIDINS Fruit 1,000 ppm Leaf 4,000
  ppm
LIMONENE Fruit
LINOLEIC-ACID Fruit 1,820–13,104 ppm Seed
  13,900 ppm
LINOLENIC-ACID Seed 200 ppm
LUTEIC-ACID Bark
LYSINE Fruit 230–1,656 ppm
MAGNESIUM Fruit 98–735 ppm
MANGANESE Fruit 1–12 ppm
MECOCYANIN Fruit
METHIONINE Plant 50–360 ppm
METHYL-CINNAMATE Fruit
METHYL-ISOPROPYLKETONE Fruit
MUFA Fruit 550–3,955 ppm
MYRICETIN Bark
MYRISTIC-ACID Fruit 120–864 ppm
NEROLIDIOL Leaf
NIACIN Fruit 12–86 ppm
OLEANOLIC-ACID Leaf
OLEIC-ACID Fruit 520–3,744 ppm Seed 27,900
  ppm
OXALIC-ACID Fruit 140 ppm
PALMITIC-ACID Fruit 1,440–10,368 ppm
PALMITOLEIC-ACID Fruit 30–216 ppm
PANTOTHENIC-ACID Fruit 2–11 ppm
PECTIN Fruit 3,000–16,000 ppm
PHENYLALANINE Fruit 20–144 ppm

PHOSPHORUS Fruit 235–1,905 ppm
PHYTIN-PHOSPHORUS Fruit 127–1,029 ppm
POTASSIUM Fruit 2,672–21,658 ppm
PROLINE Fruit 250–1,800 ppm
PROTEIN Fruit 8,200–59,000 ppm Seed
  152,000 ppm
PSIDIOLIC-ACID Leaf
PUFA Fruit 2,530–18,200 ppm
PYROGALLOL-TANNINS Bark 135,000 ppm
  Leaf 40,000–78,000 ppm
QUERCETIN Leaf
RHAMNOSE Fruit
RIBOFLAVIN Fruit 1–4 ppm
SEL-11-EN-4ALPHA-OL Leaf
SERINE Fruit 240–1,728 ppm
SESQUIGUAVENE Plant
SFA Fruit 1,720–12,375 ppm
SODIUM Fruit 26–246 ppm
STARCH Seed 132,000 ppm
STEARIC-ACID Fruit 160–1,152 ppm
SUCROSE Fruit
SUGAR Leaf
SULFUR Fruit 140 ppm
TANNIN Bark 110,000–300,000 ppm Leaf
  90,000–100,000 ppm
TANNINS Seed 14,000 ppm
THIAMIN Fruit 1–4 ppm
THREONINE Fruit 310–2,232 ppm
TRYPTOPHAN Fruit 70–504 ppm
TYROSINE Fruit 100–720 ppm
URSOLIC-ACID Leaf
VALINE Fruit 280–2,016 ppm
VIT-B-6 Fruit 1–10 ppm
WATER Fruit 854,000–868,000 ppm Seed
  103,000 ppm
WAX Leaf
XANTHOPHYLL Leaf
XYLOSE Fruit
ZINC Fruit 2–20 ppm

JACKFRUIT

Chemicals in *Artocarpus heterophyllus LAM.*
(*Moraceae*)—Jackfruit

ACETYL-CHOLINE Seed
ARTOCARPANONE Plant
ARTOCARPESINE Wood
ARTOCARPETIN Plant
ARTOCARPIN Plant

ARTOFLAVANONE Root

ARTOFLAVANONE-2',4',5,7-TETRAHYDROX-
YFLAVONE Plant

ARTOSTENONE Latex Exudate

ASCORBIC-ACID Fruit 45–435 ppm

ASH Fruit 10,000–37,355 ppm Seed
15,000–30,990 ppm

BETA-CAROTENE Fruit 0.2–8 ppm

BETULINIC-ACID Root

CALCIUM Fruit 200–1,735 ppm Seed
500–1,033 ppm

CAOUTCHOUC Latex Exudate 60,000–100,000
ppm

CARBOHYDRATES Fruit 189,000–896,900 ppm
Seed 384,000–793,400 ppm

CONCAVALIN-A Seed

COPPER Fruit 1.8–7 ppm

CYANOMACLURIN Plant

CYCLOARTOCARPESINE Wood

CYCLOARTOCARPIN Plant

DIHYDROMORIN Fruit

FAT Fruit 1,000–11,200 ppm Seed 4,000–8,265
ppm

FIBER Fruit 10,000–48,245 ppm Seed
15,000–30,990 ppm

IRON Fruit 5–22 ppm Seed 12–25 ppm

KILOCALORIES Fruit 940–3,510 /kg

MAGNESIUM Fruit 370–1,380 ppm

MANGANESE Fruit 2–7 ppm

MORIN Plant

NIACIN Fruit 4–15 ppm

NORARTOCARPETIN Wood

OXYDIHYDROARTOCARPESINE Wood

PHOSPHORUS Fruit 260–1,725 ppm Seed
1,300–2,685 ppm

POTASSIUM Fruit 1,990–15,125 ppm

PROTEIN Fruit 12,180–83,330 ppm Seed
66,000–136,360 ppm

RIBOFLAVIN Fruit 1–4 ppm

SODIUM Fruit 20–150 ppm

TANNIN Bark 33,000 ppm

THIAMIN Fruit 0.3–3 ppm

URSOLIC-ACID Root

VIT-B-6 Fruit 1–4 ppm

WATER Fruit 712,740–772,000 ppm Latex Exudate 650,000–750,000 ppm
Seed 516,000–577,000 ppm

ZINC Fruit 4–16 ppm

KIWI

Chemicals in *Actinidia chinensis PLAN-
CHON (Actinidiaceae)*—Kiwi

ACTINIDIN Fruit

ASCORBIC-ACID Fruit 750–6,370 ppm

ASH Fruit 4,500–41,600 ppm

BETA-CAROTENE Fruit 0.4–6 ppm

BETA-SITOSTEROL Plant

CALCIUM Fruit 160–1,910 ppm

CARBOHYDRATES Fruit 148,800–877,900 ppm

CAROTENOIDS Fruit 5–42 ppm

CHROMIUM Fruit

CRYPTOXANTHIN Fruit 0.037–0.185 ppm

CYANIDIN Plant

DELPHINIDIN Plant

FAT Fruit 700–38,400 ppm

FIBER Fruit 11,000–64,900 ppm

FOLACIN Fruit

GLUCOSE Fruit

IRON Fruit 3–30 ppm

KILOCALORIES Fruit 610–3,600 /kg

LEVULOSE Fruit

LUTEIN Fruit 1.8–9 ppm

MAGNESIUM Fruit 300–1,770 ppm

NEOCHROME Fruit

NEOXANTHIN Fruit

NIACIN Fruit 5–30 ppm

P-COUMARIC-ACID Plant

PECTIN Fruit 4,200–24,800 ppm

PHOSPHORUS Fruit 300–3,060 ppm

POTASSIUM Fruit 3,320–19,600 ppm

PROTEIN Fruit 7,900–62,830 ppm

QUERCETIN Plant

QUINIC-ACID Fruit

RIBOFLAVIN Fruit 0.5–3 ppm

SODIUM Fruit 50–295 ppm

SUCCINIC-ACID Plant

TANNIN Fruit 9,500 ppm

THIAMIN Fruit 0.2–1 ppm

TOCOPHEROL Fruit

VIOLAXANTHIN Fruit

WATER Fruit 812,000–837,000 ppm

ZEAXANTHIN Fruit

LEMON

Chemicals in *Citrus limon (L.) BURMAN f.
(Rutaceae)*—Lemon

1,8-CINEOLE Leaf Essent. Oil 11,000–70,000 ppm

2'-O-XYLOSYL-VITEXIN Flower

2',4',5-TRIHYDROXY-FLAVONONE-7-O-BETA-D-GLUCOSYL-RHAMNOSIDE Pericarp

3',4',5-TRIHYDROXY-FLAVONE-7-O-BETA-D-RHAMNOSYL Plant

3',4',5-TRIHYDROXY-FLAVONONE-7-O-BETA-D-RHAMNOSYL Plant

3-(4-HYDROXY-3-METHOXY-PHENYL)-1-GLU-COSYL-PROP-2-ENE Pericarp

3-HEXEN-1-OL Essential Oil

4',5,7-TRIHYDROXY-3',6,8-TRIMETHOXY-FLAVONE-3-O-BETA-D-GLUCOSIDE Plant

4',5,7-TRIHYDROXY-3',8-DIMETHOXY-FLAVONE-3-O-BETA-D-GLUCOSIDE Pericarp

4',5,7-TRIHYDROXY-3',8-DIMETHOXY-FLAVONE-3-O-BETA-D-GLUCOSYL-RHAM-NOSIDE Pericarp

4',5,7-TRIHYDROXY-FLAVONE-6,8-DI-C-GLU-COSIDE Pericarp

4',5,7-TRIHYDROXY-FLAVONE-6-O-BETA-D-RHAMNOSYL Plant

4',5,7-TRIHYDROXY-FLAVONE-8-O-BETA-D-RHAMNOSYL Plant

4',7-DIHYDROXY-3'-METHOXY-FLAVONONE-8-O-BETA-D-GLUCOSYL-RHAMNOSIDE Pericarp

4-(3-METHYL-2-BUTENOXY)-ACETOPHENONE Pericarp

5,7-DIMETHYOXYCOUMARIN Essential Oil

5-GERANOXY-7-METHOXYCOUMARIN Essential Oil 630 ppm

5-GERANOXY-7-METHOXYPSORALEN Essential Oil

5-GERANYL-OXYPSORALEN Pericarp

5-ISOPENTENOXY-7-METHOXYCOUMARIN Essential Oil

6,7-DIMETHOXYCOUMARIN Bark 162 ppm

6-8-DI-C-GLUCOSYL-DIOSMETIN Pericarp

6-C-GLUCOSYL-DIOSMETIN Pericarp

7-GLUCOSYL-APIGENIN Flower

7-PENTAHYDROXY-2',3',5,5'-PENTAHYDROXY-FLAVANONE-7-(6-O-ALPHA-L-RHAMNOSY) L-BETA-D-GLUCOSIDE Pericarp

7-RHAMNO-GLUCOSYL-DIOSMETIN Flower

7-RHAMNO-GLUCOSYL-LUTEOLIN Flower

8-C-GLUCOSYL-DIOSMETIN Pericarp

8-GERAN-OXYPSORALEN Pericarp

ACETIC-ACID Essential Oil

ADENOSINE Pericarp

ALPHA,ALPHA-P-TRIMETHYLBENZYL-ALCO-HOL Plant

ALPHA-AMINO-BUTYRIC-ACID Plant

ALPHA-BERGAMOTENE Essential Oil 250 ppm

ALPHA-COPAENE Essential Oil

ALPHA-CUBEBENE Essential Oil

ALPHA-HUMULENE Essential Oil 10 ppm

ALPHA-PHELLANDRENE Essential Oil 20 ppm

ALPHA-PINENE Essential Oil 40–500 ppm Leaf Essent. Oil 500–2,000 ppm Pericarp Essent. Oil 5,000–14,000 ppm

ALPHA-TERPINENE Essential Oil 70 ppm Pericarp

ALPHA-TERPINEOL Essential Oil 6–50 ppm Leaf Essent. Oil 11,000–125,000 ppm Pericarp Essent. Oil 4,000–73,000 ppm

ALPHA-TERPINYL-PROPIONATE Essential Oil

ALPHA-THUJENE Essential Oil 16–40 ppm

APIGENIN-C-GLYCOSIDE Plant

ASCORBIC-ACID Fruit 5,208–5,566 ppm

ASH Fruit 28,000 ppm

AUREUSIDIN Plant

AUREUSIDIN-6-GLUCOSIDE Plant

AUREUSIDIN-6-RHAMNOGLUCOSIDE Plant

BERGAMOTENE Essential Oil 16–40 ppm

BERGAMOTTIN Essential Oil 649 ppm

BERGAPTEN Essential Oil 10 ppm

BETA-BISABOLENE Essential Oil 23–400 ppm

BETA-CAROTENE Fruit 2 ppm

BETA-CARYOPHYLLENE Leaf Essent. Oil 100 ppm

BETA-ELEMENE Essential Oil

BETA-HUMULENE Essential Oil 10 ppm

BETA-PHELLANDRENE Essential Oil 80 ppm

BETA-PINENE Essential Oil 40–1,270 ppm

BETA-SITOSTEROL Plant

BRAYLIN Root

BYAKANGELICIN Essential Oil 29 ppm

BYAKANGELICOL Essential Oil

CADINENE Essential Oil

CAFFEIC-ACID Fruit 21–35 ppm

CAFFEINE Flower 50 ppm

CALCIUM Fruit 700–3,227 ppm

CAMPHENE Essential Oil 2–50 ppm

CARBOHYDRATES Fruit 111,000–863,000 ppm

CARVEOL Essential Oil

CARVONE Essential Oil

CARYOPHYLLENE Essential Oil 11–28 ppm

CARYOPHYLLENE-OXIDE Leaf Essent. Oil 0.8 ppm

CHLOROPHYLL-A Leaf

CHLOROPHYLL-B Leaf

CIS-LIMONENE-1,2-OXIDE Essential Oil

CITRAL Essential Oil 250–300 ppm

CITRIC-ACID Fruit 59,500 ppm

CITRONELLAL Leaf Essent. Oil 25,000–89,000 ppm

CITRONELLOL Leaf Essent. Oil 20 ppm

CITRONELLYL-ACETATE Plant 4–20 ppm

CITRONETIN Plant

CITRONIN Plant

CITROPTEN Fruit

CITRUSIN-A Pericarp

CITRUSIN-B Pericarp

CITRUSIN-C Pericarp

CONIFERIN Pericarp

D-GALACTURONIC-ACID Fruit

DEACETYL-NOMILIN Seed

DEACETYL-NOMILIN-17-O-BETA-D-GLUCOPY-RANOSIDE Seed

DECAN-1-AL Pericarp

DECANAL Essential Oil 6–20 ppm

DECANOIC-ACID Essential Oil

DECANOL Essential Oil

DECYL-ACETATE Plant 5 ppm

DECYL-ALDEHYDE Leaf

DELTA-CARENE Essential Oil

DICONIFERYL-ALCOHOL-4-BETA-D-GLUCO-SIDE Pericarp

DIOSMETIN Plant

DIOSMIN Fruit 5 ppm

DODECANAL Essential Oil 10 ppm

DODECANOIC-ACID Essential Oil

EPIJASMONIC-ACID-METHYL-ESTER Pericarp

ERIOCITRIN Fruit 1 ppm

ERIODICTYOSIDE Fruit

FARNESENE Essential Oil

FAT Fruit 28,000 ppm Seed 300,000–400,000 ppm

FERULIC-ACID Fruit 14–40 ppm

FIBER Fruit 17,000–47,000 ppm

GAMMA-SITOSTEROL Plant

GAMMA-TERPINENE Essential Oil 290–1,400 ppm Leaf Essent. Oil 3,000–44,000 ppm Pericarp Essent. Oil 12,000–58,000 ppm

GERANIAL Essential Oil 42–236 ppm Leaf Essent. Oil 3,000–270,000 ppm

GERANIOL Essential Oil

GERANIOL-ACETATE Leaf Essent. Oil 3,000 ppm

GERANYL-ACETATE Essential Oil 12–310 ppm

GERANYL-BUTYRATE Essential Oil

GERANYL-FORMATE Essential Oil

GERANYL-OXY-PYRANOCOUMARIN Root

GLUTAMIC-ACID Plant

HEPTADECANAL Essential Oil

HEPTANAL Essential Oil 4 ppm

HESPERIDIN Fruit 44 ppm Pericarp 68,800 ppm

HESPERIDOSIDE Fruit

HEXADECANAL Essential Oil

HEXANAL Essential Oil

HEXANOL Essential Oil

IMPERATORIN Fruit

IRON Fruit 23–72 ppm

ISOIMPERATORIN Essential Oil

ISOLIMOCITROL Pericarp

ISOLIMOCITROL-3,7,4'-TRIMETHYL-ETHER Plant

ISOLIMOCITROL-3-BETA-D-GLUCOSIDE Plant

ISOPIMPINELLIN Plant

ISOPULEGOL Leaf Essent. Oil 40,000 ppm

ISOPULEGOLE Leaf Essent. Oil 18,000–114,000 ppm

ISORHAMNETIN Flower

ISORHAMNETIN-3-ARABINOGLUCOSIDE Plant

ISORHOIFOLIN Leaf

ISOVITEXIN Pericarp

JASMONIC-ACID-METHYL-ESTER Pericarp

KILOCALORIES Fruit 2,640 /kg

LAURALDEHYDE Fruit

LIMETTIN Essential Oil 295 ppm

LIMOCITRIN Pericarp

LIMOCITRIN-3-(6-O-ALPHA-L-RHAMNOSYL-BETA-D-GLUCOSIDE) Pericarp

LIMONENE Essential Oil 2,796–8,000 ppm Leaf Essent. Oil 284,000–754,000 ppm Pericarp Essent. Oil 512,000–774,000 ppm

LIMONIN Fruit Seed

LIMONIN-17-O-BETA-D-GLUCOPYRANOSIDE Seed

LIMONOATE-A-RING-LACTONE Fruit

LINALOL Essential Oil 8–30 ppm Leaf Essent. Oil 17,000–81,000 ppm Pericarp Essent. Oil 7,000–110,000 ppm

LINALYL-ACETATE Essential Oil

LUTEIN Fruit 0.12–1.2 ppm

LUTEOLIN Flower

LUTEOLIN-7-O-BETA-RUTINOSIDE Leaf

MENTH-1-EN-9-OL Essential Oil

METHYL-HEPTANONE Essential Oil

METHYL-HEPTENONE Leaf Essent. Oil 6,000 ppm

MUCILAGE Fruit

MYRCENE Essential Oil 65–1,270 ppm Leaf Essent. Oil 13,000 ppm

N-METHYL-TYRAMINE Leaf

NARINGIN Pericarp

NARINGOSIDE Fruit

NARIRUTIN Pericarp

NEOHESPERIDIN Pericarp

NEOXANTHIN Leaf

NERAL Essential Oil 27–130 ppm Leaf Essent. Oil 4,000–270,000 ppm

NEROL Leaf Essent. Oil 18,000–76,000 ppm

NEROL-ACETATE Essential Oil 16–310 ppm Leaf Essent. Oil 40 ppm

NERYL-FORMATE Essential Oil 20 ppm

NIACIN Fruit

NOMILIN Seed

NOMILIN-17-O-BETA-D-GLUCOPYRANOSIDE Seed

NONAN-1-AL Essential Oil 3–7 ppm

NONANAL Essential Oil 9–30 ppm

NONYL-ACETATE Plant

NONYL-ALDEHYDE Essential Oil

NOOTKATONE Plant

O-PHENYLPHENOL Essential Oil

OBACUNONE Seed

OBACUNONE-17-O-BETA-D-GLUCOPYRA-NOSIDE Seed

OCIMENE Leaf Essent. Oil 10,000 ppm

OCTAN-1-AL Pericarp

OCTANOIC-ACID Essential Oil

OCTANOL Essential Oil 10–15 ppm

OCTOPAMINE Leaf

OCTYL-ACETATE Essential Oil

OCTYL-ALDEHYDE Essential Oil

OSTHOLE Root

OXYPEUCEDANIN Essential Oil 207 ppm

OXYPEUCEDANIN-HYDRATE Essential Oil 64 ppm

P-ALPHA-DIMETHYLSTYRENE Plant

P-COUMARIC-ACID Fruit 6–102 ppm

P-CYMENE Essential Oil 12–31 ppm

P-CYMOL Essential Oil

P-MENTHA-1,8-DIEN-9-YL-ACETATE Essential Oil

P-MENTHA-2,8-DIEN-1-OL Essential Oil

PE Plant

PECTIN Pericarp

PENTADECANAL Essential Oil

PENTADECANE Plant

PERILLALDEHYDE Fruit

PHELLOPTERIN Essential Oil

PHLORIN Plant

PHOSPHORUS Fruit 100–1,979 ppm

PONCIRIN Plant

POTASSIUM Fruit 14,700 ppm

PROTEIN Fruit 10,000–111,000 ppm

QUERCETIN Flower

QUERCETIN-3,5-DIGLUCOSIDE Plant

RIBOFLAVIN Fruit 2–3 ppm

RUTIN Fruit 1–2 ppm Leaf

SABINENE Essential Oil 50–175 ppm Leaf Essent. Oil 2,700 ppm

SALICYLATES Fruit

SCOPOLETIN Shoot

SELINENE Essential Oil

SESELIN Root

SINAPIC-ACID Fruit 14–18 ppm

SODIUM Fruit 470 ppm

STACHYDRINE Plant

SUBEROSIN Root

SYNEPHRINE Leaf

SYRINGIN Pericarp

TERPINEN-4-OL Essential Oil 1–40 ppm Leaf Essent. Oil 10,000 ppm Pericarp Essent. Oil 1,000–11,000 ppm

TERPINOLENE Essential Oil 14–120 ppm

TETRADECANAL Essential Oil

TETRADECANE Essential Oil

TETRAHYDROGERANIOL Essential Oil 10 ppm

THIAMIN Fruit 4–6 ppm

THYMOL Leaf Essent. Oil 400 ppm Pericarp Essent. Oil 53,000–111,000 ppm
TRANS-LIMONENE-1,2–OXIDE Essential Oil
TRIDECANAL Essential Oil
TYRAMINE Leaf
UMBELLIFERONE Shoot
UNDECANAL Essential Oil
VICENIN-2 Pericarp
VIOLAXANTHIN Leaf
WATER Fruit 850,000–894,000 ppm
XANTHOXYLETIN Root
XANTHYLETIN Root
XYLOSYL-VITEXIN Flower
ZEAXANTHIN Leaf

LIME

Chemicals in *Tilia sp.* (*Tiliaceae*)—Basswood, Lime, Linden

2-PHENYLETHANOL Flower
2-PHENYLETHYL-BENZOATE Flower
2-PHENYLETHYLPHENYLACETATE Flower
AFZELIN Flower
ALANINE Flower
ALPHA-PINENE Flower
ASCORBIC-ACID Leaf
ASH Fruit 21,000–130,000 ppm
ASPARAGINE Fruit
ASTRAGALIN Flower
BETA-AMYRIN Leaf
BETA-SITOSTEROL Wood
CAFFEIC-ACID Flower
CARBOHYDRATES Fruit 232,000–727,000 ppm Leaf 575,000–653,000 ppm
CHLOROGENIC-ACID Flower
CIS-TRANS-FARNESOL Flower
CIS-TRANS-FARNESYL-ACETATE Flower
CYSTEINE Flower
CYSTINE Flower
DOCOSANE Flower
EICOSANE Flower
EUGENOL Flower
FAT Fruit 30,000–580,000 ppm Leaf 29,000–33,000 ppm
FIBER Fruit 135,000–423,000 ppm Leaf 132,000–150,000 ppm
GERANIOL Flower

GERANYL-ACETATE Flower
GLUTAMIC-ACID Fruit
GLYCINE Fruit
HENEICOSANE Flower
HENTRIACONTANE Flower
HEPTACOSANE Flower
HESPERIDIN Flower
HEXACOSANE Flower
ISOLEUCINE Flower
ISOQUERCITRIN Flower
KAEMPFERITRIN Flower
KAEMPFEROL-3(P-COUMAROYLGLUCOSIDE) Flower
KAEMPFEROL-3,7-DIRHAMNOSIDE Flower
KAEMPFEROL-3-GLUCO-7-RHAMNOSIDE Flower
LEUCINE Flower
LIMONENE Flower
LINALOL Flower
LINALYL-ACETATE Flower
LINARIN Leaf
LINOLEIC-ACID Wood
LINOLENIC-ACID Wood
MUCILAGE Flower
NEROL Flower
NEROLIDOL Flower
NONADECANE Flower
OCTACOSANE Flower
OCTADECANE Flower
OLEIC-ACID Wood
P-COUMARIC-ACID Flower
PALMITIC-ACID Wood
PENTACOSANE Flower
PHENYLALANINE Flower
PHLOBAPHENE Leaf
PROTEIN Fruit 36,000–113,000 ppm Leaf 162,000–184,000 ppm
QUERCETIN Flower
QUERCETIN-3-GLUCOSIDE-7-RHAMNOSIDE Flower
QUERCETIN-RHAMNOSIDE-XYLOSIDE Flower
QUERCITRIN Flower
SAPONIN Flower
SERINE Flower
SQUALENE Wood
STIGMASTANOL Wood
STIGMASTEROL Wood
SUCROSE Wood

SUGAR Flower
TANNIN Flower
TARAXEROL Bark
TERPINEOL Flower
TETRACOSANE Flower
TILIROSIDE Flower
TOCOPHEROL Flower
TRIACONTANE Flower
TRICOSANE Flower
TYROSINE Fruit
VALINE Fruit
VANILLIN Flower
WATER Fruit 681,000 ppm Leaf 120,000 ppm
XANTHOPHYLL Leaf

LINGONBERRY

Chemicals in *Vaccinium vitis-iddaea var. minus LODD. (Ericaceae)*—Cowberry, Lingen, Lingonberry

(+)-CATECHIN Fruit 3,500 ppm
1-AMINOCYCLOPROPAN-1-CARBONIC-ACID Fruit
2-O-CAFFEOYL-ARBUTIN Leaf
4-HYDROXY-PHENYL-BETA-GENTIOBIOSIDE Leaf
5-HYDROXY-PIPECOLIC-ACID Fruit
ALUMINUM Fruit 5–53 ppm
ARBUTIN Leaf 40,000–90,000 ppm
ARSENIC Fruit
ASCORBIC-ACID Fruit 280–1,865 ppm
ASH Fruit 2,500–18,000 ppm
AVICULARIN Leaf
BENZOIC-ACID Fruit 1,360 ppm
BETA-CAROTENE Plant
BETA-HYDROXY-KETO-BUTYRIC-ACID Fruit
BORON Fruit 1.4–11 ppm
BROMINE Fruit
CADMIUM Fruit 0.001–0.07 ppm
CAFFEIC-ACID Leaf
CALCIUM Fruit 180–1,730 ppm
CATECHIN-TANNINS Leaf 80,000 ppm
CHROMIUM Fruit 0.01–0.13 ppm
CITRIC-ACID Fruit
COBALT Fruit
COPPER Fruit 0.7–5.2 ppm
CYANIDIN-3-GALACTOSIDE Fruit
EPICATECHIN Leaf

FLUORINE Fruit 0.1–0.7 ppm
FRUCTOSE Fruit 50,000 ppm
GALLIC-ACID Leaf
GALLOCATECHIN Leaf
GLUCOSE Fruit 40,000 ppm
HYDROQUINONE Leaf
HYPEROSIDE Fruit Leaf
IRON Fruit 4–31 ppm Leaf 250 ppm
ISOQUERCITRIN Leaf
KAEMPFEROL Fruit
KETOGLUTARIC-ACID Fruit
LEAD Fruit 0.05–0.4 ppm
LYCOPENE Fruit
MAGNESIUM Fruit 80–600 ppm
MALIC-ACID Fruit
MANGANESE Fruit 28–250 ppm Leaf 2,500 ppm
MERCURY Fruit 0.07 ppm
MOLYBDENUM Fruit
N-NONACOSANE Fruit
PECTIN Fruit 4,000 ppm
PHOSPHORUS Fruit 150–1,130 ppm
POTASSIUM Fruit 720–6,200 ppm
PYROSIDE Leaf
QUERCETIN Leaf
QUINIC-ACID Fruit
RUBIDIUM Fruit 2.7–22 ppm
SALICYLIC-ACID Fruit
SALIDROSIDE Leaf
SELENIUM Fruit 0.013 ppm
SILICON Fruit 5–133 ppm
SUCROSE Fruit 5,300 ppm
SUGAR Fruit 80,000 ppm
SULFUR Fruit 130–1,075 ppm
TANNIN Leaf 60,000–200,000 ppm
URSOLIC-ACID Fruit 7,500 ppm
VACCINIIN Fruit 410 ppm
WATER Fruit 800,000–932,000 ppm
ZEAXANTHIN Fruit
ZINC Fruit 1.7–14 ppm

MANDARIN

Chemicals in *Citrus reticulata BLANCO (Rutaceae)*—Mandarin, Tangerine

1,8-CINEOLE Fruit 76 ppm
3,5,5-TRIMETHYLBENZYL-ALCOHOL Fruit 3 ppm

ACETALDEHYDE Fruit 2 ppm
ALANINE Fruit 70–2,740 ppm
ALPHA-CAROTENE Fruit 0.2–2 ppm
ALPHA-COPAENE Fruit 1–2 ppm
ALPHA-LINOLENIC-ACID Fruit 100–806 ppm
ALPHA-PHELLANDRENE Fruit 3–32 ppm
ALPHA-PINENE Fruit 30–393 ppm
ALPHA-SELINENE Fruit 2 ppm
ALPHA-SINESAL Fruit 1–32 ppm
ALPHA-TERPINENE Fruit 4–42 ppm
ALPHA-TERPINEOL Fruit 2–110 ppm
ALPHA-TERPINYL-ACETATE Fruit 1–5 ppm
ALPHA-THUJENE Fruit 46–58 ppm
ALPHA-TOCOPHEROL Fruit 3–31 ppm
ALPHA-YLANGENE Fruit 1 ppm
ALUMINUM Fruit 1–15 ppm
ARGININE Fruit 440–3,546 ppm
ARSENIC Fruit 0.04–0.3 ppm
ASCORBIC-ACID Fruit 280–3,684 ppm
ASH Fruit 3,900–31,525 ppm
ASPARAGINE Fruit 180–850 ppm
ASPARTIC-ACID Fruit 240–6,206 ppm
BENZYL-ALCOHOL Fruit 1–2 ppm
BETA-APOCAROTENOL Fruit
BETA-CAROTENE Fruit 1–44 ppm
BETA-CITRAURIN Fruit
BETA-ELEMENE Fruit 1–80 ppm
BETA-PINENE Fruit 90–210 ppm
BETA-SESQUIPHELLANDRENE Fruit 20 ppm
BETA-TERPINEOL Fruit 40 ppm
BORON Fruit 1–14 ppm
BROMINE Fruit 1 ppm
CADMIUM Fruit
CALAMIN Plant
CALCIUM Fruit 140–3,077 ppm
CAMPHENE Fruit 1–40 ppm
CARBOHYDRATES Fruit 102,000–901,914 ppm
CARVONE Fruit 3 ppm
CARYOPHYLLENE Fruit 2–9 ppm
CHLORINE Fruit 24 ppm
CHROMIUM Fruit 0.01–0.08 ppm
CIS-3-HEXENOL Fruit 1 ppm
CIS-CARVEOL Fruit 1–4 ppm
CITRIC-ACID Fruit 8,600–12,200 ppm
CITRONELLAL Fruit 1–20 ppm
CITRONELLIC-ACID Fruit
CITRONELLOL Fruit 1–50 ppm
CITRONELLYL-ACETATE Fruit 4–10 ppm

COBALT Fruit
COPPER Fruit 4.8 ppm
CYCLOCALAMIN Plant
CYSTINE Fruit 70–564 ppm
DECANAL Fruit 3–90 ppm
DECANOIC-ACID Fruit 3 ppm
DECANOL Fruit 4 ppm
DECYL-ACETATE Fruit 1–5 ppm
DELTA-3-CARENE Fruit 1–6 ppm
DELTA-CADINENE Fruit 20 ppm
DELTA-ELEMENE Fruit 6–10 ppm
DIMETHYL-ANTHRALINATE Fruit 90 ppm
DODECANAL Fruit 1–15 ppm
DODECANOIC-ACID Fruit 1 ppm
DODECANOL Fruit 1 ppm
EO Fruit 10,000 ppm
ETHANOL Fruit 183 ppm
EUPATILIN Fruit
FAT Fruit 1,900–22,000 ppm
FERULOYL-PUTRESCINE Fruit
FIBER Fruit 1,890–43,000 ppm
FLUORINE Fruit 0.1–0.76 ppm
FOLACIN Fruit 2 ppm
GAMMA-AMINOBUTYRIC-ACID Fruit 180 ppm
GAMMA-CADANINE Fruit 2 ppm
GAMMA-ELEMENE Fruit 15–20 ppm
GAMMA-SELINENE Fruit 1 ppm
GAMMA-TERPINENE Fruit 210–2,014 ppm
GERANIAL Fruit 6–30 ppm
GERANIOL Fruit 1–4 ppm
GERANYL-ACETATE Fruit 1–18 ppm
GLUTAMIC-ACID Fruit 160–5,158 ppm
GLYCINE Fruit 20–5,158 ppm
HEPTANOIC-ACID Fruit 1 ppm
HEPTANOL Fruit 1–2 ppm
HESPERIDIN Plant
HISTIDINE Fruit 440–3,546 ppm
HUMULENE Fruit 5 ppm
IRON Fruit 1–79 ppm
ISOLEUCINE Fruit 170–1,370 ppm
ISOPULEGOL Fruit 1–5 ppm
LEUCINE Fruit 50–1,290 ppm
LIMONENE Fruit 6,500–9,400 ppm
LINALOL Fruit 3–610 ppm
LINOLEIC-ACID Fruit 270–2,176 ppm
LONGIFOLENE Fruit 1 ppm
LUTEIN Fruit 0.2–2 ppm
LYSINE Fruit 40–2,579 ppm

MAGNESIUM Fruit 111–1,416 ppm
MALIC-ACID Fruit 1,800–2,100 ppm
MALONIC-ACID Fruit
MANGANESE Fruit 4.6 ppm
MERCURY Fruit
METHIONINE Fruit 130–1,048 ppm
METHYL-HEPTENONE Fruit 1 ppm
METHYL-N-METHYL-ANTHRALINATE Fruit 1–33 ppm
METHYL-THYMOL Fruit 10 ppm
MOLYBDENUM Fruit
MYRCENE Fruit 46–760 ppm
MYRISTIC-ACID Fruit 10–80 ppm
N-METHYL-TYRAMINE Fruit 58 ppm
NERAL Fruit 2–6 ppm
NEROL Fruit 1–5 ppm
NERYL-ACETATE Fruit 1–10 ppm
NIACIN Fruit 1–35 ppm
NICKEL Fruit 0.01–0.3 ppm
NITROGEN Fruit 1,600–13,075 ppm
NOBELITIN Fruit
NONANAL Fruit 1–8 ppm
NONANOIC-ACID Fruit 1 ppm
NONANOL Fruit 2–10 ppm
NOOTKATONE Fruit 1 ppm
OCIMENE Fruit 8 ppm
OCTANAL Fruit 4–30 ppm
OCTANOIC-ACID Fruit 4 ppm
OCTANOL Fruit 9 ppm
OCTOPAMINE Fruit 1–2 ppm
OCTYL-ACETATE Fruit 2–4 ppm
OLEIC-ACID Fruit 300–2,418 ppm
OXALIC-ACID Fruit
P-CYMENE Fruit 14–820 ppm
P-MENTHA-1-EN-9-YL-ACETATE Fruit
PALMITIC-ACID Fruit 200–1,612 ppm
PALMITOLEIC-ACID Fruit 40–320 ppm
PANTOTHENIC-ACID Fruit 2–16 ppm
PERILLALDEHYDE Fruit 10 ppm
PERILLYL-ACETATE Fruit 1–10 ppm
PHENYLALANINE Fruit 50–1,693 ppm
PHOSPHORUS Fruit 90–1,385 ppm
POTASSIUM Fruit 1,200–13,127 ppm
PROLINE Fruit 310–2,499 ppm
PROTEIN Fruit 6,130–80,228 ppm
QUINIC-ACID Fruit
RETICULAXANTHIN Fruit
RETROCALAMIN Plant

RIBOFLAVIN Fruit 4 ppm
RUBIDIUM Fruit 0.25–2.4 ppm
SABINENE Fruit 40–210 ppm
SABINENE-HYDRATE Fruit 1–20 ppm
SALICYLATES Fruit 5–50 ppm
SELENIUM Fruit
SERINE Fruit 120–1,773 ppm
SILICON Fruit 3–23 ppm
SODIUM Fruit 8–154 ppm
STEARIC-ACID Fruit 10–80 ppm
SUGARS Fruit 69,400–113,600 ppm
SULFUR Fruit 130–1,000 ppm
SYNEPHERINE Fruit 50–280 ppm
TANGERAXANTHIN Fruit
TANGERITIN Fruit
TERPINEN-4-OL Fruit 2–110 ppm
TERPINEOLENE Fruit 4–110 ppm
TETRADECANAL Fruit 5 ppm
THIAMIN Fruit 1–8 ppm
THREONINE Fruit 100–806 ppm
THYMOL Fruit 1–20 ppm
THYMYL-METHYL-ETHER Fruit 10 ppm
TRANS-CARVEOL Fruit 4 ppm
TRYPTOPHAN Fruit 60–484 ppm
TYRAMINE Fruit 1 ppm
TYROSINE Fruit 110–887 ppm
UNDECANOIC-ACID Fruit 1 ppm
UNDECANOL Fruit 1 ppm
VALINE Fruit 20–2,176 ppm
VIT-B-6 Fruit 1–5 ppm
WATER Fruit 879,720–886,000 ppm
ZEAXANTHIN Fruit
ZINC Fruit 0.8–8 ppm

MANGO

Chemicals in *Mangifera indica L. (Anacardiaceae)*—Mango

2-OCTENE Flower
ALANINE Fruit 510–5,650 ppm
ALPHA-PHELLANDRENE Flower
ALPHA-PINENE Flower
AMBOLIC-ACID Plant
AMBONIC-ACID Plant
ARGININE Fruit 190–3,400 ppm
ASCORBIC-ACID Fruit 30–1,760 ppm Leaf 530–2,430 ppm

ASH Fruit 4,700–29,140 ppm Leaf 19,000–133,000 ppm Seed 36,600 ppm

ASPARTIC-ACID Fruit 420–4,100 ppm

BETA-CAROTENE Fruit 11–96 ppm Leaf 6–44 ppm

BETA-PINENE Flower

BORON Fruit 0.5–17.5 ppm

CALCIUM Fruit 92–1,400 ppm Leaf 290–29,300 ppm

CARBOHYDRATES Fruit 170,000–929,390 ppm Leaf 165,000–540,000 ppm

CARBONATE Seed 900 ppm

CAROTENOIDS Fruit 10–165 ppm

CATALASE Fruit

CHLORINE Fruit 205 ppm

CITRIC-ACID Fruit

COPPER Fruit 1.1–16.6 ppm

CYSTINE Fruit 70–350 ppm

DIPENTENE Flower

EO Flower 400 ppm

FAT Fruit 1,000–16,890 ppm Leaf 4,000–38,000 ppm Seed 107,000 ppm

FIBER Fruit 8,000–49,000 ppm Leaf 16,000–211,000 ppm

FRUCTOSE Fruit 25,700–48,300 ppm

FURFUROL Resin, Exudate, Sap 18,000 ppm

GABA Fruit

GALLIC-ACID Flower 90,000 ppm

GALLOTANNIC-ACID Flower 150,000 ppm

GERANIOL Flower

GLUCOSE Fruit 10,000–43,200 ppm

GLUTAMIC-ACID Fruit 600–6,800 ppm

GLYCINE Fruit 210–1,900 ppm

HISTIDINE Fruit 120–1,200 ppm

IODINE Fruit 0.016 ppm

IRON Fruit 1–243 ppm Leaf 62 ppm

ISOLEUCINE Fruit 180–2,000 ppm

ISOMANGIFEROLIC-ACID Plant

KAEMPFEROL Plant

KILOCALORIES Fruit 590–3,554 /kg

LAURIC-ACID Fruit 10–55 ppm

LEUCINE Fruit 310–2,950 ppm

LIMONENE Flower

LINOLEIC-ACID Fruit 140–765 ppm

LINOLENIC-ACID Fruit 370–2,023 ppm

LYSINE Fruit 410–3,200 ppm

MAGNESIUM Fruit 84–875 ppm

MALIC-ACID Fruit 6,700–36,600 ppm

MANGANESE Fruit 0.2–12.2 ppm

MANGIFERIC-ACID Fruit

MANGIFERINE Fruit

MANGIFEROL Bark

MANGIFEROLIC-ACID Plant

MANGIFERONIC-ACID Plant

METHIONINE Fruit 50–550 ppm

MUFA Fruit 1,010–5,522 ppm

MYRISTIC-ACID Fruit 90–492 ppm

NEO-BETA-CAROTENE-B Fruit 19.2 ppm

NEO-BETA-CAROTENE-U Fruit 7.3 ppm

NEOXANTHOPHYLL Fruit

NEROL Flower

NERYL-ACETATE Flower

NIACIN Fruit 6.5–63 ppm Leaf 22–100 ppm

OLEIC-ACID Fruit 540–2,950 ppm

OXALIC-ACID Fruit 300 ppm

P-COUMARIC-ACID Plant

PALMITIC-ACID Fruit 520–2,843 ppm

PALMITOLEIC-ACID Fruit 480–2,625 ppm

PANTOTHENIC-ACID Fruit 1.6–8.8 ppm

PEROXIDASE Fruit

PHENYLALANINE Fruit 170–3,700 ppm

PHOSPHORUS Fruit 103–1,050 ppm Leaf 720–3,800 ppm

PHYTIN Fruit

POTASSIUM Fruit 1,080–9,475 ppm

PROLINE Fruit 180–2,000 ppm

PROTEIN Fruit 5,000–60,000 ppm Leaf 30,000–78,000 ppm Seed 95,000 ppm

PUFA Fruit 510–2,788 ppm

QUERCETIN Plant

RIBOFLAVIN Fruit 0.5–3.3 ppm Leaf 0.6–2.7 ppm

SERINE Fruit 220–3,150 ppm

SFA Fruit 660–3,608 ppm

SILICA Seed 4,100 ppm

SODIUM Fruit 13–143 ppm

STARCH Seed 728,000 ppm

STEARIC-ACID Fruit 30–164 ppm

SUCCINIC-ACID Fruit

SUCROSE Fruit 66,700–125,800 ppm

SUGARS Fruit 112,000–205,000 ppm Seed 10,700 ppm

SULFUR Fruit 70–615 ppm Seed 2,300 ppm

TANNIN Flower 150,000 ppm Seed 1,100 ppm

THIAMIN Fruit 0.4–3.4 ppm Leaf 0.4–1.8 ppm

THREONINE Fruit 190–2,250 ppm

TRYPTOPHAN Fruit 80–700 ppm
TYROSINE Fruit 100–1,600 ppm
VALINE Fruit 260–2,700 ppm
VIT-B-6 Fruit 1.3–7.3 ppm
WATER Fruit 754,300–900,000 ppm Leaf
782,000 ppm
XANTHOPHYLL Fruit 42 ppm
ZINC Fruit 0.4–11.4 ppm

MELON

Chemicals in *Cucumis melo subsp. ssp melo var.cantalupensis NAUDIN (Cucurbitaceae)* — Cantaloupe, Melon, Muskmelon, Netted Melon, Nutmeg Melon, Persian Melon

2,4-METHYLENE-CHOLESTEROL Seed
22-DIHYDRO-SPINASTEROL Seed
22-DIHYDROBRASSICASTEROL Seed
24-BETA-ETHYL-25(27)-DEHYDROLATHOS-
TEROL Seed
24-METHYL-25(27)-DEHYDROCYCLOAR-
TANOL Seed
24-METHYL-LATHOSTEROL Seed
24-METHYLENE-24-DIHYDROPARKEOL Seed
24-METHYLENE-24-DIHYDROLANASETOL
Seed
24-METHYLENE-CYCLOARTANOL Seed
25(27)-DEHYDRO-CHONDRILLASTEROL Seed
25(27)-DEHYDRO-FUNGISTEROL Seed
25(27)-DEHYDRO-PORIFERASTEROL Seed
3,4-DIMETHOXY-ACETOPHENONE-ISOMER
Petiole
3-PHENYL-PROPYL-ACETATE Petiole
ACETALDEHYDE Petiole
ADENOSINE Fruit
ALPHA-AMYRIN Seed
ALPHA-CAROTENE Fruit
ALPHA-SPINASTEROL Stem
ALPHA-TOCOPHEROL Fruit 1.4–14 ppm
ALUMINUM Fruit 26–77 ppm
ARACHIDIC-ACID Cotyledon 10,200–55,300
ppm Seed 2,700–4,014 ppm
ARSENIC Fruit 0.004–0.006 ppm
ASCORBIC-ACID Fruit 397–4,370 ppm
ASH Fruit 6,950–110,000 ppm
AVENASTEROL Seed
BARIUM Fruit 1.3–7.7 ppm
BEHENIC-ACID Leaf

BENZALDEHYDE Petiole
BENZYL-ACETATE Petiole
BENZYL-PROPIONATE Petiole
BETA-AMYRIN Seed
BETA-CAROTENE Fruit 0.2–201 ppm
BETA-CRYPTOXANTHIN Fruit
BETA-IONONE Petiole
BETA-PYRAZOL-1-YL-ALANINE Fruit
BORON Fruit 1–16.5 ppm
BUTYL-ACETATE Petiole
CADMIUM Fruit 0.017–0.044 ppm
CAFFEIC-ACID Plant
CALCIUM Fruit 96–3,080 ppm
CAMPESTEROL Seed
CAPRIC-ACID Seed 2,400–3,570 ppm
CAPROIC-ACID Seed 3,000–5,350 ppm
CAPRYLIC-ACID Seed 6,000–8,920 ppm
CARBOHYDRATES Fruit 83,600–818,026 ppm
CERYL-ALCOHOL Seed
CHROMIUM Fruit 0.13–0.165 ppm
CINNAMIC-ACETATE Petiole
CIS,CIS-3,6-NONADIEN-1-OL Fruit
CIS-3-NONEN-1-OL Fruit
CIS-6-NONEN-1-OL Fruit
CIS-6-NONENAL Fruit
CIS-CIS-NONA-3,6-DIENYL-ACETATE Petiole
CITRIC-ACID Leaf
CITRULLINE Fruit 142–241 ppm
CLEROSTEROL Seed
COBALT Fruit 0.087–0.11 ppm
CODISTEROL Seed
COPPER Fruit 0.4–7.7 ppm
CUCURBITACIN-B Fruit
CUCURBITACIN-E Fruit
CUCURBITIN Seed
CYCLOARTENOL Seed
EPSILON-CAROTENE Fruit
ETHANOL Petiole
ETHYL-(METHYLTHIO)-ACETATE Petiole
ETHYL-2-METHYL-BUTYRATER Petiole
ETHYL-ACETATE Petiole
ETHYL-DECANOATE Petiole
EUGENOL-METHYL-ETHER Plant
EUPHOL Seed
FAT Fruit 2,600–29,355 ppm Seed
300,000–446,000 ppm
FERULIC-ACID Plant
FIBER Fruit 3,180–39,357 ppm

FOLACIN Fruit 0.1–1.9 ppm

GAMMA-GLUTAMYL-BETA-PYRAZOL-1-YL-ALA-NINE Fruit

GLOBULIN Fruit 26,000 ppm

HEPTYL-ACETATE Petiole

HEXADECENOIC-ACID Seed 2,190–3,255 ppm

HEXYL-ACETATE Petiole

HISTAMINE Juice

IRON Fruit 2–55 ppm

ISOBUTYL-ACETATE Petiole

ISOFRAXIDIN Plant

KILOCALORIES Fruit 350–3,425 /kg

LAURIC-ACID Seed 360–8,920 ppm

LEAD Fruit 1.74–2.2 ppm

LINOLEIC-ACID Cotyledon 56,100–726,700 ppm Seed 99,600–246,192 ppm

LINOLENIC-ACID Cotyledon 200,500–219,000 ppm

LITHIUM Fruit 0.348–0.44 ppm

LUPEOL Seed

MAGNESIUM Fruit 92–3,300 ppm

MALONIC-ACID Leaf

MANGANESE Fruit 0.4–7.7 ppm

MARGARIC-ACID Stem

MELONIN Seed

MELOSIDE Leaf

MELOSIDE-A-CAFFEOYL-ESTER Leaf

MERCURY Fruit

MOLYBDENUM Fruit 0.609–0.77 ppm

MULTIFLORENOL Seed

MYRISTIC-ACID Fruit 1,500–8,920 ppm

NIACIN Fruit 4.6–68 ppm

NICKEL Fruit 0.87–1.1 ppm

NONAN-1-OL Fruit

NONANAL Fruit

NONYL-ACETATE Petiole

OCTYL-ACETATE Petiole

OLEIC-ACID Cotyledon 40,500–195,300 ppm Seed 81,000–200,700 ppm

P-HYDROXY-BENZOIC-ACID Plant

PALMITIC-ACID Cotyledon 122,000–532,300 ppm Seed 9,600–58,400 ppm

PANTOTHENIC-ACID Fruit 1.2–14 ppm

PENTADECANOIC-ACID Leaf

PHOSPHORUS Fruit 121–2,640 ppm

PHYSETOLIC-ACID Cotyledon

PHYTOSTEROLS Fruit 100–978 ppm

POTASSIUM Fruit 3,018–44,000 ppm

PROPYL-ACETATE Petiole

PROTEIN Fruit 8,410–89,924 ppm Seed 358,000 ppm

RIBOFLAVIN Fruit 0.2–2.4 ppm

RUTIN Plant

SELENIUM Fruit 0.003–0.004 ppm

SILVER Fruit 0.087–0.11 ppm

SITOSTEROL Seed

SODIUM Fruit 66–1,115 ppm

STEARIC-ACID Cotyledon 10,100–61,400 ppm Seed 10,080–35,145 ppm

STIGMAST-7-EN-3-BETA-OL Stem

STIGMASTEROL Seed

STRONTIUM Fruit 2.6–16.5 ppm

SUGAR Fruit 20,000–30,000 ppm

SULFUR Fruit 139–198 ppm

TARAXEROL Seed

THIAMIN Fruit 0.3–4.4 ppm

TIRUCALLOL Seed

TITANIUM Fruit 0.435–2.2 ppm

TRANS,CIS-2,6-NONADIEN-1-OL Fruit

TRANS,CIS-2,6-NONADIENAL Fruit

TRANS-2-NONEN-1-OL Fruit

TRANS-2-NONENAL Fruit

TRIDECANOIC-ACID Root

TRIGONELLINE Seed 2–6 ppm

VIT-B-6 Fruit 1–13 ppm

WATER Fruit 896,000–938,000 ppm

ZINC Fruit 1.5–31 ppm

ZIRCONIUM Fruit 1.7–2.2 ppm

ORANGE

Chemicals in *Citrus sinensis* (*L.*) *OSBECK* (*Rutaceae*)—Orange

2'-TRANS-O-FERULOYL-GALACTARIC-ACID Pericarp

2'-TRANS-O-P-COUMAROYL-GALACTARIC-ACID Pericarp

2'-TRANS-O-P-COUMAROYL-GLUCARIC-ACID Pericarp

2,4-TRANS,TRANS-O-FERULOYL-GLUCARIC-ACID Pericarp

2-METHYL-1-PROPANOL Fruit Juice 0.07 ppm

2-TRANS-O-FERULOYL-GLUCARIC-ACID Pericarp

3,3',4,5,6,7,8-HEPTAMETHOXY-FLAVONE Fruit

3-HYDROXY-ETHYL-HEXANOATE Fruit

3-METHYL-BUT-1-ENE Essential Oil

3-METHYL-BUTAN-1-OL Fruit

4-(3-METHYL-2-BUTENOXY)-ISO-NITROSO-
ACETOPHENONE Pericarp 48 ppm

5,6-DIHYDRO-BETA-BETA-CAROTENE-3,3′,5,6-
TETROL Fruit Juice

5,8-EPOXY-5,5′,8-TETRAHYDRO-BETA,BETA-
CAROTENE-3,3′,5′,6′-TETROL Plant

5,8-EPOXY-5,8-DIHYDRO-8′-APO-BETA-
CAROTENE-3,10–DIOL Fruit Juice

6,7-DIMETHOXYCOUMARIN Bark 162 ppm

ACETALDEHYDE Fruit Juice 3–15 ppm

ACETIC-ACID Plant

ALANINE Fruit 30–3,775 ppm

ALPHA-BERGAMOTENE Fruit 6 ppm

ALPHA-CAROTENE Fruit 0.19–1.9 ppm

ALPHA-COPAENE Pericarp

ALPHA-HYDROXY-CAROTENE Pericarp

ALPHA-LINOLENIC-ACID Fruit 70–528 ppm

ALPHA-PINENE Fruit 10–60 ppm Plant

ALPHA-SINESAL Fruit 3 ppm Pericarp

ALPHA-TERPINEOL Fruit 10–50 ppm Fruit
Juice 0.09–1.1 ppm

ALPHA-TOCOPHEROL Fruit 4–29 ppm

ALUMINUM Fruit 1–165 ppm

ANTHERAXANTHIN Fruit

APIGENIN-7-O-ALPHA-L-RHAMNO-GLUCO-
SIDE Leaf

APOVIOLAXANTH-10′-AL Pericarp

ARABAN Fruit

ARGININE Fruit 230–4,908 ppm

ARSENIC Fruit 0.001–0.154 ppm

ASCORBIC-ACID Fruit 500–4,071 ppm

ASH Fruit 4,100–36,920 ppm

ASPARAGINE Fruit 200–1,800 ppm

ASPARTIC-ACID Fruit 70–8,607 ppm

AURAPTENE Fruit

AURAXANTHIN Fruit 4 ppm

BARIUM Fruit 0.54–16.5 ppm

BERGAPTOL Fruit

BETA-APO-8′-CAROTINAL Pericarp

BETA-APO-CAROTEN-8-AL Pericarp

BETA-CAROTENE Fruit 1–28 ppm

BETA-CITRAURIN Pericarp

BETA-CRYTOXANTHIN Fruit

BETA-CUBEBENE Fruit 10 ppm

BETA-ELEMENE Fruit 5 ppm

BETA-SINESAL Fruit 6 ppm Pericarp

BETA-SITOSTEROL Fruit

BETA-ZEACAROTENE Pericarp

BETAINE Fruit 390–630 ppm

BORON Fruit 1.89–27.5 ppm

BRAYLIN Root

BROMINE Fruit

BUTYRIC-ACID Fruit

CADMIUM Fruit 0.001–0.138 ppm

CAFFEIC-ACID Fruit 36–50 ppm

CAFFEINE Bud 0.3 ppm Flower 62 ppm Leaf 6
ppm

CALCIUM Fruit 210–5,615 ppm

CAMPESTEROL Fruit

CAPRIC-ACID Fruit

CAPROIC-ACID Fruit

CAPRYLIC-ACID Fruit

CARBOHYDRATES Fruit 99,000–887,125 ppm

CAROTENOIDS Fruit 12–35 ppm

CARVONE Fruit 2–10 ppm

CARYOPHYLLENE Pericarp

CHLORINE Fruit 12–32 ppm

CHOLESTEROL Fruit

CHOLINE Fruit 70–160 ppm

CHROMIUM Fruit 0.005–0.385 ppm

CITFLAVANONE Root Bark

CITRABASINE Root Bark 14 ppm

CITRACRIDONE-I Root Bark 400 ppm

CITRIC-ACID Fruit 5,600–9,800 ppm

CITRONELLAL Fruit 55 ppm

CITRUNOBIN Root Bark

CITRUSININE-I Root Bark 80 ppm

CITRUSININE-II Root Bark 40 ppm

CITRUSINS Plant

COBALT Fruit 0.001–0.055 ppm

CONIFERIN Pericarp

COPPER Fruit 0.44–5.5 ppm

CRENULATIN Root Bark 60 ppm

CRYPTOFLAVIN Pericarp

CRYPTOXANTHIN Fruit

CRYPTOXANTHIN-5,5′,6,6′-DIEPOXIDE Pericarp

CYANIDIN-3-GLUCOSIDE Fruit

CYSTINE Fruit 100–755 ppm

DEACETYL-NOMILIN Seed

DECANAL Fruit 10–60 ppm Fruit Juice 0.15
ppm

DELPHINIDIN-3-GLUCOSIDE Fruit

DELTA-CADINENE Pericarp

DIHYDROKAEMPFEROL-4'-METHYL-ETHER-7-O-RHAMNOSIDE Fruit

DIOSMETIN-7-O-ALPHA-L-RHAMNO-GLUCO-SIDE Leaf

DIOSMIN Pericarp

DODECANAL Fruit 5–20 ppm

ELEMOL Root Bark 28,200 ppm

EO Fruit 10,000 ppm

EPOXY-NOOTKATONE Pericarp

EPOXY-VALENCENE Fruit

ETA-CAROTENE Pericarp

ETHANOL Fruit Juice 64–900 ppm

ETHYL-ACETATE Fruit Juice 0.01–0.58 ppm

ETHYL-BUTYRATE Fruit Juice 0.08–1.02 ppm

ETHYL-SUBERENOL Root Bark 700 ppm

ETROGOL Root

FARNESENE Fruit 2–7 ppm

FAT Fruit 1,100–16,000 ppm

FERULIC-ACID Fruit 10–19 ppm

FERULOYL-PUTRESCINE Fruit 5 ppm

FIBER Fruit 3,740–47,000 ppm

FLAVOXANTHIN Pericarp

FLUORINE Fruit 0.04–0.76 ppm

FOLACIN Fruit 2 ppm

FR Juice

FRUCTOSE Fruit 23,800 ppm

GALACTAN Fruit

GALACTOSE Fruit

GALACTURONIC-ACID Fruit

GAMMA-AMINOBUTYRIC-ACID Fruit 40–730 ppm

GAMMA-TERPINENE Fruit 10 ppm Fruit Juice 0.04–0.46 ppm

GERANIAL Fruit 6–350 ppm

GERANIOL Fruit 50 ppm

GERANYL-OXY-PYRANOCOUMARIN Root

GLUCOSAN Fruit

GLUCOSE Fruit 23,600 ppm

GLUTAMIC-ACID Fruit 60–7,097 ppm

GLUTAMINE Fruit 30–630 ppm

GLYCINE Fruit 50–7,097 ppm

HEPTANAL Fruit 3–5 ppm

HEPTULOSE Fruit

HESPERIDIN Pericarp 40,600–63,500 ppm

HESPERIDIN-7-O-ALPHA-L-RHAMNO-GLUCO-SIDE Fruit

HEXANAL Fruit 1–2 ppm Fruit Juice 0.02–0.65 ppm

HEXANOL Fruit Juice 0.02–0.22 ppm

HISTIDINE Fruit 180–1,359 ppm

HORDENINE Fruit

HYDROXYPROLINE Leaf

IRON Fruit 1–8 ppm

ISOCAPROIC-ACID Fruit

ISOLEUCINE Fruit 250–1,888 ppm

ISOLUTEIN Pericarp

ISOPENTENYL-PSORALENS Fruit

ISOPRENE Essential Oil

ISORHOIFOLIN Pericarp

ISOSAKURANETIN Fruit

JASMONIC-ACID Fruit

LEAD Fruit 0.02–1.1 ppm

LEUCINE Fruit 230–1,136 ppm

LIMONENE Fruit 8,300–9,700 ppm Fruit Juice 1–278 ppm

LIMONEXIC-ACID Fruit

LIMONIN Fruit

LIMONOATE-A-RING-LACTONE Fruit

LINALOL Fruit 30–530 ppm Fruit Juice 0.15–4.69 ppm

LINOLEIC-ACID Fruit 180–1,359 ppm

LITHIUM Fruit 0.108–1.54 ppm

LOCHNOCARPOL-A Root

LUTEIN Fruit 3 ppm

LUTEOLIN-7-O-ALPHA-L-RHAMNO-GLUCO-SIDE Fruit

LUTEOLIN-7-O-BETA-D-RUTINOSIDE Leaf

LUTEOXANTHINS Fruit 6 ppm

LYSINE Fruit 470–3,548 ppm

MAGNESIUM Fruit 98–1,075 ppm

MALIC-ACID Fruit 600–2,000 ppm

MALONIC-ACID Plant

MANGANESE Fruit 8 ppm

MANNOSE Fruit

MERANZINE Fruit

MERCURY Fruit 0.001 ppm

METHANOL Fruit Juice 0.8–80 ppm

METHIONINE Fruit 200–1,510 ppm

METHYL-BUTYRATE Fruit Juice 0.01–0.1 ppm

MEVALONIC-ACID Fruit 0.5 ppm Pericarp 6 ppm

MOLYBDENUM Fruit 0.1–0.385 ppm

MUTATOCHROME Fruit

MUTATOXANTHIN Fruit 2 ppm

MYRCENE Fruit 69–210 ppm

N-METHYL-TYRAMINE Fruit 2 ppm

NARINGENIN Pericarp 35,000–45,800 ppm
NARINGENIN-4-BETA-D-GLUCOSIDE Plant
NARINGENIN-RUTINOSIDE Fruit
NARINGENIN-RUTINOSIDE-4-BETA-D-GLU-
  COSIDE Fruit
NARINGIN Fruit
NARINGIN-7-O-ALPHA-L-RHAMNO-GLUCO-
  SIDE Fruit
NARIRUTIN Pericarp
NEO-BETA-CAROTENE Pericarp
NEOCHROME-A Pericarp
NEOCHROME-B Pericarp
NEOHESPERIDIN Pericarp 28,000 ppm
NEOHESPERIDIN-DIHYDROCHALCONE Peri-
  carp
NEOPONCIRIN Pericarp
NEOXANTHIN-A Pericarp
NEOXANTHIN-B Pericarp
NERAL Fruit 1–20 ppm
NEROLIDOL Flower
NERYL-ACETATE Fruit 10 ppm
NERYL-FORMATE Fruit 10 ppm
NEUROSPORIN Pericarp
NIACIN Fruit
NICKEL Fruit 0.01–0.55 ppm
NITROGEN Fruit 500–13,845 ppm
NOBELITIN Fruit
NOMILIN Seed
NONANAL Fruit 6–20 ppm
NONANOL Fruit 10 ppm
NOOTKATOL Fruit
NOOTKATONE Fruit 1 ppm
NORDENTATIN Root Bark 300 ppm
OBACUNONE Seed
OCTAN-1-AL Fruit
OCTANAL Fruit 20–280 ppm Fruit Juice 0.28
  ppm
OCTOPAMINE Fruit 1 ppm
OCTYL-ACETATE Fruit 10 ppm
OLEIC-ACID Fruit 20–1,510 ppm
OSTHOLE Root
OXALIC-ACID Fruit 87 ppm
P-COUMARIC-ACID Fruit 5–17 ppm
P-CYMENE Fruit 20 ppm
P-HYDROQUINONE Root Bark 80 ppm
PALMITIC-ACID Fruit 130–982 ppm
PALMITOLEIC-ACID Fruit 30–226 ppm
PANTOTHENIC-ACID Fruit 2–19 ppm

PECTIN Fruit 1,300–5,900 ppm
PECTINESTERASE Fruit
PERILLALDEHYDE Fruit 2 ppm
PHENYLALANINE Fruit 310–2,340 ppm
PHLORIN Plant
PHOSPHORUS Fruit 136–1,980 ppm
PHYTOENE Fruit 2 ppm
PHYTOFLUENE Fruit 4 ppm
POLYGALACTURONIC-ACID Fruit
PONCITRIN Root
POTASSIUM Fruit 1,400–13,772 ppm
PROLINE Fruit 60–3,473 ppm
PROPIONIC-ACID Plant
PROTEIN Fruit 9,260–78,000 ppm
QUINIC-ACID Fruit
RIBOFLAVIN Fruit 3 ppm
RUBIDIUM Fruit 0.1–7.7 ppm
RUTIN Leaf 9,000 ppm Pericarp 6,100 ppm
SABINENE Fruit 10–60 ppm Fruit Juice 0.15
  ppm
SCOPARONE Bark
SCUTELLAREIN Fruit
SELENIUM Fruit 0.002 ppm
SERINE Fruit 40–2,410 ppm
SESELIN Root
SESLIN Root
SILICON Fruit
SILVER Fruit 0.027–0.055 ppm
SINAPIC-ACID Fruit 7–19 ppm
SINENSETIN Fruit
SINENSIAXANTHIN Fruit
SINESETIN Plant
SODIUM Fruit 29 ppm
STACHYDRINE Fruit
STIGMASTEROL Fruit
STRONTIUM Fruit 0.054–110 ppm
SUBAPHYLLIN Fruit Leaf
SUBERENOL Root Bark 700 ppm
SUBEROSIN Root
SUCCINIC-ACID Fruit
SUCROSE Fruit 47,000 ppm
SUGARS Fruit 39,600–119,800 ppm
SULFUR Fruit 46–1,000 ppm
SYNEPHRINE Fruit 15–43 ppm
TANGERETIN Fruit
TAU-CAROTENE Pericarp
TERPINEN-4-OL Fruit 6–550 ppm
TERPINOLENE Fruit 10 ppm

TETRA-O-METHYL-SCUTELLAREIN Fruit
TETRADECANAL Fruit 5–9 ppm
THIAMIN Fruit 1–7 ppm
THREONINE Fruit 150–1,132 ppm
TITANIUM Fruit 0.135–3.85 ppm
TRANS-2-HEXENOL Fruit Juice 0.1 ppm
TRYPTOPHAN Fruit 90–680 ppm
TYRAMINE Fruit 1 ppm
TYROSINE Fruit 160–1,208 ppm
URONIC-ACID Fruit
VALENCENE Fruit 10–20 ppm Fruit Juice
   0.04–15.3 ppm
VALENCIACHROME Plant
VALENCIAXANTHIN Fruit 3 ppm
VALENCIC-ACID Root
VALINE Fruit 100–3,020 ppm
VIOLAXANTHIN Fruit
VIT-B-6 Fruit 1–5 ppm
VITEXIN-XYLOSIDE Fruit
WATER Fruit 839,000–898,000 ppm
XANTHOXYLETIN Root Bark 24,000 ppm
XANTHYLETIN Root Bark 45,000 ppm
XYLAN Fruit
XYLOSE Fruit
XYLOSYL-VITEXIN Leaf
ZEAXANTHIN Fruit 2 ppm
ZETA-CAROTENE Fruit 2 ppm
ZINC Fruit 0.9–13 ppm
ZIRCONIUM Fruit 0.5–1.1 ppm

PAPAYA

Chemicals in *Carica papaya* L. (*Cari-caceae*)—Papaya

(E)-BETA-OCIMENE Fruit
(Z)-BETA-OCIMENE Fruit
3-METHYL-BUTYL-BENZOATE Fruit
4-HYDROXY-4-METHYL-PENTAN-2-ONE Fruit
4-TERPINEOL Fruit
5,6-MONOEPOXI-BETA-CAROTENE Fruit
6-METHYLKEPT-5-EN-2-ONE Fruit
ALANINE Fruit 140–1,253 ppm
ALKALOIDS Leaf 1,300–1,500 ppm
ALPHA-LINOLENIC-ACID Fruit 250–2,238
   ppm
ALPHA-PHELLANDRENE Fruit
ALPHA-TERPINENE Fruit
AMYL-ACETATE Fruit

ARGININE Fruit 100–895 ppm
ASCORBIC-ACID Fruit 330–5,732 ppm Leaf
   1,400–6,222 ppm
ASH Fruit 5,800–57,280 ppm Leaf
   22,000–154,000 ppm Seed 88,000 ppm
ASPARTIC-ACID Fruit 490–4,387 ppm
BEHENIC-ACID Seed
BENZALDEHYDE Fruit
BENZYL-ISOTHIOCYANATE Fruit
BENZYLSENEVOL Seed
BETA-CAROTENE Fruit 10–123 ppm Leaf
   116–514 ppm
BETA-PHELLANDRENE Fruit
BORON Fruit 5–15 ppm
BUTYL-ALCOHOL Fruit
BUTYL-BENZOATE Fruit
BUTYL-HEXANOATE Fruit
CALCIUM Fruit 100–2,792 ppm Leaf
   3,440–23,800 ppm
CALLOSE Latex Exudate
CAOUTCHOUC Latex Exudate 45,000 ppm
CARBOHYDRATES Fruit 95,000–991,000 ppm
   Leaf 113,000–556,000 ppm Seed 155,000
   ppm
CARICIN Seed
CARPAINE Bark Leaf 1,000–1,500 ppm Root
   Seed
CARPASEMINE Seed
CARPOSIDE Leaf
CARYOPHYLLENE Fruit
CHRYSANTHEMEXANTHIN Fruit
CHYMOPAPAIN-A Latex Exudate
CHYMOPAPAIN-B Latex Exudate
CITRIC-ACID Fruit
COPPER Fruit 0.1–5 ppm
COTININE Plant
D-GALACTOSE Fruit
D-GALACTURONIC-ACID Fruit
DECANAL Fruit
DEHYDROCARPAINES Leaf 1,000 ppm
DEHYDROCARPAMINES Plant
EO Seed 900 ppm
EPSILON-CAROTENE Fruit
ETHYL-ACETATE Fruit
ETHYL-ALCOHOL Fruit
ETHYL-BENZOATE Fruit
ETHYL-BUTYRATE Fruit
ETHYL-OCTANOATE Fruit

FAT Fruit 980–22,000 ppm Latex Exudate
24,000 ppm Leaf 8,000–136,000 ppm Seed
253,000 ppm
FIBER Fruit 6,960–75,538 ppm Leaf
18,000–145,000 ppm Seed 170,000 ppm
FLAVONOLS Leaf 2,000 ppm
GAMMA-CAROTENE Fruit
GAMMA-OCTALACTONE Fruit
GAMMA-TERPINENE Fruit
GERANYL-ACETONE Fruit
GERMACRENE-D Fruit
GLUCOTROPAEOLIN Plant
GLUTAMIC-ACID Fruit
GLYCINE Fruit 180–1,611 ppm
HEPTAN-2-ONE Fruit
HEPTANAL Fruit
HEXADECENOIC-ACID Seed
HEXANAL Fruit
HISTIDINE Fruit 50–448 ppm
IRON Fruit 0.8–38 ppm Leaf 8–38 ppm
ISOAMYL-ACETATE Fruit
ISOLEUCINE Fruit 80–716 ppm
KILOCALORIES Fruit 390–3,491 /kg Leaf 740
/kg
KRYPTOFLAVIN Fruit
KRYPTOXANTHIN Fruit
LAURIC-ACID Fruit 10–90 ppm Seed
LEUCINE Fruit 160–1,432 ppm
LINALOL Fruit
LINALOL-OXIDE-A Fruit
LINALOL-OXIDE-B Fruit
LINOLEIC-ACID Fruit 60–537 ppm Seed 5,389
ppm
LYCOPENE Fruit
LYSINE Fruit 250–2,238 ppm
MAGNESIUM Fruit 82–1,058 ppm
MALIC-ACID Fruit Latex Exudate 4,400 ppm
MANGANESE Fruit 0.1–1.1 ppm
METHIONINE Fruit 20–179 ppm
METHYL-ACETATE Fruit
METHYL-ALCOHOL Fruit
METHYL-GERANATE Fruit
METHYL-HEXANOATE Fruit
METHYL-OCTANOATE Fruit
METHYL-SALICYLATE Fruit
METHYL-THIOCYANATE Fruit
MUFA Fruit 380–3,402 ppm
MUTATOCHROM Fruit

MYOSMINE Plant
MYRCENE Fruit
MYRISTIC-ACID Fruit 70–627 ppm Seed
MYROSIN Seed
N-ACETYL-HEXOSAMIDASE Latex Exudate
NEOXANTHIN Fruit
NIACIN Fruit 3–33 ppm Leaf 21–93 ppm
NICOTINE Plant
NONANAL Fruit
OCTANAL Fruit
OLEIC-ACID Fruit 180–1,611 ppm Seed
193,545–202,400 ppm
PALMITIC-ACID Fruit 320–2,865 ppm Seed
28,791–30,107 ppm
PALMITOLEIC-ACID Fruit 200–1,790 ppm
PANTOTHENIC-ACID Fruit 2–19 ppm
PAPAIN Fruit Latex Exudate 53,000 ppm
PENTADECANE Fruit
PENTAN-2,4-DIONE Fruit
PHENYLACETONITRILE Fruit
PHENYLALANINE Fruit 90–806 ppm
PHOSPHORUS Fruit 45–1,260 ppm Leaf
1,420–6,311 ppm
PHYTOENE Fruit
PHYTOFLUENE Fruit
POTASSIUM Fruit 2,294–25,469 ppm Leaf
6,520–28,978 ppm
PROLINE Fruit 100–895 ppm
PROP-2-YL-BUTYRATE Fruit
PROPYL-ALCOHOL Fruit
PROTEIN Fruit 5,000–57,370 ppm Leaf
70,000–326,000 ppm Seed 243,000 ppm
PSEUDOCARPAINE Leaf 100 ppm
PUFA Fruit 310–2,775 ppm
RESIN Latex Exudate 28,000 ppm
RIBOFLAVIN Fruit 0.3–3 ppm Leaf 5–21 ppm
SERINE Fruit 150–1,343 ppm
SFA Fruit 430–3,850 ppm
SODIUM Fruit 26–554 ppm Leaf 160–711 ppm
STEARIC-ACID Fruit 20–179 ppm Seed
12,650–13,282 ppm
SUCROSE Fruit
SULFUR Fruit 300–900 ppm
TANNINS Leaf 5,000–6,000 ppm
TARTARIC-ACID Fruit
TERPINOLENE Fruit
THIAMIN Fruit 0.2–2.6 ppm Leaf 1–4 ppm
THREONINE Fruit 110–985 ppm

TRIACETIN Fruit

TRYPTOPHAN Fruit 80–716 ppm

TYROSINE Fruit 50–448 ppm

VALINE Fruit 100–895 ppm

VIOLAXANTHIN Fruit

VIT-B-6 Fruit 0.2–1.7 ppm

WATER Fruit 865,000–918,300 ppm Latex Exudate 750,000 ppm Leaf 697,000–703,000 ppm

ZEAXANTHIN Fruit

ZINC Fruit 1.8–5.4 ppm

PASSIONFRUIT

Chemicals in *Passiflora edulis* SIMS (*Passifloraceae*)—Maracuya, Passionfruit

ALKALOIDS Fruit 120–7,000 ppm

ARACHIDIC-ACID Seed 780 ppm

ASCORBIC-ACID Fruit 300–1,205 ppm

ASH Fruit 8,000–32,000 ppm Seed 18,400 ppm

BETA-CAROTENE Fruit 4–17 ppm

CALCIUM Fruit 130–1,190 ppm Seed 800 ppm

CARBOHYDRATES Fruit 212,000–851,000 ppm

CAROTENOIDS Fruit 580–11,600 ppm

CATALASE Fruit

CITRIC-ACID Fruit 20,000–45,600 ppm

EO Fruit Juice 23–43 ppm

ETHYL-BUTYRATE Fruit

ETHYL-CAPROATE Fruit Juice 14–30 ppm

FAT Fruit 7,000–28,000 ppm Seed 230,000–238,000 ppm

FIBER Fruit Juice 500–12,000 ppm Seed 537,000 ppm

FLAVONOIDS Fruit 10,000–10,600 ppm

HARMAN Fruit 7,001 ppm

IRON Fruit 16–64 ppm Seed 180 ppm

KILOCALORIES Fruit 900–3,610 /kg

LINOLEIC-ACID Seed 137,770 ppm

LINOLENIC-ACID Seed 12,420 ppm

MALIC-ACID Fruit 1,200–3,800 ppm

N-HEXYL-BUTYRATE Fruit Juice 3–6 ppm

N-HEXYL-CAPROATE Fruit Juice 14–30 ppm

NIACIN Fruit 15–60 ppm

NITROGEN Plant 960–1,920 ppm

OLEIC-ACID Seed 43,700 ppm

PALMITIC-ACID Seed 15,595 ppm

PASSIFLORINE Leaf

PECTIN Petiole 24,000–140,000 ppm

PECTIN-METHYL-ESTERASE Fruit

PELARGONIDIN-3-DIGLUCOSIDE Petiole 14 ppm

PHENOLASE Fruit

PHOSPHORUS Fruit 480–2,570 ppm Seed 6,400 ppm

POTASSIUM Fruit 3,480–13,975 ppm

PROTEIN Fruit 22,000–88,000 ppm Seed 111,000 ppm

RIBOFLAVIN Fruit 1–5 ppm

SFA Seed 20,470 ppm

SODIUM Fruit 280–1,124 ppm

STEARIC-ACID Seed 4,050 ppm

THIAMIN Fruit 1.4 ppm

WATER Fruit 751,000–790,000 ppm Seed 54,000 ppm

XANTHOPHYLLS Fruit 60–2,495 ppm

PEACH

Chemicals in *Prunus persica* (*L.*) BATSCH (*Rosaceae*)—Peach

(+)-ABSCISIC-ACID Plant

24-METHYLENE-CYCLOARTANOL Seed

3′,5′-DIHYDROXY-4′,7-DIMETHOXY-FLAVANONE Plant

4-ALPHA-METHYLSTIGMASTA-7,Z,24(28)-DIEN-3-BETA-OL Seed

A-DECALACTONE Fruit

ACETALDEHYDE Plant

ACETIC-ACID Fruit

AFZELIN Flower

ALANINE Fruit 420–3,402 ppm

ALPHA-TOCOPHEROL Fruit 10–86 ppm

ALUMINUM Bark 43 ppm Fruit 2.25–1,050 ppm

AMANDIN Seed

AMYGDALIN Leaf 10,000 ppm Seed 25,500–60,000 ppm

ANTHOCYANIDIN Fruit

ARGININE Fruit 180–1,458 ppm

ARSENIC Fruit 0.001–0.053 ppm

ASCORBIC-ACID Fruit 14–1,127 ppm

ASH Bark 63,000 ppm Fruit 4,000–150,000 ppm

ASPARTIC-ACID Fruit 1,170–8,586 ppm

BARIUM Fruit 0.045–30 ppm

BENZALDEHYDE Fruit Seed

BENZALDEHYDECYANHYDRIN Seed
BENZYL-ACETATE Fruit
BENZYL-ALCOHOL Fruit
BETA-CAROTENE Fruit 30 ppm
BETA-SITOSTEROL Leaf
BORON Fruit 1–150 ppm
BROMINE Fruit
CADMIUM Fruit 0.45 ppm
CAFFEIC-ACID Leaf
CAFFEIC-ACID-ESTER Leaf
CALCIUM Fruit 18–8,850 ppm Seed 970 ppm
CAMPESTEROL Seed
CAMPESTEROL-3-O-BETA-(6-O-OLEYL)-GLU-
  COPYRANOSIDE Seed
CAMPESTEROL-3-O-BETA-(6-O-PALMITYL)-
  GLUCOPYRANOSIDE Seed
CAMPESTEROL-3-O-BETA-D-GLUCOPYRA-
  NOSIDE Seed
CAPRONIC-ACID Plant
CARBOHYDRATES Fruit 111,000–910,000 ppm
CHLOROGENIC-ACID Flower Leaf
CHROMIUM Bark 35 ppm Fruit 0.01–2.25 ppm
CITRIC-ACID Fruit
COBALT Bark 20 ppm Fruit 0.005–0.45 ppm
COPPER Fruit 0.3–30 ppm Seed 10 ppm
CRYPTOXANTHIN Plant 0.5–10 ppm
CYANIDIN-3-MONOGLUCOSIDE Fruit
CYSTINE Fruit 60–486 ppm
D-AFZELECHIN Root
D-GALACTOSE Gum
D-GLUCURONIC-ACID Plant
D-XYLOSE Gum
ETHANOL Fruit
ETHYL-ACETATE Fruit
ETHYL-BENZOATE Fruit
FAT Fruit 860–18,000 ppm Seed
  399,000–456,000 ppm
FERULIC-ACID Plant
FIBER Fruit 6,210–162,000 ppm Seed 148,000
  ppm
FLAVONOL-GLYCOSIDES Fruit 10 ppm
FLAVONOL-GLYCOSIDES Leaf 7,500–10,400
  ppm
FLUORINE Fruit 0.1–0.8 ppm
FOLACIN Fruit 0.031–0.303 ppm
FORMIC-ACID Fruit
GAMMA-HEPTALACTONE Fruit
GAMMA-HEXALACTONE Fruit

GAMMA-NONALACTONE Fruit
GAMMA-OCTALACTONE Plant
GIBBERELLIN-A-32 Seed
GIBBERELLIN-A-32-ACETONIDE Plant
GIBBERELLIN-A-5 Plant
GLUCOSE Seed
GLUTAMIC-ACID Fruit 1,060–8,586 ppm
GLYCINE Fruit 240–1,944 ppm
HCN Leaf
HENTRIACONTANE Leaf
HEXANOIC-ACID Fruit
HEXYL-ACETATE Fruit
HEXYL-FORMATE Fruit
HISTIDINE Fruit 130–1,053 ppm
IRON Bark 117 ppm Fruit 1–99 ppm Seed 80
  ppm
ISOLEUCINE Fruit 200–1,620 ppm
ISOVALERIANIC-ACID Fruit
KAEMPFEROL Leaf
KAEMPFEROL-3-0-GALACTOSIDE Plant
KAEMPFEROL-3-0-GLUCOSIDE Plant
KAEMPFEROL-3-RHAMNOSIDE Plant
L-ARABINOSE Gum
L-MALIC-ACID Fruit
L-RHAMNOSE Gum
LEAD Fruit 0.3–3 ppm
LEUCINE Fruit 400–3,240 ppm
LINOLEIC-ACID Fruit 440–3,565 ppm Seed
LINOLENIC-ACID Fruit 10–80 ppm
LITHIUM Fruit 0.06–0.6 ppm
LUTEIN Fruit 0.14–2.8 ppm
LYCOPENE Fruit
LYSINE Fruit 230–1,863 ppm
MAGNESIUM Bark 4,220 ppm Fruit 68–850
  ppm Seed 3,810 ppm
MALONIC-ACID Fruit
MANGANESE Bark 54 ppm Fruit 22.5 ppm
  Seed 17 ppm
MERCURY Fruit 0.007 ppm
METHIONINE Fruit 170–1,377 ppm
METHYL-ACETATE Fruit
METHYL-FRUCTOFURANOSIDE Seed
METHYL-GALLATE Flower
METHYL-GLUCOPYRANOSIDE Seed
MOLYBDENUM Fruit 0.1–1.05 ppm
MUCIC-ACID Plant
MUFA Fruit 340–2,755 ppm
MULTIFLORIN-A Flower

MULTIFLORIN-B Flower

MULTINOSIDE-A Flower

MULTINOSIDE-B Flower

NARINGENIN Plant

NIACIN Fruit 10–82 ppm

NICKEL Fruit 0.15–4.5 ppm

NITROGEN Fruit 1,400–13,075 ppm

OLEIC-ACID Fruit 340–2,755 ppm Seed

OXALIC-ACID Hh 10 ppm

P-COUMARIC-ACID Leaf

P-COUMARIC-ACID-ESTER Leaf

PALMITIC-ACID Fruit 90–730 ppm Seed

PALMITOLEIC-ACID Fruit 10–80 ppm

PANTOTHENIC-ACID Fruit 2–14 ppm

PECTINS Fruit 8,600 ppm

PENTANOIC-ACID Fruit

PENTYL-ACETATE Fruit

PHENYLALANINE Plant 220–1,782 ppm

PHOSPHORUS Bark 3,150 ppm Fruit 90–2,000
ppm

PHYTIN-PHOSPHORUS Fruit 10 ppm

PHYTOSTEROLS Fruit 100–810 ppm

POTASSIUM Bark 19,400 ppm Fruit
1,275–22,072 ppm Seed 7,010 ppm

PROLINE Fruit 290–2,349 ppm

PROTEIN Fruit 6,850–63,000 ppm Seed
239,000–312,000 ppm

PRUNASIN Seed

PUFA Fruit 450–3,645 ppm

QUERCETIN Plant

QUERCETIN-3'-GLUCOSIDE Fruit Leaf

QUERCETIN-3-0–GALACTOSIDE Fruit Leaf

QUERCETIN-3-0–RHAMNOSIDE Fruit Leaf

QUERCETIN-3-0–RUTINOSIDE Fruit

QUERCETIN-3-DIGLUCOSIDE Fruit Leaf

QUERCITRIN Flower

QUINIC-ACID Leaf

RIBOFLAVIN Fruit 1–4 ppm

SELENIUM Bark Fruit 0.003 ppm

SERINE Fruit 320–2,592 ppm

SFA Fruit 100–810 ppm

SILICON Bark Fruit 4–30 ppm

SILVER Fruit 0.015–0.3 ppm

SODIUM Bark Fruit 366 ppm Seed 29 ppm

SQUALENE Seed

STARCH Seed 36,000 ppm

STEARIC-ACID Fruit 10–80 ppm Seed

STIGMASTEROL Seed

STRONTIUM Fruit 0.225–45 ppm

SUCROSE Fruit 20,000–100,000 ppm

SULFUR Fruit 3–700 ppm

TANNIN Fruit 8,000 ppm Leaf 8,000 ppm

THIAMIN Fruit 1–2 ppm

THREONINE Fruit 270–2,187 ppm

TIN Bark 9.4 ppm

TITANIUM Fruit 0.075–30 ppm

TRANS-2-HEXENYL-ACETATE Fruit

TRIFOLIN Flower

TRIOLEIN Seed

TRYPTOPHAN Fruit 20–162 ppm

TYROSINE Fruit 180–1,458 ppm

URSOLIC-ACID Leaf

VALINE Fruit 380–3,078 ppm

VIT-B-6 Fruit 0.2–1.6 ppm

WATER Bark 792,000 ppm Fruit
835,000–964,000 ppm

ZEAXANTHIN Fruit

ZINC Bark Fruit 0.45–37.5 ppm Seed 31 ppm

ZIRCONIUM Fruit 0.3–4.5 ppm

PEAR

Chemicals in *Pyrus communis L.*
(*Rosaceae*)—Pear

4'-DIHYDROPHASEIC-ACID Seed

4-HYDROXYMETHYLPROLINE Fruit

6-O-ACETYLARBUTIN Plant

ABSCISSIC-ACID Seed

ACETIC-ACID Plant

ACETIC-ACID-ISOBUTYL-ESTER Plant

ACETONE Plant

ACETYLARBUTIN Plant

ALANINE Fruit 130–803 ppm

ALPHA-LINOLENIC-ACID Fruit 10–62 ppm

ALPHA-PYRUFURAN Plant

ALPHA-TOCOPHEROL Fruit 0.6–31 ppm

ALUMINUM Fruit 1–105 ppm

AMYGDALIN Seed

ARBUTIN Plant

ARGININE Fruit 70–432 ppm

ARSENIC Fruit 0.001–0.06 ppm

ASCORBIC-ACID Fruit 40–250 ppm

ASH Fruit 2,720–40,000 ppm

ASPARTIC-ACID Fruit 770–4,756 ppm

BARIUM Fruit 0.045–11 ppm

BETA-CAROTENE Fruit 0.17–1.7 ppm

BETA-PHENYLETHYLAMINE Fruit
BETA-PYRUFURAN Plant
BORON Fruit 1–82 ppm
BROMINE Fruit
CADMIUM Fruit 0.125 ppm
CAFFEIC-ACID Fruit 43–19,700 ppm
CALCIUM Fruit 68–1,776 ppm
CARBOHYDRATES Fruit 151,000–933,292 ppm
CATECHIN Plant
CHROMIUM Fruit 0.002–0.555 ppm
CIS-4-DECADIENIC-ACID-ETHYL-ESTER Plant
CIS-4-DECADIENIC-ACID-METHYL-ESTER
  Plant
CIS-CHLOROGENIC-ACID Plant
CIS-ISOCHLOROGENIC-ACID Plant
CIS-P-COUMAROYLQUINIC-ACID Plant
CITRIC-ACID Fruit
COBALT Fruit 0.015–0.111 ppm
COPPER Fruit 0.45–11.1 ppm
CYANIDIN-3-GALACTOSIDE Epidermis
CYSTINE Fruit 40–247 ppm
EPICATECHIN Plant
EPIFRIEDELIN Fruit
FAT Fruit 2,790–32,198 ppm
FIBER Fruit 14,000–86,473 ppm
FLUORINE Fruit
FOLACIN Fruit 0.06–0.5 ppm
FORMALDEHYDE Plant
FRIEDELIN Fruit
GADOLEIC-ACID Fruit 10–62 ppm
GIBBERELLIN-A-25 Seed
GIBBERELLIN-A-45 Seed
GLUTAMIC-ACID Fruit 280–1,729 ppm
GLYCINE Fruit 110–679 ppm
HEXANAL Plant
HISTIDINE Fruit 40–247 ppm
HYDROQUINONE Plant
IRON Fruit 0.9–37 ppm
ISOAMYL-ALCOHOL Plant
ISOLEUCINE Fruit 110–679 ppm
ISORHAMNETIN-3-GLUCOSIDE Plant
ISORHAMNETIN-3-RHAMNOSYLGALACTO-
  SIDE Plant
ISORHAMNETIN-3-RHAMNOSYLGLUCOSIDE
  Plant
KAEMPFEROL-3-0-GALACTOSIDE Plant
KAEMPFEROL-3-0-GLUCOSIDE Plant
KAEMPFEROL-3-0-RUTINOSIDE Plant

KAEMPFEROL-3-ARABINOSIDE Plant
LEAD Fruit 0.02–1.11 ppm
LEUCINE Fruit 200–1,235 ppm
LINOLEIC-ACID Fruit 930–5,744 ppm
LITHIUM Fruit 0.06–0.185 ppm
LUTEIN Fruit 1–11 ppm
LYSINE Fruit 140–865 ppm
MAGNESIUM Fruit 54–1,110 ppm
MALIC-ACID Fruit
MANGANESE Fruit 0.3–5.55 ppm
MERCURY Fruit 0.019 ppm
METHIONINE Fruit 50–309 ppm
METHYL-ETHYL-KETONE Plant
METHYL-N-PROPYL-KETONE Plant
MOLYBDENUM Fruit 0.1–0.26 ppm
MUFA Fruit 840–5,188 ppm
NIACIN Fruit 1–6 ppm
NICKEL Fruit 0.1–1.11 ppm
NITROGEN Fruit 480–3,000 ppm
OLEIC-ACID Fruit 810–5,003 ppm
PALMITIC-ACID Fruit 170–1,050 ppm
PALMITOLEIC-ACID Fruit 20–124 ppm
PANTOTHENIC-ACID Fruit 0.7–4 ppm
PECTIN Fruit 40,000 ppm
PHLORORRHIZIN Plant
PHOSPHORUS Fruit 90–1,332 ppm
PHYTOSTEROLS Fruit 80–494 ppm
POTASSIUM Fruit 1,200–11,250 ppm
PROLINE Fruit 110–679 ppm
PROPIONALDEHYDE Plant
PROTEIN Fruit 3,690–25,400 ppm
PUFA Fruit 940–5,806 ppm
QUERCETIN Pericarp 28 ppm
QUERCETIN-3'-GLUCOSIDE Plant
QUERCETIN-3-0-GALACTOSIDE Plant
QUERCETIN-3-0-RUTINOSIDE Plant
QUERCETIN-3-ARABINOSIDE Plant
QUINIC-ACID Fruit
RIBOFLAVIN Fruit 0.4–2.4 ppm
RUBIDIUM Fruit 1.6–20 ppm
SELENIUM Fruit 0.001 ppm
SERINE Fruit 140–865 ppm
SFA Fruit 220–1,359 ppm
SHIKIMIC-ACID Fruit
SILICON Fruit 2–20 ppm
SILVER Fruit 0.015–0.037 ppm
SODIUM Fruit 407 ppm
STRONTIUM Fruit 0.45–18.5 ppm

SULFUR Fruit 3–300 ppm

THIAMIN Fruit 0.2–1.2 ppm

THREONINE Fruit 100–618 ppm

TITANIUM Fruit 0.075–7.4 ppm

TRANS-2,TRANS-4-DECADIENIC-ACID-ETHYL-ESTER Plant

TRANS-2,TRANS-4-DECADIENIC-ACID-METHYL-ESTER Plant

TRANS-2-DECADIENIC-ACID-ETHYL-ESTER Plant

TRANS-2-DECADIENIC-ACID-METHYL-ESTER Plant

TRANS-CAFFEOYLARBUTIN Plant

TRANS-CAFFEOYLCALLERYANIN Plant

TRANS-CHLOROGENIC-ACID Plant

TRANS-ISOCHLOROGENIC-ACID Plant

TRANS-NEOCHLOROGENIC-ACID Plant

TRANS-P-COUMAROYLQUINIC-ACID Plant

TYROSINE Fruit 30–185 ppm

URSOLIC-ACID Fruit

VALINE Fruit 140–865 ppm

VANADIUM Fruit 0.225–0.555 ppm

VIT-B-6 Fruit 0.1–1.1 ppm

WATER Fruit 817,000–891,000 ppm

ZINC Fruit 0.15–26.6 ppm

ZIRCONIUM Fruit 0.3–1.11 ppm

PINEAPPLE

Chemicals in *Ananas comosus (L.) MERR.* (*Bromeliaceae*)—Pineapple

2,5-DIMETHYL-4-HYDROXY-3(2H)-FURA-NONE Plant 1.2 ppm

5-HYDROXYTRYPTAMINE Plant

ACETALDEHYDE Fruit 0.61–1.4 ppm

ACETIC-ACID Fruit 0.49 ppm

ACETONE Fruit

ACETOXYACETONE Fruit

ACRYLIC-ACID Plant

ALANINE Fruit 170–1,259 ppm

ALPHA-LINOLENIC-ACID Fruit 620–4,592 ppm

ALPHA-TOCOPHEROL Fruit 1–7 ppm

AMYL-CAPROATE Fruit

ANANASIC-ACID Plant

ARGININE Fruit 46–1,333 ppm

ASCORBIC-ACID Fruit 148–4,178 ppm

ASH Fruit 2,800–36,000 ppm

ASPARAGINE Fruit 1,251 ppm

ASPARTIC-ACID Fruit 293–4,222 ppm

BETA-CAROTENE Fruit 3 ppm

BETA-METHYL-THIOPROPIONIC-ACID-ETHYL-ESTER Plant

BETA-METHYL-THIOPROPIONIC-ACID-METHYL-ESTER Plant

BIACETYL Fruit

BORON Fruit 0.2 ppm

BROMELAIN Fruit

BROMELIN Fruit

BUTYL-FORMATE Fruit

CALCIUM Fruit 62–1,308 ppm

CARBOHYDRATES Fruit 116,000–938,000 ppm

CELLULOSE Fruit 4,300–5,400 ppm

CHAVICOL Fruit 0.27 ppm

CHLORINE Fruit 460 ppm

CITRIC-ACID Fruit 3,200–86,000 ppm

COPPER Fruit 1–8.8 ppm

CYSTINE Fruit 20–148 ppm

DELTA-OCTALACTONE Fruit 0.3 ppm

DIMETHYL-MALONATE Fruit 0.06 ppm

ERGOSTEROL-PEROXIDE Plant

ESTERS Fruit 1–250 ppm

ETHYL-ACETATE Fruit 3–120 ppm

ETHYL-ACRYLATE Fruit 0.77 ppm

ETHYL-ALCOHOL Fruit 60 ppm

ETHYL-BETA-ACETOXYHEXANOATE Fruit 0.006 ppm

ETHYL-BETA-HYDROXYHEXANOATE Fruit 0.03 ppm

ETHYL-BETA-METHYLTHIOPROPIONATE Fruit 0.09 ppm

ETHYL-BUTYRATE Fruit

ETHYL-CAPROATE Fruit 0.77 ppm

ETHYL-CAPRYLATE Fruit

ETHYL-FORMATE Fruit

ETHYL-ISOBUTYRATE Fruit

ETHYL-ISOVALERATE Fruit 0.39 ppm

ETHYL-LACTATE Fruit

ETHYL-PROPIONATE Fruit

FAT Fruit 1,000–42,772 ppm

FERULIC-ACID Plant 200–760 ppm

FIBER Fruit 3,000–45,000 ppm

FRUCTOSE Fruit 6,000–23,000 ppm

GABA Fruit 124 ppm

GAMMA-BUTYROLACTONE Fruit

GAMMA-CAPROLACTONE Fruit 0.12 ppm

GAMMA-OCTALACTONE Fruit 0.3 ppm
GLUCOSE Fruit 10,000–32,000 ppm
GLUTAMIC-ACID Fruit 90–3,333 ppm
GLUTAMINE Fruit 256 ppm
GLYCINE Fruit 65–1,259 ppm
HEXOSANS Fruit 1,000–1,500 ppm
HISTIDINE Fruit 48–667 ppm
INDOLE-ACETIC-ACID-OXIDASE Fruit
IODINE Fruit 1 ppm
IRON Fruit 3–73 ppm
ISOBUTANOL Fruit
ISOBUTYL-ACETATE Fruit
ISOBUTYL-FORMATE Fruit
ISOCAPRONIC-ACID Fruit
ISOLEUCINE Fruit 23–963 ppm
ISOPROPYL-ISOBUTYRATE Fruit
L-MALIC-ACID Fruit
LEUCINE Fruit 24–1,407 ppm
LINOLEIC-ACID Fruit 840–6,222 ppm
LYSINE Fruit 46–1,852 ppm
MAGNESIUM Fruit 110–1,075 ppm
MALIC-ACID Fruit 1,000–4,700 ppm
MANGANESE Fruit 12–209 ppm
METHANOL Fruit
METHIONINE Fruit 110–815 ppm
METHYL-ACETATE Fruit
METHYL-BETA-ACETOXYHEXANOATE Fruit
  0.03 ppm
METHYL-BETA-HYDROXYBUTYRATE Fruit
  0.006 ppm
METHYL-BETA-HYDROXYHEXANOATE Fruit
  0.021 ppm
METHYL-BETA-METHYLTHIOPROPIONATE
  Fruit 0.12–1.1 ppm
METHYL-BUTYRATE Fruit
METHYL-CAPROATE Fruit
METHYL-CAPRYLATE Fruit 0.75 ppm
METHYL-CIS-(4?)-OCTENOATE Fruit 0.001
  ppm
METHYL-ISOBUTYRATE Fruit
METHYL-ISOCAPROATE Fruit 1.4 ppm
METHYL-ISOVALERATE Fruit 0.6 ppm
METHYL-N-PROPYL-KETONE Fruit
MUFA Fruit 480–3,556 ppm
N-VALERIANIC-ACID Fruit
NIACIN Fruit 2–33 ppm
NITRATE Fruit 1,200 ppm
NITROGEN Fruit 450–1,150 ppm

OLEIC-ACID Fruit 450–3,333 ppm
OXALIC-ACID Fruit 50–58 ppm
P-AMINOBENZOIC-ACID Fruit 1 ppm
P-COUMARIC-ACID Plant 330–730 ppm
PALMITIC-ACID Fruit 190–1,407 ppm
PALMITOLEIC-ACID Fruit 30–220 ppm
PANTOTHENIC-ACID Fruit 1–11 ppm
PECTIN Fruit 600–1,600 ppm
PENTANOL Fruit
PENTOSANS Fruit 3,300–4,300 ppm
PEROXIDASE Fruit
PHENYLALANINE Fruit 40–889 ppm
PHOSPHATASE Fruit
PHOSPHORUS Fruit 60–923 ppm
PHYTOSTEROLS Fruit 60–444 ppm
POTASSIUM Fruit 110–9,932 ppm
PROLINE Fruit 31–963 ppm
PROPANOL Fruit
PROPYL-ACETATE Fruit
PROPYL-FORMATE Fruit
PROTEIN Fruit 4,000–55,000 ppm
PUFA Fruit 1,460–10,815 ppm
RIBOFLAVIN Fruit 3 ppm
SERINE Fruit 250–1,852 ppm
SEROTONIN Fruit 19–60 ppm
SFA Fruit 320–2,370 ppm
SILICON Fruit 110–690 ppm
SODIUM Fruit 10–180 ppm
STARCH Fruit 19 ppm
STEARIC-ACID Fruit 110–815 ppm
STIGMAST-5-ENE-3-BETA-7-ALPHA-DIOL Plant
SUCROSE Fruit 59,000–150,000 ppm
SULFUR Fruit 70 ppm
THIAMIN Fruit 7 ppm
THREONINE Fruit 78–859 ppm
TRANS-TETRAHYDRO-ALPHA-ALPHA-5-
  TRIMETHYL-5-VINYLFURFURYL-ALC Plant
TYROSINE Fruit 58–889 ppm
VALINE Fruit 39–1,185 ppm
VANILLIN Fruit
VIT-B-6 Fruit 0.9–6 ppm
WATER Fruit 812,000–890,000 ppm
ZINC Fruit 0.7–6 ppm

PLUM

Chemicals in *Prunus domestica L.*
(*Rosaceae*)—Plum

4-O-METHYL-GLUCURONIC-ACID Fruit

ALANINE Fruit 290–1,959 ppm

ALPHA-TOCOPHEROL Fruit 8–62 ppm

ALUMINUM Fruit 1–255 ppm

AMYGDALIN Seed 25,000 ppm

ARACHIDIC-ACID Seed 21,450–23,100 ppm

ARGININE Fruit 130–878 ppm

ARSENIC Fruit 0.001–0.51 ppm

ASCORBIC-ACID Fruit 86–699 ppm

ASH Fruit 3,810–170,000 ppm

ASPARTIC-ACID Fruit 2,490–16,824 ppm

BARIUM Fruit 0.154–25.5 ppm

BETA-CAROTENE Fruit 1.4–43 ppm

BORON Fruit 1–255 ppm

BROMINE Fruit

CADMIUM Fruit 0.001–0.068 ppm

CAFFEIC-ACID Plant

CALCIUM Fruit 38–2,040 ppm

CARBOHYDRATES Fruit 130,100–879,054 ppm

CHLOROGENIC-ACID Fruit

CHROMIUM Fruit 0.005–1.19 ppm

CITRIC-ACID Fruit

COBALT Fruit 0.005–0.34 ppm

COPPER Fruit 0.33–34 ppm

CRYPTOCHLOROGENIC-ACID Fruit

CYANIDIN Plant

CYSTINE Fruit 40–270 ppm

D-GALACTOSE Fruit

D-MANNOSE Fruit

D-XYLOSE Fruit

DIHYDROKAEMPFERIDE Wood

DIHYDROKAEMPFEROL Wood

FAT Fruit 6,000–43,243 ppm Seed
390,000–420,000 ppm

FERULIC-ACID Fruit

FIBER Fruit 6,000–40,540 ppm Seed 122,000 ppm

FLUORINE Fruit 0.1–0.6 ppm

FOLACIN Fruit 0.019–0.167 ppm

FRUCTOSE Fruit 27,000–61,000 ppm

GLUCOSE Fruit 30,000–62,000 ppm

GLUTAMIC-ACID Fruit 370–2,500 ppm

GLYCINE Fruit 120–811 ppm

HCN Seed 500 ppm

HEXURONIC-ACID Resin, Exudate, Sap

HISTIDINE Fruit 130–878 ppm

IRON Fruit 0.8–85 ppm

ISOCHLOROGENIC-ACID Fruit

ISOLEUCINE Fruit 160–1,081 ppm

KAEMPFERIDE Wood

KAEMPFEROL Wood

KILOCALORIES Fruit 550–3,716 /kg

LANTHANUM Fruit 1.5–12 ppm

LAURIC-ACID Seed 3,510–3,780 ppm

LEAD Fruit 0.02–11.9 ppm

LECITHIN Seed 1,500 ppm

LEUCINE Fruit 210–1,419 ppm

LINOLEIC-ACID Fruit 1,340–9,054 ppm Seed
54,600–83,160 ppm

LITHIUM Fruit 0.088–0.68 ppm

LUTEIN Fruit 2.4–24 ppm

LYSINE Fruit 170–1,149 ppm

MAGNESIUM Fruit 68–3,400 ppm

MALIC-ACID Fruit 15,000 ppm

MANGANESE Fruit 0.22–25.5 ppm

MERCURY Fruit 0.013 ppm

METHIONINE Fruit 60–405 ppm

MOLYBDENUM Fruit 0.1–1.7 ppm

MUFA Fruit 4,060–27,432 ppm

MYRISTIC-ACID Seed 14,820–15,960 ppm

NEO-CHLOROGENIC-ACID Fruit

NIACIN Fruit 5–34 ppm

NICKEL Fruit 0.03–1.7 ppm

NITROGEN Fruit 960–10,000 ppm

OLEIC-ACID Fruit 4,000–27,027 ppm Seed
254,280–306,600 ppm

P-COUMARIC-ACID Fruit

PALMITIC-ACID Fruit 410–2,770 ppm Seed
2,340–2,520 ppm

PALMITOLEIC-ACID Fruit 50–338 ppm

PANTOTHENIC-ACID Fruit 1.8–13 ppm

PECTIN Fruit 8,000–40,000 ppm

PERSICAXANTHIN Plant

PHENYLALANINE Fruit 170–1,149 ppm

PHOSPHATIDES Seed 3,000 ppm

PHOSPHORUS Fruit 70–4,080 ppm

POTASSIUM Fruit 1,677–44,200 ppm

PROLINE Fruit 340–2,297 ppm

PROTEIN Fruit 7,660–55,000 ppm Seed
202,000 ppm

PRUDOMESTIN Wood

PUFA Fruit 1,340–9,054 ppm

QUERCETIN Plant

QUINIC-ACID Fruit

RHAMNOSE Fruit

RIBOFLAVIN Fruit 0.9–6.5 ppm

RUBIDIUM Fruit 0.5–15 ppm

SELENIUM Fruit 0.013 ppm
SERINE Fruit 200–1,351 ppm
SEROTONIN Fruit
SFA Fruit 490–3,310 ppm
SILICON Fruit 2–62 ppm
SILVER Fruit 0.022–0.51 ppm
SODIUM Fruit 54 ppm
STEARIC-ACID Fruit 90–608 ppm Seed 16,380–17,640 ppm
STRONTIUM Fruit 0.33–51 ppm
SUCCINIC-ACID Fruit
SUCROSE Fruit 7,000–48,000 ppm
SUGAR Fruit 100,000–200,000 ppm
SULFUR Fruit 4–400 ppm
TANNIN Bark 68,000 ppm
TARTARIC-ACID Fruit
THIAMIN Fruit 0.4–2.9 ppm
THREONINE Fruit 160–1,081 ppm
TITANIUM Fruit 0.11–25.5 ppm
TRYPTAMINE Fruit
TYRAMINE Fruit
TYROSINE Fruit 60–405 ppm
VALINE Fruit 190–1,284 ppm
VIT-B-6 Fruit 0.7–6 ppm
WATER Fruit 840,000–933,000 ppm
ZINC Fruit 0.66–131 ppm
ZIRCONIUM Fruit 0.44–3.4 ppm

POMEGRANATE

Chemicals in *Punica granatum L.* (*Punicaceae*)—Pomegranate

1,2,3,4,6–PENTA-O-GALLOYL-BETA-D-GLU-COSE Leaf
1,2,4,6-TETRA-O-GALLOYL-BETA-D-GLUCOSE Leaf
2-(2-PROPENYL)-DELTA'-PIPERIDEINE Leaf
2-O-GALLOYLPUNICALIN Leaf
ALKALOIDS Root Bark 1,000–7,000 ppm
ARACHIDIC-ACID Seed
ASCORBIC-ACID Fruit 40–636 ppm
ASH Fruit 5,000–35,858 ppm
ASIATIC-ACID Flower
BETA-SITOSTEROL Bark
BETULINIC-ACID Bark Leaf
BORIC-ACID Fruit 50 ppm
CALCIUM Fruit 30–650 ppm
CALCIUM-OXALATE Petiole 40,000 ppm

CARBOHYDRATES Fruit 162,000–927,000 ppm
CAROTENE Fruit 2 ppm
CASUARIIN Bark Plant
CEREBROSIDE Seed
CHLORINE Fruit 20 ppm
CHLOROGENIC-ACID Fruit
CIS-9,TRANS-11,CIS-13-TRIENE-ACID Seed
CITRIC-ACID Fruit Juice 8,100–12,300 ppm
COPPER Fruit 2 ppm
CORILAGIN Leaf
CYANIDIN-3,5–DIGLUCOSIDE Fruit
CYANIDIN-3-GLUCOSIDE Fruit
D-MANNITOL Bark Leaf Root Seed Stem
DELPHINIDIN-3,5–DIGLUCOSIDE Pericarp
DELPHINIDIN-3-GLUCOSIDE Fruit
ELAIDIC-ACID Pericarp 5,500 ppm
ELLAGIC-ACID Bark
ELLAGITANNIN Bark
ESTRADIOL Seed
ESTRONE Seed 17 ppm
FAT Fruit 1,000–38,000 ppm Seed 50,000–200,000 ppm
FIBER Fruit 2,000–232,000 ppm Seed 224,000 ppm
FLAVOGALLOL Pericarp
FRIEDELIN Bark
FRUCTOSE Fruit
GALLIC-ACID Pericarp 900–40,000 ppm
GLUCOSE Fruit
GRANATIN-A Pericarp
GRANATIN-B Pericarp
GRANATINS Leaf 15,000 ppm
GUM Petiole 32,000 ppm
INULIN Petiole 10,000 ppm
IRON Fruit 3–16 ppm
ISOPELLETIERINE Bark
ISOQUERCETRIN Pericarp
LINOLEIC-ACID Seed
MAGNESIUM Fruit 120 ppm
MALIC-ACID Fruit
MALTOSE Fruit
MALVIDIN Fruit
MALVIDIN-PENTOSE-GLYCOSIDE Fruit Juice
MANNITOL Pericarp 18,000 ppm
MASLINIC-ACID Flower
METHYL-ISOPELLETIERINE Bark
METHYL-PELLETIERINE Bark
MUCILAGE Petiole 6,000–340,000 ppm

NEO-CHLOROGENIC-ACID Fruit

NIACIN Fruit 3–50 ppm

OLEIC-ACID Seed

OXALIC-ACID Fruit 140 ppm

P-COUMARINIC-ACID Fruit

PALMITIC-ACID Seed

PANTOTHENIC-ACID Fruit 6–31 ppm

PECTIN Fruit 2,700 ppm Pericarp
  20,000–40,000 ppm

PELARGONIDIN-3,5-DIGLUCOSIDE Flower

PELARGONIDIN-3–GLUCOSIDE Seed

PELLETIERINE Bark

PHOSPHATIDYL-CHOLINE Seed

PHOSPHATIDYL-INOSITOL Seed

PHOSPHATIDYL-SERINE Seed

PHOSPHORUS Fruit 80–3,182 ppm

PHYTOSTEROLS Fruit 170–892 ppm

POLYPHENOLS Fruit 2,200–10,500 ppm

POTASSIUM Fruit 1,330–18,950 ppm

PROTEIN Fruit 7,700–73,000 ppm Seed 25,000
  ppm

PROTOCATECHUIC-ACID Fruit

PSEUDOPELLETIERINE Bark

PUNICACORTEINS Bark

PUNICAFOLIN Plant

PUNICALAGIN Pericarp

PUNICALIN Pericarp

PUNICIC-ACID Seed 35,000–140,000 ppm

PUNIGLUCONIN Bark

RESINS Pericarp 45,000 ppm

RIBOFLAVIN Fruit 4 ppm

SODIUM Fruit 9–350 ppm

SORBITOL Plant

STARCH Seed

STEARIC-ACID Seed

STRICTININ Leaf

STYPTIC-ACID Flower

SULFUR Fruit 120 ppm

TANNIN Fruit Juice 1,700 ppm Leaf 110,000
  ppm Pericarp 104,000–336,000 ppm Root
  Bark 280,000 ppm Stem Bark 100,000–
  250,000 ppm

THIAMIN Fruit 4 ppm

URSOLIC-ACID Fruit Leaf

VIT-B-6 Fruit 1–5 ppm

WATER Fruit 780,000–823,220 ppm Seed
  350,000 ppm

WAX Pericarp 8,000 ppm

RED CURRANT

Chemicals in *Ribes rubrum L. (Grossulari-aceae)*—Red Currant, White Currant

ACETIC-ACID Fruit

ALPHA-LINOLENIC-ACID Fruit 350–2,180
  ppm

ALPHA-TOCOPHEROL Fruit 8–59 ppm

ALUMINUM Fruit 3–100 ppm

ARSENIC Fruit 0.01–0.18 ppm

ASCORBIC-ACID Fruit 300–2,554 ppm

ASH Fruit 6,000–75,000 ppm

BETA-CAROTENE Fruit 0.25–4 ppm

BORIC-ACID Fruit

BORON Fruit 1–80 ppm

BROMINE Fruit

CADMIUM Fruit 0.003–0.03 ppm

CALCIUM Fruit 298–2,875 ppm

CARBOHYDRATES Fruit 138,000–859,740 ppm

CHLORINE Fruit 146–910 ppm

CHROMIUM Fruit 0.01–0.125 ppm

CITRIC-ACID Fruit 20,200 ppm

COBALT Fruit

COPPER Fruit 0.5–7 ppm

CYANIDIN-3-GLUCOSYL-RUTINOSIDE Fruit

CYANIDIN-3-RUTINOSIDE Fruit

CYANIDIN-3-SAMBUBIOSIDE Fruit

CYANIDIN-3-SOPHOROSIDE Fruit

CYANIDIN-3-XYLOSYLRUTINOSIDE Fruit

CYANIN Fruit

DELPHINIDIN-3-GLUCOSIDE Fruit

FAT Fruit 2,000–12,460 ppm Seed
  160,000–250,000 ppm

FIBER Fruit 34,000–211,820 ppm

FLUORINE Fruit 0.05–1.8 ppm

FRUCTOSE Fruit 19,300 ppm

GLUCOSE Fruit 22,800 ppm

HCN Leaf

INDOLE-ACETIC-ACID Seed

IRON Fruit 9–68 ppm

ISOCITRIC-ACID Fruit

LEAD Fruit 0.02–0.5 ppm

LINOLEIC-ACID Fruit 530–3,302 ppm

LUTEIN Fruit 0.47–2.3 ppm

MAGNESIUM Fruit 122–935 ppm

MALIC-ACID Fruit 2,600 ppm

MANGANESE Fruit 1–15 ppm

MERCURY Fruit 0.006 ppm

METHYL-SALICYLATE Fruit

MOLYBDENUM Fruit 0.1–0.6 ppm
NIACIN Fruit 1–6 ppm
NICKEL Fruit 0.03–0.6 ppm
NITROGEN Fruit 1,600–20,000 ppm
OLEIC-ACID Fruit 280–1,744 ppm
OXALIC-ACID Fruit
P-HYDROXY-BENZOIC-ACID Fruit
PALMITIC-ACID Fruit 100–623 ppm
PALMITOLEIC-ACID Fruit 10–62 ppm
PANTOTHENIC-ACID Fruit 1–4 ppm
PECTIN Fruit 8,000 ppm
PHOSPHORUS Fruit 418–3,310 ppm
POTASSIUM Fruit 2,585–21,250 ppm
PROTEIN Fruit 14,000–87,220 ppm
PROTOPECTIN Fruit
RIBOFLAVIN Fruit 1–3 ppm
RUBIDIUM Fruit 0.9–23 ppm
SALICYLIC-ACID Fruit
SELENIUM Fruit
SILICON Fruit 10–312 ppm
SODIUM Fruit 8–72 ppm
STEARIC-ACID Fruit 30–187 ppm
SUCCINIC-ACID Fruit
SUCROSE Fruit 1,500 ppm
SUGARS Fruit 6,000–83,200 ppm
SULFUR Fruit 130–1,782 ppm
TARTARIC-ACID Fruit
THIAMIN Fruit 1–2 ppm
VIT-B-6 Fruit 1–4 ppm
WATER Fruit 834,000–845,000 ppm
ZINC Fruit 2–16 ppm

RED RASPBERRY

Chemicals in *Rubus idaeus L.* (*Rosaceae*)—
Raspberry, Red Raspberry

1-PENTANOL Fruit
1-PENTEN-3-OL Plant
2-HEXEN-4-OLIDE Plant
3-METHYL-2-BUTEN-1-OL Plant
5-METHYL-FURFURAL Fruit
ACETIC-ACID Plant
ACETOIN Fruit
ALPHA-CAROTENE Fruit 0.13–0.6 ppm
ALPHA-FURANCARBONIC-ACID Plant
ALPHA-TOCOPHEROL Fruit 9–56 ppm
ALUMINUM Leaf 392 ppm

ASCORBIC-ACID Leaf 3,670 ppm Seed 300 ppm
ASH Leaf 80,000 ppm
BENZALDEHYDE Plant
BENZOIC-ACID Plant
BETA-CAROTENE Fruit 0.06–0.3 ppm Leaf 114 ppm
BETA-IONONE Plant
BETA-PHENYLETHYLALCOHOL Fruit
BORON Fruit 1–13 pp
BUTYRIC-ACID Fruit
CAFFEIC-ACID Fruit
CALCIUM Leaf 12,100 ppm
CAPRONIC-ACID Fruit
CAPRYLIC-ACID Fruit
CARBOHYDRATES Leaf 790,000 ppm
CHROMIUM Leaf 13 ppm
CINNAMYL-ALCOHOL Plant
CIS-HEXEN-3-OL Plant
COBALT Leaf 34 ppm
CYANIDIN-3-GLUCOSIDE Plant
CYANIDIN-3-GLUCOSYL-RUTINOSIDE Plant
CYANIDIN-3-RUTINOSIDE Plant
CYANIDIN-3-SOPHOROSIDE Plant
CYANIDIN-5-MONOGLYCOSIDE Plant
CYANIN Fruit
DAMASCENE Plant
DEXTROSE Fruit 35,000 ppm
DIACETYL Fruit
DIHYDRO-BETA-IONONE Plant
ELLAGIC-ACID Leaf
EPOXY-BETA-IONONE Plant
ETHANOL Plant
ETHYL-ACETATE Plant
FARNESOL Plant
FAT Leaf 17,000 ppm Seed 145,000–240,000 ppm
FERULIC-ACID Fruit
FIBER Leaf 82,000 ppm
FORMIC-ACID Fruit
FURFURAL Fruit
GALLIC-ACID Leaf
GERANIOL Fruit
HEXEN-2-ACID Fruit
HEXEN-3-ACID Fruit
IRON Leaf 1,010 ppm
ISOAMYL-ALCOHOL Fruit
SOBUTYRIC-ACID Fruit

ISOVALERIANIC-ACID Fruit
KAEMPFEROL-3-BETA-GLUCURONIDE Plant
KILOCALORIES Leaf 2,750 /kg
LACTIC-ACID Leaf
LEVULOSE Fruit 35,000 ppm
LUTEIN Fruit 0.76–4 ppm
MAGNESIUM Leaf 3,190 ppm
MALIC-ACID Fruit
MALTOL Fruit
MANGANESE Fruit 16–18 ppm Leaf 146 ppm
NIACIN Leaf
O-PHTHALIC-ACID Plant
ORGANIC-ACIDS Plant 15,000–20,000 ppm
OXYBENZOIC-ACID Fruit
P-CRESOL Plant
P-ETHYL-PHENOL Plant
P-HYDROXYPHENYLETHYLALCOHOL Plant
PECTIN Fruit 14,500 ppm
PELARGONIN-3,2-GLUCOSYL-RUTINOSIDE
 Fruit
PELARGONIN-3,5-DIGLYCOSIDE Fruit
PHOSPHORUS Leaf 2,340 ppm
POTASSIUM Leaf 13,400 ppm
PROPIONIC-ACID Fruit
PROTEIN Leaf 113,000 ppm
QUERCETIN-3-BETA-GLUCURONIDE Plant
RIBOFLAVIN Leaf
SALICYLIC-ACID Fruit
SELENIUM Leaf
SILICON Leaf 13 ppm
SODIUM Leaf 77 ppm
SUCCINIC-ACID Fruit Leaf
TANNIN Fruit 6,200 ppm Leaf
 100,000–120,000 ppm
THEASPIRANE Plant
THIAMIN Leaf 3.4 ppm
TRANS-2-PHENYLBUTANONE Plant
VALERIANIC-ACID Fruit
WATER Leaf 831,000 ppm
ZINC Leaf

STAR FRUIT

Chemicals in *Averrhoa carambola L.* (*Oxalidaceae*)—Carambola, Star Fruit

ALANINE Fruit 370–2,075 ppm
ALPHA-KETO-GLUTARIC-ACID Fruit
 3,900–22,000 ppm

ALUMINUM Fruit 3–41 ppm
ARGININE Fruit 110–1,210 ppm
ASCORBIC-ACID Fruit 200–4,935 ppm
ASH Fruit 2,600–52,000 ppm
ASPARTIC-ACID Fruit 510–5,615 ppm
BETA-APO-8'-CAROTENE Fruit
BETA-CAROTENE Fruit 0.03–75 ppm
BETA-CRYPTOFLAVIN Fruit 0.6–75 ppm
BETA-DAMASCENONE Fruit
BETA-IONONE Fruit
BORON Fruit 0.6–8 ppm
CALCIUM Fruit 29–1,040 ppm
CARBOHYDRATES Fruit 67,000–936,000 ppm
CAROTENOIDS Fruit 3–220 ppm
CITRIC-ACID Fruit 13,200 ppm
COPPER Fruit 1–15 ppm
CRYPTOCHROME Fruit
CRYPTOXANTHIN Fruit
CYANIDIN Plant
FAT Fruit 800–52,000 ppm
FIBER Fruit 6,000–130,000 ppm
FUMARIC-ACID Fruit 3,100 ppm
GLUTAMIC-ACID Fruit 770–8,480 ppm
GLYCINE Fruit 260–2,860 ppm
HISTIDINE Fruit 40–440 ppm
IRON Fruit 1–165 ppm
ISOLEUCINE Fruit 230–2,530 ppm
KILOCALORIES Fruit 280–3,920 /kg
LEUCINE Fruit 400–4,400 ppm
LUTEIN Fruit
LYSINE Fruit 400–4,400 ppm
MAGNESIUM Fruit 80–1,200 ppm
MALIC-ACID Fruit 12,100 ppm
MANGANESE Fruit 1–11 ppm
METHIONINE Fruit 110–1,210 ppm
MUTATOXANTHIN Fruit 0.3–30 ppm
NIACIN Fruit 3–53 ppm
NITROGEN Fruit 10,200–12,800 ppm
OXALIC-ACID Fruit 50,000–95,800 ppm
P-COUMARIC-ACID Plant
PHENYLALANINE Fruit 190–2,090 ppm
PHOSPHORUS Fruit 140–2,100 ppm
PHYTOFLUENE Fruit 0.3–37 ppm
POTASSIUM Fruit 1,400–23,500 ppm
PROLINE Fruit 260–2,860 ppm
PROTEIN Fruit 3,000–73,000 ppm
RIBOFLAVIN Fruit 0.2–5.2 ppm
SERINE Fruit 430–4,735 ppm

SINAPIC-ACID Plant
SODIUM Fruit 17–351 ppm
SUCCINIC-ACID Fruit 2,200 ppm
SULFUR Fruit 1,000–1,300 ppm
TARTARIC-ACID Fruit 9,100–43,700 ppm
THIAMIN Fruit 0.2–6.57 ppm
THREONINE Fruit 230–2,530 ppm
TRYPTOPHAN Fruit 40–440
TYROSINE Fruit 230–2,530 ppm
VALINE Fruit 260–2,860 ppm
WATER Fruit 874,000–923,000 ppm
ZINC Fruit 1–12 ppm

STRAWBERRY

Chemicals in *Fragaria spp* (*Rosaceae*)—
Strawberry

(+)-ABSCISIC-ACID Plant
2-HEXEN-1-AL Plant
2-METHYL-NAPHTHALENE Plant
ALANINE Fruit 310–3,677 ppm
ALPHA-LINOLENIC-ACID Fruit 780–9,253
  ppm
ALPHA-TERPINEOL Leaf
ALPHA-TOCOPHEROL Fruit 1–54 ppm
ALUMINUM Fruit 3–70 ppm
ANTHOCYANIN Plant
ARBUTIN Leaf
ARGININE Fruit 260–3,084 ppm
ARSENIC Fruit
ASCORBIC-ACID Fruit 400–6,948 ppm Leaf
  3,190–4,350 ppm
ASH Fruit 3,900–52,065 ppm
ASPARAGINE Plant
ASPARAGINIC-ACID Plant
ASPARTIC-ACID Fruit 1,380–16,370 ppm
BETA-CAROTENE Fruit 0.089–7 ppm
BORON Fruit 1–160 ppm
BROMINE Fruit
CADMIUM Fruit 0.004–0.18 ppm
CAFFEIC-ACID Fruit 15–34 ppm
CALCIUM Fruit 135–2,900 ppm
CARBOHYDRATES Fruit 70,200–850,000 ppm
CATECHIN Fruit
CATECHOL Fruit
CHLOROGENIC-ACID Fruit
CHROMIUM Fruit 0.005–0.18 ppm
CINNAMIC-ACID-METHYL-ESTER Plant

CIS-3-HEXEN-1-OL Plant
CITRAL Leaf
CITRIC-ACID Fruit 3,500–8,000 ppm
COBALT Fruit 0.004–2 ppm
COPPER Fruit 0.4–17 ppm
CYANIDIN Plant
CYSTINE Fruit 50–593 ppm
DIHYDROTRIMETHYLNAPHTHALENE Leaf
ELLAGIC-ACID Fruit 430–8,430 ppm Leaf
  8,080–32,300 ppm Seed 1,370–
  21,650 ppm
ELLAGITANNIN Leaf
EO Plant
FAT Fruit 2,350–59,893 ppm Seed 190,000
  ppm
FIBER Fruit 5,300–181,000 ppm
FLUORINE Fruit 0.03–0.9 ppm
FOLACIN Fruit 0.1–0.2 ppm
FURFURAL Leaf
GALLIC-ACID Fruit 80–121 ppm
GALLOCATECHIN Fruit
GAMMA-AMINOBUTYRIC-ACID Plant
GENTISIC-ACID Fruit
GLUTAMIC-ACID Fruit 900–10,676 ppm
GLUTAMINE Plant
GLYCINE Fruit 240–2,847 ppm
HISTIDINE Fruit 120–1,423 ppm
IODINE Plant 0.157–0.23 ppm
IRON Fruit 3–100 ppm
ISOLEUCINE Fruit 140–1,661 ppm
KAEMPFEROL Leaf
KAEMPFEROL-3-BETA-GLUCURONIDE Plant
KAEMPFEROL-3-BETA-MONOGLUCOSIDE
  Fruit
KAEMPFEROL-7-MONOGLUCOSIDE Fruit
KILOCALORIES Fruit 300–3,559 /kg
LECITHIN Fruit 620 ppm
LEUCINE Fruit 310–3,667 ppm
LEUCOANTHOCYANIN Leaf
LINALOL Leaf
LINOLEIC-ACID Fruit 1,080–12,811 ppm Seed
  153,900 ppm
LINOLENIC-ACID Seed 9,975 ppm
LUTEIN Fruit 0.3–3 ppm
LUTEOFOROL Leaf
LYSINE Fruit 250–2,966 ppm
MAGNESIUM Fruit 98–1,545 ppm
MALIC-ACID Fruit 3,500–8,000 ppm

MALVIDIN-3,5-DIGLUCOSIDE Fruit

MANGANESE Fruit 1.4–125 ppm

MERCURY Fruit 0.009 ppm

METHIONINE Fruit 10–119 ppm

METHYL-FURFURAL Plant

METHYL-SALICYLATE Leaf

MOLYBDENUM Fruit

MUFA Fruit 520–6,168 ppm

N-NONAL Leaf

N-NONANOL Leaf

N-OCTANOL Leaf

NEO-CHLOROGENIC-ACID Fruit

NIACIN Fruit 2.3–27 ppm

NICKEL Fruit 0.03–0.36 ppm

NICOTINIC-ACID Plant 2 ppm

NITROGEN Fruit 880–10,000 ppm

OLEIC-ACID Fruit 510–6,050 ppm Seed 9,975 ppm

P-COUMARIC-ACID Fruit 63–125 ppm

P-HYDROXY-BENZOIC-ACID Fruit 19–108 ppm

PALMITIC-ACID Fruit 140–1,661 ppm

PALMITOLEIC-ACID Fruit 10–119 ppm

PANTOTHENIC-ACID Fruit 3.4–40 ppm

PECTIN Fruit 5,400 ppm

PELARGONIC-ACID Leaf

PELARGONIDIN-3-MONOGLUCOSIDE Fruit

PHOSPHORUS Fruit 185–3,191 ppm

PHYTOSTEROLS Fruit 120–1,423 ppm

POTASSIUM Leaf 1,400–22,500 ppm

POTASSIUM-OXIDE Plant

PROLINE Fruit 190–1,898 ppm

PROTEIN Fruit 5,840–85,000 ppm

PROTOCATECHUIC-ACID Fruit

PUFA Fruit 1,860–22,064 ppm

QUERCETIN Leaf

QUERCETIN-3-BETA-GLUCURONIDE Fruit

QUERCETIN-3-BETA-MONOGLUCOSIDE Fruit

QUERCITRIN Leaf

RIBOFLAVIN Fruit 0.7–8 ppm

RUBIDIUM Fruit 0.2–6.5 ppm

SALICYLIC-ACID Fruit

SELENIUM Fruit 0.002 ppm

SERINE Fruit 230–2,728 ppm

SFA Fruit 200–2,372 ppm

SILICON Fruit 10–270 ppm

SODIUM Fruit 8–106 ppm

STEARIC-ACID Fruit 40–475 ppm

SULFUR Fruit 77–1,270 ppm

TANNIN Leaf

THIAMIN Fruit 0.2–4 ppm

THREONINE Fruit 190–2,254 ppm

TRYPTOPHAN Fruit 70–830 ppm

VALINE Fruit 180–2,135 ppm

VANILLIC-ACID Fruit 3–25 ppm

VIT-B-6 Fruit 0.6–7 ppm

WATER Fruit 870,000–917,000 ppm

ZINC Fruit 1.1–17 ppm

TANGERINE-SEE MANDARIN

WATERMELON

Chemicals in *Citrullus lanatus* (*THUNB.*) *MATSUM. & NAKAI* (*Cucurbitaceae*)— Watermelon

(+)-VALINE Plant

ALANINE Fruit 2,000 ppm Seed 15,000 ppm

ALPHA-AMINO-BETA-(1-IMIDAZOYL)-PROPI-ONIC-ACID Plant

ARGININE Fruit 6,949 ppm Seed 46,600 ppm

ASH Fruit 30,600 ppm Seed 62,000 ppm

ASPARTIC-ACID Fruit 4,594 ppm Seed 25,500 ppm

BETA-CAROTENE Fruit 2–48 ppm

BORON Fruit 1–4 ppm

CALCIUM Fruit 100–3,400 ppm Seed 1,294–1,300 ppm

CAPRIC-ACID Seed 2,200–4,840 ppm

CAPRYLIC-ACID Seed 400–880 ppm

CARBOHYDRATES Fruit 3,800–859,000 ppm Seed 44,000–48,000 ppm

CIS,CIS-3,6-NONADIEN-1-OL Fruit

CITRULLIC-ACID Plant

CITRULLINE Fruit 1,627 ppm

CITRULLOL Fruit

COPPER Fruit 4 ppm

CUCURBITACIN-E Fruit Leaf

CUCURBITOCITRIN Seed

CYSTEINE Fruit 236 ppm Seed 5,742 ppm

FAT Fruit 200–89,000 ppm Seed 200,000–571,000 ppm

FIBER Fruit 35,300–257,000 ppm Seed 67,000–316,000 ppm

FOLACIN Fruit 0.259 ppm

GLOBULIN Seed

GLUTAMIC-ACID Fruit 7,420 ppm Seed 53,000 ppm
GLUTELIN Seed
GLYCINE Fruit 1,178 ppm
HENTRIACONTANE Fruit
HISTIDINE Fruit 707 ppm Seed 7,018 ppm
HYDROXYPROLINE Fruit
IRON Fruit 2–143 ppm Seed 75 ppm
ISOLEUCINE Fruit 2,238 ppm Seed 12,100 ppm
KILOCALORIES Fruit 3,513 /kg Seed 6,500 /kg
L-(+)-ISOLEUCINE Plant
L-(−)-PHENYLALANINE Plant
L-(−)-THREONINE Plant
L-(−)-TYROSINE Plant
L-BETA-(PYRAZOL-1-YL)-ALANINE Fruit Seed
L-GLUTAMIC-ACID Seed
LAURIC-ACID Seed 1,600–3,250 ppm
LEUCINE Fruit 2,120 ppm Seed 21,100 ppm
LINOLEIC-ACID Seed 52,000–210,280 ppm
LUTEIN Fruit 0.14–3 ppm
LYCOPENE Fruit 45–900 ppm
LYSINE Fruit 7,303 ppm Seed 8,932 ppm
MAGNESIUM Fruit 1,081–1,500 ppm
MANGANESE Fruit 4 ppm
METHIONINE Fruit 707 ppm Seed 5,742 ppm
MYRISTIC-ACID Seed 400–800 ppm
N-OCTACOSANOL Fruit
NEOLYCOPENE Fruit
NEUROSPORIN Fruit
NIACIN Fruit 15–27 ppm
OLEIC-ACID Seed 71,000–189,000 ppm
OXYSILVINE Seed
PALMITIC-ACID Seed 15,200–55,000 ppm

PANTOTHENIC-ACID Fruit 25 ppm
PECTIN Fruit
PHENYLALANINE Fruit 1,767 ppm Seed 16,600 ppm
PHOSPHORUS Fruit 1–2,900 ppm Seed 8,300–14,600 ppm
PHYSETOLIC-ACID Plant
PHYTOFLUIN Fruit
PHYTOIN Fruit
PHYTOSTEROLS Fruit 236 ppm
POLY-CIS-LYCOPENE Fruit
POTASSIUM Fruit 13,514–18,000 ppm
PRO-BETA-CAROTENE Fruit
PROLINE Fruit 2,827 ppm Seed 11,800 ppm
PRONEUROSPORIN Fruit
PROTEIN Fruit 1,000–100,000 ppm Seed 198,000–343,000 ppm
RIBOFLAVIN Fruit 2–8 ppm Seed 1 ppm
SERINE Fruit 1,885 ppm Seed 13,700 ppm
SODIUM Fruit 135–236 ppm
STEARIC-ACID Seed 12,200–66,000 ppm
STIGMAST-7-EN-3BETA-OL-BETA-D-GLUCOPY-RANOSIDE Plant
THIAMIN Fruit 4–9 ppm
THREONINE Fruit 3,180 ppm Seed 15,300 ppm
TRYPTOPHAN Fruit 825 ppm
TYROSINE Fruit 1,413 ppm Seed 10,200 ppm
UREASE Seed
VALINE Fruit 1,885 ppm Seed 10,200 ppm
WATER Fruit 915,100–957,000 ppm Seed 71,000–81,000 ppm
ZINC Fruit 8 ppm

Appendix C

Vegetable Phytochemicals

ALFALFA

Chemicals in *Medicago sativa subsp. sativa* (*Fabaceae*)—Alfalfa, Lucerne

11,12-DIMETHOXY-7-HYDROXYCOUMESTIN Plant
2-METHYL-PROPANOL Essential Oil
3'-METHOXYCOUMESTROL Plant
3-METHYL-BUTANOL Essential Oil
4-0-METHYLCOUMESTROL Plant
4-AMINO-BUTYRIC-ACID Root
ACETONE Essential Oil
ADENINE Plant
ADENOSINE Plant
ALFALFONE Plant
ALPHA-SPINASTEROL Plant
ALPHA-TOCOPHEROL Plant 26–257 ppm
ALUMINUM Plant 135 ppm
AMYLASE Plant
ARABINOSE Plant
ASCORBIC-ACID Plant 1,470–9,364 ppm
ASH Plant 14,000–100,000 ppm Seed 44,000–49,830 ppm
BETA-CAROTENE Leaf 0.06–394 ppm

BETA-SITOSTEROL Plant
BETAINE Plant
BIOCHANIN-A Plant
BIOTIN Plant 0.18 ppm
BORON Leaf 25 ppm Plant 17–45 ppm Stem 14 ppm
BUTANONE Essential Oil
CALCIUM Plant 120–17,200 ppm
CAMPESTEROL Plant
CARBOHYDRATES Plant 95,000–717,000 ppm Seed 401,000–454,135 ppm
CHLOROPHYLLIDE-A Plant
CHOLINE Plant
CHROMIUM Plant 9 ppm
CITRIC-ACID Plant
COAGULASE Plant
COBALT Plant 115 ppm
COUMESTROL Plant
CRYPTOXANTHIN Plant
CYCLOARTENOL Plant
CYTIDINE Plant
DAIDZEN Plant
DAPHNORETIN Plant
EREPSIN Plant

ppm = parts per million
tr = trace

502

FAT Plant 4,000–43,000 ppm Seed 101,000–123,000 ppm
FIBER Plant 31,000–423,000 ppm Seed 81,000–91,732 ppm
FOLACIN Plant
FORMONONETIN Plant
FRUCTOSE Plant
FUMARIC-ACID Plant
GENISTEIN Leaf Plant
GUANINE Plant
GUANOSINE Plant
HEDERAGENIN Plant
HENTRIACONTANE Plant
HYDROGEN-CYANIDE Plant
HYPOXANTHINE Plant
INOSINE Plant
INOSITOL Plant
INVERTASE Plant
IRON Plant 54–333 ppm
ISOCYTOSINE Plant
L-HOMOSTACHYDRINE Seed
L-STACHYDRINE Hay 1,400 ppm
LIMONENE Essential Oil
LUCERNOL Plant
LUTEIN Plant
MAGNESIUM Plant 2,300–4,400 ppm
MALIC-ACID Plant
MALONIC-ACID Plant
MANGANESE Plant 25.3 ppm
MEDICAGENIC-ACID Plant
MEDICAGOL Plant
MOLYBDENUM Leaf 0.028 ppm Stem 0.015 ppm
MYRISTONE Plant
NEOXANTHIN Plant
NIACIN Plant
OCTACOSANOL Plant
OXALIC Plant
PANTOTHENIC Plant
PECTIN Plant
PECTINASE Plant
PENTANAL Essential Oil
PEROXIDASE Plant
PHAEOPHORBIDE-A Plant
PHOSPHORUS Plant 510–3,100 ppm
POTASSIUM Plant 12,000–20,300 ppm
PROPANAL Plant
PROTEIN Leaf 60,000–347,000 ppm Seed 332,000–385,000 ppm

PYRIDOXINE Plant
QUINIC-ACID Plant
RIBOFLAVIN Plant 1.4–16.1 ppm
RIBOSE Plant
SAPONIN Plant 5,000–20,000 ppm
SATIVOL Plant
SELENIUM Leaf 0.026 ppm Plant Stem 0.015 ppm
SHIKIMIC-ACID Plant
SILICON Plant
SODIUM Plant 170 ppm
SOYASAPOGENOLS Plant
STACHYDRINE Seed
STARCH Plant 30,000–80,000 ppm
STIGMASTEROL Plant
SUCCINIC-ACID Plant
SUCROSE Plant
TANNIN Hay 27,000–28,000 ppm
THIAMIN Plant 1.3–7.5 ppm
TIN Plant
TRIACONTANOL Plant
TRICIN Plant
TRIFOLIOL Plant
TRIGONELLINE Plant
TRIMETHYLAMINE Plant
TRYPTOPHAN Plant
VIOLAXANTHIN Plant
VIT-E Plant
VIT-K Plant
WATER Plant 812,000–827,000 ppm Seed 117,000 ppm
XANTHOPHYLLS Plant
XYLOSE Plant
ZEAXANTHIN Plant
ZINC Plant

ARTICHOKE

Chemicals in *Cynara cardunculus subsp. cardunculus* (*Asteraceae*)—Artichoke

1,3-DI-O-CAFFEOYLQUINIC-ACID Flower
1,4-DICAFFEOYLQUINIC-ACID Flower
1,5-DI-O-CAFFEOYLQUINIC-ACID Flower
1-CAFFEOYLQUINIC-ACID Flower
3-CAFFEOYLQUINIC-ACID Flower
4-CAFFEOYLQUINIC-ACID Flower
5-CAFFEOYLQUINIC-ACID Flower
ASCORBIC-ACID Flower 828 ppm

ASH Flower 10,600–106,000 ppm
BETA-CAROTENE Flower 1–20 ppm
BETA-SELINENE Essential Oil
BETA-SITOSTEROL Leaf
BORON Flower 2–5 ppm
CAFFEIC-ACID Flower
CAFFEOYL-4-QUINIC-ACID Flower
CALCIUM Flower 120–5,286 ppm
CARBOHYDRATES Flower 105,000–755,000 ppm
CARYOPHYLLENE Essential Oil
CHLOROGENIC-ACID Flower
COPPER Flower 2–24 ppm
CYANIDOL-3-CAFFEYLGLUCOSIDE Plant
CYANIDOL-3-CAFFEYLSOPHOROSIDE Plant
CYANIDOL-5-GLUCOSIDE-3-CAFFEYL-
  SOPHOROSIDE Plant
CYANIDOL-DICAFFEYLSOPHOROSIDE Plant
CYANIDOL-GLUCOSIDE Plant
CYANIDOL-SOPHOROSIDE Plant
CYNARAGENIN Leaf
CYNARAPICRIN Leaf
CYNARATRIOL Flower
CYNARIN Leaf 200–300 ppm
CYNAROLIDE Plant
DECANAL Essential Oil
EUGENOL Essential Oil
FAT Flower 1,000–20,000 ppm
FERULIC-ACID Plant
FIBER Flower 11,400–224,000 ppm
FLAVONOIDS Flower 1,000–10,000 ppm
FOLACIN Flower 0.7–4.7 ppm
GLYCERIC-ACID Flower
GLYCOLIC-ACID Flower
HETEROSIDE-B Flower
HEX-1-EN-3-ONE Flower
INULIN Flower
IRON Flower 11–101 ppm
ISOAMERBOIN Plant
KILOCALORIES Flower 470–3,120 /kg
LAURIC-ACID Flower 20–135 ppm
LINOLEIC-ACID Flower 460–3,055 ppm
LINOLENIC-ACID Flower 170–1,130 ppm
LUTEOLIN-4-BETA-D-GLUCOSIDE Flower
LUTEOLIN-7-BETA-D-GLUCOSIDE Flower
LUTEOLIN-7-BETA-RUTINOSIDE Flower
LUTEOLIN-7-RUTINOSIDE-4'-GLUCOSIDE
  Plant
MAGNESIUM Flower 555–4,275 ppm

MANGANESE Flower 2–17 ppm
MUCILAGE Plant
MUFA Flower 50–330 ppm
MYRISTIC-ACID Flower 20–135 ppm
NEO-CHLOROGENIC-ACID Plant
NIACIN Flower 10–82 ppm
NON-TRANS-2-EN-AL Flower
O-DIPHENOLICS Flower 20,000 ppm
OCT-1-EN-3-ONE Flower
OLEIC-ACID Flower 50–330 ppm
PALMITIC-ACID Flower 290–1,925 ppm
PANTOTHENIC-ACID Flower 3–23 ppm
PHENYL-ACETALDEHYDE Flower
PHOSPHORUS Flower 860–6,240 ppm
POTASSIUM Flower 3,500–29,780 ppm
PROTEIN Flower 31,000–276,000 ppm
PSEUDOTARAXASTEROL Leaf
PUFA Flower 630–4,185 ppm
RIBOFLAVIN Flower 0.6–7 ppm
SCOLYMOSIDE Flower
SFA Flower 350–2,325 ppm
SODIUM Flower 850–6,840 ppm
STEARIC-ACID Flower 30–200 ppm
STIGMASTEROL Leaf
TANNIN Plant
TARAXASTEROL Leaf
THIAMIN Flower 0.7–6 ppm
VIT-B-6 Flower 1–8 ppm
WATER Flower 773,000–854,870 ppm
ZINC Flower 4–36 ppm

ASPARAGUS

Chemicals in *Asparagus officinalis* L. (*Liliaceae*)—Asparagus

22-SPIROSTAN-3BETA-OL Shoot
4-VINYL-GUAIACOL Shoot
4-VINYL-PHENOL Shoot
ALANINE Seed 1,440–18,581 ppm
ALPHA-AMINODIMETHYL-GAMMA-BUTY-
  ROTHETIN Rhizome
ALPHA-CAROTENE Plant
ALPHA-LINOLENIC-ACID Shoot 50–645 ppm
ALUMINUM Shoot 13–700 ppm
ARGININE Shoot 1,430–18,452 ppm
ARSENIC Shoot 0.005–0.006 ppm
ASCORBIC-ACID Shoot 100–5,714 ppm
ASH Shoot 6,000–171,000 ppm

ASPARAGINE Shoot

ASPARAGOSIDES Shoot

ASPARAGUSIC-ACID Shoot

ASPARASAPONINS Plant

ASPARTIC-ACID Shoot 3,550–45,805 ppm

BARIUM Shoot 2–70 ppm

BETA-CAROTENE Shoot 0.3–120 ppm

BORON Shoot 6–104 ppm

CADMIUM Shoot 0.018–0.07 ppm

CALCIUM Shoot 160–3,840 ppm

CARBOHYDRATES Shoot 36,000–602,000 ppm

CHOLINE Rhizome

CHROMIUM Shoot 0.135–0.7 ppm

COBALT Shoot 0.09–0.12 ppm

CONIFERIN Shoot

COPPER Shoot 1–24 ppm

CYANIDIN-3,5-DIGLUCOSIDE Shoot

CYANIDIN-3-MONOGLUCOSIDE Shoot

CYANIDIN-3-RHAMNOSYLGLUCOSIDE Shoot

CYANIDIN-3-RHAMNOSYLGLUCOSYLGLUCO-
SIDE Shoot

CYSTINE Shoot 360–4,645 ppm

DIOSGENIN Shoot

FAT Shoot 2,000–41,000 ppm

FIBER Shoot 7,000–141,000 ppm

FOLACIN Shoot 1–18 ppm

FRUCTOSE Rhizome

GLUCOSE Shoot

GLUTAMIC-ACID Shoot 5,010–64,645 ppm

GLYCINE Shoot 990–12,774 ppm

GUAIACOL Shoot

HISTIDINE Shoot 470–6,065 ppm

INOSITOL Shoot

INULIN Root

IRON Shoot 6–240 ppm

ISOLEUCINE Shoot 1,120–14,452 ppm

JAMOGENIN Shoot

KAEMPFEROL Root

KILOCALORIES Shoot 210–3,130 /kg

LAURIC-ACID Shoot 10–129 ppm

LEAD Shoot 1.5–30 ppm

LEUCINE Shoot 1,330–17,161 ppm

LINOLEIC-ACID Shoot 910–11,742 ppm

LITHIUM Shoot 0.36–0.6 ppm

LUTEIN Plant

LYSINE Shoot 1,450–18,710 ppm

M-CRESOL Shoot

MAGNESIUM Shoot 165–7,000 ppm

MANGANESE Shoot 2–100 ppm

MANNAN Rhizome

MERCURY Shoot 0.001–0.001 ppm

METHIONINE Shoot 290–3,742 ppm

MOLYBDENUM Shoot 0.63–1.8 ppm

MUFA Shoot 70–903 ppm

MYRISTIC-ACID Shoot 10–129 ppm

NIACIN Shoot 11–366 ppm

NICKEL Shoot 0.9–1.8 ppm

O-CRESOL Shoot

OFFICINALISIN-II Root

OLEIC-ACID Shoot 60–774 ppm

P-CRESOL Shoot

PAEONIDIN-3-GLUCOSYLRHAMNOSYLGLU-
COSIDE Shoot

PAEONIDINRHAMNOSYLGLUCOSIDE Shoot

PALMITIC-ACID Shoot 450–5,806 ppm

PALMITOLEIC-ACID Shoot 10–129 ppm

PANTOTHENIC-ACID Shoot 2–22.4 ppm

PENTOSANS Shoot 70,000 ppm

PHENOL Shoot

PHENYLALANINE Shoot 720–9,290 ppm

PHILOTHION Shoot

PHOSPHORUS Shoot 390–10,244 ppm

PHYTOSTEROLS Shoot 246–3,097 ppm

POTASSIUM Shoot 2,210–55,200 ppm

PROLINE Shoot 1,620–20,903 ppm

PROTEIN Shoot 22,000–394,840 ppm

PSEUDOASPARAGOSE Rhizome

PUFA Shoot 960–12,387 ppm

QUERCETIN Root

RHAMNOSE Shoot

RIBOFLAVIN Shoot 1–36 ppm

RUTIN Root

SARSAPOGENIN Shoot

SELENIUM Shoot 0.041–0.078 ppm

SERINE Shoot 1,160–14,968 ppm

SFA Shoot 500–6,452 ppm

SILVER Shoot 0.09–0.12 ppm

SODIUM Shoot 18–685 ppm

STEARIC-ACID Shoot 30–387 ppm

STRONTIUM Shoot 19–200 ppm

SUCCINIC-ACID Shoot

SUCROSE Rhizome

SUGAR Shoot 15,000 ppm

SULFUR Shoot 56–864 ppm

THIAMIN Shoot 1–26 ppm

THREONINE Shoot 850–10,968 ppm

TITANIUM Shoot 0.45–180 ppm

TOCOPHEROL Shoot 19.8–256 ppm

TRYPTOPHAN Shoot 300–3,871 ppm

TYROSINE Shoot 480–6,194 ppm

VALINE Shoot 1,180–15,226 ppm

VANADIUM Shoot 0.3–2 ppm

WATER Plant 914,000–950,000 ppm

ZEAXANTHIN Plant

ZINC Shoot 12–124 ppm

ZIRCONIUM Shoot 1.8–2.4 ppm

BEET

Chemicals in *Beta vulgaris L.* (*Chenopodiaceae*)—Beet, Swiss Chard

3-HYDROXYTYRAMINE Root

ACETAMIDE Root

ACONITIC-ACID Plant

ADENINE Root

ADIPIC-ACID Root

ALANINE Root 560–4,338 ppm

ALLANTOIN Root

ALPHA-LINOLENIC-ACID Leaf 316–3,160 ppm
Root 40–315 ppm

ALPHA-SPINASTERYLGLUCOSIDE Root

ALPHA-TOCOPHEROL Leaf 321–439 ppm
Root 0.5–3.6 ppm

ALUMINUM Root 1–420 ppm

ARGININE Root 380–2,997 ppm

ARSENIC Root 0.01–0.08 ppm

ASCORBIC-ACID Leaf 120–3,696 ppm Root
50–868 ppm

ASH Leaf 15,000–250,000 ppm Root
7,600–140,000 ppm

ASPARTIC-ACID Root 1,060–8,360 ppm

BARIUM Root 17–70 ppm

BETA-CAROTENE Root 438 ppm

BETA-INDOLEACETIC-ACID Root

BETA-SITOSTEROL Leaf

BETAINE Root

BETANIDINE Root

BETANIN Plant

BETANINE Root

BORON Root 1–80 ppm

BROMINE Root 2–16 ppm

CADMIUM Root 0.01–0.33 ppm

CAFFEIC-ACID Leaf

CALCIUM Leaf 700–17,368 ppm Root
120–4,200 ppm

CARBOHYDRATES Leaf 36,000–609,000 ppm
Root 95,000–794,000 ppm

CHLOROGENIC-ACID Leaf

CHROMIUM Root 0.001–0.33 ppm

CITRIC-ACID Root

COBALT Root 0.001–0.42 ppm

CONIFERIN Plant Root Seed

COPPER Root 0.6–17 ppm

CYSTINE Root 180–1,420 ppm

D-ALPHA-OXYGLUTARIC-ACID Root

D-RIBULOSE Leaf

DAUCIC-ACID Plant

DIOXYMALONIC-ACID Root

FARNESOL Root Essent. Oil

FAT Leaf 2,000–58,000 ppm Root
1,000–16,000 ppm Seed 28,000–70,000
ppm

FERULIC-ACID Leaf

FIBER Leaf 4,000–279,000 ppm Root
8,000–90,000 ppm

FOLACIN Root 0.8–8 ppm

FORMALDEHYDE Root

GABA Root

GALACTOSE Root

GLUCOSE Root

GLUTAMIC-ACID Root 3,930–30,994 ppm

GLUTARIC-ACID Root

GLYCINE Root 290–2,287 ppm

GLYCOCEREBROSIDE Root

GLYOXALIC-ACID Sprout Seedling

GUANINE Root

GUANOSINE Root

HETEROXANTHIN Root

HEXOSANS Root

HISTIDINE Root 200–1,577 ppm

HOMOGENTISINIC-ACID Root

HYDANTOIN Sprout Seedling

HYDROCAFFEIC-ACID Root

HYPOXANTHIN Root

INVERTASE Root

IRON Leaf 7–392 ppm Root 5–165 ppm

ISOLEUCINE Root 440–3,470 ppm

KAEMPFEROL Plant

KAEMPFEROL-GLYCOSIDE Leaf

KILOCALORIES Leaf 210–3,310 /kg Root
430–3,610 /kg

L-ARABINOSE Root
LEAD Root 0.01–3.5 ppm
LEUCINE Root 630–4,968 ppm
LINOLEIC-ACID Root 460–3,628 ppm
LITHIUM Root 0.36–0.6 ppm
LYSINE Root 530–4,180 ppm
MAGNESIUM Root 130–4,200 ppm
MANGANESE Root 3–90 ppm
MELILOTIC-ACID Root
MERCURY Root 0.016 ppm
METHIONINE Root 170–1,341 ppm
MOLYBDENUM Root
MUFA Root 270–2,219 ppm
NEOBETANIN Plant
NIACIN Leaf 4–68 ppm Root 2–32 ppm
NICKEL Root 2.5 ppm
NITROGEN Root 2,600–35,830 ppm
OLEANOLIC-ACID-3-O-BETA-D-GLUCOPYRA-
 NOSIDE Root
OLEIC-ACID Root 270–2,129 ppm
ORNITHINE Root
OXALIC-ACID Root 404 ppm
OXYCITRONIC-ACID Root
P-COUMARIC-ACID Plant
P-HYDROXY-BENZOIC-ACID Root
PALMITIC-ACID Root 210–1,656 ppm
PANTOTHENIC-ACID Root 1.5–11.8 ppm
PENTOSANS Root
PHENYLALANINE Root 420–3,312 ppm
PHOSPHORUS Leaf 290–5,946 ppm Root
 260–45,580 ppm
PHYTOSTEROLS Root 250–1,972 ppm
POTASSIUM Leaf 4,380–61,798 ppm Root
 3,033–50,000 ppm
PRAEBETANINE Root
PROLINE Root 380–2,997 ppm
PROTEIN Leaf 16,000–270,000 ppm Root
 12,850–143,000 ppm Seed 110,000 –150,000
 ppm
PROTOPORPHYRIN Root
PUFA Root 500–3,943 ppm
QUERCETIN Plant
QUERCETIN-GLUCOSIDE Leaf
QUINIC-ACID Leaf
RAFFINOSE Root
RAPHANOL Plant Root Seed
RIBOFLAVIN Leaf 1.7–26 ppm Root 0.2–3.9
 ppm

RUBIDIUM Root 0.76–32 ppm
SALICYLIC-ACID Root
SEDOHEPTULOSE Leaf
SELENIUM Root
SERINE Root 540–4,259 ppm
SFA Root 220–1,735 ppm
SILICON Root 1–83 ppm
SODIUM Leaf 1,300–16,571 ppm Root
 590–6,705 ppm
STEARIC-ACID Root 10–79 ppm
STRONTIUM Root 16–70 ppm
SUCROSE Root 270,000 ppm
SULFUR Root 130–2,000 ppm
SYRINGIC-ACID Root
TARTARIC-ACID Root
THIAMIN Leaf 0.6–14 ppm Root 0.1–2.4 ppm
THREONINE Root 440–3,470 ppm
TIN Root 0.8–2.8 ppm
TITANIUM Root 0.5–9.8 ppm
TRICARBALLYL-ACID Leaf
TRYPTOPHAN Root 170–1,341 ppm
TYROSINE Root 350–2,760 ppm
VALINE Root 520–4,100 ppm
VANILLIC-ACID Leaf
VANILLIN Root
VIT-B-6 Root 0.5–3.6 ppm
VULGAXANTHIN-I Plant
VULGAXANTHIN-II Plant
WATER Leaf 864,000–926,000 ppm Root
 865,000–881,340 ppm
XYLOSE Leaf
ZINC Root 3–70 ppm
ZIRCONIUM Plant

BELL PEPPER

Chemicals in *Capsicum annuum L.*
(*Solanaceae*)—Bell Pepper, Cherry Pepper,
Cone Pepper, Green Pepper, Paprika, Sweet
Pepper

1-HEXANOL Fruit
1-O-CAFFEOYL-BETA-D-GLUCOSE Fruit
1-O-FERRULOYL-BETA-D-GLUCOSE Fruit
2,3,5-TRIMETHYLPYRAZINE Fruit
2,3-BUTANEDIOL Fruit
2,3-DIMETHYL-5-ETHYLPYRAZINE Fruit
2,3-DIMETHYL-PYRAZINE Fruit
2-BUTANONE Fruit

2-HEXANOL Fruit

2-HEXANONE Fruit

2-METHOXY-3-ISOBUTYL-PYRAZINE Fruit

2-METHYL-5-ETHYLPYRAZINE Fruit

2-METHYL-BUTAN-1-OL Fruit

2-METHYL-BUTAN-2-OL Fruit

2-METHYL-BUTANAL Fruit

2-METHYL-BUTYRIC-ACID Fruit

2-METHYL-PENTAN-2-OL Fruit

2-METHYL-PROPIONIC-ACID Fruit

2-PENTYL-FURAN Fruit

2-PENTYLPYRIDINE Fruit

24-®-ETHYL-LOPHENOL Seed

24-METHYL-LANOST-9(11)-EN-3-BETA-OL Seed

24-METHYL-LOPHENOL Seed

24-METHYLENE-CYCLOARTANOL Seed

3,6-EPOXIDE-5-HYDROXY-5,6-DIHYDRO-ZEAXANTHIN Fruit

3-(SEC-BUTYL)-2-METHOXYPYRAZINE Fruit

3-HEXANOL Fruit

3-HYDROXY-ALPHA-CAROTENE Fruit

3-ISOBUTYL-2-METHOXYPYRAZINE Fruit

3-ISOPROPYL-2-METHOXYPYRAZINE Fruit

3-METHYL-1-PENTYL-3-METHYL-BUTYRATE Fruit

3-METHYL-BUTANAL Fruit

3-METHYL-BUTYRIC-ACID Fruit

3-METHYL-PENTAN-3-OL Fruit

31-NOR-LANOST-8-EN-3-BETA-OL Seed

31-NOR-LANOST-9(11)-EN-3-BETA-OL Seed

31-NOR-LANOSTEROL Seed

31-NORCYCLOARTANOL Seed

4-ALPHA-14-ALPHA-24-TRIMETHYL-CHOLESTA-8(24)-DIEN-3-BETA-OL Seed

4-ALPHA-24-DIMETHYL-CHOLESTA-7,24-DIEN-3-BETA-OL Seed

4-ALPHA-METHYL-5-ALPHA-CHOLEST-8(14)-EN-3-BETA-OL Seed

4-METHYL-1-PENTYL-2-METHYL-BUTYRATE Fruit

4-METHYL-3-PENTEN-2-ONE Fruit

4-METHYL-HEPTADECANE Fruit

4-METHYL-HEXADECANE Fruit

4-METHYL-PENTANOIC-ACID Fruit

4-METHYLPENTADECANE Fruit

4-METHYLTETRADECANE Fruit

4-METHYLTRIDECANE Fruit

5,6-DIHYDROXY-5,6-DIHYDRO-ZEAXANTHIN Fruit

5-HYDROXY-CAPSANTHIN-5,6-EPOXIDE Fruit

5-METHYL-2-FURFURAL Fruit

ACETYL-CHOLINE Pericarp Seed

ACETYLFURAN Fruit

ALANINE Fruit 350–4,774 ppm

ALPHA-CAROTENE Fruit

ALPHA-COPAENE Fruit

ALPHA-CRYPTOXANTHIN Plant

ALPHA-LINOLENIC-ACID Fruit 220–3,001 ppm

ALPHA-PHELLANDRENE Fruit

ALPHA-PINENE Fruit

ALPHA-TERPINEOL Fruit

ALPHA-THUJENE Fruit

ALPHA-TOCOPHEROL Fruit 22–284 ppm

ALUMINUM Fruit 1–44 ppm

AMMONIA(NH3) Fruit 382 ppm

ANTHERAXANTHIN Fruit

APIIN Fruit

ARACHIDIC-ACID Fruit

ARGININE Fruit 410–5,592 ppm

ARSENIC Fruit 0.004–0.015 ppm

ASCORBIC-ACID Fruit 230–20,982 ppm

ASH Fruit 5,000–122,000 ppm

ASPARAGINE Fruit

ASPARTIC-ACID Fruit 1,200–16,504 ppm

AUROCHROME Fruit

BARIUM Fruit 2–8 ppm

BEHENIC-ACID Fruit

BETA-AMYRIN Seed

BETA-APO-8'-CAROTENAL Fruit

BETA-CAROTENE Fruit 462 ppm

BETA-CAROTENE-EPOXIDE Fruit

BETA-CRYPTOXANTHIN Fruit

BETA-PINENE Fruit

BETA-SITOSTEROL Plant

BETAINE Fruit

BORON Fruit 1–18 ppm

BROMINE Fruit 0.1–111 ppm

CADMIUM Fruit 0.005–0.33 ppm

CAFFEIC-ACID Fruit 11 ppm

CALCIUM Fruit 36–1,956 ppm

CAMPESTEROL Fruit

CAMPHENE Fruit

CAPSAICIN Fruit 100–4,000 ppm

CAPSANTHIN Fruit

CAPSANTHIN-5,6-EPOXIDE Fruit

CAPSIAMIDE Fruit 20–200 ppm
CAPSIANOSIDE-A Fruit 33–250 ppm
CAPSIANOSIDE-B Fruit 2–18 ppm
CAPSIANOSIDE-C Fruit 35–103 ppm
CAPSIANOSIDE-D Fruit 21–38 ppm
CAPSIANOSIDE-E Fruit 15 ppm
CAPSIANOSIDE-F Fruit 5 ppm
CAPSIANOSIDE-I Fruit 18 ppm
CAPSIANOSIDE-II Fruit 43–138 ppm
CAPSIANOSIDE-III Fruit 15–105 ppm
CAPSIANOSIDE-IV Fruit 9 ppm
CAPSIANOSIDE-V Fruit 2 ppm
CAPSIANSIDE-A Fruit 300 ppm
CAPSICOSIDE-A-1 Root 530 ppm
CAPSICOSIDE-B-1 Root 620 ppm
CAPSICOSIDE-C-1 Root 600 ppm
CAPSIDIOL Fruit 29 ppm
CAPSOCHROME Fruit
CAPSOLUTEIN Fruit
CAPSORUBIN Fruit
CARBOHYDRATES Fruit 53,100–813,000 ppm
CARNAUBIC-ACID Seed
CARYOPHYLLENE Fruit
CHLOROGENIC-ACID Fruit
CHOLINE Pericarp 297 ppm Seed 360 ppm
CHROMIUM Fruit 0.546 ppm
CINNAMIC-ACID Tissue Culture
CIS-13'-CAPSANTHIN Fruit
CIS-9'-CAPSANTHIN Fruit
CIS-9,10-DIHYDRO-CAPSENONE Tissue Culture 1 ppm
CITRIC-ACID Fruit
CITROSTADIENOL Seed
CITROXANTHIN Fruit
CITRULLIN Fruit
COBALT Fruit 0.001–0.1 ppm
COPPER Fruit 0.5–20 ppm
CRYPTOCAPSIN Fruit
CRYPTOXANTHIN Fruit
CYCLOARTANOL Seed
CYCLOARTENOL Seed
CYCLOEUCALENOL Seed
CYCLOHEXANONE Fruit
CYCLOPENTANOL Fruit
CYSTINE Fruit 160–2,182 ppm
DECANOIC-ACID-VANILLYLAMIDE Fruit 1–68 ppm
DEHYDROASCORBIC-ACID Fruit 20,000 ppm

DELTA-3-CARENE Fruit
DIHYDROCAPSAICIN Fruit 75–1,628 ppm
DIN-N-PROPYL-AMINE Fruit 0.3 ppm
EO Fruit 16,000 ppm
ERIODICTIN Fruit
ETHYL-3-METHYLBUTYRATE Fruit
EUGENOL Fruit
FAT Fruit 2,000–144,000 ppm Seed 100,000–150,000 ppm
FIBER Fruit 12,000–351,000 ppm
FLUORINE Fruit 0.05–1 ppm
FOLACIN Fruit 3 ppm
FOLIAXANTHIN Fruit
FUNKIOSIDE Root
GALACTOSAMINE Fruit
GALACTOSE Fruit
GAMMA-TERPINENE Fruit
GLUCOSAMINE Fruit
GLUCOSE Fruit
GLUTAMIC-ACID Fruit 1,120–15,277 ppm
GLUTAMINASE Fruit
GLYCINE Fruit 310–4,228 ppm
GRAMISTEROL Seed
GROSSAMIDE Root 3 ppm
HENEICOSANE Fruit
HEPTADECANE Fruit
HESPERIDIN Fruit
HEXADECANE Fruit
HEXAN-1-AL Fruit
HEXANAL Fruit
HEXANOIC-ACID Fruit
HISTIDINE Fruit 170–2,319 ppm
HOMOCAPSAICIN Fruit 2–90 ppm
HOMODIHYDROCAPSAICIN Fruit 2–90 ppm
HYDROXY-ALPHA-CAROTENE Fruit
HYDROXY-BENZOIC-ACID-4-BETA-D-GLUCO-SIDE Fruit
IRON Fruit 4–286 ppm
ISOHEXYL-ISOCAPROATE Fruit
ISOLEUCINE Fruit 270–3,683 ppm
L-ASPARIGINASE Fruit
LANOST-8-EN-3-BETA-OL Seed
LANOSTENOL Plant
LANOSTEROL Seed
LEAD Fruit 0.004–2 ppm
LEUCINE Fruit 440–6,002 ppm
LIMONENE Fruit
LINALOL Fruit

LINOLEIC-ACID Fruit 2,190–29,871 ppm

LITHIUM Fruit 0.284–0.4 ppm

LOPHENOL Seed

LUPEOL Seed

LUTEIN Fruit

LUTEOLIN-7-O-BETA-APIOGLUCOSIDE Leaf

LUTEOLIN-7-O-BETA-D-GLUCOSIDE Leaf

LUTEOLIN-7-O-BETA-DIGLUCOSIDE Leaf

LYSINE Fruit 380–5,183 ppm

MAGNESIUM Fruit 118–2,340 ppm

MALONIC-ACID Fruit Leaf

MANGANESE Fruit 0.7–39 ppm

MARGARIC-ACID Fruit

MERCURY Fruit 0.001–0.001 ppm

METHIONINE Fruit 100–1,364 ppm

MOLYBDENUM Fruit 15 ppm

MYRCENE Fruit

MYRISTIC-ACID Fruit 10–136 ppm

N-(13-METHYLTETRADECYL)ACETAMIDE Fruit 300–400 ppm

N-CIS-FERULOYL-TYRAMINE Root 2 ppm

N-HEXANAL Fruit

N-METHYL-ANILINE Fruit 13.1 ppm

N-NITROSO-DIMETHYLAMINE Fruit

N-NITROSO-PYRROLIDINE Fruit

N-PENTYL-AMINE Fruit 3 ppm

N-PROPYL-AMINE Fruit 2.3 ppm

N-TRANS-FERULOYL-OCTOPAMINE Root 1–2 ppm

N-TRANS-FERULOYL-TYRAMINE Root 12 ppm

N-TRANS-P-COUMAROYL-OCTOPAMINE Root 1 ppm

N-TRANS-P-COUMAROYL-TYRAMINE Root 2 ppm

NEO-BETA-CAROTENE Plant

NEOXANTHIN Fruit

NIACIN Fruit 4–172 ppm

NICKEL Fruit 0.05–5.5 ppm

NITROGEN Fruit 1,900–23,330 ppm

NONADECANE Fruit

NONANOIC-ACID-VANILLYLAMIDE Fruit 2–45 ppm

NORCAPSAICINE Fruit

NORDIHYDROCAPSAICIN Fruit 15–335 ppm

OBTUSIFOLIOL Seed

OCTANE Fruit

OCTANOIC-ACID Fruit

OLEIC-ACID Fruit 270–3,582 ppm Seed

OXALIC-ACID Fruit 257–1,171 ppm

P-AMINO-BENZALDEHYDE Root 6 ppm

P-COUMARIC-ACID Fruit 79 ppm

P-CYMENE Fruit

P-XYLENE Fruit

PALMITIC-ACID Fruit 500–6,820 ppm Seed

PALMITOLEIC-ACID Fruit 30–409 ppm

PANTOTHENIC-ACID Fruit 5 ppm

PENTADECANE Fruit

PENTADECANOIC-ACID Fruit

PHENYLALANINE Fruit 260–3,546 ppm

PHOSPHATIDYL-GLYCEROL Fruit

PHOSPHODIESTERASE Tissue Culture

PHOSPHORUS Fruit 186–3,885 ppm

PHYTOENE Fruit

PHYTOFLUENE Fruit

PIPERIDINE Fruit 5.2 ppm

PORPHOBILINOGEN-OXYGENASE Leaf

POTASSIUM Fruit 1,862–35,000 ppm

PROLINE Fruit 370–5,047 ppm

PROTEIN Fruit 8,000–184,000 ppm

PULEGONE Fruit

PYRROLIDINE Fruit 1.4 ppm

RIBOFLAVIN Fruit 19 ppm

RUBIDIUM Fruit 0.38–10 ppm

SABINENE Fruit

SCOPOLETIN Fruit

SELENIUM Fruit 0.001–0.002 ppm

SERINE Fruit 340–4,638 ppm

SILICON Fruit 1–33 ppm

SILVER Fruit 0.071–0.1 ppm

SKATOLE-PYRROLO-OXYGENASE Leaf

SODIUM Fruit 25–625 ppm

SOLANIDINE Fruit

SOLANINE Fruit Leaf 500 ppm

SOLASODINE Fruit

STEARIC-ACID Fruit 160–2,180 ppm Seed

STIGMASTEROL Fruit

STRONTIUM Fruit 2–12 ppm

SULFOQUINOVOSYL-DIACYL-GLYCEROL Fruit

SULFUR Fruit 190–2,440 ppm

TERPINEN-4-OL Fruit

TERPINOLENE Fruit

TETRADECANE Fruit

TETRAMETHYL-PYRAZINE Fruit

THIAMIN Fruit 1–15 ppm

THREONINE Fruit 310–4,228 ppm

TIN Fruit 5 ppm

TITANIUM Fruit 0.355–16 ppm
TOCOPHEROL Fruit 24 ppm
TOLUENE Fruit
TRIGONELLINE Seed 0.6 ppm
TRYPTOPHAN Fruit 110–1,500 ppm
TRYPTOPHAN-PYRROLO-OXYGENASE Leaf
TYROSINE Fruit 180–2,455 ppm
VALINE Fruit 360–4,910 ppm
VANILLOYL-GLUCOSE Fruit
VANILLYL-CAPROYLAMIDE Fruit
VANILLYL-DECANAMIDE Fruit
VANILLYL-OCTANAMIDE Fruit
VIOLAXANTHIN Fruit
VIT-B-6 Fruit 2–22 ppm
WATER Fruit 742,000–937,000 ppm
XANTHOPHYLL Plant
XANTHOPHYLL-EPOXIDE Fruit
XYLOSE Fruit
ZEAXANTHIN Fruit
ZETA-CAROTENE Fruit
ZINC Fruit 1–77 ppm
ZIRCONIUM Fruit 1.4–2 ppm

BROCCOLI

Chemicals in *Brassica oleracea var. botrytis L.* (*Brassicaceae*)—Broccoli, Cauliflower

1-METHOXY-GLUCOBRASSICIN Leaf
1-METHOXY-INDOLE-3-CARBALDEHYDE Plant
1-O-FERULOYL-BETA-D-GLUCOSE Leaf
1-O-P-COUMAROYL-BETA-D-GLUCOSE Leaf
1-O-SINAPOYL-BETA-D-GLUCOSE Leaf
24-METHYLENE-CYCLOARTENOL Leaf
3,3'-DIINDOYL-METHANE Leaf
3-METHYL-SULFINYL-PROPYL-GLUCOSINO-LATE Flower
3-METHYLTHIOPROPYL-GLUCOSINOLATE Flower
4-HYDROXY-GLUCOBRASSICIN Flower 7–390 ppm Leaf 3–325 ppm
4-METHOXY-GLUCOBRASSICIN Flower 15–355 ppm Leaf 8–580 ppm
4-METHOXY-INDOL-3-YL-METHYL-GLUCOSI-NOLATE Flower Leaf
4-METHYL-SULFINYL-BUTYL-GLUCOSINO-LATE Flower

4-METHYL-THIO-BUTYL-GLUCOSINOLATE Flower
4-VINYL-GUAIACOL Plant
5-HYDROXY-GLUCOBRASSICIN Leaf Tissue Culture
5-METHOXY-GLUCOBRASSICIN Leaf Tissue Culture
ABSCISIC-ACID Flower
ACETONE Flower Leaf
ALANINE Flower 1,050–13,565 ppm Leaf 1,180–12,673 ppm
ALLYL-ISOTHIOCYANATE Leaf
ALPHA-AMYRIN Bud Flower
ALPHA-CAROTENE Plant
ALPHA-LINOLENIC-ACID Leaf 1,290–13,855 ppm
ALPHA-TOCOPHEROL Flower 0.3–4 ppm Leaf 7–439 ppm
ALUMINUM Flower 1–150 ppm Leaf 1–27 ppm
AMMONIA(NH3) Flower 6,376 ppm
ANILINE Flower 22 ppm
ARGININE Flower 960–12,400 ppm Leaf 1,450–15,573 ppm
ARSENIC Flower Leaf
ASCORBIC-ACID Flower 660–9,300 ppm Leaf 911–10,360 ppm
ASH Flower 6,600–121,250 ppm Leaf 2,800–101,708 ppm
ASPARTIC-ACID Leaf 2,130–22,876 ppm
BENZYL-AMINE Flower 1.4 ppm
BETA-AMYRIN Bud Flower
BETA-CAROTENE Flower 4 ppm Leaf 9–138 ppm
BETA-CRYPTOXANTHIN Plant
BETA-SITOSTEROL Plant
BORON Flower 1–76 ppm Leaf 1–85 ppm Stem 21 ppm
BROMINE Flower Leaf
CADMIUM Flower 0.003–0.25 ppm Leaf 0.01–0.18 ppm
CAFFEIC-ACID Leaf 8 ppm
CALCIUM Flower 210–4,040 ppm Leaf 360–54,247 ppm
CARBOHYDRATES Flower 49,200–635,660 ppm Leaf 52,400–562,776 ppm
CHLOROGENIC-ACID Leaf
CHLOROPHYLL Leaf

CHROMIUM Flower 0.001–0.125 ppm Leaf
0.005–0.18 ppm
CINNAMIC-ACID Leaf
CITRIC-ACID Flower Plant
COBALT Flower 0.001–0.125 ppm Leaf
0.02–0.6 ppm
COPPER Flower 0.3–8 ppm Leaf 0.68–52 ppm
CYSTINE Flower 230–2,970 ppm Leaf
200–2,148 ppm
DIMETHYL-AMINE Flower 14 ppm
DIMETHYL-DISULFIDE Plant
ETHANOL Flower Plant
FAT Flower 1,800–29,400 ppm Leaf
3,160–41,242 ppm
FERULIC-ACID Leaf 13 ppm
FIBER Flower 8,000–132,000 ppm Leaf
10,760–122,866 ppm
FLUORINE Flower 0.02–2.5 ppm Leaf 0.03–0.9
ppm
FOLACIN Leaf 0.64–8.4 ppm
FUMARIC-ACID Flower Plant
GLUCOBRASSICIN Flower 60–1,670 ppm Leaf
30–580 ppm
GLUCOERUCIN Flower 210 ppm Leaf 15,020
ppm
GLUCOIBERIN Flower 1,600 ppm Leaf 248
ppm
GLUCONAPOLEIFERIN Flower 80 ppm Leaf
9–135 ppm
GLUCONASTURTIN Flower Leaf 145 ppm
GLUCORAPHANIN Flower 990 ppm Leaf
255–8,990 ppm
GLUCOSINOLATES Flower 20–1,140 ppm Leaf
70–2,120 ppm
GLUTAMIC-ACID Flower 2,650–34,240 ppm
Leaf 3,750–40,275 ppm
GLYCINE Flower 640–8,270 ppm Leaf
950–10,203 ppm
HEX-CIS-3-EN-1-OL Plant
HEX-CIS-3-ENOL-ACETATE Plant
HEXYL-ACETATE Plant
HISTIDINE Flower 400–5,165 ppm Leaf
500–5,370 ppm
INDOLE-3-ACETONITRILE Leaf
INDOLE-3-CARBINOL Leaf
INDOLE-3-CARBOXYLIC-ACID Plant
INDOYL-3-METHYL-GLUCOSINOLATE Flower
IRON Flower 5–122 ppm Leaf 8–109 ppm

ISOLEUCINE Flower 760–9,820 ppm Leaf
1,090–11,707 ppm
KAEMPFEROL Flower 30 ppm Leaf
KILOCALORIES Leaf 280–3,007 /kg Plant
240–3,100 /kg
LEAD Flower Leaf 0.01–1 ppm
LEUCINE Flower 1,160–15,000 ppm Leaf
1,310–14,069 ppm
LINOLEIC-ACID Flower 190–2,455 ppm Leaf
380–4,081 ppm
LINOLENIC-ACID Flower 640–8,270 ppm
LYSINE Flower 1,070–13,825 ppm Leaf
1,410–15,143 ppm
MAGNESIUM Flower 115–2,250 ppm Leaf
214–3,072 ppm
MALIC-ACID Flower Plant
MANGANESE Flower 1.5–48 ppm Leaf 2–80
ppm
MERCURY Flower 0.025 ppm Leaf 0.002–0.09
ppm
METHANOL Flower Plant
METHIONINE Flower 280–3,615 ppm Leaf
340–3,652 ppm
METHYL-AMINE Flower 65 ppm
MOLYBDENUM Flower 0.1 ppm Leaf 0.1–3.76
ppm Stem 1.76 ppm
MUFA Flower 120–1,550 ppm
N-METHYL-BETA-PHENETHYLAMINE Flower
1.6 ppm Plant 1.6 ppm
N-METHYL-PHENETHYLAMINE Flower 1.6
ppm
N-PENTYL-AMINE Flower 3.3 ppm
NEOGLUCOBRASSICIN Flower 8–450 ppm
Leaf 10–900 ppm Tissue Culture
NIACIN Flower 5–85 ppm Leaf
NICKEL Flower 0.03–12 ppm Leaf 0.3–7 ppm
NITROGEN Flower 3,100–47,500 ppm Leaf
7,000–71,800 ppm
OLEIC-ACID Flower 120–1,550 ppm Leaf
240–2,578 ppm
OXALATE Leaf 1,900–20,406 ppm
OXALIC-ACID Plant 68 ppm
P-COUMARIC-ACID Flower 35 ppm Leaf 13
ppm
P-HYDROXY-BENZOIC-ACID Leaf
PALMITIC-ACID Flower 240–3,100 ppm Leaf
470–5,048 ppm

PANTOTHENIC-ACID Flower 1.4–18 ppm Leaf
 5.35–63 ppm
PENTAN-3-ONE Plant
PENTEN-1-OL Plant
PHENETHYL-ISOTHIOCYANATE Leaf
PHENETHYLAMINE Flower 1.8 ppm
PHENYLALANINE Flower 710–9,175 ppm Leaf
 840–9,022 ppm
PHOSPHORUS Flower 385–7,375 ppm Leaf
 644–9,090 ppm
PHYTIC-ACID Leaf
PHYTOSTEROLS Flower 180–2,325 ppm Plant
POTASSIUM Flower 3,300–49,080 ppm Leaf
 3,178–37,270 ppm
PROGOITRIN Flower 60 ppm Leaf
PROLINE Flower 860–11,110 ppm Leaf
 1,140–12,244 ppm
PROP-2-ENYL-GLUCOSINOLATE Flower
PROTEIN Flower 18,680–300,000 ppm Leaf
 28,710–331,159 ppm
PUFA Flower 830–10,725 ppm
QUERCETIN Flower 6 ppm Leaf
QUERCITRIN Leaf
QUINIC-ACID Flower Leaf
RIBOFLAVIN Flower 0.3–11 ppm Leaf 1.1–21
 ppm
RUBIDIUM Flower 0.43–11 ppm Leaf 1–23
 ppm
RUTIN Leaf
SALICYLIC-ACID Leaf
SEC-BUTYL-ISOTHIOCYANATE Seed
SELENIUM Flower Leaf 0.024 ppm Stem 0.015
 ppm
SERINE Flower 1,040–13,440 ppm Leaf
 1,000–10,740 ppm
SFA Flower 270–3,490 ppm
SILICON Flower 2–125 ppm Leaf 1–90 ppm
SINAPIC-ACID Leaf 40 ppm
SINIGRIN Flower 325 ppm Plant
SODIUM Flower 120–2,300 ppm Leaf
 252–3,091 ppm
SQUALENE Plant
STEARIC-ACID Flower 30–390 ppm Leaf
 70–752 ppm
STIGMASTEROL Plant
SUCCINIC-ACID Flower Plant
SULFUR Leaf 1,200–11,800 ppm
THIAMIN Flower 0.6–12 ppm Leaf 0.6–8 ppm

THREONINE Flower 720–9,300 ppm Leaf
 910–9,773 ppm
TRANS-FERULIC-ACID Leaf
TRYPTOPHAN Flower 260–3,360 ppm Leaf
 290–3,115 ppm
TYROSINE Flower 430–5,555 ppm Leaf
 630–6,766 ppm
VALINE Flower 1,000–12,920 ppm Leaf
 1,280–13,747 ppm
VANILLIC-ACID Plant
VIT-B-6 Flower 2–30 ppm Leaf 1.6–18 ppm
WATER Leaf 890,000–910,230 ppm Plant
 894,000–926,000 ppm
ZINC Flower 3–97 ppm Leaf 4–118 ppm

BRUSSELS SPROUTS

Chemicals in *Brassica oleracea var. gemmifera DC* (*Brassicaceae*)—Brussels Sprouts

1-O-FERULOYL-BETA-D-GLUCOSE Leaf
1-O-P-COUMAROYL-BETA-D-GLUCOSE Leaf
1-O-P-SINAPOYL-BETA-D-GLUCOSE Leaf
2-HYDROXY-BUT-3-ENYL-GLUCOSINOLATE
 Leaf
4-METHOXY-INDOL-3-YL-METHYL-GLUCOSI-
 NOLATE Leaf
ALLYL-ISOTHIOCYANATE Seed
ALPHA-LINOLENIC-ACID Leaf 990–7,069 ppm
ALPHA-TOCOPHEROL Leaf 4–63 ppm
ANTEISO-HEPTACOSAN-1-OL Flower
ANTEISO-MONTANYL-ALCOHOL Leaf
ANTEPENTACOSAN-1-OL Leaf
ARACHIDONIC-ACID Leaf 10–71 ppm
ARGININE Leaf 2,030–14,494 ppm
ASCORBIC-ACID Leaf 720–6,069 ppm
ASH Leaf 13,700–97,818 ppm
BETA-CAROTENE Leaf 5–41 ppm
BORON Leaf 57 ppm Stem 21 ppm
CAFFEIC-ACID Leaf 34 ppm
CALCIUM Leaf 395–3,177 ppm
CARBOHYDRATES Leaf 89,600–639,744 ppm
CITRIC-ACID Leaf
COPPER Leaf 1–5 ppm
COUMESTROL Shoot 400 ppm
CYSTINE Leaf 220–1,571 ppm
FAT Leaf 2,000–28,560 ppm
FERULIC-ACID Leaf 10 ppm
FIBER Leaf 15,100–107,814 ppm

FOLACIN Leaf 0.56–4 ppm
FUMARIC-ACID Leaf
HEPTACOSAN-1-OL Flower
HEXACOSAN-1-OL Leaf
HISTIDINE Leaf 760–5,426 ppm
INDOLE-3-ACETONITRILE Shoot
INDOLE-3-CARBINOL Shoot
INDOLE-3-CARBOXALDEHYDE Shoot
INDOLE-3-CARBOXYLIC-ACID Shoot
INDOYL-3,3'-DIMETHANE-CARBOXYLIC-ACID
  Shoot
IRON Leaf 9–136 ppm
ISOHEXACOSAN-1-OL Leaf
ISOLEUCINE Leaf 1,320–9,425 ppm
ISOOCTACOSAN-1-OL Leaf
KILOCALORIES Leaf 430–3,070 /kg
LEUCINE Leaf 1,520–10,853 ppm
LINOLEIC-ACID Leaf 450–3,213 ppm
LYSINE Leaf 1,540–10,996 ppm
MAGNESIUM Leaf 230–1,642 ppm
MALIC-ACID Leaf
MANGANESE Leaf 3–24 ppm
METHIONINE Leaf 320–2,285 ppm
MOLYBDENUM Leaf 0.9 ppm Stem 0.36 ppm
MONTANYL-ALCOHOL Leaf
NIACIN Leaf 6–64 ppm
OCTACOSAN-1-OL Leaf
OLEIC-ACID Leaf 190–1,357 ppm
OXALATE Leaf 3,600–25,704 ppm
P-COUMARIC-ACID Leaf 12 ppm
PALMITIC-ACID Leaf 530–3,784 ppm
PALMITOLEIC-ACID Leaf 20–142 ppm
PANTOTHENIC-ACID Leaf 3.1–22 ppm
PENTACOSAN-1-OL Leaf
PHENYLALANINE Leaf 980–6,997 ppm
PHOSPHORUS Leaf 690–4,927 ppm
PHYTOSTEROLS Leaf 240–1,710 ppm
POTASSIUM Leaf 3,670–29,343 ppm
PROP-2-ENYL-GLUCOSINOLATE Leaf
PROTEIN Leaf 32,580–250,000 ppm
QUERCETIN Sprout Seedling 25 ppm
QUINIC-ACID Leaf
RIBOFLAVIN Leaf 0.4–10 ppm
RUTIN Shoot 20 ppm
SEC-BUTYL-ISOTHIOCYANATE Seed
SELENIUM Leaf 0.024 ppm Stem 0.012 ppm
SINAPIC-ACID Leaf 107 ppm
SODIUM Leaf 221–1,990 ppm

STEARIC-ACID Leaf 30–214 ppm
SUCCINIC-ACID Leaf
TETRACOSAN-1-OL Leaf
THIAMIN Leaf 1.3–11 ppm
THREONINE Leaf 1,200–8,568 ppm
TRIACONTAN-1-OL Leaf
TRYPTOPHAN Leaf 370–2,642 ppm
VALINE Leaf 1,550–11,067 ppm
VIT-B-6 Leaf 2.2–16 ppm
WATER Leaf 846,000–945,500 ppm
ZINC Leaf 10–157 ppm

CABBAGE

Chemicals in *Brassica oleracea var. capitata
L. (Brassicaceae)*—Cabbage

METHOXYBRASSITIN Leaf 30 ppm
1-CYANO-2,3-EPITHIOPROPANE Plant
1-CYANO-2-HYDROXY-3-BUTENE Plant
1-CYANO-3,4-EPITHIOBUTANE Plant
1-CYANO-3,4-EPITHIOPENTANE Plant
1-CYANO-3-METHYL-SULFINYL-PROPANE
  Plant
1-CYANO-3-METHYL-THIO-PROPANE Leaf
1-CYANO-4-METHYL-SULFINYL-BUTANE Plant
1-CYANO-4-METHYL-THIO-BUTANE Leaf
1-METHOXY-3-INDOYL-METHYL Plant
1-METHOXY-GLUCOBRASSICIN Leaf
1-O-FERULOYL-BETA-D-GLUCOSE Leaf
1-O-P-COUMAROYL-BETA-D-GLUCOSE Leaf
1-O-SINAPOYL-BETA-D-GLUCOSE Leaf
2-HYDROXY-1-CYANO-BUT-3-ENE Leaf
2-HYDROXY-3-BUTENYL-GLUCOSINOLATE
  Leaf
2-METHOXY-PHENOL Plant
2-METHYL-THIO-PROPYL-GLUCOSINOLATE
  Leaf
2-PHENYL-ETHYL-GLUSOSINOLATE Leaf
2-PROPENYL-GLUCOSINOLATE Plant
3-(METHYLTHIO)-PROPYL-ISOTHIOCYANATE
  Leaf
3-BUTENYL-GLUCOSINOLATE Leaf
3-BUTENYL-ISOTHIOCYANATE Leaf
3-INDOYL-METHYL-GLUCOSINOLATE Plant
3-METHYL-SULFINYL-PROPYL-GLUCOSINO-
  LATE Leaf
3-METHYL-SULFINYL-PROPYL-ISOTHIO-
  CYANATE Leaf

3-O-(2-O-{BETA-D-GLUCOPYRANOSYL}-6-O-
(4-O-{BETA-D-GLUCOPYRANOSYL}-5-O-BE
TA-D-GLUCOPYRANOSYL) . . . CYANIDIN Leaf
16 ppm
3-O-(2-O-{BETA-D-GLUCOPYRANOSYL}-6-O-
(4-O-{BETA-D
GLUCOPYRANOSYL}TRANS-F
ERULYL) . . . CYANIDIN Leaf 0.5 ppm
3-O-(2-O-{BETA-D-GLUCOPYRANOSYL}-6-O-
(4-O-{BETA-D
GLUCOPYRANOSYL}TRANS-P
COUMARYL) . . . CYANIDIN Leaf 0.3 ppm
3-O-(6-O-{TRANS-FERULYL)-2-O-BETA-D-GLU-
COPYRANOSYL} . . . CYANIDIN Leaf 0.2
ppm
3-O-(6-O-{TRANS-P-COUMAROYL)-2-O-BETA-
D
GLUCOPYRANOSYL} . . . CYANIDIN Leaf 27
ppm
3-O-(6-O-{TRANS-SINAPL}-2-O-(BETA-D-GLU-
COPYRANOSYL)-BETA-D
GLUCOPYRANOSY
L5-O-(BETA-D-GLUCOPYRANOSYL)-CYANIDIN
Leaf 0.1 ppm
4-(METHYLTHIO)-BUTYL-ISOTHIOCYANATE
Leaf
4-CAFFOYLQUINIC-ACID Plant
4-HYDROXY-GLUCOBRASSICIN Leaf
4-HYDROXY-INDO-3-YL-METHYL-GLUCOSI-
NOLATE Seed
4-HYDROXY-INDOYL-3-YL-METHYL-GLUCOSI-
NOLATE Leaf
4-METHOXYBRASSININ Leaf 1 ppm
4-METHYL-SULFINYL-BUTYL-GLUCOSINO-
LATE Leaf
4-METHYL-SULFINYL-BUTYL-ISOTHIO-
CYANATE Leaf
4-METHYL-THIO-BUTYL-GLUCOSINOLATE
Leaf
4-P-COUMAROYLQUINIC-ACID Plant
4-PENTENYL-ISOTHIOCYANATE Plant
5-FERULOYLQUINIC-ACID Plant
5-P-COUMAROYLQUINIC-ACID Plant
5-VINYLOXAZOLIDINE-2-THIONE Plant
ALANINE Leaf 420–5,615 ppm
ALLYL-CYANIDE Plant
ALLYL-GLUCOSINOLATE Seed
ALLYL-ISOTHIOCYANATE Leaf 20 ppm

ALPHA-LINOLENIC-ACID Leaf 460–6,150 ppm
ALPHA-TOCOPHEROL Leaf 0.4–7 ppm
ALUMINUM Plant
AMMONIA(NH3) Leaf 3,800–11,060 ppm
ANILINE Leaf 1–4 ppm
ANTHERAXANTHIN Leaf
ANTHOXANTHINS Sprout Seedling
ARGININE Leaf 690–9,225 ppm
ARSENIC Leaf 0.004–0.007 ppm
ASCORBIC-ACID Leaf 190–6,774 ppm
ASH Leaf 6,000–98,072 ppm
ASPARTIC-ACID Leaf 1,190–15,910 ppm
BARIUM Leaf 1–87 ppm
BENZYL-AMINE Leaf 2.8–3.3 ppm
BENZYL-GLUCOSINOLATE Leaf
BENZYL-ISOTHIOCYANATE Leaf
BETA-CAROTENE Leaf 0.6–12 ppm
BETA-SITOSTEROL Leaf
BORON Leaf 1–145 ppm
BRASSININ Leaf 1.3 ppm
BROMINE Leaf 0.2–37 ppm
BUTYL-GLUCOSINOLATE Plant
CADMIUM Leaf 0.005–0.39 ppm
CAFFEIC-ACID Leaf 0.5–77 ppm
CAFFEIC-ACID-4-O-BETA-GLUCOSIDE Leaf
CALCIUM Leaf 290–7,500 ppm
CARBOHYDRATES Leaf 53,700–717,969 ppm
CARVONE Plant
CHLOROGENIC-ACID Plant
CHROMIUM Leaf 0.001–8.7 ppm
CITRIC-ACID Leaf
COBALT Leaf 0.001–2.9 ppm
COPPER Leaf 0.3–87 ppm
CROCETIN Leaf
CYANIDIN-3,5-DIGLUCOSIDE Sprout Seedling
229 ppm
CYANIDIN-3-(DI-P-COUMAROYL)-SOPHORO-
SIDE-5-GLUCOSIDE Sprout Seedling 229
ppm
CYANIDIN-3-(DIFERULYL)-SOPHOROSIDE-5-
GLUCOSIDE Sprout Seedling 214 ppm
CYANIDIN-3-(DISINAPYL)-SOPHOROSIDE-5-
GLUCOSIDE Sprout Seedling 257 ppm
CYANIDIN-3-(P-COUMAROYL)-SOPHORO-
SIDE-5-GLUCOSIDE Sprout Seedling 200
ppm
CYANIDIN-3-FERULYL-SOPHOROSIDE-5-GLU-
COSIDE Sprout Seedling 243 ppm

CYANIDIN-3-MALONYL-SOPHOROSIDE-5-
GLUCOSIDE Sprout Seedling 171 ppm
CYANIDIN-3-SINAPYL-SOPHOROSIDE-5-GLU-
COSIDE Sprout Seedling 200 ppm
CYANIDIN-3-SOPHOROSIDE-5-GLUCOSIDE
Sprout Seedling 257 ppm
CYCLOBRASSININ Leaf 4.3 ppm
CYSTINE Leaf 100–1,337 ppm
DEHYDROASCORBIC-ACID Shoot
DIINDOLYLMETHANE Plant
DIMETHYL-AMINE Leaf 2–2.8 ppm
ERYTHRO-1-CYANO-2-HYDROXY-3,4-EP-
ITHIOBUTANE Plant
ETHYL-AMINE Leaf 1.3 ppm
ETHYL-METHYL-AMINE Leaf 0.9 ppm
FAT Leaf 1,090–33,559 ppm
FERULIC-ACID Leaf 4–20 ppm
FERULIC-ACID-B-BETA-D-GLUCOSIDE Leaf
FIBER Leaf 6,000–106,960 ppm
FLUORINE Leaf 0.02–2.5 ppm
FOLACIN Leaf 0.45–9 ppm
FUMARIC-ACID Leaf
GLUCOBRASSICANAPIN Seed
GLUCOBRASSICIN Plant
GLUCOIBERIN Leaf
GLUCONAPIN Seed
GLUCORAPHANIN Leaf
GLUTAMIC-ACID Leaf 2,700–36,099 ppm
GLYCINE Leaf 270–3,610 ppm
GOITRIN Plant
HISTIDINE Leaf 250–3,343 ppm
INDOLE-3-ACETONITRILE Plant
INDOLE-3-CARBINOL Plant
INDOLE-3-CARBOXALDEHYDE Shoot
INDOYL-3,3'-DIMETHANE Shoot
IRON Leaf 4–151 ppm
ISOLEUCINE Leaf 610–8,156 ppm
ISOMENTHOL Plant
JASMONIC-ACID Leaf
KAEMPFEROL Leaf 100–300 ppm
KAEMPFEROL-3-0-SOPHOROSIDE Leaf
KAEMPFEROL-3-FERULOYL-SOPHOROSIDE
Leaf
KAEMPFEROL-3-SINAPOYL-SOPHOROSIDE
Leaf
KAEMPFEROL-3-SOPHOROSIDE-7-GLUCO-
SIDE Leaf
KAEMPFEROL-7-GLUCOSIDE Leaf

KILOCALORIES Leaf 240–3,209 /kg
LANTHANUM Leaf 6.7–20.3 ppm
LEAD Leaf 0.002–5.8 ppm
LEUCINE Leaf 630–8,423 ppm
LINOLEIC-ACID Leaf 350–4,680 ppm
LITHIUM Leaf 0.28–1.4 ppm
LUTEIN Leaf
LYSINE Leaf 570–7,621 ppm
MAGNESIUM Leaf 120–2,228 ppm
MALIC-ACID Leaf
MANGANESE Leaf 1–45 ppm
MENTHOL Plant
MERCURY Leaf 0.013 ppm
METHIONINE Leaf 120–1,604 ppm
METHYL-AMINE Leaf 3.4–22.7 ppm
MEVALONIC-ACID Leaf
MOLYBDENUM Leaf 0.1–8.7 ppm
N-(1)-METHOXYBRASSININ Leaf 63 ppm
N-METHYL-ANILINE Leaf 0.3 ppm
N-METHYL-BETA-PHENETHYLAMINE Leaf
0.5–2 ppm
N-METHYL-PHENETHYLAMINE Leaf 0.5–3.7 ppm
N-NONACOSANE Leaf
N-PENTYL-AMINE Leaf 0.6–1.4 ppm
NAPOLEIFERIN Seed
NARCOTINE Leaf
NEO-CHLOROGENIC-ACID Plant
NEOGLUCOBRASSICIN Plant
NEOMENTHOL Plant
NEOXANTHIN Leaf
NIACIN Leaf 3–40 ppm
NICKEL Leaf 0.02–8.7 ppm
NITROGEN Leaf 2,100–37,500 ppm
NONACOSAN-15-ONE Leaf
OLEIC-ACID Leaf 130–1,738 ppm
OXALATE Leaf 1,000–13,370 ppm
OXALIC-ACID Leaf 59–350 ppm
P-COUMARIC-ACID Leaf 0.5–9 ppm
P-COUMARIC-ACID-O-BETA-D-GLUCOSIDE
Leaf
PALMITIC-ACID Leaf 190–2,540 ppm
PANTOTHENIC-ACID Leaf 1.4–19 ppm
PHENETHYL-CYANIDE Leaf
PHENETHYLAMINE Leaf 2.1–8.6 ppm
PHENYLALANINE Leaf 390–5,214 ppm
PHENYLETHYL-ISOTHIOCYANATE Leaf
PHEOPHYTIN-A Leaf
PHOSPHORUS Leaf 214–6,500 ppm

PHYTOSTEROLS Leaf 110–1,471 ppm
POTASSIUM Leaf 2,368–42,500 ppm
PROGOITRIN Leaf Seed
PROLINE Leaf 2,380–31,821 ppm
PROP-2-ENYL-ISOTHIOCYANATE Plant
PROPYL-GLUCOSINOLATE Plant
PROTEIN Leaf 10,780–179,425 ppm
PROTOCATECHUIC-ACID Plant
QUERCETIN Leaf 2–100 ppm
QUERCETIN-3'-GLUCOSIDE Leaf
QUERCETIN-3-SINAPOYL-SOPHOROSIDE Leaf
QUERCETIN-3-SOPHOROSIDE Leaf
QUERCETIN-3-SOPHOROSIDE-7-GLUCOSIDE
  Leaf
QUINIC-ACID Leaf
RIBOFLAVIN Leaf 4 ppm
RUBIDIUM Leaf 0.4–27.5 ppm
S-METHYL-CYSTEINE-SULFOXIDE Leaf
SEC-BUTYL-ISOTHIOCYANATE Seed
SELENIUM Leaf 0.003–0.25 ppm
SERINE Leaf 710–9,493 ppm
SILICON Leaf 1–25 ppm
SILVER Leaf 0.07–0.58 ppm
SINAPIC-ACID Leaf 13–67 ppm
SINIGRIN Seed
SODIUM Leaf 163–4,510 ppm
SPIROBRASSININ Leaf 35 ppm
STEARIC-ACID Leaf 10–134 ppm
STRONTIUM Leaf 3–870 ppm
SUCCINIC-ACID Leaf
SULFUR Leaf 385–8,750 ppm
THIAMIN Leaf 0.5–10 ppm
THREO-1-CYANO-2-HYDROXY-3,4-EP-
  ITHIOBUTANE Plant
THREONINE Leaf 420–5,615 ppm
TITANIUM Leaf 0.35–203 ppm
TRYPTOPHAN Leaf 120–1,604 ppm
TYROSINE Leaf 210–2,807 ppm
VALINE Leaf 520–6,952 ppm
VANADIUM Leaf 0.48–14.5 ppm
VIOLAXANTHIN Leaf
VIT-B-6 Leaf 0.8–14 ppm
VIT-U Leaf 2–25 ppm
WATER Leaf 891,000–950,000 ppm
YTTERBIUM Leaf 0.19–8.7 ppm
YTTRIUM Leaf 0.48–29 ppm
ZINC Leaf 2–36 ppm
ZIRCONIUM Leaf 1.4–203 ppm

CARROT

Chemicals in *Daucus carota L. (Apiaceae)*—
Carrot

2-METHOXY-3-SEC-BUTYL-PYRAZINE Root
2-OCTANONE Seed
3'-NUCLEOTIDASE Tissue Culture
3,4-DIMETHOXY-ALLYL-BENZENE Root
3-METHOXY-4,5-METHYLENEDIOXY-PROPYL-
  BENZENE Root
4-(BETA-D-GLUCOPYRANOSYLOXY)-BEN-
  ZOIC-ACID Seed 65 ppm
4-HYDROXY-PROLINE Plant
4-METHYL-ISO-PROPENYL-BENZENE Seed
5,7-DIHYDROXY-2-METHYL-CHROMONE
  Root
5-METHOXY-PSORALEN Plant
6-(GAMMA,GAMMA-DIMETHYL-ALLYL-
  AMINO)-PURINE Tissue Culture
6-HYDROXY-MELLEIN Root
6-METHOXY-MELLEIN Root
8-HYDROXY-6-METHOXY-3-METHYL-3,4-DI-
  HYDRO-ISOCOUMARIN Tissue Culture
ACETALDEHYDE Root
ACETONE Root
ACETYL-CHOLINE Root
ACORENONE Seed
ALANINE Root 590–4,830 ppm
ALDOLASE Tissue Culture
ALPHA-AMYRIN Root
ALPHA-BERGAMOTENE Root 2,000 ppm
ALPHA-CAROTENE Root 17–25 ppm
ALPHA-CARYOPHYLLENE Root
ALPHA-CURCUMENE Seed
ALPHA-GLUCOSIDASE Tissue Culture
ALPHA-GURJUNENE Seed
ALPHA-HUMULENE Root 12 ppm
ALPHA-IONONE Root
ALPHA-KETO-GLUTARIC-ACID Root
ALPHA-LINOLENIC-ACID Seed 270–935 ppm
ALPHA-PHELLANDRENE Root
ALPHA-PINENE Root 48 ppm Seed 12–1,300
  ppm Shoot 12 ppm
ALPHA-TERPINENE Root 28 ppm Seed 20–40
  ppm
ALPHA-TERPINEOL Root 28 ppm
ALPHA-THUJENE Shoot 12 ppm
ALPHA-TOCOPHEROL Leaf 788 ppm Root
  4–36 ppm

ALUMINUM Root 1–1,050 ppm
AMMONIA(NH3) Root 3,970 ppm
AMYLASE Tissue Culture
ANILINE Root 31 ppm
ANTHERAXANTHIN Leaf
APIGENIN Fruit
APIGENIN-4'-O-BETA-D-GLUCOSIDE Seed
APIGENIN-7-O-BETA-D-GALACTOMANNO-
  SIDE Plant
APIGENIN-7-O-BETA-D-GALACTOPYRANOSYL-
  (1,4)-O-BETA-D-MANN . . . Plant
APIGENIN-7-O-BETA-D-GLUCOSIDE Seed
APIGENIN-7-O-BETA-D-RUTINOSIDE Seed
ARABINOSIDE Root
ARACHIC-ACID Seed 270–936 ppm
ARACHIDONIC-ACID Plant
ARGININE Root 430–3,520 ppm
ARSENIC Root 0.003–1 ppm
ASARALDEHYDE Seed
ASARONE Seed 400 ppm
ASCORBIC-ACID Root 91–775 ppm
ASH Root 56,000–79,000 ppm
ASPARTIC-ACID Root 1,370–11,220 ppm
ASTRAGALIN Seed
AZULENE Seed
BARIUM Root 1.7–150 ppm
BENZOIC-ACID-4-O-BETA-D-GLUCOSIDE
  Root 11 ppm
BENZYL-AMINE Root 2.8 ppm
BERGAMOTENE Seed 200–700 ppm
BERGAPTEN Root 0.3 ppm
BETA-AMYRIN Root
BETA-BISABOLENE Root 116 ppm Seed
  100–3,500 ppm Shoot 38 ppm
BETA-CAROTENE Root 27–673 ppm
BETA-CARYOPHYLLENE Seed 55–170 ppm
  Shoot 24 ppm
BETA-CRYPTOXANTHIN Root
BETA-ELEMENE Plant
BETA-FARNESENE Root 12 ppm
BETA-GALACTOSIDASE Tissue Culture
BETA-GLUCOSIDASE Tissue Culture
BETA-GLUCURONIDASE Tissue Culture
BETA-IONONE Seed 300 ppm
BETA-PHELLANDRENE Shoot 177 ppm
BETA-PINENE Root 4 ppm Seed 50–5,500 ppm
  Shoot 44 ppm
BETA-SELINENE Seed 118–410 ppm

BETA-SITOSTEROL Root
BETA-SITOSTEROL-GLYCOSIDE Plant
BETAINE Root 35 ppm
BIPHENYL Root 4 ppm
BORNEOL Root
BORNYL-ACETATE Plant Root 24 ppm
BORON Root 1–36 ppm
BROMINE Root 1–9 ppm
BUTYRIC-ACID Root
CADMIUM Root 0.012–0.6 ppm
CAFFEIC-ACID Root
CAFFEIC-ACID-4-O-BETA-D-GLUCOSIDE Plant
CAFFEOYLQUINIC-ACID Root
CALCIUM Root 210–5,710 ppm
CAMPESTEROL Root
CAMPHENE Seed 1–70 ppm
CAMPHOR Seed
CAPRIC-ACID Seed 1,360–7,065 ppm
CAR-6-ENE Seed 56–112 ppm
CARBOHYDRATES Root 101,000–850,000 ppm
CAROTA-1,4-BETA-OXIDE Seed 0.2–0.5 ppm
CAROTATOXIN Root
CAROTOL Root 8 ppm Seed 1,150–8,000 ppm
  Shoot 1,450 ppm
CARVONE Seed
CARYOPHYLLENE Root 200 ppm Seed
  134–1,000 ppm
CARYOPHYLLENE-OXIDE Root 310–350 ppm
  Seed 310–350 ppm
CHLOROGENIC-ACID Root
CHLOROPHYLL Plant
CHOLESTEROL Leaf
CHOLINE Root 36 ppm Shoot 73 ppm
CHROMIUM Root 0.005–1.5 ppm
CHRYSIN Seed
CINNAMIC-ACID Tissue Culture
CIS-BETA-BERGAMOTENE Root
CIS-GAMMA-BISABOLENE Root 8 ppm
CITRAL Seed 200 ppm
CITRIC-ACID Root
CITRONELLYL-ACETATE Seed 150–200 ppm
COBALT Root 0.005–0.058 ppm
COPPER Root 0.3–18 ppm
COSMOSIIN Leaf
COUMARIN Root
CROCETIN Leaf
CUMINALDEHYDE Seed
CYANIDIN-3,5-DIGALACTOSIDE Tissue Culture

CYANIDIN-3-(SINAPOYL-XYLOSYL-GLUCO-SYL)-GALACTOSIDE Leaf

CYANIDIN-3-GALACTOSIDE Tissue Culture

CYANIDIN-3-GLUCOGALACTOSIDE Tissue Culture

CYANIDIN-3-O-BETA-D-GLUCOSIDE Tissue Culture

CYANIDIN-DIGLYCOSIDE Root

CYSTEINE Tissue Culture

CYSTINE Root 80–655 ppm

D-GLUCOSE Root 80,000 ppm

DAUCARIN Seed

DAUCENE Seed 200 ppm

DAUCIC-ACID Root

DAUCINE Plant

DAUCOL Seed 60–1,960 ppm Shoot 535 ppm

DAUCOSTEROL Root

DEC-2-EN-1-AL Root 1.6 ppm

DECA-TRANS-2,TRANS-4-DIEN-1-AL Plant Root

DEHYDROASCORBIC-ACID Root

DEHYDROXYDAUCOL Seed

DELTA-3-CARENE Seed 12–120 ppm

DEOXY-RIBONUCLEASE Tissue Culture

DIOSGENIN Root 5,400–6,000 ppm Tissue Culture 5,400–6,000 ppm

DIPENTENE Root

DODECAN-1-AL Root

ELEMICIN Seed 2,000 ppm

EO Root 4,000 ppm Seed 4,000–8,000 ppm Shoot 4,000 ppm

EPOXYDIHYDROCARYOPHYLLENE Seed 250–2,000 ppm

EPSILON-CAROTENE Root

ESCULETIN Leaf

ETHANOL Root

ETHYL-AMINE Root 1 ppm

ETHYL-METHYL-AMINE Root 7 ppm

ETHYLENE Tissue Culture

EUGENIN Tissue Culture

EUGENOL Seed 7,000 ppm

FALCARINDIOL Root 88 ppm

FALCARINOL Root 10–47 ppm

FAT Root 1,700–29,000 ppm Seed 87,000–302,000 ppm

FERULIC-ACID Root

FERULIC-ACID-O-BETA-D-GLUCOSIDE Shoot

FIBER Root 10,000–134,000 ppm

FLUORINE Root 0.03–1.8 ppm

FOLACIN Root 0.1–1.2 ppm

FORMIC-ACID Plant

FRUCTOSE Root

FUMARASE Tissue Culture

FUMARIC-ACID Root

GALACTOSE Root

GAMMA-BISABOLENE Root 264 ppm

GAMMA-CAROTENE Root

GAMMA-DECALACTOSE Seed

GAMMA-DECANOLACTONE Root

GAMMA-LINOLENIC-ACID Seed 540–1,870 ppm

GAMMA-MUUROLENE Root 3,000 ppm

GAMMA-TERPINENE Root 216 ppm

GENTISIC-ACID Tissue Culture

GERANIOL Root 10–8,120 ppm Seed 10–8,120 ppm

GERANYL-2-METHYL0BUTYRATE Seed 3,000 ppm

GERANYL-ACETATE Shoot 265 ppm

GERANYL-ACETONE Seed 300 ppm

GERANYL-FORMATE Seed

GERANYL-ISOBUTYRATE Seed 500 ppm

GLUTAMATE-OXALACETATE-TRANSAMINASE Tissue Culture

GLUTAMATE-PYRUVATE-TRANSAMINASE Tissue Culture

GLUTAMIC-ACID Root 2,020–16,545 ppm

GLUTAMINE Root

GLYCINE Root 300–2,455 ppm

HCN Root

HEPTAN-1-AL Root 2 ppm

HERACLENIN Root

HISTIDINE Root 160–1,310 ppm

INDOLE-ACETIC-ACID Tissue Culture

INVERTASE Tissue Culture

IONENE Root

IRON Root 3–300 ppm

ISOBUTYRIC-ACID Plant

ISOCHLOROGENIC-ACID Leaf

ISOCITRIC-ACID Root

ISOLEUCINE Root 410–3,360 ppm

ISOPIMPINELLIN Root

ISOPRENE Root

KAEMPFEROL Seed

KAEMPFEROL-3-O-BETA-D-GLUCOSIDE Root

KILOCALORIES Resin, Exudate, Sap 2,710 /kg
  Root 430–3,520 /kg
LAURIC-ACID Root 20–165 ppm Seed
  1,810–6,280 ppm
LEAD Root 0.01–2 ppm
LECITHIN Root
LECITHINASE Plant
LEUCINE Root 430–3,520 ppm
LIMONENE Root 150 ppm Seed 20–1,500 ppm
  Shoot 26 ppm
LINALOL Root 32 ppm Seed 4–600 ppm
LINOLEIC-ACID Root 670–5,485 ppm Seed
  9,360–43,400 ppm
LINOLENIC-ACID Root 100–820 ppm
LITHIUM Root 0.23–0.6 ppm
LUPEOL Root
LUTEIN Root
LUTEOLIN Plant
LUTEOLIN-4'-O-BETA-D-DIGLUCOSIDE Seed
LUTEOLIN-4'-O-BETA-GLUCOSIDE Seed
LUTEOLIN-7-O-(6''-O-MALONYL)-BETA-D-
  DIGLUCOSIDE Plant
LUTEOLIN-7-O-BETA-D-DIGLUCOSIDE Seed
LUTEOLIN-7-O-BETA-GLUCOSIDE Root 100
  ppm Seed
LUTEOLIN-7-O-BETA-GLUCURONIDE Plant
LUTEOLIN-7-O-BETA-RUTINOSIDE Seed
LYCOPENE Root 80–140 ppm
LYSINE Root 400–3,275 ppm
MAGNESIUM Root 100–1,980 ppm
MALIC-ACID Root
MALTOSE Root
MALVIDIN-3,5-DIGLUCOSIDE Root
MANGANESE Root 1–62 ppm
MANNOSE Root
MERCURY Root 0.001–0.045 ppm
METHIONINE Root 70–575 ppm
METHYL-AMINE Root 3,970 ppm
METHYL-PENTOSANS Plant
MEVALONIC-ACID Root 4 ppm
MOLYBDENUM Root 0.1–0.7 ppm
MUFA Root 80–655 ppm
MYRCENE Seed 10–250 ppm
MYRICETIN Fruit
MYRISTIC-ACID Root 10–80 ppm Seed
  10,470–36,300 ppm
MYRISTICIN Root 0.5–34 ppm
MYRISTOLEIC-ACID Seed

N-HENTRIACONTANE Seed
N-HEPTACOSANE Seed
N-METHYL-ANILINE Root 0.8 ppm
N-METHYL-BENZYLAMINE Root 16 ppm
N-METHYL-PHENETHYLAMINE Root 2 ppm
N-NONACOSANE Seed
N-OCTACOSANE Seed
NEOXANTHIN Leaf
NEUROSPORENE Root
NIACIN Root
NICKEL Root 2 ppm
NITROGEN Root 1,400–20,000 ppm
NON-2-EN-1-AL Root 12 ppm
NONAN-1-AL Root 0.8 ppm
NOPOL Root
OCTAN-1-AL Root 8 ppm
OLEIC-ACID Root 60–490 ppm Seed
  55,800–230,300 ppm
OSTHOLE Plant 610 ppm Root
OXALIC-ACID Root 56 ppm
OXYPEUCEDANIN Root
P-COUMARIC-ACID Root
P-COUMARIC-ACID-O-BETA-D-GLUCOSIDE
  Shoot
P-CYMEN-8-OL Seed 9,000 ppm
P-CYMENE Root 12 ppm Seed 10–160 ppm
P-HYDROXY-BENZOIC-ACID Root
P-VINYL-GUAIACOL Seed 4,000 ppm
PALMITIC-ACID Root 230–1,885 ppm Seed
  3,265–11,500 ppm
PALMITOLEIC-ACID Root 20–165 ppm Seed
  270–1,725 ppm
PANTOTHENIC-ACID Root 2–17 ppm
PECTIN Root 100,000–188,000 ppm
PECTINESTERASE Root
PENTOSANS Plant
PEROXIDASE Root
PETROSELINIC-ACID Seed 712,000 ppm
PHENYLALANINE Root 320–2,620 ppm
PHENYLALANINE-AMMONIA-LYASE Tissue
  Culture
PHOSPHATIDYL-CHOLINE Tissue Culture
PHOSPHATIDYL-ETHANOLAMINE Tissue Cul-
  ture
PHOSPHATIDYL-GLYCEROL Tissue Culture
PHOSPHATIDYL-INOSITOL Tissue Culture
PHOSPHOFRUCTOKINASE Root
PHOSPHORUS Root 340–5,090 ppm

PHYTIN Root 52,700 ppm

PHYTOENE Plant

PHYTOFLUENE Root

PHYTOSTEROLS Root 120–980 ppm

PIPECOLIC-ACID Plant

POTASSIUM Root 3,000–46,360 ppm

PROLINE Root 290–2,375 ppm

PROTEIN Root 72,000–106,000 ppm

PSORALEN Root 0.3 ppm Shoot 0.8 ppm

PUFA Root 770–6,300 ppm

PUTRESCINE Tissue Culture

PYRROLIDINE Plant

QUERCETIN Seed

QUERCETIN-3-O-BETA-GLUCOSIDE Seed

QUERCITRIN Plant

QUINIC-ACID Root

RHAMNOSE Root

RIBOFLAVIN Root 0.6–5 ppm

RIBONUCLEASE Tissue Culture

RUBIDIUM Root 0.42–12.7 ppm

SABINENE Root 160 ppm Seed 50–2,000 ppm

SAKURANETIN Fruit

SCOPOLETIN Root

SELENIUM Root 0.001–0.02 ppm

SERINE Plant Root 350–2,865 ppm

SFA Root 300–2,455 ppm

SHIKIMIC-ACID Root

SILICON Root 1–91 ppm

SODIUM Root 340–9,504 ppm

STARCH Root 14,800–25,200 ppm

STEARIC-ACID Root 10–80 ppm Seed
   285–1,240 ppm

STIGMASTEROL Root

STRONTIUM Root 1–148 ppm

SUBERIN Root

SUCCINIC-ACID Root

SUCROSE Root 60,000–339,000 ppm

SULFUR Root 52–1,635 ppm

SYRINGIC-ACID Root

TARAXASTEROL Shoot

TARTARIC-ACID Root

TERPINEN-4-OL Root 28 ppm

TERPINEOL-ACETATE Shoot 746 ppm

TERPINOLENE Root 1,520 ppm Seed 10 ppm

TETRADECENOIC-ACID Root

THERMOPSOSIDE Leaf

THIAMIN Root 1–6 ppm

THREONINE Root 380–3,110 ppm

TIGLIC-ACID Seed

TIN Root 3 ppm

TITANIUM Root 0.017–30 ppm

TOLUIDENE Root 7.2 ppm

TRANS-1,10-HEPTADECADIENE-5,7-DIYN-3-OL
   Plant

TRANS-2(7)-2,6-DIMETHYLOCTA-4,6-DIENE
   Plant

TRANS-BETA-BERGAPTENE Seed 170 ppm

TRANS-CHLOROGENIC-ACID Shoot

TRANS-CINNAMIC-ACID Tissue Culture

TRANS-GAMMA-BISABOLENE Root 268 ppm

TRANS-ISOASARONE Plant

TRYPTOPHAN Root 110–900 ppm

TYROSINE Root 200–1,640 ppm

UBIQUINONE-100 Tissue Culture

UMBELLIFERONE Leaf

UMBELLIFEROSE Plant

URONIC-ACID Root

VALINE Root 440–3,600 ppm

VANILLIC-ACID Tissue Culture

VIOLAXANTHIN Leaf

VIT-B-6 Root 1–13 ppm

VIT-D Plant

VIT-E Plant

WATER Root 858,000–907,000 ppm

XANTHOPHYLLS Root 12–16 ppm

XANTHOTOXIN Root 0.3 ppm Shoot 1.6 ppm

XYLITOL Root

XYLOSE Root

ZINC Root 2–79 ppm

ZIRCONIUM Root 1–2 ppm

ZOSIMIN Plant

CAULIFLOWER—SEE BROCCOLI

CELERY

Chemicals in *Apium graveolens* L. (*Apiaceae*)—Celery

3-BUTYLHEXAHYDROPHTHALIDE Root

3-BUTYLPHTHALIDE Seed 40–120 ppm

3-ISOBUTYLIDENE-3-A,4-DIHYDROPH-
   THALIDE Seed 133–1,500 ppm

3-ISOBUTYLIDENE-PHTHALIDE Plant 0.001
   ppm

3-ISOVALERIDENE-3A,4-DIHYDROPHTHALIDE
   Leaf

3-ISOVALERIDENE-PHTHALIDE Leaf

3-ISOVALIDENE-3A,4-DIHYDROPHTHALIDE Essential Oil 255 ppm Leaf 0.003 ppm

3-ISOVALIDENE-PHTHALIDE Plant

3-METHYL-4-ETHYL-HEXANE Root Essent. Oil 124,000 ppm

3-N-BUTYL-4,5-DIHYDROPHTHALIDE Seed

3-N-BUTYL-PHTHALIDE Fruit Essent. Oil 108,000 ppm Leaf Essent. Oil 40,000 ppm Seed

4-DIHYDROPHTHALIDE Seed 57–1,500 ppm

5-ALPHA-ANDROST-16-EN-3-ONE Plant 0.009 ppm

5-METHOXY-8-O-BETA-D-GLUCOSYL-OXYPSO-RALEN Seed 2.9 ppm

5-METHOXY-PSORALEN Fruit 7 ppm Leaf Wax 2 ppm

8-HYDROXY-5-METHOXY-PSORALEN Seed 375 ppm

8-HYDROXYFALCARINONE Root 8.3 ppm

8-METHOXY-PSORALEN Leaf 1 ppm

ACETALDEHYDE Leaf

ACETIC-ACID Plant

ADENINE Plant

ADENOSINE Plant

ALANINE Pt 220–4,665 ppm

ALLOOCIMENE-I Leaf Essent. Oil 1,000 ppm

ALLOOCIMENE-II Leaf Essent. Oil 1,000 ppm

ALPHA-EUDESMOL Seed 76–225 ppm

ALPHA-HUMULENE Leaf 266–2,500 ppm

ALPHA-IONONE Plant

ALPHA-LINOLENIC-ACID Seed 1,600–2,554 ppm

ALPHA-P-DIMETHYL-STYRENE Seed 170–270 ppm

ALPHA-PHELLANDRENE Fruit 2,000 ppm

ALPHA-PINENE Et 12,000–14,000 ppm Fruit Essent. Oil 10,000 ppm Leaf Essent. Oil 2,000 ppm Root Essent. Oil 179,000 ppm Seed 38–60 ppm

ALPHA-SELINENE Seed 95–250 ppm

ALPHA-TERPINENE Fruit Essent. Oil 1,000 ppm Leaf

ALPHA-TERPINEOL Fruit Essent. Oil 3,000–14,000 ppm Leaf Essent. Oil 2,000 ppm Root Essent. Oil 69,000 ppm Seed 1 ppm

ALPHA-TERPINYL-ACETATE Leaf

ALPHA-TERPINYL-PROPIONATE Leaf

ALPHA-TOCOPHEROL Plant 64 ppm Pt 3–67 ppm

ALUMINUM Root 0.3–9 ppm

ANGELIC-ACID Plant

ANILINE Pt 0.7 ppm

APIGENIN Plant

APIGENIN-7-BETA-APIOSYL-GLUCOSIDE Leaf

APIGRAVIN Seed

APIIN Plant 2,000 ppm

APIOLE Essential Oil

APIUMETIN Seed 12.5 ppm

APIUMETRIN Seed

APIUMOSIDE Seed

ARABINOSE Plant

ARGININE Pt 200–4,105 ppm

ARSENIC Root 0.01–0.09 ppm

ARSENIC-OXIDE Plant

ASCORBIC-ACID Plant 17–129 ppm Pt 58–2,778 ppm Seed 171–182 ppm

ASH Pt 6,000–219,000 ppm Root 8,300–100,000 ppm Seed 85,500–106,294 ppm

ASPARAGINE Root

ASPARTIC-ACID Pt 1,130–23,880 ppm

BENTONITE Plant

BENZOIC-ACID-4-O-BETA-D-GLUCOSIDE Root 3 ppm Seed 56 ppm

BENZOYL-BENZOATE Leaf

BENZYL-AMINE Stem 3.4 ppm

BERGAPTEN Plant 1–520 ppm Pt 0.04–0.35 ppm Seed 1 ppm

BETA-CAROTENE Pt 1–144 ppm

BETA-CARYOPHYLLENE Fruit Essent. Oil 5,000–43,000 ppm Leaf Essent. Oil 5,000 ppm Seed 95–1,075 ppm

BETA-ELEMENE Fruit Essent. Oil 35,000 ppm Leaf Seed 1–875 ppm

BETA-EUDESMOL Seed 76–225 ppm

BETA-HUMULENE Seed

BETA-PHELLANDRENE Fruit 2,000 ppm

BETA-PINENE Fruit Essent. Oil 5–15,000 ppm Seed 57–210 ppm

BETA-SELINENE Fruit Essent. Oil 55,000–325,000 ppm Leaf Essent. Oil 30,000 ppm Seed 209–8,125 ppm Stem Essent. Oil 10,000 ppm

BORON Root 4–103 ppm Seed 43–61 ppm

BROMINE Root
BUTYLIDENE-NAPHTHALIDE Essential Oil
BUTYLIDENE-PHTHALIDE Et 12,000 ppm Fruit
Essent. Oil 4,000 ppm Leaf Essent. Oil 15,000
ppm
BUTYLPHENYL-KETONE Plant
CADMIUM Root 0.001–0.364 ppm
CAFFEIC-ACID Leaf
CALCIUM Pt 313–11,918 ppm Root 340–3,635
ppm Seed 15,814–20,776 ppm
CAMPHENE Leaf Essent. Oil 1,000 ppm
CAPRIC-ACID Leaf 200–213 ppm
CAR-3-ENE Essential Oil
CARBOHYDRATES Pt 36,300–684,980 ppm
Seed 413,500–439,964 ppm
CAROTENES Leaf 80–145 ppm
CARVEOL-ACETATE Plant
CARVONE Essential Oil 2,000–5,000 ppm Fruit
Essent. Oil 550,000 ppm Leaf 1 ppm Seed
19–75 ppm
CARVYL-ACETATE Leaf
CELEREOIN Seed 13.3 ppm
CELEREOSIDE Seed
CELERIN Seed
CELEROSIDE Seed
CHLOROGENIC-ACID Leaf
CHOLINE Root
CHOLINE-ASCORBATE Leaf
CHROMIUM Root 0.002–0.045 ppm
CHRYSOERIOL-7-APIOSYL-GLUCOSIDE Seed
CIS-1(7),8-DIEN-2-OL Plant
CIS-3-HEXEN-1-YL-PYRUVATE Leaf
CIS-3-HEXENOL Essential Oil
CIS-3-HEXENOL-PYRUVATE Plant
CIS-3-HEXENYL-ACETATE Plant
CIS-CARVEOL Fruit Essent. Oil 1,000 ppm
CIS-CARVYL-ACETATE Leaf
CIS-DIHYDRO-ISOCARVONE Fruit Essent. Oil
15,000 ppm
CIS-DIHYDROCARVONE Seed 1 ppm
CIS-LIMONENE-OXIDE Seed
CIS-OCIMENE Et 78,000 ppm Leaf 2,000–2,500
ppm Leaf Essent. Oil 145,000 ppm Root Es-
sent. Oil 68,000 ppm
CIS-P-MENTHA-1(7),8-DIEN-2-YL-ACETATE
Plant
CIS-P-MENTHA-2,8-DIEN-1-OL Seed
CITRIC-ACID Pt

CITRONELLAL Leaf
CITRONELLYL-ACETATE Leaf
CNIDILIDE Root
COBALT Root
COPPER Pt 0.4–7 ppm Root 0.7–11 ppm Seed
14 ppm
COUMARIN Plant
CYSTINE Pt 40–755 ppm
D-SELINENE Seed 2,000–3,000 ppm
DECYL-ACETATE Leaf
DEHYDROASCORBIC-ACID Plant
DI-N-PROPYL-AMINE Pt 0.9 ppm
DIACETYL Leaf
DIHYDROCARVEOL Fruit Essent. Oil 2,000
ppm Leaf
DIHYDROCARVONE Essential Oil 5,000 ppm
Seed 19–75 ppm
DIHYDROCARVYL-ACETATE Plant
DIHYDRONEOCARVEOL Fruit Essent. Oil 1,000
ppm
DIHYDRONEOISOCARVEOL Fruit Essent. Oil
2,000 ppm
DIMETHYL-AMINE Pt 5.1 ppm
DODECANAL Leaf
E-BUTYLIDENEPHTHALIDE Plant
E-LIGUSTILIDE Plant 1 ppm
EO Seed 19,000–30,000 ppm
EUDESMOL Fruit Essent. Oil 5,000–10,000 ppm
EUGENOL Plant
FALCARINDIOL Root 3.3 ppm
FALCARINONE Root 1.7 ppm
FAT Leaf 1,300–42,000 ppm Seed
242,730–279,483 ppm
FERULIC-ACID Root
FIBER Pt 6,900–158,000 ppm Seed
106,750–138,586 ppm
FOLIACIN Pt 0.3–5.6 ppm
FORMALDEHYDE Plant
FRUCTOSE Plant
FUMARIC-ACID Pt
GALACTOSE Plant
GALACTURONIC-ACID Plant
GAMMA-SELINENE Plant
GAMMA-TERPINEOL Fruit Essent. Oil
3,000–5,000 ppm Seed 57–125 ppm
GENTISIC-ACID Leaf
GERANYL-ACETATE Leaf
GERANYL-BUTYRATE Leaf

GLUCOSE Plant

GLUCOSIDASE Plant

GLUTAMIC-ACID Pt 860–18,285 ppm

GLUTAMINE Root

GLYCINE Pt 210–4,290 ppm

GLYCOLIC-ACID Root

GRAVEOBIOSIDE-A Seed

GRAVEOBIOSIDE-B Seed

GUAIACOL Leaf Seed

HEPTANAL Leaf

HEPTANOL Leaf

HEXANAL Leaf

HEXANOL Leaf

HISTIDINE Pt 110–2,425 ppm

HYPOXANTHINE Plant

INDOSTEROL Pt 300 ppm

INOSINE Plant

INOSITOL Leaf

IRON Pt 3–347 ppm Root 3.6–47 ppm Seed
    361–571 ppm

ISOAMYL-ALCOHOL Leaf

ISOBUTYLIDENE Leaf 32 ppm

ISOBUTYLIDENE-3-A,4-DIHYDROPHTHALIDE
    Et 21,000 ppm Fruit Essent. Oil 17,000 ppm
    Leaf Essent. Oil 40,000 ppm

ISOBUTYRIC-ACID Leaf Plant

ISOCHLOROGENIC-ACID Leaf

ISOCITRIC-ACID Root

ISOIMPERATORIN Seed

ISOLEUCINE Pt 200–4,290 ppm

ISOPIMPINELLIN Plant 4–122 ppm Pt
    0.05–0.41 ppm

ISOQUERCITRIN Seed

ISOVALERIC-ACID Seed 1 ppm

ISOVALERIC-ACID-ETHYL-ESTER Plant

KETO-ALCOHOL Seed 2,140–3,390 ppm

LAURIC-ACID Seed 200–213 ppm

LEAD Root 0.01–2 ppm

LEUCINE Pt 310–6,530 ppm

LIGUSTILIDE Essential Oil 2,000–5,000 ppm

LIMONENE Et 695,000 ppm Fruit Essent. Oil
    350,000–706,000 ppm Root Essent. Oil
    117,000 ppm Seed 530–24,000 ppm

LINALOL Seed 1 ppm

LINALYL-ACETATE Leaf

LINASE Plant

LINOLEIC-ACID Leaf 60–1,132 ppm Pt
    690–12,875 ppm Seed 31,310–41,592 ppm

LUTEOLIN Leaf

LUTEOLIN-7-APIOSYL-GLUCOSIDE Fruit

LUTEOLIN-7-O-BETA-GLUCOSIDE Plant

LUTEOLIN-GLYCOSIDE Plant

LYSINE Pt 260–5,410 ppm

MAGNESIUM Leaf 99–2,650 ppm Root
    140–1,635 ppm Seed 4,192–4,903 ppm

MALIC-ACID Pt

MANGANESE Pt 1–33 ppm Root 0.74–23 ppm
    Seed 76 ppm

MANNITOL Root 50,000 ppm Stem
    10,000–20,000 ppm

MENTHONE Essential Oil

MERCURY Root 0.027 ppm

METHIONINE Pt 50–1,120 ppm

METHYL-AMINE Pt 6.4 ppm

MOLYBDENUM Root

MUCILAGE Plant

MUFA Pt 270–5,035 ppm

MYRCENE Et 18,000 ppm Fruit Essent. Oil
    2,000–61,000 ppm Leaf Essent. Oil 14,000
    ppm Root Essent. Oil 18,000 ppm Seed
    190–300 ppm

MYRISTIC-ACID Pt 10–190 ppm Seed 200–213
    ppm

MYRISTICIN Plant

N-6-BENZYL-ADENINE Seed

N-6-BENZYL-ADENINE-RIBOSIDE Seed

N-6-ISOPENT-2-ENYL-ADENOSINE Seed

N-BUTYLPHTHALIDE Fruit Essent. Oil
    50,000–72,000 ppm Root 30 ppm Seed
    190–1,800 ppm

N-METHYL-ANILINE Pt 7 ppm

N-METHYL-PHENETHYLAMINE Pt 0.5 ppm

N-PENTYL-AMINE Pt 0.8 ppm

N-PENTYL-BENZENE Seed 190–300 ppm

N-PENTYL-CYCLOHEXADIENE Fruit Essent. Oil
    3,000 ppm Leaf Essent. Oil 17,000 ppm

N-PROPYL-AMINE Pt 2.7 ppm

NEOCNIDILIDE Plant 70–260 ppm

NEOCNIDOLIDE Root 17 ppm

NERAL Leaf

NERYL-ACETATE Leaf

NIACIN Pt 3–57 ppm

NICKEL Root 0.04–0.9 ppm

NICOTINE Plant

NITROGEN Root 2,000–19,090 ppm

NODAKENETIC Seed

NODAKENIN Seed
OCTANAL Leaf
OLEIC-ACID Pt 230–4,850 ppm Seed
  146,440–162,560 ppm
OSTHENOL Seed
OXALIC-ACID Plant
P-COUMARIC-ACID Root
P-COUMAROYL-QUINIC-ACID Leaf
P-CYMENE Et 17,000 ppm Fruit Essent. Oil
  2,000–31,000 ppm Root Essent. Oil 31,000
  ppm Seed 190–775 ppm
P-HYDROXYCINNAMIC-ACID Plant
P-MENTH-8(9)-ENE-1,2-DIOL Essential Oil
P-MENTHA-8(9)-EN-1,2-DIOL Seed
P-METHOXY-CINNAMIC-ACID Seed 7.5 ppm
PALMITIC-ACID Pt 280–5,970 ppm Seed
  9,470–17,375 ppm
PALMITOLEIC-ACID Pt 10–190 ppm
PANTOTHENIC-ACID Pt 1–36 ppm
PECTIN Leaf 3,000 ppm
PENTOSANE Root 1,600 ppm
PENTYL-BENZENE Fruit Essent. Oil 9,000 ppm
  Leaf Essent. Oil 2,000 ppm
PERILLALDEHYDE Seed 1 ppm
PEROXIDASE Plant
PETROSELINIC-ACID Seed 2,400–2,554 ppm
PHENYLALANINE Leaf 190–4,105 ppm
PHOSPHORUS Pt 201–6,849 ppm Root
  470–7,900 ppm Seed 4,509–6,843 ppm
PHYTOSTEROLS Pt 60–1,120 ppm
PINOCARVYL-ACETATE Plant
PIPERIDINE Pt 1 ppm
PIPERITONE Fruit
POLYACETYLENES Root
POTASSIUM Pt 2,689–57,800 ppm Root
  3,900–56,360 ppm Seed 13,592–15,330 ppm
PROLINE Leaf 170–3,208 ppm
PROPIONALDEHYDE Leaf 3 ppm
PROTEIN Pt 6,030–194,000 ppm Seed
  170,250–203,385 ppm
PROTOCATECHUIC-ACID Plant
PSORALEN Plant Pt 0.03–0.15 ppm
PUFA Pt 690–12,875 ppm
PYRROLIDINE Pt 0.4–2.6 ppm
PYRUVIC-ACID Plant
QUERCETIN-3-0-GALACTOSIDE Plant
QUERCETIN-3-O-BETA-GLUCOSIDE Plant
QUINIC-ACID Pt

RIBOFLAVIN Pt 34 ppm
RUBIDIUM Root 0.24–9 ppm
RUTARETIN Seed 10 ppm
RUTIN Plant 170 ppm
S-METHYL-METHIONINE Plant
SABINENE Seed
SANTALOL Seed 874–1,150 ppm
SCOPOLETIN Plant
SCOPOLIN Leaf
SEDANENOLIDE Seed 95–900 ppm
SEDANOIC-ACID Plant
SEDANOIC-ALDEHYDE Plant
SEDANOIC-ANHYDRIDE Essential Oil
  30,000–80,000 ppm
SEDANOLIDE Seed
SEDANOLINE Plant
SEDANONIC-ANHYDRIDE Leaf 570–15,750
  ppm
SELANOLIDE Plant
SELENIUM Root
SENKYUNOLIDE Root 30–240 ppm
SERINE Pt 200–4,105 ppm
SESALIN Seed
SFA Pt 370–6,900 ppm
SHIKIMIC-ACID Root
SILICON Root 2 ppm
SINAPIC-ACID Plant
SODIUM Pt 774–17,135 ppm Seed
  1,424–1,900 ppm
SPINOSTEROL Plant
STEARIC-ACID Pt 30–560 ppm Seed
  3,100–5,000 ppm
SUCCINIC-ACID Pt
SUCCINIC-ACID-DEHYDROGENASE Plant
SUCROSE Plant
SULFUR Root 100–1,000 ppm
TARTARIC-ACID Pt
TERPINEN-4-OL Leaf Essent. Oil 1,000 ppm
  Seed 1–1,400 ppm
TERPINEOLENE Root Essent. Oil 33,000 ppm
TERPINOLENE Fruit Essent. Oil 2,000 ppm Leaf
  Essent. Oil 2,000 ppm
THIAMIN Pt 10 ppm
THREONINE Pt 190–4,105 ppm
THYMOL Plant
TIGLIC-ACID Plant
TOLUIDINE Pt 1.1 ppm
TRANS-1,2-EPOXYLIMONENE Seed 1 ppm

TRANS-2-HEXENOL Essential Oil

TRANS-3-HEXENOL Essential Oil

TRANS-ANETHOLE Plant 1 ppm

TRANS-CARVEOL Fruit Essent. Oil 1,000 ppm

TRANS-CARVYL-ACETATE Plant 1 ppm

TRANS-DIHYROCARVONE Fruit Essent. Oil 14,000 ppm

TRANS-FARNESENE Essential Oil

TRANS-LIMONENE-OXIDE Seed

TRANS-OCIMENE Et 67,000 ppm Fruit Essent. Oil 3,000 ppm Leaf Leaf Essent. Oil 20,000 ppm Root Essent. Oil 201,000 ppm

TRANS-P-MENTHA-1(7),8-DIEN-2-OL Seed

TRANS-P-MENTHA-2,8-DIEN-1-OL Seed

TRYPTOPHAN Pt 90–1,865 ppm

TYROSINE Pt 90–1,865 ppm

UMBELLIFERONE Seed

UNDECANAL Leaf

URONIC-ACID Root

VALERIC-ACID Flower

VALINE Pt 260–5,600 ppm

VELLEIN Seed

VIT-B-6 Leaf 6 ppm

VIT-U Pt 41–96 ppm

WATER Pt 927,000–947,000 ppm Root 890,000 ppm Seed 60,400 ppm

XANTHOTOXIN Plant 6–183 ppm Pt 0.04–0.61 ppm

XYLOSE Plant

Z-BUTYLIDENEPHTHALIDE Plant

Z-LIGUSTILIDE Plant 1–5 ppm

ZEATIN Seed

ZEATIN-RIBOSIDE Seed

ZINC Leaf 1–44 ppm Root 2.8–70 ppm Seed 54–89 ppm

CHICORY

Chemicals in *Cichorium intybus L.* (*Asteraceae*)—Chicory, Succory, Witloof

11(S),13-DIHYDRO-8-DEOXYLACTUCIN Root

11(S),13-DIHYDROLACTUCIN Root

11(S),13-DIHYDROLACTUCOPICRIN Root

8-DEOXYLACTUCIN Root

ACETOPHENONE Root

ALPHA-LINOLENIC-ACID Leaf 60–1,224 ppm Root 130–650 ppm

ARGININE Leaf 730–14,892 ppm

ASCORBIC-ACID Leaf 100–2,040 ppm Root 50–250 ppm

ASH Leaf 6,000–180,000 ppm Root 8,900–44,500 ppm

BETA-CAROTENE Leaf 228 ppm

BETAINE Root

BORON Root 20 ppm

CAFFEIC-ACID Leaf 767 ppm

CALCIUM Leaf 790–18,900 ppm Root 410–2,050 ppm

CARBOHYDRATES Leaf 32,000–654,000 ppm Root 175,100–875,500 ppm

CELLULOSE Root

CHOLINE Root

CICHORIC-ACID Leaf

CICHORIIN Flower 1,000–2,000 ppm

ESCULETIN Flower

ESCULIN Flower

FAT Leaf 1,000–29,000 ppm Root 2,000–10,000 ppm

FERULIC-ACID Plant

FIBER Plant 9,000–153,000 ppm Root 19,500–97,500 ppm

FRUCTOSE Root 45,000–220,000 ppm

GLUCOSE Root 11,000 ppm

HARMAN Root

HISTIDINE Leaf 170–3,468 ppm

INOSITOL Root

INULIN Root 110,000–580,000 ppm

IRON Leaf 5–246 ppm Root 8–40 ppm

ISOLEUCINE Leaf 600–12,240 ppm

JACQUINELIN Root

KAEMPFEROL Plant

LACTUCIN Latex Exudate

LACTUCIN-P-OXYPHENYLACETICACID-ESTER Root

LACTUCOPICRIN Root

LEUCINE Leaf 440–8,976 ppm

LINOLEIC-ACID Leaf 370–7,548 ppm Root 750–3,750 ppm

LYSINE Leaf 390–7,956 ppm

MAGNESIUM Leaf 130–2,652 ppm Root 220–1,100 ppm

MANNAN Root

MANNITOL Plant

MANNOSE Root

METHIONINE Leaf 60–1,224 ppm

MYRISTIC-ACID Leaf 10–204 ppm Root 30–150 ppm

NIACIN Leaf 5–102 ppm Root 4–20 ppm

NORHARMAN Root

OLEIC-ACID Leaf 20–408 ppm Root 40–200 ppm

P-HYDROXY-BENZOIC-ACID Leaf 11 ppm

PALMITIC-ACID Leaf 210–4,284 ppm Root 410–2,050 ppm

PALMITOLEIC-ACID Root 750–3,750 ppm

PECTIN Root

PENTOSANE Root 47,000–65,000 ppm

PHENYLALANINE Leaf 240–4,896 ppm

PHOSPHORUS Leaf 210–4,284 ppm Root 610–3,050 ppm

POTASSIUM Leaf 1,820–37,128 ppm Root 2,900–14,500 ppm

PROTEIN Leaf 10,000–246,000 ppm Root 14,000–70,000 ppm

PROTOCATECHUIC-ALDEHYDE Seed

QUERCETIN Plant

RIBOFLAVIN Leaf 1–29 ppm Root 2 ppm

SCOPOLETIN Flower

SINAPIC-ACID Plant

SODIUM Leaf 70–1,428 ppm Root 500–2,500 ppm

STEARIC-ACID Leaf 10–204 ppm Root 20–100 ppm

TANNIN Plant

TARAXASTEROL Root

THIAMIN Leaf 1–14 ppm Root 2 ppm

THREONINE Leaf 280–5,712 ppm

TRYPTOPHAN Leaf 180–3,672 ppm

UMBELLIFERONE Flower

VALINE Leaf 450–9,180 ppm

VANILLIC-ACID Leaf 0.5 ppm

WATER Leaf 931,000–951,000 ppm Root 777,000–800,000 ppm

CHIVES

Chemicals in *Allium schoenoprasum L.* (*Liliaceae*)—Chives

1-O-FERULOYL-BETA-D-GLUCOSE Leaf

1-O-P-COUMAROYL-BETA-D-GLUCOSE Leaf

2-METHYL-2-BUTENAL Plant

2-METHYL-2-PENTENAL Plant

3,5-DIETHYL-1,2,4-TRITHIOLANE Leaf

ALANINE Leaf 1,260–15,750 ppm

ALLITHIAMINE Plant

ALLYL-DISULFIDE Plant

ALLYL-MERCAPTAN Plant

ALPHA-LINOLENIC-ACID Leaf 130–1,625 ppm

ARGININE Leaf 2,020–25,250 ppm

ASCORBIC-ACID Leaf 57–9,875 ppm

ASH Leaf 4,000–100,000 ppm

ASPARTIC-ACID Leaf 2,590–32,375 ppm

BETA-CAROTENE Leaf 34–475 ppm

CAFFEIC-ACID Leaf

CALCIUM Leaf 690–10,375 ppm

CARBOHYDRATES Leaf 38,000–667,000 ppm

CIS-PENTYL-HYDRO-DISULFIDE Essential Oil

CIS-PROPENYL-PROPYL-DISULFIDE Plant

CITRIC-ACID Leaf

DESOXYRIBONUCLEIC-ACID Plant

DIPROPYL-DISULFIDE Essential Oil

DOTRIACONTANAL Plant

FAT Leaf 3,000–75,000 ppm

FERULIC-ACID Leaf

FIBER Leaf 7,000–137,500 ppm

FUMARIC-ACID Leaf

GALACTOSE Plant

GAMMA-GLUTAMYL-PEPTIDASE Plant

GAMMA-GLUTAMYL-PEPTIDE Plant

GAMMA-GLUTAMYL-S-ALLYLCYSTEINE Plant

GAMMA-GLUTAMYL-TRIPEPTIDE Plant

GLUCOSE Plant

GLUTAMIC-ACID Leaf 5,790–72,385 ppm

GLYCINE Leaf 1,390–17,375 ppm

HISTIDINE Leaf 480–6,000 ppm

IRON Leaf 8–200 ppm

ISOLEUCINE Leaf 1,190–14,875 ppm

ISORHAMNETIN-GLYCOSIDE Plant

KAEMPFEROL Leaf 6–55 ppm

KAEMPFEROL-DIGLUCOSIDE Plant

KAEMPFEROL-GLUCOSIDE Plant

KAEMPFEROL-TRIGLUCOSIDE Plant

LEUCINE Leaf 1,670–20,875 ppm

LINOLEIC-ACID Leaf 2,220–27,750 ppm

MAGNESIUM Leaf 550–6,875 ppm

MALIC-ACID Leaf

METHIONINE Leaf 300–3,750 ppm

METHYL-ALLYL-ALLITHIAMINE Plant

METHYL-DISULFIDE Plant

METHYL-PENTYL-DISULFIDE Essential Oil

METHYL-PROPYL-DISULFIDE Plant

MYRISTIC-ACID Leaf 30–375 ppm
NIACIN Leaf 5–88 ppm
OCTACOSANOL Plant
OLEIC-ACID Leaf 840–10,500 ppm
OXALIC-ACID Plant
P-COUMARIC-ACID Leaf 21 ppm
PALMITIC-ACID Leaf 910–11,375 ppm
PANTOTHENIC-ACID Leaf 2–22 ppm
PENTYL-HYDRO-DISULFIDE Essential Oil 25,000 ppm
PHENYLALANINE Leaf 900–11,250 ppm
PHOSPHORUS Leaf 410–6,437 ppm
POTASSIUM Leaf 2,500–31,250 ppm
PROLINE Leaf 1,850–23,125 ppm
PROPYL-ALLYL-ALLITHIAMINE Plant
PROTEIN Leaf 18,000–350,000 ppm
QUERCETIN Leaf 4–9 ppm
QUINIC-ACID Leaf
RIBOFLAVIN Leaf 1–22 ppm
S-(PROPENYL-1-YL)-CYSTEINE-SULFOXIDE Plant
SAPONIN Leaf
SCORDININE Plant
SERINE Leaf 1,260–15,750 ppm
SODIUM Leaf 60–750 ppm
STEARIC-ACID Leaf 80–1,000 ppm
SUCCINIC-ACID Leaf
THIAMIN Leaf 1–12 ppm
THREONINE Leaf 1,110–13,875 ppm
TRANS-PENTYL-HYDRO-DISULFIDE Essential Oil
TRANS-PROPENYL-PROPYL-DISULFIDE Plant
TRIACONTANAL Plant
TRYPTOPHAN Leaf 310–3,875 ppm
TYROSINE Leaf 810–10,125 ppm
VALINE Leaf 1,240–15,500 ppm
VIT-B-6 Leaf 2–22 ppm
WATER Leaf 913,000–920,000 ppm

COLLARDS

Chemicals in *Brassica oleracea L.* (*Brassicaceae*)—Collards

ALANINE Leaf 670–10,981 ppm
ALPHA-LINOLENIC-ACID Plant
ARGININE Leaf 800–13,112 ppm
ASCORBIC-ACID Leaf 233–3,819 ppm

ASH Leaf 5,500–90,145 ppm
ASPARTIC-ACID Leaf 1,200–19,668 ppm
BETA-CAROTENE Leaf 20–328 ppm
CALCIUM Leaf 1,170–19,180 ppm
CARBOHYDRATES Leaf 37,600–616,264 ppm
COPPER Leaf 2–43 ppm
CYSTINE Leaf 160–2,624 ppm
FAT Leaf 2,200–36,058 ppm
FIBER Leaf 5,700–93,423 ppm
FOLACIN Leaf 0.83–2.4 ppm
GLUCOBRASSICANAPIN Seed
GLUCONAPIN Seed
GLUTAMIC-ACID Leaf 1,310–21,471 ppm
GLYCINE Leaf 600–9,834 ppm
HISTIDINE Leaf 300–4,917 ppm
IRON Leaf 6–102 ppm
ISOLEUCINE Leaf 640–10,490 ppm
KILOCALORIES Leaf 190–3,112 /kg
LEUCINE Leaf 970–15,900 ppm
LINOLEIC-ACID Plant
LYSINE Leaf 750–12,293 ppm
MAGNESIUM Leaf 170–2,786 ppm
MANGANESE Leaf 4–60 ppm
METHIONINE Leaf 210–3,442 ppm
MYRISTIC-ACID Plant
NAPOLEIFERIN Seed
NIACIN Leaf 3.7–61 ppm
OLEIC-ACID Plant
OXALATE Leaf 4,500–73,755 ppm
PALMITIC-ACID Plant
PALMITOLEIC-ACID Plant
PANTOTHENIC-ACID Leaf 0.64–10.5 ppm
PHENYLALANINE Leaf 560–9,178 ppm
PHOSPHORUS Leaf 160–2,622 ppm
PHYTOSTEROLS Plant
POTASSIUM Leaf 1,480–24,257 ppm
PROGOITRIN Seed
PROLINE Leaf 670–10,981 ppm
PROTEIN Leaf 15,700–257,323 ppm
RIBOFLAVIN Leaf 0.6–10.5 ppm
SERINE Leaf 500–8,195 ppm
SINIGRIN Seed
SODIUM Leaf 280–4,589 ppm
STEARIC-ACID Plant
THIAMIN Leaf 0.3–4.75 ppm
THREONINE Leaf 550–9,014 ppm
TRYPTOPHAN Leaf 200–3,278 ppm
TYROSINE Leaf 420–6,884 ppm

VALINE Leaf 770–12,620 ppm

VIT-B-6 Leaf 0.7–11 ppm

WATER Leaf 932,500–945,500 ppm

ZINC Leaf 10–157 ppm

CORN

Chemicals in *Zea mays L.* (*Poaceae*)—Corn

1,1-DIPHENYL-ETHANE Leaf

1,2,3-TRIMETHYL-BENZENE Silk Stigma Style

1,2,4-TRIMETHYL-BENZENE Silk Stigma Style

1,2-DIMETHOXY-BENZENE Hull Husk

1,2-DIMETHYL-4-ETHYL-BENZENE Silk Stigma Style

1,3-AMINO-PROPYL-PYRROLINIUM Sprout Seedling

1,3-DIMETHYL-4-ETHYL-BENZENE Silk Stigma Style

1,8-CINEOLE Silk Stigma Style

1-(3-METHYL-2-FURYL)PROPANE Leaf

1-ACETO-METHYL-NAPTHONE Leaf

1-ACETO-NAPTHONE Leaf

1-O-FERULOYL-BETA-D-GLUCOSE Leaf

1-O-SINAPOYL-BETA-D-GLUCOSE Leaf

1-P-HYDROXY-TRANS-CINNAMOYL)-GLYC-EROL Seed 45 ppm 1.2 Seed

2"-O-ALPHA-RHAMNOSYL-6C-(6-DEOXO-XYLO-HEXOS-4-ULOSYL)-APIGENIN Plant

2"-O-ALPHA-RHAMNOSYL-6C-(6-DEOXO-XYLO-HEXOS-4-ULOSYL)-CHRYSOERIOL Plant

2(3)-BENZOXAZOLINONE Sprout Seedling

2,3-DIHYDRO-2-PYRAN-2-CARBOXALDEHYDE Leaf

2,4-DIHYDROXY-6,7-DIMETHOXY-2H,1,4-BEN-ZOXAZIN-3-ONE Sprout Seedling

2,4-METHYLENE-CHOLESTEROL Pollen Or Spore

2-(2,4-DIHYDROXY-1,4(2H)-BENZOXAZIN-3(4H)-ON-BETA-D-GLUCOSIDE Sprout Seedling

2-(2,4-DIHYDROXY-7-METHOXY-1,4(2H)-BEN-ZOXAZIN-3(4H9 Plant

2-(2,4-DIHYDROXY-7-METHOXY-1,4-BENZOX-AZIN-3-ONE-BETA-D-GLUCOPYRANOSIDE Sprout Seedling

2-(2-HYDROXY-1,4(2H)-BENZOXAZIN-3(4H)-ON-BETA-D-GLUCOSIDE Sprout Seedling

2-(2-HYDROXY-7-METHOXY-1,4(2H)-BENZOX-AZIN-3(4H)-ON-BETA-D-GLUCOSIDE Sprout Seedling

2-(2-HYDROXY-7-METHOXY-1,4-BENZOX-AZIN-3-ONE-BETA-D-GLUCOPYRANOSIDE Root

2-(5-CHLORO-2-HYDROXY-7-METHOXY-1,4(2H)-BENZOXAZIN-3(4H0)-ONE-BETA-D-GLU COPYRANOSIDE Root

2-ACETO-NAPTHONE Leaf

2-ETHYL-1-CYCLOHEXEN-1-YL Essential Oil

2-ETHYL-HEX-AN-1-OL Plant

2-METHYL-BUTAN-1-AL Silk Stigma Style

2-METHYL-BUTAN-1-OL Silk Stigma Style

2-METHYL-NAPHTHALENE Silk Essent. Oil

2-METHYL-PENT-2-EN-1-AL Silk Stigma Style

2-METHYL-PENTAN-3-ONE Silk Stigma Style

2-METHYL-PROPAN-1-OL Silk Stigma Style

2-O-CAFFEOYLHYDROXY-CITRIC-ACID Shoot

2-O-FERULOYL-HYDROXY-CITRIC-ACID Shoot

2-O-P-COUMAROYL-HYDROXY-CITRIC-ACID Shoot

2-PENTYL-FURAN Essential Oil 10,000 ppm Plant Silk Essent. Oil 3,000 ppm

2-PHENYLALDEHYDE Leaf

2-THIOPHENE-ACETALDEHYDE Leaf

24-ETHYL-CHOLESTEROL Root

24-ETHYLIDENE-LOPHENOL Shoot

24-METHYL-23-DEHYDRO-CHOLESTEROL Seed Oil

24-METHYL-CHOLESTEROL Root

24-METHYLENE-CYCLOARTENOL Plant

24-METHYLENE-LOPHENOL Shoot

3'-NUCLEOTIDASE Tissue Culture

3'-O-METHYL-MAYSIN Silk Stigma Style

3,7-DIHYDROXY-INDOLIN-2-ONE-3-ACETIC-ACID-7'-O-BETA-D-GLUCOSIDE Plant

3-FERULOYLQUINIC-ACID Leaf

3-METHYL-BUTAN-1-OL Silk Stigma Style

3-METHYL-INDOLE Leaf

3-O-CAFFEOYLQUINIC-ACID Plant

3-O-COUMARYLQUINIC-ACID Plant

4-ETHYL-GUAIACOL Seed

4-HYDROXY-BENZOIC-ACID Tissue Culture

4-METHYL-GUAIACOL Seed

4-VINYL-4-DEETHYL-CHLOROPHYLL-A Plant

4-VINYL-GUAIACOL Seed

4-VINYL-PHENOL Seed

5,6-DIHYDRO-2-PYRAN-2-CARBOXALDEHYDE Leaf

5-DEHYDRO-AVENASTEROL Seed

5-HYDROXY-TRANS-FERULIC-ACID Plant

5-O-CAFFEOYLQUINIC-ACID Plant

5-O-COUMARYLQUINIC-ACID Plant

5-O-FERULOYLQUINIC-ACID Plant

6,7-DIMETHOXY-2-BENZOXAZOLIN-2-ONE Plant

6-METHOXY-2-(3)-BENZOXAZOLINONE Shoot

6-METHOXY-BENZOXAZOLIN-2-ONE Plant

7-DEHYDRO-AVENASTEROL Seed

8-HYDROXY-QUINOL-2-ONE-4-CARBOXYLIC-ACID-8'-O-BETA-D-GLUCOSIDE Plant

ABSCISIC-ACID Flower

ABSCISSIN-II Seed

ACETOIN Plant

ACONITIC-ACID Root

ADENINE Seed

ADENOSINE Seed

ALANINE Seed 2,950–12,272 ppm

ALDOBIOURONIC-ACID Plant

ALLANTOIN Seed

ALPHA-AMYLASE Plant

ALPHA-AMYRIN Plant

ALPHA-CAROTENE Seed 0.5–2.5 ppm

ALPHA-COPAENE Leaf

ALPHA-GLUCOSIDASE Plant

ALPHA-LINOLENIC-ACID Seed 160–666 ppm

ALPHA-MUUROLENE Plant

ALPHA-PINENE Husk Essent. Oil

ALPHA-SITOSTEROL Plant

ALPHA-TERPINEOL Silk Stigma Style

ALPHA-TOCOPHEROL Oil 90–257 ppm

ALPHA-YLANGENE Essential Oil 17,000 ppm

ALPHA-ZEACAROTENE Plant

ALPHA-ZEIN Seed

ALUMINUM Seed 1–275 ppm Silk Stigma Style 213 ppm

AMINO-ADIPIC-ACID Plant

AMMONIA(NH3) Seed 1,030 ppm

ANILINE Seed

ANTHERAXANTHIN Leaf

ANTHRANILIC-ACID Leaf

ANTHRANILIC-ACID-BETA-D-GLUCOSIDE Leaf

APIFOROL Silk Stigma Style

APIGENIDIN Silk Stigma Style

APIGENIN-GLYCOSIDE Plant

ARABINOSE Plant

ARACHIDIC-ACID Plant

ARGININE Seed 1,310–5,450 ppm

ARSENIC Seed 0.001–0.211 ppm

ASCORBIC-ACID Seed 85 ppm Silk Stigma Style 11 ppm

ASH Seed 10,000–90,000 ppm Silk Stigma Style 33,000 ppm

ASPARTIC-ACID Seed 2,440–10,150 ppm

ASTRAGALIN Pollen Or Spore

BARIUM Seed 14 ppm

BAZZANENE Root

BENZALDEHYDE Silk Essent. Oil 1,000 ppm

BENZOTHIAZOLE Leaf

BENZOXAZIONE Sprout Seedling

BENZYL-AMINE Seed 3.4 ppm

BENZYL-FORMATE Leaf

BETA-AMYLASE Plant

BETA-AMYRIN Shoot

BETA-CAROTENE Seed 0.5–2.5 ppm Silk Stigma Style

BETA-CARYOPHYLLENE Root

BETA-COPAENE Leaf

BETA-IONONE Leaf Plant Silk Essent. Oil 1,000 ppm

BETA-PINENE Silk Essent. Oil 3,000 ppm

BETA-SITOSTEROL Silk Stigma Style 1,300 ppm

BETA-ZEACAROTENE Plant

BETA-ZEIN Plant

BETAINE Root 59 ppm Shoot 234 ppm Silk Stigma Style

BIOTIN Cob 0.02–0.06 ppm

BIPHENYL Silk Stigma Style

BISABOLOL Essential Oil

BORON Seed 15 ppm

BUTAN-1-OL Silk Stigma Style

BUTENYL-ISOTHIOCYANATE Seed

CADAVERINE Plant

CADMIUM Seed 1 ppm

CAFFEIC-ACID Shoot 0.7 ppm

CAFFEIC-ACID-ESTER Leaf

CALCIUM Seed 10–181 ppm Silk Stigma Style 2,520 ppm

CAMPESTEROL Seed

CARBOHYDRATES Seed 190,209–838,000 ppm Silk Stigma Style 825,000 ppm

CARVACROL Seed Silk Stigma Style 144–216 ppm

CARYOPHYLLENE Leaf

CASTASTERONE Pollen Or Spore 0.12 ppm

CELLULOSE Plant

CHELIDONIC-ACID Shoot 158 ppm

CHLORINE Fruit 330 ppm

CHOLESTEROL Seed

CHOLINE Root 36 ppm Seed 430 ppm Shoot 85 ppm

CHROMIUM Seed 1.65 ppm Silk Stigma Style 13 ppm

CINNAMIC-ACID-ETHYL-ESTER Silk Stigma Style

CITRONELLOL Leaf

COBALT Fruit 0.01–0.8 ppm Silk Stigma Style 64 ppm

COIXOL Plant

COPPER Fruit 20 ppm

COUMARIC-ACID-ESTER Leaf

COUMARIN Leaf

CROCETIN Leaf

CRYPTOXANTHIN Plant

CUBEBENOL Leaf

CYANIDIN Silk Stigma Style

CYANIDIN-3-(6'-MALONYL-GLUCOSIDE) Leaf

CYANIDIN-3-DIMALONYL-GLUCOSIDE Leaf

CYANIDIN-3-GALACTOSIDE-P-COUMARIC-ACID-ESTER Plant

CYANIDIN-3-MONOSIDE Plant

CYANIN Cob

CYCLOARTENOL Shoot

CYCLOEUCALENOL Shoot

CYCLOSADOL Seed

CYCLOSATIVENE Leaf

CYSTATHIONE Plant

CYSTINE Seed 260–1,082 ppm

D-GLUCURONIC-ACID Plant

DAUCOSTEROL Silk Stigma Style 440 ppm

DEC-TRANS-2-CIS-4-DIEN-1-AL Plant Silk Essent. Oil 7,000 ppm

DEC-TRANS-2-EN-1-AL Silk Essent. Oil 3,000 ppm

DEC-TRANS-2-TRANS-4-DIEN-1-AL Plant Silk Essent. Oil 6,000–20,000 ppm

DECA-TRANS-2-TRANS-7-TRIEN-1-AL Plant

DECAN-1-AL Silk Essent. Oil 10,000–90,000 ppm

DECAN-1-OL Silk Stigma Style

DECAN-2-OL Essential Oil 15,000 ppm

DECAN-2-ONE Essential Oil

DELTA-AMINO-LEVULINIC-ACID Sprout Seedling

DELTA-CADINENE Leaf

DIAMINO-PROPANE Sprout Seedling

DIETHYL-AMINE Seed

DIGALACTOSYL-DIGLYCERIDE Seed

DIHYDRO-PHASEIC-ACID Flower

DIHYDROSITOSTEROL Plant

DIMETHYL-AMINE Seed 1.1–3.5 ppm

DIOXYCINNAMIC-ACID Plant

DODECAN-1-AL Silk Essent. Oil

EO Silk Stigma Style 800–1,200 ppm

ERGOSTEROL Root Silk Stigma Style

ESTRONE Seed Oil 0.04 ppm

ETHANOL Silk Stigma Style

ETHYL-ACETATE Silk Stigma Style

ETHYL-AMINE Seed 2.4 ppm

ETHYL-METHYL-AMINE Seed

ETHYL-PHENYLACETATE Silk Essent. Oil 250,000–740,000 ppm

EUGENOL Seed

FAT Seed 10,480–54,579 ppm Silk Stigma Style 43,000 ppm

FERREDOXIN Leaf 37 ppm

FERULIC-ACID Leaf Seed 6–27 ppm Sprout Seedling

FERULOYLQUINIC-ACID Sprout Seedling

FIBER Silk Stigma Style 81,000 ppm

FLUORENE Silk Stigma Style

FOLACIN Fruit 1–2 ppm Seed 0.142–0.4 ppm

FRIEDELIN Shoot

FRUCTOSE Fruit 1,000–4,000 ppm

FUCOSE Root

FURFURAL Plant

GALACTOSE Plant

GALACTOXYLASE Plant

GALLIC-ACID Tissue Culture

GAMMA-NONALACTONE Silk Stigma Style

GAMMA-SITOSTEROL Plant

GAMMA-TOCOPHEROL Oil 752 ppm

GEOSMIN Essential Oil 4,000 ppm Plant

GERANIAL Hull Husk

GERANIOL Silk Stigma Style

GERANYL-ACETONE Seed

GIBBERELLINS Flower

GLOBULIN Seed 4,500–6,000 ppm

GLUCOSE Fruit 2,000–5,000 ppm

GLUTAMIC-ACID Seed 6,360–26,457 ppm

GLUTAMIC-ACID-DECARBOXYLASE Plant

GLUTATHIONE Seed 54–169 ppm

GLUTELIN Fruit 14,685–67,325 ppm

GLYCEROL Plant

GLYCINE Seed 1,270–5,283 ppm

GLYCOLIC-ACID Silk Stigma Style

GUAIACOL Seed

GUANIDINE Plant

HEMICELLULOSE Cob

HEPT-4-EN-2-ONE Essential Oil 15,000 ppm

HEPT-4-EN-OL Essential Oil 120,000 ppm
Plant

HEPT-CIS-4-EN-2-OL Silk Essent. Oil 10,000
ppm

HEPT-CIS-4-EN-2-ONE Leaf

HEPTA-TRANS-2-CIS-4-DIEN-1-AL Husk Essent.
Oil 19,000–21,000 ppm Silk Essent. Oil 3,000
ppm

HEPTA-TRANS-2-EN-1-AL Silk Essent. Oil 5,000
ppm

HEPTA-TRANS-2-TRANS-4-DIEN-1-AL Silk Essent. Oil 3,000 ppm

HEPTAN-1-AL Plant Silk Essent. Oil
20,000–50,000 ppm

HEPTAN-1-OL Silk Essent. Oil 20,000–30,000
ppm

HEPTAN-2-OL Essential Oil 250,000 ppm Plant
Silk Essent. Oil 10,000–20,000 ppm

HEX-1-EN-3-OL Silk Stigma Style

HEX-CIS-3-EN-1-AL Leaf

HEX-CIS-3-EN-1-OL Husk Essent. Oil 52,000
ppm Silk Essent. Oil 5,000 ppm

HEX-TRANS-2-EN-1-AL Plant

HEX-TRANS-2-TRANS-4-DIEN-1-AL Silk Essent.
Oil 3,000 ppm

HEX-TRANS-3-EN-1-OL Silk Essent. Oil

HEXADECENOIC-ACID Seed

HEXAN-1-AL Plant Silk Essent. Oil
2,000–10,000 ppm

HEXAN-1-OL Plant Silk Essent. Oil
2,000–10,000 ppm

HEXAN-2-OL Silk Stigma Style

HEXAN-2-ONE Essential Oil Husk Essent. Oil

HEXENYL-ISOTHIOCYANATE Seed

HISTIDINE Seed 890–3,702 ppm

HORDENINE Silk Stigma Style

HYDROXAMIC-ACID Leaf

INDOLE Leaf

INDOLE-3-ACETIC-ACID Seed

INDOLE-3-ACETIC-ACID-CELLULOSIGLUCAN
Seed

INDOLE-3-ACETIC-ACID-MYOINOSITOL Seed

INOSITOL Plant

IODINE Seed 0.012 ppm

IRON Seed 5–41 ppm Silk Stigma Style 504
ppm

ISOAMYL-AMINE Sprout Seedling

ISOBEHENIC-ACID Seed 80 ppm

ISOLEUCINE Seed 1,290–5,366 ppm

ISOPROPYL-AMINE Seed 2.3 ppm

ISOQUERCITRIN Plant

ISORHAMNETIN-3,4'-O-DIGLUCOSIDE Pollen
Or Spore

ISORHAMNETIN-3-O-BETA-D-GLUCOSIDE
Pollen Or Spore

ISORHAMNETIN-3-O-GLUCOSIDE-4'-O-
DIGLUCOSIDE Pollen Or Spore

ISORHAMNETIN-3-O-NEOHESPEROSIDE
Pollen Or Spore

KAEMPFEROL-3-O-ALPHA-L-GALACTOSIDE
Pollen Or Spore

KILOCALORIES Silk Stigma Style 3,690 /kg

LACTIC-ACID Plant

LANOSTEROL Plant

LEAD Seed 14 ppm

LEUCINE Seed 3,480–14,477 ppm

LEUCOCYANIDIN Plant

LEUCOPELARGONIDIN Plant

LIGNIN Stem 213,000–245,000 ppm

LIGNOCERIC-ACID Fruit

LIMONENE Silk Essent. Oil 7,000 ppm

LINALOL Plant

LINGIFOLENE Root

LINOLEIC-ACID Seed 5,420–22,547 ppm

LIPOXIDASE Plant

LITHIUM Seed 0.048–0.22 ppm

LONGIFOLENE Root

LOPHENOL Shoot

LUTEIN Leaf

LUTEIN_+_ZEAXANTHIN Seed 7.3–22 ppm

LUTEOFOROL Silk Stigma Style

LUTEOLINIDIN Silk Stigma Style

LYSINE Seed 1,370–5,699 ppm

MAGNESIUM Seed 100–1,600 ppm Silk Stigma Style 1,790 ppm

MALEIC-ACID Plant

MALIC-ACID Plant

MALIC-ACID-DEHYDROGENASE Plant

MALONIC-ACID Plant

MALTOSYL-TRANSFERASE Plant

MANGANESE Seed 0.84–63 ppm Silk Stigma Style 34 ppm

MANNOSE Plant 1–7 ppm

MAYSIN Silk Stigma Style 9,000 ppm

MENTHOL Leaf Silk Stigma Style

MERCURY Seed 0.072 ppm

MESO-INOSITOL Pollen Or Spore

METHIONINE Seed 670–2,787 ppm

METHYL-2-THIENYL-KETONE Leaf

METHYL-AMINE Seed 27 ppm

METHYL-PHENYLACETATE Silk Essent. Oil 30,000–40,000 ppm

METHYL-PYRAN-2-CARBOXALDEHYDE Leaf

MEVALONIC-ACID Seed 14 ppm

MOLYBDENUM Seed 0.084–6.3 ppm

MONOGALACTOSYL-DIGLYCERIDE Plant

MYO-INOSITOL Plant

MYRCENE Seed

MYRECITIN-GLUCOSIDE Plant

MYRISTIC-ACID Seed

N-METHYL-BETA-PHENETHYLAMINE Seed 1.1 ppm

N-PROPYL-GALLATE Seed

NAPHTHALENE Silk Essent. Oil 3,000 ppm

NEOCRYPTOXANTHIN Plant

NEOXANTHIN Leaf

NEROLIDOL Leaf

NIACIN Cob 4–16 ppm Seed 16–71 ppm Silk Stigma Style

NICKEL Seed 0.12–6.3 ppm

NICOTIANAMINE Leaf

NON-CIS-3-EN-1-OL Essential Oil 30,000 ppm

NON-TRANS-2-EN-1-AL Husk Essent. Oil 10,000 ppm Silk Essent. Oil 10,000 ppm

NONA-TRANS-2-TRANS-4-DIEN-1-AL Silk Essent. Oil 3,000 ppm

NONAL-N-2-OL Silk Stigma Style

NONAN-1-AL Silk Essent. Oil 80,000–28,000 ppm

NONAN-1-OL Essential Oil 30,000 ppm

NONAN-2-OL Essential Oil 260,000 ppm Plant Silk Essent. Oil 2,000 ppm

NONAN-2-ONE Essential Oil 20,000 ppm

O-DIETHYL-PHTHALATE Silk Stigma Style

OBTUSIFOLIOL Shoot

OCT-1-EN-3-OL Plant Silk Essent. Oil 1,000 ppm

OCT-TRANS-2-EN-1-AL Plant Silk Essent. Oil 1,000 ppm

OCT-TRANS-2-EN-1-OL Plant

OCTA-3-5-DIENE-2-ONE Silk Stigma Style

OCTA-TRANS-2-TRANS-5-DIEN-2-ONE Silk Essent. Oil 2,000 ppm

OCTADECADIENOIC-ACID Seed

OCTADECATRIENOIC-ACID Seed

OCTADECENOIC-ACID Seed

OCTAN-1-OL Silk Essent. Oil 5,000–10,000 ppm

OCTAN-2-OL Essential Oil 20,000 ppm Plant

OCTAN-2-ONE Essential Oil Husk Essent. Oil

OLEIC-ACID Seed 3,470–14,435 ppm

ORIENTIN Silk Stigma Style

OXALIC-ACID Fruit 99 ppm

P-COUMARIC-ACID Seed 4–46 ppm Shoot 1 ppm

P-HYDROXYBENZALDEHYDE Cob

P-VINYL-GUAIACOL Husk Essent. Oil

PALMITIC-ACID Seed 1,710–7,114 ppm

PALMITOLEIC-ACID Fruit

PANTOTHENIC-ACID Cob 3–7 ppm Seed 4–34 ppm

PECTIN Leaf 10,000–17,000 ppm

PECTINS Plant 5,900 ppm

PELARGONIDIN Silk Stigma Style

PELARGONIDIN-3-GLUCOSIDE Plant

PENT-1-EN-2-OL Silk Stigma Style

PENTAN-1-OL Silk Stigma Style

PENTAN-2-OL Silk Stigma Style

PENTAN-3-ONE Silk Stigma Style

PEROXIDASE Anther

PHENANTHRENE Leaf

PHENETHYL-ALCOHOL Silk Stigma Style

PHENYL-ACETALDEHYDE Plant Silk Essent. Oil 1,000 ppm

PHENYLALANINE Seed 1,500–6,240 ppm

PHENYLALANINE-AMMONIA-LYASE Plant

PHOSPHATIDYL-CHOLINE Plant

PHOSPHATIDYL-ETHANOLAMINE Plant

PHOSPHATIDYL-INOSITOL Plant

PHOSPHOENOL-PYRUVATE Sprout Seedling

PHOSPHOLIPIDS Seed

PHOSPHORUS Seed 600–4,066 ppm Silk
Stigma Style 287 ppm

PHYTIN Plant

PHYTOFLUENE Plant

PHYTOHAEMAGGLUTININ Silk Stigma Style

POTASSIUM Seed 2,400–11,450 ppm Silk
Stigma Style 12,200 ppm

PROLAMINE Seed 45,000–55,000 ppm

PROLINE Root 69 ppm Seed 2,920–12,147
ppm Shoot 11 ppm

PROPAN-1-OL Silk Stigma Style

PROTEIN Seed 22,520–132,000 ppm Silk
Stigma Style 99,000 ppm

PROTOCATECHUIC-ACID Tissue Culture

PUTRESCINE Sprout Seedling

PYRIDOXINE Cob 1–3 ppm

PYRROLIDINE Seed

PYRUVIC-ACID Sprout Seedling

QUERCETIN Plant

QUERCETIN-3,3'-O-BETA-D-GLUCOSIDE
Pollen Or Spore

QUERCETIN-3,7-DI-O-BETA-D-GLUCOSIDE
Pollen Or Spore

QUERCETIN-3-O-ALPHA-D-RHAMNOSYL-O-
BETA-L-GALACTOSIDE? Pollen Or Spore

QUERCETIN-3-O-BETA-D-GLUCOSIDE Pollen
Or Spore

QUERCETIN-3-O-BETA-D-GLUCOSYL-O-
ALPHA-L-GALACTOSIDE? Pollen Or Spore

QUERCETIN-3-O-BETA-D-NEOHESPEROSIDE
Pollen Or Spore

QUERCETIN-DIGLUCOSIDE Plant

QUINIC-ACID Plant

RAFFINOSE Fruit 1,000–3,000 ppm

RHAMNOGALACTURONAN-I Tissue Culture

RIBOFLAVIN Cob 1–3 ppm Fruit 1–4 ppm Silk
Stigma Style 1.5 ppm

RIBONUCLEASE Tissue Culture

RICINOLEIC-ACID Plant

SABINOL Leaf

SALICYLIC-ACID-METHYL-ESTER Leaf

SAPONIN Silk Stigma Style 23,000–32,000 ppm

SD Plant

SELENIUM Seed 0.5 ppm Silk Stigma Style

SERINE Seed 1,530–6,365 ppm

SEROTIN Plant

SI Plant

SILICON Silk Stigma Style 237 ppm

SILVER Seed 0.012–0.055 ppm

SODIUM Seed 757 ppm Silk Stigma Style 130
ppm

SPERMIDINE Seed

SPERMINE Seed

SQUALENE Seed

STARCH Seed

STEARIC-ACID Seed 110–457 ppm

STIGMASTEROL Seed

STRONTIUM Seed 0.12–14 ppm

SUCCINIC-ACID Plant

SUCROSE Fruit 9,000–19,000 ppm

SULFUR Fruit 6–1,140 ppm

SYRINGALDEHYDE Seed

SYRINGIC-ACID Tissue Culture

TEASTERONE Pollen Or Spore 0.041 ppm

THIAMIN Fruit 2–8 ppm Silk Stigma Style 2.1
ppm

THREONINE Seed 1,290–5,366 ppm

THYMOL Seed Silk Stigma Style

TIN Seed 1–1.8 ppm Silk Stigma Style

TITANIUM Seed 0.06–63 ppm

TOCOPHEROLS Seed 900–1,000 ppm

TRANS-24-METHYL-23-DEHYDRO-LOPHENOL
Seed

TRANS-BETA-FARNESENE Leaf

TRANS-FERULIC-ACID Plant

TRANS-ISO-MENTH-5-EN-2-OL Plant

TRANS-SINAPIC-ACID Plant

TRICARBALLYL-ACID Plant

TRICIN-GLYCOSIDE Plant

TRIDECAN-1-AL Husk Essent. Oil

TRIGONELLINE Seed 4 ppm

TRYPTOPHAN Seed 230–957 ppm

TYPHASTEROL Pollen Or Spore 0.066 ppm

TYROSINE Seed 1,230–5,117 ppm

UNDEC-TRANS-2-EN-1-AL Silk Essent. Oil
2,000 ppm

UNDECAN-1-AL Husk Essent. Oil

UNDECAN-2-OL Essential Oil 45,000 ppm
Husk Essent. Oil

UNDECAN-2-ONE Husk Essent. Oil

UREASE Plant

URIDINE Seed

URONIC-ACID Plant

VALINE Seed 1,850–7,696 ppm
VANADIUM Seed 0.05–1.35 ppm
VANILLIC-ACID Sprout Seedling
VANILLIN Seed 4–31 ppm
VINYL-ETHYL-PHENETHYL-KETONE Leaf
VIOLAXANTHIN Leaf
VIT-B-6 Seed 1–3 ppm
VIT-D-3 Leaf
VITEXIN Silk Stigma Style
WATER Seed 100,000–885,000 ppm Silk Stigma Style 620,000 ppm
XANTHOTOXIN Root
XYLENE Husk Essent. Oil
XYLOARABINOSE Plant
XYLOSE Plant
YTTERBIUM Seed 0.02–4.5 ppm
ZEANIN Seed
ZEANOSIDE-B Seed
ZEANOSIDE-C Seed 1.2 ppm
ZEATIN Plant 0.014 ppm
ZEAXANTHIN Plant
ZEINOXANTHIN Plant
ZINC Seed 4–20 ppm
ZIRCONIUM Seed 0.2–1.8 ppm

CUCUMBER

Chemicals in *Cucumis sativus L.* (*Cucurbitaceae*)—Cucumber

1,3-DIAMINO-PROPANE Seed
2,4-METHYLENE-CHOLESTEROL Seed
22-DIHYDRO-SPINASTEROL Leaf
22-DIHYDROBRASSICASTEROL Seed
24®-14ALPHA-METHYL-24-ETHYL-5ALPHA-CHOLEST-9(11)-EN-3BETA-OL Plant
24-BETA-ETHYL-25(27)-DEHYDROLATHOS-TEROL Seed
24-EPSILON-ETHYL-25(27)-DEHYDROLOPHE-NOL Seed
24-EPSILON-ETHYL-31-NORLANOSTA-8,25(27)-DIEN-3-BETA-OL Seed Oil 11 ppm
24-ETHYL-5ALPHA-CHOLESTA-7,22-DIEN-3BETA-OL Plant
24-ETHYLCHOLESTA-5-EN-7BETA-OL Plant
24-METHYL-25(27)-DEHYDROCYCLOAR-TANOL Seed
24-METHYL-CHOLEST-7-EN-3-BETA-OL Seed
24-METHYL-LATHOSTEROL Seed

24-METHYLENE-24-DIHYDRO-LANOSTEROL Seed
24-METHYLENE-24-DIHYDRO-PARKEOL Seed
24-METHYLENE-CYCLOARTENOL Seed
24-METHYLENEPOLLINASTEROL Plant
25(27)-DEHYDRO-CHONDRILLASTEROL Seed
25(27)-DEHYDRO-FUNGISTEROL Seed
25(27)-DEHYDRO-PORIFERASTEROL Seed
7,22-STIGMASTADIEN-3BETA-OL Plant
7-DEHYDRO-AVENASTEROL Seed
7-STIGMASTEN-3BETA-OL Plant
ALANINE Fruit 180–4,557 ppm
ALPHA-AMYRIN Seed
ALPHA-LINOLENIC-ACID Fruit 290–7,342 ppm
ALPHA-SPINASTEROL Leaf
ALPHA-TOCOPHEROL Fruit 0.4–38 ppm
ALUMINUM Fruit 0.4–21,000 ppm
ARGININE Fruit 340–8,608 ppm
ARSENIC Fruit 0.003–0.25 ppm
ASH Fruit 3,670–140,000 ppm
ASPARTIC-ACID Fruit 320–8,101 ppm
AVENASTEROL Seed
BARIUM Fruit 2–70 ppm
BETA-AMYRIN Fruit
BETA-CAROTENE Fruit 0.3–8 ppm
BETA-PYRAZOL-1-YL-ALANINE Seed
BETA-SITOSTEROL Fruit
BORON Fruit 1–46 ppm
BUTYRIC-ACID Seed 1,200–1,700 ppm
CADMIUM Fruit 0.001–0.56 ppm
CAFFEIC-ACID Fruit
CALCIUM Fruit 129–10,000 ppm
CAMPESTEROL Seed
CARBOHYDRATES Fruit 29,100–736,709 ppm
CHLOROGENIC-ACID Fruit
CHROMIUM Fruit 0.002–0.98 ppm
CITRULLINE Fruit 146 ppm
CLADOCHROMES Sprout Seedling
COBALT Fruit 0.14 ppm
COPPER Fruit 0.3–42 ppm
CUCURBITACIN-A Fruit
CUCURBITACIN-B Fruit
CUCURBITACIN-C Fruit
CUCURBITACIN-D Sprout Seedling
CUCURBITACIN-E Fruit
CUCURBITACIN-I Sprout Seedling
CUCURBITIN Seed
CYCLOARTENOL Seed

CYCLOEUCALENOL Seed

CYSTINE Fruit 30–759 ppm

D-GLUCOSE Petiole

EUPHOL Seed

FAT Fruit 900–43,037 ppm Seed 300,000–425,000 ppm

FERULIC-ACID Fruit

FIBER Fruit 6,000–151,896 ppm

FLUORINE Fruit

FOLACIN Fruit 0.12–4 ppm

GAMMA-GLUTAMYL-BETA-PYRAZOL-1-YL-ALA-NINE Seed

GLUTAMIC-ACID Fruit 1,540–38,987 ppm

GLYCINE Fruit 190–4,810 ppm

GRAMISTEROL Seed

HEXANAL Fruit

HEXEN-(2)-AL-(1) Fruit

HISTIDINE Fruit 80–2,025 ppm

IRON Fruit 2.6–420 ppm

ISOLEUCINE Fruit 170–4,303 ppm

ISOMULTIFLORINEOL Seed

ISOORIENTIN Leaf

LEAD Fruit 0.002–2.8 ppm

LEUCINE Fruit 230–5,822 ppm

LINOLEIC-ACID Cotyledon 35,100–486,700 ppm Fruit 220–5,570 ppm Seed 66,900–170,468 ppm

LINOLENIC-ACID Cotyledon 312,200 ppm

LITHIUM Fruit 0.236–0.56 ppm

LUPEOL Seed

LYSINE Fruit 220–5,570 ppm

LYSOLECITHIN Seed

MAGNESIUM Fruit 101–7,000 ppm

MANGANESE Fruit 0.5–98 ppm

MELOSIDE-A Leaf

MERCURY Fruit 0.05 ppm

METHIONINE Fruit 40–1,012 ppm

MEVALONIC-ACID Fruit 3 ppm

MOLYBDENUM Fruit 0.1–2.8 ppm

MUFA Fruit 30–759 ppm

MULTIFLORINEOL Seed

MYRISTIC-ACID Fruit 10–253 ppm

NIACIN Fruit 3–76 ppm

NICKEL Fruit 0.01–1.25 ppm

NITROGEN Fruit 1,400–80,000 ppm

NON-TRANS-2-EN-AL Fruit

NONA-TRANS-2,CIS-6-DIEN-1-AL Plant

NONADIEN-2,6-AL-1 Fruit

NONADIEN-2,6-OL-2 Fruit

NONEN-2-AL-1 Fruit

OBTUSIFOLIOL Seed

OLEIC-ACID Cotyledon 55,200–241,000 ppm Fruit 20–506 ppm Seed 116,100–180,000 ppm

PALMITIC-ACID Cotyledon 213,200–504,700 ppm Fruit 270–6,835 ppm Seed 12,420–20,400 ppm

PANTOTHENIC-ACID Fruit 2.5–63 ppm

PENTADEC-CIS-8-EN-1-AL Fruit

PHOSPHATIDIC-ACID Seed

PHOSPHATIDYL-CHOLINE Seed

PHOSPHATIDYL-ETHANOLAMINE Seed

PHOSPHATIDYL-GLYCEROL Seed

PHOSPHATIDYL-INOSITOL Seed

PHOSPHORUS Fruit 158–12,600 ppm

PHYTOSTEROLS Fruit 14–3,544 ppm

PL Plant

POTASSIUM Fruit 1,465–72,500 ppm

PROLINE Fruit 120–3,038 ppm

PROPANAL Fruit

PROTEIN Fruit 5,120–142,772 ppm

PUFA Fruit 510–12,911 ppm

RIBOFLAVIN Fruit 0.2–5.1 ppm

RUBIDIUM Fruit 0.4–19 ppm

SELENIUM Fruit 0.001–2.8 ppm

SERINE Fruit 160–4,051 ppm

SFA Fruit 330–8,354 ppm

SILICON Fruit 10–1,000 ppm

SILVER Fruit 0.01–0.14 ppm

SODIUM Fruit 16–714 ppm

SPERMIDINE Seed

SQUALENE Fruit

STEARIC-ACID Cotyledon 28,800–59,100 ppm Fruit 30–759 ppm Seed 11,100–69,785 ppm

STELLASTEROL Seed

STIGMAST-7,22,25-TRIEN-3-BETA-OL Seed

STIGMAST-7,25-DIEN-3-BETA-OL Seed

STIGMAST-7-EN-3-BETA-OL Leaf

STIGMASTEROL Plant

STRONTIUM Fruit 4–98 ppm

SUGAR Fruit 10,000 ppm

SULFOQUINOVOSYL-DIACYL-GLYCEROL Petiole

SULFUR Fruit 140–5,250 ppm

TARAXEROL Seed

THIAMIN Fruit 0.3–7.6 ppm

THREONINE Fruit 150–3,797 ppm

TIRUCALLOL Seed

TITANIUM Fruit 0.3–18 ppm

TRYPTOPHAN Fruit 40–1,012 ppm

TYROSINE Fruit 90–2,278 ppm

VALINE Fruit 170–4,304 ppm

VIT-B-6 Fruit 0.5–13 ppm

WATER Fruit 944,000–971,000 ppm

ZINC Fruit 2–157 ppm

ZIRCONIUM Fruit 1.18–2.8 ppm

DANDELION

Chemicals in *Taraxacum officinale WEBER EX F. H. WIGG.* (*Asteraceae*)—Dandelion

11,13-DIHYDROTARAXIN-ACID-BETA-D-GLU-
COPYRANOSYL-ESTER Plant

14-TARAXEREN-3BETA-OL Plant

3,4-DIHYDROXYCINNAMIC-ACID Plant

31-NORCYCLOARTENOL Plant

ALPHA-AMYLASE Plant

ALUMINUM Root 656 ppm

ANDROSTEROL Plant

ANEURINE Plant

APIGENIN-7-GLUCOSIDE Leaf

ARABINOSE Plant

ARNIDIOL Flower

ARSENIC Leaf

ASCORBIC-ACID Leaf 350–2,430 ppm Root
376 ppm

ASH Root 80,000 ppm

ASPARAGINIC-ACID Plant

BARIUM Leaf 50–80 ppm

BETA-AMYRIN Flower

BETA-CAROTENE Root 84 ppm

BETA-SITOSTEROL Plant

BORON Leaf 4–125 ppm

BROMINE Leaf 30–80 ppm

CAFFEIC-ACID Plant

CALCIUM Leaf 1,870–13,000 ppm Plant
12,000–21,000 ppm Root 6,140 ppm

CAOUTCHOUC Latex Exudate 3,000 ppm

CARBOHYDRATES Leaf 92,000–486,000 ppm
Root 749,000 ppm

CEROTIC-ACID Root

CERYL-ALCOHOL Latex Exudate

CHLORINE Leaf 5,300–22,000 ppm

CHOLINE Root

CHROMIUM Leaf 11–50 ppm Root 9 ppm

CHRYSANTHEMUMXANTHIN Flower

CLUYTIANOL Root

COBALT Root 80 ppm

COPPER Leaf 9–12 ppm

COUMESTROL Plant

CRYPTOXANTHIN Flower

CRYPTOXANTHIN-EPOXIDE Flower

CYCLOARTANOL Plant

CYCLOARTENOL Plant

D-GLUCURONIC-ACID Plant

FARADIOL Plant

FAT Leaf 7,000–48,600 ppm Root 16,000
ppm

FIBER Leaf 4,400–111,110 ppm Root 89,000
ppm

FLAVOXANTHIN Flower

FRUCTOSE Root

GERMACRANOLIDE Plant

GLUCOSE Root 5,000 ppm

GLUTAMIC-ACID Leaf

GLYCEROL Latex Exudate

HOMOANDROSTEROL Root

HOMOTARAXASTEROL Root

INULIN Root 250,000–400,000 ppm

IODINE Leaf

IRON Leaf 31–5,000 ppm Root 960 ppm

KILOCALORIES Root 2,650 /kg

LACTUCEROL Plant

LEAD Plant

LECITHIN Flower 29,700 ppm

LEVULIN Plant

LEVULOSE Plant

LINOLEIC-ACID Root

LINOLENIC-ACID Root

LUTEIN Flower

LUTEOLIN-7-GLUCOSIDE Leaf

MAGNESIUM Leaf 360–2,500 ppm Root 1,570
ppm

MANGANESE Plant 100–130 ppm Root 68
ppm

MANNITOL Root

MELISSIC-ACID Root

MOLYBDENUM Plant

MUCILAGE Root 85,000 ppm

NIACIN Root

NICKEL Plant

NICOTINIC-ACID Root

OLEIC-ACID Root

P-COUMARIC-ACID Plant

P-HYDROXYPHENYLACETIC-ACID Plant

PALMITIC-ACID Root

PECTINS Root 78,000 ppm

PHLOBAPHENE Root

PHOSPHORUS Leaf 591–4,583 ppm Root 3,100–3,620 ppm

POLLINASTANOL Plant

POTASSIUM Leaf 3,970–27,569 ppm Root 12,000–75,000 ppm

PROTEIN Leaf 27,000–187,500 ppm Root 36,000–165,000 ppm

PSEUDOTARAXASTEROL Plant

RESIN Root

RIBOFLAVIN Leaf 1–18 ppm Root 2.1 ppm

RUBIDIUM Plant 19–50 ppm

SACCHAROSE Root 11,000 ppm

SAPONIN Plant

SELENIUM Root

SILICON Root 47 ppm

SODIUM Leaf 760–5,278 ppm Root 1,130 ppm

STIGMASTEROL Root

STRONTIUM Plant 64–120 ppm

SUCROSE Plant

SULFUR Plant 2,600–3,300 ppm

TANNIN Root

TARAXACERINE Root

TARAXACINE Root

TARAXACOSIDE Plant

TARAXANTHIN Plant

TARAXASTEROL Latex Exudate

TARAXEROL Root

TARAXIN-ACID Plant

TARAXIN-ACID-BETA-D-GLUCOPYRANOSYL-ESTER Plant

TARAXOL Root

TARTARIC-ACID Plant

THIAMIN Leaf 1–13 ppm Root

TIN Root 13 ppm

TITANIUM Plant 58–330 ppm

TYROSINASE Root

VIOLAXANTHIN Flower

WATER Leaf 356,000–880,000 ppm Root 857,000 ppm

XANTHOPHYLL Plant

ZINC Root 13–60 ppm

DILL

Chemicals in *Anethum graveolens L.* (*Apiaceae*)—Dill, Garden Dill

1,4-TERPINENOL Plant

1,5-CINEOLE Plant

1-METHYL-4-ISOPROPENYL-BENZENE Fruit

2-NONANOL Plant

3,6-DIMETHYL-2,3,4,5,8,9-HEXAHYDROBEN-ZOFURAN Plant

3,6-DIMETHYL-3A,4,5,7A-TETRAHYDRO-COUMARAN Fruit

3,6-DIMETHYLCOUMARAN Plant

3,7-DIMETHYL-4,5,6,9-TETRAHYDRO-COUMARAN Fruit

4-ALPHA-DIMETHYLSTYRENE Root

6,7-DIHYDRO-8,8,DIMETHYL-2H,8H-BENZO-(1,2B5,4')-DIPYRAN-2,6-DIONE Plant

6-OCTADECENOIC-ACID Plant

7-OCTADECENOIC-ACID Plant

ALPHA,ALPHA-BETA-TRIMETHYLBENZYL-AL-COHOL Root

ALPHA-LINOLENIC-ACID Fruit 1,500–1,624 ppm

ALPHA-PINENE Fruit 24–1,001 ppm

ALPHA-TERPINEOL Plant

ALPHA-THUJENE Fruit 36–231 ppm

ALPHA-TOCOPHEROL Leaf 16–147 ppm

ALUMINUM Plant 4–210 ppm

ANETHOLE Plant

ANISIC-ALDEHYDE Plant

APIOLE Root

ARGINASE Plant

ARGININE Fruit 12,630–13,678 ppm

ARSENIC Plant 0.01–0.06 ppm

ASCORBIC-ACID Plant 1,440 ppm

ASH Fruit 64,000–84,000 ppm Plant 26,000–205,880 ppm

BENZYL-ETHER Plant

BERGAPTEN Fruit

BETA-CARYOPHYLLENE Plant

BETA-ELEMENE Fruit 12–77 ppm

BETA-MYRCENE Plant

BETA-PHELLANDRENE Fruit 168–1,925 ppm Root 168–1,925 ppm

BETA-PINENE Plant

BETA-SITOSTEROL Plant

BETA-SITOSTEROL-GLUCOSIDE Plant

BETA-SITOSTEROL-GLYCOSIDE Fruit

BETA-TERPINEOL Fruit Plant

BORON Plant 4–35 ppm Seed 28–50 ppm

BROMINE Plant 1–6 ppm

BUTYL-PHTHALIDE Root

CADMIUM Plant 0.02–1 ppm

CAFFEIC-ACID Fruit

CALCIUM Fruit 14,003–17,671 ppm Plant
1,900–21,453 ppm

CAMPHENE Plant

CAMPHOR Root

CARBOHYDRATES Fruit 551,700–597,491 ppm
Plant 558,200–602,000 ppm

CAROTENOIDS Leaf 465 ppm

CARVACROL Plant

CARVONE Plant

CARVOTANACETONE Fruit

CHLOROGENIC-ACID Fruit

CHROMIUM Plant 0.01–0.29 ppm

CINEOLE Plant

CIS-CARVEOL Fruit

CIS-DIHYDROCARVONE Fruit 36–12,782 ppm

COBALT Plant 0.002–0.29 ppm

COPPER Fruit 8 ppm Plant 1.7–17 ppm

D-(+)-CARVONE Fruit 5,196–37,653 ppm

D-(+)-DIHYDROCARVONE Fruit 168–1,925
ppm

D-(+)-LIMONENE Fruit 3,972–31,416 ppm

D-ALPHA-PHELLANDRENE Fruit 516–7,469
ppm

DECANAL Fruit 24–154 ppm

DELTA-5,6-OCTADECENOIC-ACID Plant

DIHYDROCARVEOL Plant

DILLANOSIDE Plant

DILLAPIOLE Fruit 1,440–40,425 ppm

DIPENTENE Plant

EICOSANE Root

ELEMICIN Plant

EO Fruit 12,000–77,000 ppm Plant
5,600–15,000 ppm Root 300–500 ppm

ESCULETIN Fruit

EUGENOL Plant

FAT Fruit 68,000–180,200 ppm Plant
43,000–47,000 ppm

FERULIC-ACID Fruit

FIBER Fruit 177,230–264,869 ppm Leaf
119,300–128,000 ppm

FLAVONE Plant

FLUORINE Plant 0.1–5.3 ppm

FURFURAL Plant

GAMMA-PINENE Plant

GAMMA-SITOSTEROL Fruit

GAMMA-TERPINENE Fruit 12–77 ppm

GERANIOL Fruit 24–154 ppm

HEXADECANE Root

HISTIDINE Fruit 3,200–3,466 ppm

IRON Fruit 114–230 ppm Plant 23–755 ppm

ISOEUGENOL Plant

ISOLEUCINE Fruit 7,670–8,307 ppm

ISORHAMNETIN Plant

ISORHAMNETIN-3-GLUCURONIDE Plant

KAEMPFEROL Fruit

KAEMPFEROL-3-GLUCURONIDE Leaf

LAURIC-ACID Fruit 100–108 ppm

LEAD Plant 0.05–0.8 ppm

LEUCINE Fruit 9,250–10,018 ppm

LIMONENE Plant

LINALOL Plant

LINOLEIC-ACID Fruit 9,600–10,397 ppm

LUTEOLIN-7-GLUCOSIDE Plant

LYSINE Fruit 10,380–11,242 ppm

MAGNESIUM Fruit 2,449–2,893 ppm Plant
560–6,470 ppm

MANGANESE Fruit 18 ppm Plant 8–435 ppm

MERCURY Plant 0.003–0.06 ppm

METHIONINE Fruit 1,430–1,549 ppm

METHYL-BENZOATE Plant

METHYL-CHAVICOL Fruit

MOLYBDENUM Plant

MYRCENE Fruit 84–924 ppm

MYRISTIC-ACID Fruit 100–108 ppm

MYRISTICIN Fruit Root

NEOCNIDOLIDE Root

NIACIN Fruit 28–30 ppm Plant 28–30 ppm

NICKEL Plant 0.1–4.7 ppm

NITROGEN Plant 6,800–55,300 ppm

NONADECANE Root

NONANAL Fruit

OCTANOL Root

OLEIC-ACID Fruit 93,600–101,369 ppm

P-CYMENE Fruit 336–3,773 ppm

PALMITIC-ACID Fruit 5,800–6,281 ppm

PALMITOLEIC-ACID Fruit 500–542 ppm

PARAFFIN Plant

PENTADECANE Root

PETROSELINIC-ACID-TRIGYLCERIDE Plant

PHENYLALANINE Fruit 6,700–7,256 ppm

PHOSPHORUS Fruit 2,102–3,723 ppm Plant
600–7,625 ppm
POTASSIUM Fruit 10,680–14,122 ppm Plant
8,700–76,450 ppm
PROTEIN Fruit 147,680–226,000 ppm Plant
199,600–216,000 ppm
QUERCETIN Plant
QUERCETIN-3-0-RUTINOSIDE Plant
QUERCETIN-3-GLUCURONIDE Leaf
QUERCITRIN Plant
RIBOFLAVIN Fruit 3 ppm Plant 3 ppm
RUBIDIUM Plant 1.1–28 ppm
SABINENE Plant
SAFROLE Plant
SALICALDEHYDE Plant
SCOPOLETIN Fruit
SELENIUM Plant 0.001–0.012 ppm
SENKYUNOLIDE Root
SILICON Plant 30–700 ppm
SODIUM Fruit 158–262 ppm Plant
1,097–3,308 ppm
STEARIC-ACID Fruit 1,000–1,083 ppm
STIGMASTEROL Plant
SULFUR Plant 1,400–11,175 ppm
TANNINS Plant
TERPINEN-4-OL Fruit 12–77 ppm
TETRADECANE Root
TETRAHYDROCOUMARANE Plant
THIAMIN Fruit 4–5 ppm Plant 4–5 ppm
THREONINE Fruit 5,750–6,227 ppm
TRANS-ANETHOLE Fruit 12–539 ppm
TRANS-CARVEOL Fruit 42–270 ppm
TRANS-DIHYDROCARVONE Fruit 24–154 ppm
TRIDECENE Root
UMBELLIFERONE Fruit
UMBELLIPRENIN Fruit
UREASE Plant
VALINE Fruit 11,200–12,130 ppm
VICENIN Fruit
WATER Fruit 70,310–83,690 ppm Plant
73,000–830,000 ppm
XANTHOPHYLL Fruit
Z-LIGUSTILIDE Root
ZINC Fruit 43–66 ppm Plant 11–150 ppm

DULSE

Chemicals in *Rhodymenia palmata*—Dulse

ALPHA-CAROTENE Plant
ALPHA-CRYPTOXANTHIN Plant
ALUMINUM Plant 615 ppm
ARSENIC Plant 33 ppm
ASCORBIC-ACID Plant 120 ppm
ASH Plant 182,000 ppm
BETA-CAROTENE Plant
BETA-CRYPTOXANTHIN Plant
CALCIUM Plant 6,320 ppm
CHROMIUM Plant 27 ppm
COBALT Plant 150 ppm
IRON Plant 792 ppm
LEAD Plant 3.5 ppm
LUTEIN Plant
MAGNESIUM Plant 5,930 ppm
MANGANESE Plant 37 ppm
MERCURY Plant 26 ppm
NIACIN Plant
PHOSPHORUS Plant 3,860 ppm
POTASSIUM Plant 22,700 ppm
PROTEIN Plant 133,000 ppm
RIBOFLAVIN Plant 1.1 ppm
SELENIUM Plant
SILICON Plant 368 ppm
SODIUM Plant 99,170 ppm
THIAMIN Plant 1.6 ppm
TIN Plant 33 ppm
ZEAXANTHIN Plant
ZINC Plant 39 ppm

EGGPLANT

Chemicals in *Solanum melongena L.*
(*Solanaceae*)—Aubergine, Eggplant

5-HYDROXYTRYPTAMINE Fruit
9-OXO-NEROLIDOL Plant
ALANINE Fruit 420–6,815 ppm
ALPHA-LINOLENIC-ACID Fruit 70–867 ppm
ALUMINUM Fruit 10–16 ppm
ARACHIDIC-ACID Seed
ARGININE Fruit 610–7,559 ppm
ARSENIC Fruit 0.004–0.004 ppm
ASCORBIC-ACID Fruit 13–947 ppm Leaf
790–5,809 ppm
ASH Fruit 5,000–80,000 ppm Leaf
20,000–147,000 ppm
ASPARTIC-ACID Fruit 1,770–21,933 ppm
AUBERGENONE Plant

BARIUM Fruit 3.5–5.6 ppm

BETA-AMINO-4-ETHYL-GLYOXALINE Fruit

BETA-CAROTENE Fruit 6 ppm

BORON Fruit 1–8 ppm

CADMIUM Fruit 0.3–0.44 ppm

CAFFEIC-ACID Fruit

CALCIUM Fruit 120–5,706 ppm Leaf
  2,540–18,676 ppm

CARBOHYDRATES Fruit 56,000–811,000 ppm
  Leaf 66,000–485,000 ppm

CHLORINE Fruit 520 ppm

CHLOROGENIC-ACID Fruit

CHOLINE Fruit 520 ppm

CHROMIUM Fruit 0.1–0.12 ppm

COBALT Fruit 0.07–0.08 ppm

COPPER Fruit 0.6–20 ppm

CYANIDIN Fruit

CYSTINE Fruit 60–743 ppm

DELPHINIDIN Fruit

DELPHINIDIN-3-RUTINOSIDE-3-(4'-
  COUMAROYLRUTINOSIDE)5-GLUC . . .
  Plant

DELPHINIDIN-P-COUMAROYL-MON-
  ORHAMNOSIDE-DIGLUCOSIDE Fruit

ETHYL-CAFFEATE Root

FAT Fruit 1,000–38,000 ppm Leaf 4,000–29,000
  ppm Seed 198,300–212,000 ppm

FERULIC-ACID Root

FIBER Fruit 9,000–137,000 ppm

FOLACIN Fruit 0.1–2.6 ppm

GABA Fruit

GAMMA-HYDROXYGLUTAMIC-ACID Fruit

GLUTAMIC-ACID Fruit 2,010–24,907 ppm

GLYCINE Fruit 320–5,452 ppm

GLYCOALKALOIDS Fruit 280–470 ppm

HCN Fruit

HISTIDINE Fruit 240–3,098 ppm

IRON Fruit 3–137 ppm Leaf 155–1,140 ppm

ISOLEUCINE Fruit 480–5,948 ppm

ISOSCOPOLETIN Root

KILOCALORIES Fruit 250–3,370 /kg Leaf
  150–2,790 /kg

LEAD Fruit 1.4–1.6 ppm

LEUCINE Fruit 570–8,550 ppm

LINOLEIC-ACID Fruit 350–4,337 ppm

LITHIUM Fruit 0.28–0.32 ppm

LUBIMIN Plant

LYCOPENE Fruit

LYCOXANTHIN Fruit

LYSINE Fruit 510–6,320 ppm

MAGNESIUM Fruit 85–1,563 ppm

MANGANESE Fruit 1.4–40 ppm

MERCURY Fruit 0.001–0.001 ppm

METHIONINE Fruit 60–1,487 ppm

MOLYBDENUM Fruit 0.5–0.56 ppm

MUFA Fruit 90–1,152 ppm

N-TRANS-FERULOYL-OCTOPAMINE Root

N-TRANS-FERULOYL-TYRAMINE Root

N-TRANS-P-COUMAROYL-OCTOPAMINE
  Root

N-TRANS-P-COUMAROYL-TYRAMINE Root

NASUNIN Fruit

NEO-CHLOROGENIC-ACID Fruit

NIACIN Fruit 0.9–98 ppm

NICKEL Fruit 0.7–0.8 ppm

NITROGEN Fruit 5,400–10,250 ppm

OLEIC-ACID Fruit 80–991 ppm

OXALIC-ACID Fruit 291 ppm

PALMITIC-ACID Fruit 140–1,735 ppm

PALMITOLEIC-ACID Fruit 10–124 ppm

PANTOTHENIC-ACID Fruit 0.8–10 ppm

PECTIN Fruit 110,000 ppm

PHENYLALANINE Fruit 430–5,700 ppm

PHOSPHORUS Fruit 189–5,836 ppm Leaf
  380–2,794 ppm

PHYTOSTEROLS Fruit 70–867 ppm

PIPECOLIC-ACID Fruit

POTASSIUM Fruit 620–32,000 ppm

PROLINE Fruit 460–5,700 ppm

PROTEIN Fruit 10,000–200,000 ppm Leaf
  46,000–338,000 ppm

PUFA Fruit 420–5,204 ppm

RIBOFLAVIN Fruit 0.2–8.8 ppm

SCOPOLETIN Fruit

SELENIUM Fruit 0.001–0.002 ppm

SERINE Fruit 410–5,576 ppm

SFA Fruit 200–2,478 ppm

SILVER Fruit 0.07–0.18 ppm

SODIUM Fruit 20–2,150 ppm

SOLAMARGINE Fruit

SOLANIDINE Fruit

SOLANINE Fruit

SOLASODINE Fruit

SOLASONINE Fruit

STEARIC-ACID Fruit 50–620 ppm

STRONTIUM Fruit 2–5.6 ppm

SUCROSE Fruit

SUGAR Fruit 20,000–30,000 ppm

SULFUR Fruit 126–152 ppm

TANNIN Fruit 2,000 ppm

THIAMIN Fruit 0.4–10 ppm

THREONINE Fruit 380–4,957 ppm

TITANIUM Fruit 0.35–0.4 ppm

TRIGONELLINE Fruit

TRYPTAMINE Fruit

TRYPTOPHAN Fruit 100–1,239 ppm

TYRAMINE Fruit

TYROSINE Fruit 250–3,593 ppm

VALINE Fruit 550–7,063 ppm

VANILLIN Root

VIT-B-6 Fruit 0.9–11.6 ppm

WATER Fruit 905,000–932,000 ppm Leaf
864,000 ppm

ZINC Fruit 18–25.6 ppm

ZIRCONIUM Fruit 1.4–1.6 ppm

ENDIVE

Chemicals in *Cichorium endivia L.* (*Aster-aceae*)—Endive, Escarole

ALANINE Leaf 620–9,984 ppm

ALPHA-LINOLENIC-ACID Leaf 130–2,093 ppm

ALUMINUM Leaf 60–168 ppm

ARGININE Leaf 620–9,984 ppm

ARSENIC Leaf 0.04–0.048 ppm

ASCORBIC-ACID Leaf 462–9,302 ppm

ASH Leaf 13,590–240,000 ppm

ASPARTIC-ACID Leaf 1,300–20,934 ppm

BARIUM Leaf 14–24 ppm

BETA-CAROTENE Leaf 9.6–241 ppm

BETA-LACTUCEROL Latex Exudate

BORON Leaf 1–24 ppm

CADMIUM Leaf 0.2–0.24 ppm

CAFFEIC-ACID Leaf

CALCIUM Leaf 462–10,080 ppm

CAOUTCHOUC Latex Exudate

CARBOHYDRATES Leaf 33,500–539,452 ppm

CHROMIUM Leaf 0.3–0.48 ppm

COBALT Leaf 0.2–0.24 ppm

COPPER Leaf 1–16.8 ppm

CYSTINE Leaf 100–1,610 ppm

FAT Leaf 2,000–32,200 ppm

FIBER Leaf 9,000–144,927 ppm

FOLACIN Leaf 1.2–25 ppm

GLUTAMIC-ACID Leaf 1,660–26,731 ppm

GLYCINE Leaf 580–9,340 ppm

HISTIDINE Leaf 230–3,704 ppm

HYDROXYCINNAMIC-ACID Leaf

INULIN Root

IRON Leaf 6–360 ppm

ISOLEUCINE Leaf 720–11,594 ppm

KAEMPFEROL-3-0-GLUCOSIDE Leaf

KAEMPFEROL-GLYCOSIDES Plant

KILOCALORIES Leaf 170–2,737 /kg

LEAD Leaf 4–4.8 ppm

LEUCINE Leaf 980–15,781 ppm

LINOLEIC-ACID Leaf 750–12,077 ppm

LITHIUM Leaf 0.8–0.96 ppm

LYSINE Leaf 630–10,145 ppm

MAGNESIUM Leaf 95–2,400 ppm

MANGANESE Leaf 4–72 ppm

MERCURY Leaf 0.002–0.002 ppm

METHIONINE Leaf 140–2,254 ppm

MOLYBDENUM Leaf 1.4–1.68 ppm

MUFA Leaf 40–644 ppm

MYRISTIC-ACID Leaf 30–483 ppm

NIACIN Leaf 4–64 ppm

NICKEL Leaf 2–2.4 ppm

OLEIC-ACID Leaf 40–644 ppm

PALMITIC-ACID Leaf 410–6,602 ppm

PANTOTHENIC-ACID Leaf 9–145 ppm

PHENOLICS Leaf 32,000 ppm

PHENYLALANINE Leaf 530–8,535 ppm

PHOSPHORUS Leaf 242–5,760 ppm

POTASSIUM Leaf 2,915–96,000 ppm

PROLINE Leaf 590–9,500 ppm

PROTEIN Leaf 12,000–209,300 ppm

PUFA Leaf 870–14,010 ppm

QUERCETIN Leaf

RIBOFLAVIN Leaf 0.7–13 ppm

SELENIUM Leaf 0.008–0.024 ppm

SERINE Leaf 490–7,890 ppm

SFA Leaf 480–7,729 ppm

SILVER Leaf 0.2–0.24 ppm

SODIUM Leaf 179–4,560 ppm

STEARIC-ACID Leaf 20–322 ppm

STRONTIUM Shoot 140–240 ppm

SULFUR Shoot 740–912 ppm

TARAXASTEROL Latex Exudate

THIAMIN Leaf 0.7–14 ppm

THREONINE Leaf 500–8,051 ppm

TITANIUM Leaf 1–1.2 ppm

TRYPTOPHAN Leaf 50–805 ppm

TYROSINE Leaf 400–6,441 ppm

VALINE Leaf 630–10,145 ppm
VIT-B-6 Leaf 0.2–3.2 ppm
WATER Leaf 934,000–943,800 ppm
ZINC Leaf 8–146 ppm
ZIRCONIUM Leaf 4–4.8 ppm

FENNEL

Chemicals in *Foeniculum vulgare MILLER* (*Apiaceae*)—Fennel

1,8-CINEOLE Fruit 1–300 ppm Plant
3-CARENE Fruit 120–720 ppm
5-METHOXY-PSORALEN Fruit 5 ppm
8-METHOXY-PSORALEN Fruit 1 ppm
ALANINE Fruit 7,890–8,655 ppm
ALPHA-PHELLANDRENE Fruit 44–6,600 ppm
    Plant 135 ppm
ALPHA-PINENE Fruit 200–8,820 ppm Plant 480
    ppm
ALPHA-TERPINENE Fruit 1 ppm Plant 135 ppm
ALPHA-TERPINEOL Fruit 1–6 ppm
ALPHA-THUJENE Fruit
ALUMINUM Seed 56 ppm
ANISALDEHYDE Fruit 1–1,080 ppm
ANISIC-ACID Fruit
ANISIC-KETONE Fruit
APIOLE Fruit
ARGININE Fruit 6,800–7,460 ppm
ASCORBIC-ACID Fruit Plant 340–3,148 ppm
ASH Fruit 79,600–93,026 ppm Plant
    17,000–170,000 ppm
ASPARTIC-ACID Fruit 18,333–20,111 ppm
AVICULARIN Leaf
BENZOIC-ACID Fruit
BERGAPTEN Fruit
BETA-CAROTENE Fruit 1 ppm Plant 21–241
    ppm
BETA-PHELLANDRENE Fruit 170–1,020 ppm
BETA-PINENE Fruit 1–780 ppm Plant 10 ppm
BETA-SITOSTEROL Fruit
BORON Leaf 1–36 ppm
CAFFEIC-ACID Fruit
CALCIUM Fruit 880–13,941 ppm Leaf
    1,000–10,556 ppm
CAMPHENE Fruit 10–540 ppm
CAMPHOR Fruit 10–180 ppm
CARBOHYDRATES Fruit 522,900–577,680 ppm
    Plant 51,000–519,000 ppm

CERYL-ALCOHOL Fruit
CHOLINE Seed
CHROMIUM Fruit 4–5 ppm
CINNAMIC-ACID Fruit
CIS-ANETHOLE Fruit 10–300 ppm Plant 50
    ppm
CIS-OCIMENE Fruit 40–600 ppm
CITRIC-ACID Fruit
COBALT Fruit 1–31 ppm
COLUMBIANETIN Fruit
COPPER Fruit 8–24 ppm
CYNARIN Plant
CYSTINE Fruit 2,220–2,435 ppm
D-LIMONENE Fruit
DIANETHOLE Fruit
DILLAPIOL Root Essent. Oil
DIPENTENE Essential Oil
EO Fruit 10,000–80,000 ppm Plant 10,000 ppm
ESTRAGOLE Fruit 64,000 ppm
FAT Fruit 120,000–280,000 ppm Plant
    4,000–46,000 ppm
FENCHONE Fruit 10–24,000 ppm Plant 30
    ppm
FENCHYL-ALCOHOL Seed Essent. Oil
FERULIC-ACID Fruit
FIBER Fruit 144,250–183,338 ppm Plant
    5,000–50,000 ppm
FUMARIC-ACID Fruit
GAMMA-TERPINENE Fruit 1–342 ppm Plant
    135 ppm
GAMMA-TOCOTRIENOL Fruit
GENTISIC-ACID Fruit
GLUTAMIC-ACID Fruit 29,560–32,427 ppm
GLYCINE Fruit 11,070–12,144 ppm
GLYCOLLIC-ACID Plant
HISTIDINE Fruit 3,310–3,631 ppm
IMPERATORIN Fruit 3 ppm
IODINE Fruit 0.002 ppm
IRON Fruit 100–240 ppm Plant 27–270 ppm
ISOLEUCINE Fruit 6,950–7,624 ppm
ISOPIMPINELLIN Fruit 1 ppm
ISOQUERCITRIN Fruit
KAEMPFEROL Plant
KAEMPFEROL-3-ARABINOSIDE Leaf
KAEMPFEROL-3-GLUCURONIDE Leaf
L-LIMONENE Fruit
LIMONENE Fruit 200–9,420 ppm Plant 1,800
    ppm

LINALOL Fruit 1–2,050 ppm Plant 60 ppm

LINOLEIC-ACID Fruit 14,000–18,539 ppm

MAGNESIUM Fruit 1,730–5,012 ppm

MALIC-ACID Fruit

MANGANESE Fruit 24–721 ppm

MARMESIN Fruit

METHIONINE Fruit 3,010–3,302 ppm

METHYL-CHAVICOL Fruit 70–4,018 ppm Plant 390 ppm

MYRCENE Fruit 100–2,700 ppm

MYRISTICIN Fruit

N-DOCOSYL-ARACHIDATE Plant

N-EICOSYL-ARACHIDATE Plant

N-HEXACOSYL-ARACHIDATE Plant

N-OCTACOSYL-ARACHIDATE Plant

N-TETRACOSYL-ARACHIDATE Plant

N-TRIACONTYL-ARACHIDATE Plant

NIACIN Fruit 60–66 ppm Plant 7–65 ppm

NICKEL Fruit 1 ppm

O-COUMARIC-ACID Fruit

OLEIC-ACID Fruit 22,000–108,712 ppm

OSTHENOL Fruit

P-COUMARIC-ACID Fruit 93 ppm

P-CYMENE Fruit 20–480 ppm

P-HYDROXY-BENZOIC-ACID Fruit

P-HYDROXYCINNAMIC-ACID Fruit

PALMITIC-ACID Fruit 4,000–6,000 ppm

PECTIN Fruit

PETROSELINIC-ACID Fruit 72,000–168,000 ppm

PHENYLALANINE Fruit 6,470–7,098 ppm

PHOSPHORUS Fruit 4,449–5,960 ppm Plant 510–5,100 ppm

PHOTOANTHEOLE Fruit

POTASSIUM Fruit 14,800–19,400 ppm Plant 3,380–39,700 ppm

PROLINE Fruit 9,000–9,873 ppm

PROTEIN Fruit 148,735–200,000 ppm Plant 28,000–280,000 ppm

PROTOCATECHUIC-ACID Fruit

PSORALEN Fruit 1 ppm

QUERCETIN Fruit

QUERCETIN-3-ARABINOSIDE Plant

QUERCETIN-3-GLUCURONIDE Plant

QUERCETIN-3-L-ARABINOSIDE Plant

QUINIC-ACID Fruit

RIBOFLAVIN Fruit 4 ppm Plant 1–14 ppm

RUTIN Fruit

SABINENE Fruit 1–60 ppm

SCOPARONE Fruit

SCOPOLETIN Fruit

SELENIUM Fruit

SERINE Fruit 9,000–9,873 ppm

SESELIN Fruit

SHIKIMIC-ACID Fruit

SILICON Fruit 4.2 ppm

SINAPIC-ACID Fruit

SODIUM Fruit 50–1,980 ppm

STIGMASTEROL Fruit Root

STIGMASTEROL-PALMITATE Root

SUGAR Fruit 40,000–50,000 ppm

SYRINGIC-ACID Fruit

TARTARIC-ACID Fruit

TERPINEN-4-OL Fruit 10–60 ppm

TERPINOLENE Fruit 10–60 ppm Plant 230 ppm

THIAMIN Fruit 4–5 ppm Plant 1–11 ppm

THREONINE Fruit 6,020–6,604 ppm

TIN Fruit 11 ppm

TOCOPHEROL Fruit

TRANS-1,8-TERPIN Fruit

TRANS-ANETHOLE Fruit 3,030–72,980 ppm Plant 5,550 ppm

TRANS-OCIMENE Fruit 20–330 ppm

TRIGONELLINE Fruit

TRYPTOPHAN Fruit 2,530–2,775 ppm

TYROSINE Fruit 4,100–4,498 ppm

UMBELLIFERONE Fruit Root

UREASE Leaf Root Stem

VALINE Fruit 9,150–10,037 ppm

VANILLIC-ACID Fruit

VANILLIN Fruit

WATER Fruit 80,670–104,796 ppm Plant 842,000–900,000 ppm

XANTHOTOXIN Fruit

ZINC Fruit 7.1–33 ppm

GARDEN CRESS

Chemicals in *Lepidium sativum L.* (*Brassicaceae*)—Garden Cress

4-HYDROXY-3,5-DIMETHOXYCINNAMIC-ACID Seed

ALKALOID Seed 1,900–2,015 ppm

ALPHA-TOCOPHEROL Leaf 7–66 ppm Oil 1,830 ppm

ARACHIDIC-ACID Seed 2,450–3,925 ppm

ASCORBIC-ACID Leaf 690–6,510 ppm

ASH Leaf 18,000–169,800 ppm Seed
57,000–60,440 ppm

BEHENIC-ACID Seed 2,750–4,410 ppm

BENZYL-CYANIDE Plant

BENZYL-ISOTHIOCYANATE Plant

BENZYL-THIOCYANATE Essential Oil

BETA-CAROTENE Leaf 20–526 ppm

BETA-SITOSTEROL Seed

CALCIUM Leaf 810–20,340 ppm Seed
3,100–3,290 ppm

CARBOHYDRATES Leaf 55,000–518,870 ppm

CELLULOSE Seed 9,150 ppm

COBALT Leaf 0.012 ppm

D-GALACTURONIC-ACID Seed

D-GLUCURONIC-GALACTOSIDE Seed

D-XYLOSE Seed

DIALLYL-SULFIDE Essential Oil

EO Plant 1,150 ppm

ERUCIC-ACID Leaf 910–8,585 ppm

FAT Leaf 7,000–66,040 ppm Seed
150,000–255,000 ppm

FIBER Leaf 11,000–103,775 ppm

GADOLEIC-ACID Leaf 610–5,755 ppm

GLUCOTROPAEOLIN Plant

IODINE Leaf 0.11 ppm

IRON Leaf 13–286 ppm

KILOCALORIES Leaf 320–3,020 /kg

L-ARABINOSE Seed

L-RHAMNOSE Seed

LIGNOCERIC-ACID Seed 320–510 ppm

LINOLEIC-ACID Leaf 1,520–14,340 ppm

LINOLENIC-ACID Leaf 760–7,170 ppm Seed
44,550–71,400 ppm

MUCILAGE Seed 50,000 ppm

MUFA Leaf 2,390–22,545 ppm

MYROSIN Plant

NIACIN Leaf 10–95 ppm

NICKEL Leaf 0.04 ppm

OLEIC-ACID Leaf 870–8,210 ppm Seed
97,450–156,200 ppm

PALMITIC-ACID Leaf 160–1,510 ppm Seed
2,020–3,240 ppm

PHOSPHORUS Leaf 760–7,170 ppm Seed
16,500–17,500 ppm

POTASSIUM Leaf 6,060–57,170 ppm

PROTEIN Leaf 26,000–327,685 ppm Seed
235,000–249,180 ppm

PUFA Leaf 2,280–21,500 ppm

RIBOFLAVIN Leaf 1.7–25 ppm

SFA Leaf 230–2,170 ppm

SINAPIC-ACID Seed

SINAPIN Seed

SODIUM Leaf 140–1,320 ppm

STEARIC-ACID Leaf 70–660 ppm Seed
9,560–15,325 ppm

SULFUR Seed 9,000–9,545 ppm

THIAMIN Leaf 0.8–7.5 ppm

URIC-ACID Seed 108 ppm

VIT-B-6 Leaf 2.5–23 ppm

WATER Leaf 823,000–894,000 ppm Seed
56,900 ppm

GARLIC

Chemicals in *Allium sativum L. (Liliaceae)*—Garlic

1,2-(PROP-2-ENYL)-DISULFANE Bulb

1,2-DIMERCAPTOCYCLOPENTANE Bulb 2.4
ppm

1,2-EPITHIOPROPANE Bulb 0.1–1.66 ppm

1,3-DITHIANE Bulb 0.08–3 ppm

1-HEXANOL Bulb 0.23 ppm

1-METHYL-1,2-(PROP-2-ENYL)-DISULFANE
Bulb

1-METHYL-2-(PROP-2-ENYL)-DISULFANE Bulb

1-METHYL-3-(PROP-2-ENYL)-TRISULFANE Bulb

2,3,4-TRITHIAPENTANE Bulb

2,5-DIMETHYL-TETRAHYDROTHIOPHENE
Bulb 0.6 ppm

2-METHYL-BENZALDEHYDE Bulb 0.1 ppm

2-PROPEN-1-OL Bulb 0.1–121 ppm

2-VINYL-4H-1,3-DITHIIN Bulb 2–29 ppm

24-METHYLENE-CYCLOARTENOL Plant

3,5-DIETHYL-1,2,4-TRITHIOLANE Bulb 0.15–43
ppm

3-METHYL-2-CYCLOPENTENE-1-THIONE Bulb
0.16–1.6 ppm

3-VINYL-4H-1,2-DITHIIN Bulb 0.34–10.65 ppm

4-METHYL-5-VINYLTHIAZOLE Bulb 0.75 ppm

5-BUTYL-CYSTEINE-SULFOXIDE Bulb

ADENOSINE Bulb

AJOENE Bulb

ALANINE Bulb 1,320–3,168 ppm

ALLICIN Bulb 1,500–27,800 ppm

ALLIIN Bulb 5,000–10,000 ppm

ALLIINASE Bulb

ALLISATIN Plant

ALLISTATIN-I Bulb

ALLISTATIN-II Bulb

ALLIXIN Bulb

ALLYL-DISULFIDE Bulb

ALLYL-METHYL-DISULFIDE Bulb

ALLYL-METHYL-TRISULFIDE Bulb

ALLYL-PROPYL-DISULFIDE Bulb 36–216 ppm

ALPHA-PHELLANDRENE Bulb

ALPHA-PROSTAGLANDIN-F-1 Bulb

ALPHA-PROSTAGLANDIN-F-2 Bulb

ALPHA-TOCOPHEROL Bulb

ALUMINUM Bulb 52 ppm

ANILINE Bulb 10 ppm

ARACHIDONIC-ACID Bulb

ARGININE Bulb 6,340–15,216 ppm

ASCORBIC-ACID Bulb 100–788 ppm Flower 440–3,793 ppm Leaf 390–2,868 ppm Shoot 420–1,883 ppm

ASH Bulb 10,000–395,000 ppm Flower 6,000–52,000 ppm Leaf 10,000–74,000 ppm Shoot 7,000–31,000 ppm

ASPARTIC-ACID Bulb 4,890–11,736 ppm

BETA-CAROTENE Bulb 0.17 ppm Flower 0.6–5 ppm Leaf 9–68 ppm Shoot 2–9 ppm

BETA-PHELLANDRENE Bulb

BETA-SITOSTEROL Plant

BETA-TOCOPHEROL Bulb

BIOTIN Bulb 22 ppm

BORON Bulb 3–6 ppm

CAFFEIC-ACID Bulb 20 ppm

CALCIUM Bulb 180–4,947 ppm Flower 250–2,155 ppm Leaf 580–4,265 ppm Shoot 120–538 ppm

CALCIUM-OXALATE Bulb

CARBOHYDRATES Bulb 274,000–851,000 ppm Flower 94,000–810,000 ppm Leaf 95,000–699,000 ppm Shoot 201,000–901,000 ppm

CHLOROGENIC-ACID Plant

CHOLINE Bulb

CHROMIUM Bulb 2.5–15 ppm

CIS-AJOENE Bulb

CITRAL Bulb

COBALT Bulb 0.5–100 ppm

COPPER Bulb 4.8–9.7 ppm

CYCLOALLIIN Bulb

CYSTINE Bulb 650–1,560 ppm

DESGALACTOTIGONIN Root 400 ppm

DESOXYRIBONUCLEASE Bulb

DIALLYL-DISULFIDE Bulb 16–613 ppm

DIALLYL-SULFIDE Bulb 2–99 ppm

DIALLYL-TETRASULFIDE Bulb

DIALLYL-TRISULFIDE Bulb 10–1,061 ppm

DIGALACTOSYL-DIGLYCERIDE Bulb

DIMETHYL-DIFURAN Bulb 5–30 ppm

DIMETHYL-DISULFIDE Bulb 0.6–2.5 ppm

DIMETHYL-SULFIDE Bulb

DIMETHYL-TRISULFIDE Bulb 0.8–19 ppm

EICOSAPENTAENOIC-ACID Bulb

EO Bulb 600–3,600 ppm

FAT Bulb 2,000–12,000 ppm Flower 2,000–17,000 ppm Leaf 5,000–37,000 ppm Shoot 3,000–13,000 ppm

FERULIC-ACID Bulb 27 ppm

FIBER Bulb 7,000–39,000 ppm Flower 8,000–69,000 ppm Leaf 18,000–132,000 ppm Shoot 17,000–76,000 ppm

FOLIACIN Bulb 1 ppm

FRUCTOSE Bulb

GAMMA-L-GLUTAMYL-ISOLEUCINE Bulb

GAMMA-L-GLUTAMYL-L-LEUCINE Bulb

GAMMA-L-GLUTAMYL-L-PHENYLALANINE Bulb

GAMMA-L-GLUTAMYL-L-VALINE Plant

GAMMA-L-GLUTAMYL-METHIONINE Bulb

GAMMA-L-GLUTAMYL-S-(2-CARBOXY-1-PROPYL)-CYSTEINEGLYCINE Plant

GAMMA-L-GLUTAMYL-S-ALLYL-CYSTEINE Bulb

GAMMA-L-GLUTAMYL-S-ALLYL-MERCAPTO-CYSTEINE Bulb

GAMMA-L-GLUTAMYL-S-BETA-CARBOXY-BETA-METHYL-ETHYL-CYSTEINYL-GLYCINE Bulb

GAMMA-L-GLUTAMYL-S-METHYL-L-CYSTEINE-SULFOXIDE Bulb

GAMMA-L-GLUTAMYL-S-PROPYL-L-CYSTEINE Bulb

GERANIOL Bulb

GERMANIUM Bulb

GIBBERELLIN-A-3 Bulb

GIBBERELLIN-A-7 Bulb

GITONIN Root 300 ppm

GLUCOSE Bulb

GLUTAMIC-ACID Bulb 8,050–19,320 ppm

GLUTATHIONE Bulb

GLYCEROL-SULFOQUINOVOSIDE Bulb

GLYCINE Bulb 2,000–4,800 ppm

GUANOSINE Bulb

HEXA-1,5-DIENYL-TRISULFIDE Bulb

HEXOKINASE Bulb

HISTIDINE Bulb 1,130–2,712 ppm

IODINE Bulb

IRON Bulb 15–129 ppm Flower 9–78 ppm Leaf 6–44 ppm Shoot 17–76 ppm

ISOBUTYL-ISOTHIOCYANATE Bulb 0.14–25 ppm

ISOLEUCINE Bulb 2,170–5,208 ppm

KAEMPFEROL Plant

KILOCALORIES Bulb 1,170–3,630 /kg Flower 390–3,366 /kg Leaf 440–3,240 /kg Shoot 760–3,410 /kg

LEUCINE Bulb 3,050–7,392 ppm

LINALOL Bulb

LINOLENIC-ACID Plant

LYSINE Bulb 2,730–6,552 ppm

MAGNESIUM Bulb 240–1,210 ppm

MANGANESE Bulb 5.4–15.3 ppm

METHIONINE Bulb 760–1,824 ppm

METHYL-ALLYL-DISULFIDE Bulb 6–104 ppm

METHYL-ALLYL-SULFIDE Bulb 0.5–4.6 ppm

METHYL-ALLYL-TRISULFIDE Bulb 6–279 ppm

METHYL-PROPYL-DISULFIDE Bulb 0.03–0.66 ppm

MONOGALACTOSYL-DIGLYCERIDE Bulb

MYROSINASE Bulb

NIACIN Bulb 4–17 ppm Flower 4–34 ppm Leaf 6–44 ppm Shoot 5–22 ppm

NICKEL Bulb 1.5–1.7 ppm

NICOTINIC-ACID Bulb 4.8 ppm

OLEANOLIC-ACID Plant

OLEIC-ACID Plant

ORNITHINE Leaf

P-COUMARIC-ACID Bulb 58 ppm

P-HYDROXY-BENZOIC-ACID Plant

PEROXIDASE Bulb

PHENYLALANINE Bulb 1,830–4,392 ppm

PHLOROGLUCINOL Plant

PHOSPHATIDYL-CHOLINE Bulb

PHOSPHATIDYL-ETHANOLAMINE Bulb

PHOSPHATIDYL-INOSITOL Bulb

PHOSPHATIDYL-SERINE Bulb

PHOSPHORUS Bulb 880–5,220 ppm Flower 460–3,966 ppm Leaf 460–3,382 ppm Shoot 520–2,332 ppm

PHYTIC-ACID Plant

POTASSIUM Bulb 3,730–13,669 ppm Leaf 3,260–23,971 ppm Shoot 2,730–12,242 ppm

PROLINE Bulb 1,000–2,400 ppm

PROP-2-ENYL-DISULFANE Bulb

PROPENE Bulb 0.01–6 ppm

PROPENETHIOL Bulb 1–41 ppm

PROSTAGLANDIN-A-1 Bulb

PROSTAGLANDIN-A-2 Bulb

PROSTAGLANDIN-B-1 Bulb

PROSTAGLANDIN-B-2 Bulb

PROSTAGLANDIN-E-1 Bulb

PROSTAGLANDIN-E-2 Bulb

PROTEIN Bulb 35,000–179,000 ppm Flower 14,000–121,000 ppm Leaf 26,000–191,000 ppm Shoot 12,000–54,000 ppm

PROTODEGALACTOTIGONIN Bulb 10 ppm

PROTOERUBOSIDE-B Bulb 100 ppm

PSEUDOSCORIDININE-A Bulb

PSEUDOSCORIDININE-B Bulb

QUERCETIN Bulb 200 ppm

QUERCETIN-3-O-BETA-D-GLUCOSIDE Plant

RAFFINOSE Bulb

RIBOFLAVIN Bulb 0.5–3 ppm Flower 0.6–5.2 ppm Leaf 1.4–10.3 ppm Shoot 0.6–2.7 ppm

RUTIN Plant

S-(2-CARBOXY-PROPYL)-GLUTATHIONE Bulb 92.5 ppm

S-ALLO-MERCAPTO-CYSTEINE Bulb 2 ppm

S-ALLYL-CYSTEINE Bulb 10 ppm

S-ALLYL-CYSTEINE-SULFOXIDE Bulb

S-ETHYL-CYSTEINE-SULFOXIDE Bulb

S-METHYL-CYSTEINE Bulb

S-METHYL-CYSTEINE-SULFOXIDE Bulb

S-METHYL-L-CYSTEINE-SULFOXIDE Bulb

S-PROPENYL-CYSTEINE Bulb

S-PROPYL-CYSTEINE-SULFOXIDE Bulb

SAPONIN Bulb

SATIVOSIDE-B-1 Bulb 30 ppm

SATIVOSIDE-R-1 Root 500 ppm

SATIVOSIDE-R-2 Root 300 ppm

SCORDINE Bulb 250 ppm

SCORDININ-A Bulb 39,000 ppm

SCORODININ-A-1 Bulb 67–30,000 ppm

SCORODININ-A-2 Bulb 250–8,000 ppm

SCORODININ-B Bulb 800 ppm

SCORODININE-A-3 Bulb 333 ppm
SCORODOSE Bulb
SELENIUM Bulb
SERINE Bulb 1,900–4,560 ppm
SILICON Bulb
SINAPIC-ACID Plant 27 ppm
SODIUM Bulb 158–559 ppm Leaf 40–294 ppm
STIGMASTEROL Plant
SUCCINIC-ACID Plant
SUCROSE Bulb
TAURINE Plant
THIAMACORNINE Bulb
THIAMAMIDINE Bulb
THIAMIN Bulb 2–8 ppm Flower 1.1–9.5 ppm
  Leaf 1.1–8.1 ppm Shoot 1.4–6.3 ppm
THREONINE Bulb 1,570–3,768 ppm
TIN Bulb 6 ppm
TRANS-1-PROPENYL-METHYL-DISULFIDE Bulb
  0.9 ppm
TRANS-AJOENE Bulb 268 ppm
TRANS-S-(PROPENYL-1-YL)-CYSTEINE-DISUL-
  FIDE Bulb
TRYPTOPHAN Bulb 660–1,584 ppm
TYROSINASE Bulb
TYROSINE Bulb 810–1,944 ppm
URANIUM Bulb
VALINE Bulb 2,910–6,984 ppm
VIT-U Plant
WATER Bulb 585,000–678,000 ppm Flower
  884,000 ppm Leaf 864,000 ppm Shoot
  777,000 ppm
ZINC Bulb 15.3 ppm

GINGER

Chemicals in *Zingiber officinale* ROSCOE
(*Zingiberaceae*)—Ginger

1,8-CINEOLE Rhizome 33–5,000 ppm
1-(4-HYDROXY METHOXYPHENYL)-3,5-DI-
  ACETOXYOCTANE Rhizome
1-(4-HYDROXY-3-METHOXYPHENYL)-3,5-OC-
  TANEDIOL Rhizome
10-DEHYDROGINGERDIONE Rhizome
10-EPIZONARENE Essential Oil
10-GINGEDIOL Rhizome
10-GINGERDIONE Rhizome
10-GINGEROL Rhizome 200–1,862 ppm
10-SHOGOAL Rhizome

12-GINGEROL Rhizome
14-GINGEROL Rhizome
16-GINGEROL Rhizome
2,2,4-TRIMETHYL-HEPTANE Rhizome
3-PHENYL-BENZALDEHYDE Rhizome
4-GINGEROL Rhizome
4-PHENYL-BENZALDEHYDE Rhizome
6,10-DEHYDROGINGERDIONE Rhizome
6-DEHYDROGINGERDIONE Rhizome
6-DIHYDROGINGERDIONE Rhizome
6-GINGEDIOL Rhizome
6-GINGEDIOL-ACETATE Rhizome
6-GINGEDIOL-ACETATE-METHYL-ETHER Rhizome
6-GINGEDIOL-METHYL-ETHER Rhizome
6-GINGERDIONE Rhizome
6-GINGEROL Rhizome 130–7,138 ppm
6-METHYL-HEPT-5-EN-2-ONE Rhizome 2–50
  ppm
6-METHYLGINGEDIACETATE Rhizome
6-METHYLGINGEDIOL Rhizome
6-PARADOL Rhizome
6-SHOGAOL Rhizome 40–330 ppm
7-GINGEROL Rhizome
8-BETA-17-EPOXY-LABD-TRANS-12-ENE-15,16-
  DIAL Rhizome 40 ppm
8-GINGEDIOL Rhizome
8-GINGEROL Rhizome 200–1,069 ppm
8-SHOGAOL Rhizome
9-GINGEROL Rhizome
9-OXO-NEROLIDOL Rhizome
ACETALDEHYDE Essential Oil
ACETIC-ACID Rhizome
ACETONE Essential Oil
ALANINE Rhizome 310–1,793 ppm
ALBUMIN Rhizome 4,984–45,924 ppm
ALLO-AROMADENDRINE Rhizome 1–70
  ppm
ALPHA-CADINENE Rhizome
ALPHA-CADINOL Rhizome
ALPHA-COPAENE Rhizome
ALPHA-CURCUMENE Rhizome
ALPHA-FARNESENE Rhizome 20–1,250 ppm
ALPHA-LINOLENIC-ACID Rhizome 340–3,190
  ppm
ALPHA-MUUROLENE Rhizome
ALPHA-PHELLANDRENE Rhizome 3–200 ppm
ALPHA-PINENE Rhizome 10–1,950 ppm

ALPHA-SELINENE Rhizome

ALPHA-TERPINENE Rhizome 0.5–35 ppm

ALPHA-TERPINEOL Rhizome 8–500 ppm

ALPHA-ZINGIBERENE Rhizome 74–4,600 ppm

ALUMINUM Rhizome 663 ppm

ANTI-METHYL-10-SHOGOAL Rhizome

ANTI-METHYL-6-SHOGAOL Rhizome

ANTI-METHYL-8-SHOGOAL Rhizome

AR-CURCUMENE Rhizome 20–9,520 ppm

ARGININE Rhizome 430–2,486 ppm

AROMADENDRINE Rhizome

ASCORBIC-ACID Rhizome 317 ppm

ASH Rhizome 7,700–200,000 ppm

ASPARAGINE Rhizome 500 ppm

ASPARTIC-ACID Rhizome 2,080–11,990 ppm

BETA-BISABOLENE Rhizome 5–3,600 ppm

BETA-BISABOLOL Rhizome 5–295 ppm

BETA-CAROTENE Rhizome 4 ppm

BETA-CARYOPHYLLENE Rhizome 0.7–45 ppm

BETA-ELEMENE Rhizome 2–500 ppm

BETA-EUDESMOL Rhizome 7–465 ppm

BETA-HIMACHALENE Rhizome

BETA-IONONE Rhizome

BETA-MYRCENE Rf 2–950 ppm

BETA-PHELLANDRENE Rhizome 32–2,850
ppm

BETA-PINENE Rhizome 4–265 ppm

BETA-SELINENE Rhizome

BETA-SESQUIPHELLANDRENE Rhizome
20–6,012 ppm

BETA-SITOSTEROL Plant

BETA-THUJONE Rhizome

BETA-ZINGIBERENE Rhizome

BORNYL-ACETATE Rhizome 2–105 ppm

BORON Rhizome 1–4 ppm

CAFFEIC-ACID Rhizome

CALAMENEN Rhizome

CALCIUM Rhizome 150–3,458 ppm

CAMPHENE Rhizome 28–6,300 ppm

CAMPHENE-HYDRATE Rhizome

CAMPHOR Rhizome 1–60 ppm

CAPRIC-ACID Rhizome 1,800–1,980 ppm

CAPRYLIC-ACID Rhizome 70–380 ppm

CAPSAICIN Plant

CAR-3-ENE Rhizome

CARBOHYDRATES Rhizome 92,000–823,240
ppm

CARYOPHYLLENE Essential Oil

CEDOROL Rhizome

CHAVICOL Rhizome

CHLOROGENIC-ACID Plant

CHROMIUM Rhizome 6–20 ppm

CINEOLE Rhizome

CIS-10-SHOGOAL Rhizome

CIS-12-SHOGOAL Rhizome

CIS-6-SHOGOAL Rhizome 40 ppm

CIS-8-SHOGOAL Rhizome 40 ppm

CIS-BETA-SESQUIPHELLANDROL Essential Oil

CIS-HEXAN-3-OL Rhizome

CIS-SESQUIABINENE-HYDRATE Rhizome

CIS-SESQUISABINENE-HYDRATE Plant

CITRAL Rhizome 13,500 ppm

CITRONELLAL Rhizome 2–145 ppm

CITRONELLOL Rhizome 2–6,500 ppm

CITRONELLYL-ACETATE Rhizome

COBALT Rhizome 0.9–42 ppm

COPPER Rhizome 3–16 ppm

CUMENE Rhizome 1 ppm

CURCUMIN Plant

CYSTINE Rhizome 80–462 ppm

D-BORNEOL Rhizome 14–1,102 ppm

DECANAL Plant 5–100 ppm

DECYL-ALDEHYDE Rhizome

DELPHINIDIN Plant

DELTA-CADINENE Rhizome 1–65 ppm

DELTA-CAR-3-ENE Rhizome

DEMETHYL-HEXAHYDROCURCUMIN Rhizome

DIETHYLSULFIDE Essential Oil

DIHYDROGINGEROL Rhizome

DODECANOIC-ACID Rhizome

ELEMOL Rhizome 3–190 ppm

EO Or 800–50,000 ppm Resin, Exudate, Sap
60,000 ppm Rhizome 800–50,000 ppm

ETHYL-ACETATE Essential Oil

ETHYL-ISOPROPYL-SULFIDE Essential Oil

ETHYL-MYRISTATE Rhizome

FARNESAL Rhizome 1–100 ppm

FARNESENE Rhizome 245–4,910 ppm

FARNESOL Rhizome

FAT Rhizome 7,000–77,000 ppm

FERULIC-ACID Plant

FIBER Rhizome 9,000–171,000 ppm

FLUORINE Rhizome 2 ppm

FRUCTOSE Rhizome

FURANOGERMENONE Rhizome

FURFURAL Plant
GADOLEIC-ACID Rhizome 70–380 ppm
GAMMA-AMINOBUTYRIC-ACID Rhizome
GAMMA-EUDESMOL Rhizome 2–115 ppm
GAMMA-MUUROLENE Rhizome 7–455 ppm
GAMMA-SELINENE Rhizome 35–700 ppm
GAMMA-TERPINENE Rhizome 0.4–25 ppm
GERANIAL Rhizome 35–20,000 ppm
GERANIOL Rhizome 2–345 ppm
GERANYL-ACETATE Rhizome
GERMANIUM Rhizome 87–169 ppm
GINGEDIACETATE Rhizome
GINGERENONE-A Rhizome 118 ppm
GINGERENONE-B Rhizome 4.7 ppm
GINGERENONE-C Rhizome 14.2 ppm
GINGEROL-METHYL-ETHER Rhizome
GINGEROLS Rhizome 13,200 ppm
GINGERONE Rhizome
GLANOLACTONE Rhizome 120 ppm
GLOBULIN Rhizome 2,366–21,801 ppm
GLUCOSE Rhizome
GLUTAMIC-ACID Rhizome 1,620–9,328 ppm
GLUTELIN Rhizome 2,506–23,091 ppm
GLYCINE Rhizome 430–2,486 ppm
GLYOXAL Essential Oil
GUAIL Rhizome
HEPTAN-2-OL Rhizome 1–135 ppm
HEPTAN-2-ONE Rhizome
HEXAHYDROCURCUMIN Rhizome
HEXAN-1-AL Rhizome 2–35 ppm
HEXANOL Rhizome
HISTIDINE Rhizome 300–1,738 ppm
HUMULENE Rhizome
IRON Rhizome 4–162 ppm
ISOEUGENOL-METHYL-ETHER Rhizome
   0.6–40 ppm
ISOGINGERENONE-B Rhizome 4.7 ppm
ISOLEUCINE Rhizome 510–2,926 ppm
ISOVALERALDEHYDE Essential Oil
KAEMPFEROL Plant
KILOCALORIES Rhizome 690–3,764 /kg
LAURIC-ACID Rhizome 390–3,630 ppm
LECITHIN Rhizome
LEUCINE Rhizome 740–4,257 ppm
LIMONENE Rhizome 17–1,050 ppm
LINALOL Rhizome 2–1,500 ppm
LINOLEIC-ACID Rhizome 1,200–11,220 ppm
LYSINE Rhizome 570–3,110 ppm

MAGNESIUM Rhizome 430–2,690 ppm
MANGANESE Rhizome 106–350 ppm
MENTHOL-ACETATE Rhizome
METHIONINE Rhizome 130–737 ppm
METHYL-10-SHOGOAL Rhizome
METHYL-12-GINGEROL Rhizome
METHYL-6-GINGEROL Rhizome
METHYL-6-SHOGOAL Rhizome
METHYL-8-GINGEROL Rhizome
METHYL-8-SHOGOAL Rhizome
METHYL-ACETATE Essential Oil
METHYL-ALLYL-SULFIDE Essential Oil
METHYL-CAPRYLATE Essential Oil
METHYL-GLYOXAL Essential Oil
METHYL-HEPTENONE Rhizome
METHYL-ISOBUTYL-KETONE Essential Oil
METHYL-NONYL-KETONE Rhizome
MUFA Rhizome 1,540–8,400 ppm
MYRCENE Rf 2–950 ppm
MYRICETIN Plant
MYRISTIC-ACID Rhizome 180–1,650 ppm
MYRTENAL Rhizome 0.5–30 ppm
N-BUTYRALDEHYDE Essential Oil
N-DECANAL Essential Oil
N-HEPTANE Rhizome
N-NONANE Essential Oil
N-NONANOL Essential Oil
N-NONANONE Rhizome
N-OCTANE Essential Oil
N-PROPANOL Essential Oil
N-UNDECANONE Rhizome
NEO-ISOPULEGOL Rhizome
NERAL Rhizome 20–13,000 ppm
NEROL Rhizome
NEROLIDOL Essential Oil
NIACIN Rhizome 5–135 ppm
NICKEL Rhizome 2–5.2 ppm
NITROGEN Rhizome 16,000–24,440 ppm
NONAN-2-OL Rhizome 5–100 ppm
NONAN-2-ONE Rhizome 8–160 ppm
NONANAL Rhizome 2–50 ppm
NONYL-ALDEHYDE Rhizome
OCTAN-1-AL Rhizome 2–40 ppm
OLEIC-ACID Rhizome 1,190–11,000 ppm
OXALIC-ACID Rhizome 5,000 ppm
P-COUMARIC-ACID Rhizome 19 ppm
P-CYMEN-8-OL Rhizome 0.5–35 ppm
P-CYMENE Rhizome 2–1,300 ppm

P-HYDROXY-BENZOIC-ACID Plant

PALMITIC-ACID Rhizome 1,200–11,220 ppm

PALMITOLEIC-ACID Rhizome 210–1,145 ppm

PANTOTHENIC-ACID Rhizome 2–11 ppm

PARADOL Rhizome

PATCHOULI-ALCOHOL Rhizome

PENTOSANS Rhizome

PERILLEN Rhizome

PERILLENE Rhizome 1–95 ppm

PHENYLALANINE Rhizome 450–2,455 ppm

PHOSPHATIDIC-ACID Rhizome

PHOSPHORUS Rhizome 320–5,323 ppm

PHYTOSTEROLS Rhizome 150–913 ppm

PIPECOLIC-ACID Rhizome 320 ppm

POTASSIUM Rhizome 2,640–25,079 ppm

PROLAMINE Plant 1,540–14,190 ppm

PROLINE Rhizome 410–2,376 ppm

PROPIONALDEHYDE Essential Oil

PROTEIN Rhizome 14,000–129,000 ppm

PUFA Rhizome 1,540–8,400 ppm

QUERCETIN Plant

RAFFINOSE Rhizome

RIBOFLAVIN Rhizome 5 ppm

ROSEFURAN Rhizome 1–90 ppm

SABINENE Rhizome 0.5–35 ppm

SEC-BUTANOL Essential Oil

SELENIUM Rhizome

SELINA-3,7(11)-DIENE Rhizome 1–65 ppm

SERINE Rhizome 450–2,596 ppm

SESQUITHUJENE Essential Oil

SFA Rhizome 2,030–11,085 ppm

SHIKIMIC-ACID Leaf

SHOGAOLS Rhizome 1,800 ppm

SILICON Rhizome 285 ppm

SODIUM Rhizome 60–709 ppm

STARCH Rhizome 123,000–500,000 ppm

STEARIC-ACID Rhizome 170–1,540 ppm

SUCROSE Rhizome

TERPINEN-4-OL Rhizome

TERPINOLENE Rhizome 1–90 ppm

TERT-BUTANOL Essential Oil

THIAMIN Rhizome 3 ppm

THREONINE Rhizome 360–2,057 ppm

TIN Rhizome 13 ppm

TRAN-6-SHOGOAL Rhizome 40 ppm

TRAN-8-SHOGOAL Rhizome 40 ppm

TRANS-10-SHOGOAL Rhizome

TRANS-12-SHOGOAL Rhizome

TRANS-BETA-FARNESENE Rhizome 1–60 ppm

TRANS-BETA-SESQUIPHELLANDROL Rhizome 6–360 ppm

TRANS-LINALOL-OXIDE Rhizome

TRANS-NEROLIDOL Rhizome 5–350 ppm

TRANS-OCTEN-2-AL Rhizome

TRICYCLENE Rhizome 2–115 ppm

TRYPTOPHAN Rhizome 120–693 ppm

TYROSINE Rhizome 200–1,122 ppm

UNDECAN-2-OL Rhizome 1–25 ppm

UNDECAN-2-ONE Rhizome

VALINE Rhizome 730–4,202 ppm

VANILLIC-ACID Plant

VANILLIN Plant

VIT-B-6 Rhizome 1.6–8.7 ppm

WATER Rhizome 93,090–930,000 ppm

XANTHORRHIZOL Rhizome 1–50 ppm

ZINC Rhizome 57 ppm

ZINGERBERONE Essential Oil

ZINGERONE Rhizome

ZINGIBAIN Rhizome

ZINGIBERENE Rhizome 0.5–30 ppm

ZINGIBERENES Rhizome 890–17,836 ppm

ZINGIBERENOL Rhizome

ZINGIBEROL Rhizome 8,000 ppm

ZINGIBERONE Rhizome 0.3–20 ppm

ZONARENE Essential Oil

GREEN BEAN

Chemicals in *Phaseolus vulgaris L.* (*Fabaceae*)—Black Bean, Garden Bean, Green Bean, Haricot, String Bean

12-DICARBONIC-ACID Hull Husk

17-BETA-ESTRADIOL Flower

2-HYDROXYGENISTEIN Fruit

2-METHOXYPHASEOLINISO-FLAVAN Sprout Seedling

ALANINE Fruit 840–8,633 ppm Seed 9,050–10,171 ppm Sprout Seedling 1,740–18,710 ppm

ALLANTOIC-ACID Fruit

ALPHA-LINOLENIC-ACID Fruit 360–3,700 ppm Seed 2,780–3,124 ppm Sprout Seedling 1,690–18,172 ppm

ALPHA-TOCOPHEROL Fruit 0.2–14 ppm Leaf 698–719 ppm

ALUMINUM Fruit 1–1,050 ppm Seed 5–73 ppm

APIGENIN Plant

ARGININE Fruit 730–7,503 ppm Seed 13,370–15,026 ppm Sprout Seedling 2,280–24,516 ppm

ARSENIC Fruit 0.003–0.01 ppm Seed 0.002–0.002 ppm

ASCORBIC-ACID Fruit 10–2,389 ppm Leaf 1,100–8,333 ppm Seed 177 ppm Sprout Seedling 387–4,161 ppm

ASH Fruit 6,000–156,000 ppm Leaf 26,000–177,000 ppm Seed 17,000–62,000 ppm Sprout Seedling 5,000–53,763 ppm

ASPARAGINE Fruit

ASPARTIC-ACID Fruit 2,550–26,208 ppm Seed 26,130–29,366 ppm Sprout Seedling 5,460–58,710 ppm

BARIUM Fruit 0.4–45 ppm Seed 0.1–7.3 ppm

BETA-CAROTENE Fruit 2.2–66 ppm Leaf 32.4–245.5 ppm Seed 0.1–9.8 ppm Sprout Seedling

BIOTIN Root

BORON Fruit 0.1–45 ppm Seed 2–43 ppm

BROMINE Fruit 2–20 ppm

CADMIUM Fruit 0.002–0.2 ppm Seed 0.007–0.039 ppm

CALCIUM Fruit 356–18,000 ppm Leaf 2,740–20,758 ppm Seed 510–3,295 ppm Sprout Seedling 170–1,828 ppm

CARBOHYDRATES Fruit 56,000–733,778 ppm Leaf 66,000–500,000 ppm Seed 278,000–701,039 ppm Sprout Seedling 41,000–440,860 ppm

CEREBROSIDE Fruit

CHOLINE Fruit

CHROMIUM Fruit 0.005–1.5 ppm Seed 0.051–4.9 ppm

COBALAMINE Root

COBALT Fruit 10.5 ppm Seed 0.034–1.05 ppm

COPPER Fruit 0.62–45 ppm Seed 2–15 ppm

CYSTINE Fruit 180–1,850 ppm Seed 2,350–2,641 ppm Sprout Seedling 480–5,161 ppm

DEC-2-EN Hull Husk

ESTROL Flower

ESTRONE Flower

FAT Fruit 2,000–47,000 ppm Leaf 4,000–54,000 ppm Seed 3,000–24,000 ppm Sprout Seedling 5,000–53,763 ppm

FERRITINE Flower

FERULIC-ACID Plant

FIBER Fruit 10,000–159,000 ppm Leaf 28,000–212,000 ppm Seed 37,000–88,700 ppm

FLUORINE Fruit 0.1–2 ppm

FOLACIN Seed 4.1–5.3 ppm Sprout Seedling 0.3–4.1 ppm

GENISTEIN Fruit

GIBBERELIN-A-37 Plant

GIBBERELIN-A-38 Plant

GLUCOKININ Fruit

GLUTAMIC-ACID Fruit 1,870–19,219 ppm Seed 32,940–37,019 ppm Sprout Seedling 5,120–55,054 ppm

GLUTATHIONE Root

GLYCINE Fruit 650–6,680 ppm Seed 8,430–9,474 ppm Sprout Seedling 1,440–15,484 ppm

HISTIDINE Fruit 340–3,494 ppm Seed 6,010–6,754 ppm Sprout Seedling 1,180–12,688 ppm

INOSITOL Fruit

IRON Fruit 6–1,050 ppm Leaf 92–697 ppm Seed 24–147 ppm Sprout Seedling 8–87 ppm

ISOLEUCINE Fruit 660–6,783 ppm Seed 9,540–10,722 ppm Sprout Seedling 1,860–20,000 ppm

KAEMPFEROL-3-GLUCURONIDE Leaf

KILOCALORIES Fruit 280–3,830 /kg Leaf 360–2,730 /kg Seed 3,230–3,832 /kg Sprout Seedling 290–3,118 /kg

LEAD Fruit 0.01–10.5 ppm Seed 0.7–1 ppm

LEUCINE Fruit 1,120–11,511 ppm Seed 17,250–19,386 ppm Sprout Seedling 3,020–32,473 ppm

LIGNIN Seed 4,100–10,800 ppm

LINOLEIC-ACID Fruit 230–2,364 ppm Seed 3,320–3,731 ppm Sprout Seedling 1,070–11,505 ppm

LITHIUM Fruit 0.216–2.7 ppm Seed 0.136–2.45 ppm

LUTEOLIN Plant

LYSINE Fruit 880–9,044 ppm Seed 14,830–16,667 ppm Sprout Seedling 2,390–25,700 ppm

MAGNESIUM Fruit 210–18,000 ppm Seed

510–3,430 ppm Sprout Seedling 210–2,258 ppm

MALONIC-ACID Fruit

MANGANESE Fruit 1–150 ppm Seed 2–24 ppm

MERCURY Fruit 0.02 ppm

METHIONINE Fruit 220–2,261 ppm Seed 3,250–3,653 ppm Sprout Seedling 440–4,731 ppm

MOLYBDENUM Fruit 20 ppm Seed 0.5–14 ppm

MUFA Fruit 50–514 ppm Seed 1,230–1,382 ppm Sprout Seedling 390–4,194 ppm

NIACIN Fruit 5–77 ppm Leaf 13–98 ppm Seed 15–38 ppm Sprout Seedling 29–312 ppm

NICKEL Fruit 15 ppm Seed 0.5–7 ppm

NITROGEN Fruit 3,600–41,000 ppm

OLEIC-ACID Fruit 40–411 ppm Seed 1,230–1,382 ppm Sprout Seedling 390–4,194 ppm

OXALIC-ACID Fruit 312 ppm

P-COUMARIC-ACID Plant

PALMITIC-ACID Fruit 220–2,261 ppm Seed 3,430–3,855 ppm Sprout Seedling 640–6,882 ppm

PANTOTHENIC-ACID Fruit 0.9–10 ppm Seed 9–10 ppm

PHASELIC-ACID Plant

PHASEOLIDES Plant

PHASEOLLIDIN Plant

PHASEOLLIN Plant

PHASEOLLIN-ISOFLAVONE Plant

PHENYLALANINE Fruit 670–6,886 ppm Seed 11,680–13,127 ppm Sprout Seedling 2,120–22,796 ppm

PHOSPHORUS Fruit 370–13,500 ppm Leaf 750–5,682 ppm Seed 2,130–5,880 ppm Sprout Seedling 370–3,978 ppm

PHYTIC-ACID Seed 4,800 ppm

PHYTOSTEROLS Seed

PIPECOLIC-ACID Fruit

POTASSIUM Fruit 1,960–58,500 ppm Seed 9,840–21,070 ppm Sprout Seedling 1,870–20,108 ppm

PROLINE Fruit 680–6,989 ppm Seed 9,160–10,294 ppm Sprout Seedling 1,690–18,172 ppm

PROTEIN Fruit 17,700–224,000 ppm Leaf 36,000–297,000 ppm Seed 98,000–394,000 ppm Sprout Seedling 42,000–451,613 ppm

PUFA Fruit 590–6,064 ppm Seed 6,100–6,855 ppm Sprout Seedling 2,760–29,677 ppm

PYRROLIDINONCARBONIC-ACID Fruit

QUERCETIN-3-GLUCURONIDE Leaf

RIBOFLAVIN Fruit 1–12 ppm Leaf 0.6–4.5 ppm Seed 1.2–3 ppm Sprout Seedling 2.5–27 ppm

RUBIDIUM Fruit 0.47–7 ppm

SELENIUM Fruit 0.001–0.008 ppm Seed 0.01 ppm

SERINE Fruit 990–10,175 ppm Seed 11,750–13,205 ppm Sprout Seedling 2,240–24,086 ppm

SFA Fruit 260–2,672 ppm Seed 3,660–4,113 ppm Sprout Seedling 720–7,742 ppm

SILICON Fruit 80–1,200 ppm

SILVER Fruit 0.3 ppm Seed 0.034–0.147 ppm

SODIUM Fruit 5.4–707 ppm Seed 0.85–112 ppm

STEARIC-ACID Fruit 40–411 ppm Seed 220–247 ppm Sprout Seedling 90–968 ppm

STRONTIUM Fruit 2–105 ppm Seed 0.7–34 ppm

SUCCINIC-ACID Fruit

SULFUR Fruit 54–875 ppm Seed 54–137 ppm

THIAMIN Fruit 0.5–8.8 ppm Leaf 1.8–13.6 ppm Seed 3.7–10 ppm Sprout Seedling 3.7–40 ppm

THREONINE Fruit 790–8,119 ppm Seed 9,090–10,216 ppm Sprout Seedling 1,760–18,925 ppm

TITANIUM Fruit 0.1–105 ppm Seed 0.17–7.4 ppm

TRAUMATINIC-ACID Hull Husk

TRIGONELLINE Fruit

TRYPTOPHAN Fruit 190–1,953 ppm Seed 2,560–2,877 ppm Sprout Seedling 440–4,731 ppm

TYROSINE Fruit 420–4,317 ppm Seed 6,080–6,833 ppm Sprout Seedling 1,440–15,484 ppm

VALINE Fruit 900–9,250 ppm Seed 11,300–12,699 ppm Sprout Seedling 2,160–23,226 ppm

VANADIUM Fruit 0.24–105 ppm

VIT-B-6 Fruit 0.74–7.6 ppm Seed 2.8–3.3 ppm

WATER Fruit 688,000–942,000 ppm Leaf 868,000 ppm Seed 63,000–604,000 ppm Sprout Seedling 907,000 ppm

ZINC Fruit 2–150 ppm Seed 19–50 ppm

ZIRCONIUM Fruit 1–22 ppm Seed 0.68–1.47 ppm

GREEN PEPPER

Chemicals in *Capsicum annuum L. (Solanaceae)*—Bell Pepper, Cherry Pepper, Cone Pepper, Green Pepper, Paprika, Sweet Pepper

1-HEXANOL Fruit
1-O-CAFFEOYL-BETA-D-GLUCOSE Fruit
1-O-FERRULOYL-BETA-D-GLUCOSE Fruit
2,3,5-TRIMETHYLPYRAZINE Fruit
2,3-BUTANEDIOL Fruit
2,3-DIMETHYL-5-ETHYLPYRAZINE Fruit
2,3-DIMETHYL-PYRAZINE Fruit
2-BUTANONE Fruit
2-HEXANOL Fruit
2-HEXANONE Fruit
2-METHOXY-3-ISOBUTYL-PYRAZINE Fruit
2-METHYL-5-ETHYLPYRAZINE Fruit
2-METHYL-BUTAN-1-OL Fruit
2-METHYL-BUTAN-2-OL Fruit
2-METHYL-BUTANAL Fruit
2-METHYL-BUTYRIC-ACID Fruit
2-METHYL-PENTAN-2-OL Fruit
2-METHYL-PROPIONIC-ACID Fruit
2-PENTYL-FURAN Fruit
2-PENTYLPYRIDINE Fruit
24-®-ETHYL-LOPHENOL Seed
24-METHYL-LANOST-9(11)-EN-3-BETA-OL Seed
24-METHYL-LOPHENOL Seed
24-METHYLENE-CYCLOARTANOL Seed
3,6-EPOXIDE-5-HYDROXY-5,6-DIHYDRO-ZEAXANTHIN Fruit
3-(SEC-BUTYL)-2-METHOXYPYRAZINE Fruit
3-HEXANOL Fruit
3-HYDROXY-ALPHA-CAROTENE Fruit
3-ISOBUTYL-2-METHOXYPYRAZINE Fruit
3-ISOPROPYL-2-METHOXYPYRAZINE Fruit
3-METHYL-1-PENTYL-3-METHYL-BUTYRATE Fruit
3-METHYL-BUTANAL Fruit
3-METHYL-BUTYRIC-ACID Fruit
3-METHYL-PENTAN-3-OL Fruit
31-NOR-LANOST-8-EN-3-BETA-OL Seed
31-NOR-LANOST-9(11)-EN-3-BETA-OL Seed

31-NOR-LANOSTEROL Seed
31-NORCYCLOARTANOL Seed
4-ALPHA-14-ALPHA-24-TRIMETHYL-CHOLESTA-8(24)-DIEN-3-BETA-OL Seed
4-ALPHA-24-DIMETHYL-CHOLESTA-7,24-DIEN-3-BETA-OL Seed
4-ALPHA-METHYL-5-ALPHA-CHOLEST-8(14)-EN-3-BETA-OL Seed
4-METHYL-1-PENTYL-2-METHYL-BUTYRATE Fruit
4-METHYL-3-PENTEN-2-ONE Fruit
4-METHYL-HEPTADECANE Fruit
4-METHYL-HEXADECANE Fruit
4-METHYL-PENTANOIC-ACID Fruit
4-METHYLPENTADECANE Fruit
4-METHYLTETRADECANE Fruit
4-METHYLTRIDECANE Fruit
5,6-DIHYDROXY-5,6-DIHYDRO-ZEAXANTHIN Fruit
5-HYDROXY-CAPSANTHIN-5,6-EPOXIDE Fruit
5-METHYL-2-FURFURAL Fruit
ACETYL-CHOLINE Pericarp Seed
ACETYLFURAN Fruit
ALANINE Fruit 350–4,774 ppm
ALPHA-CAROTENE Fruit
ALPHA-COPAENE Fruit
ALPHA-CRYPTOXANTHIN Plant
ALPHA-LINOLENIC-ACID Fruit 220–3,001 ppm
ALPHA-PHELLANDRENE Fruit
ALPHA-PINENE Fruit
ALPHA-TERPINEOL Fruit
ALPHA-THUJENE Fruit
ALPHA-TOCOPHEROL Fruit 22–284 ppm
ALUMINUM Fruit 1–44 ppm
AMMONIA(NH3) Fruit 382 ppm
ANTHERAXANTHIN Fruit
APIIN Fruit
ARACHIDIC-ACID Fruit
ARGININE Fruit 410–5,592 ppm
ARSENIC Fruit 0.004–0.015 ppm
ASCORBIC-ACID Fruit 230–20,982 ppm
ASH Fruit 5,000–122,000 ppm
ASPARAGINE Fruit
ASPARTIC-ACID Fruit 1,200–16,504 ppm
AUROCHROME Fruit
BARIUM Fruit 2–8 ppm
BEHENIC-ACID Fruit
BETA-AMYRIN Seed

BETA-APO-8'-CAROTENAL Fruit

BETA-CAROTENE Fruit 462 ppm

BETA-CAROTENE-EPOXIDE Fruit

BETA-CRYPTOXANTHIN Fruit

BETA-PINENE Fruit

BETA-SITOSTEROL Plant

BETAINE Fruit

BORON Fruit 1–18 ppm

BROMINE Fruit 0.1–111 ppm

CADMIUM Fruit 0.005–0.33 ppm

CAFFEIC-ACID Fruit 11 ppm

CALCIUM Fruit 36–1,956 ppm

CAMPESTEROL Fruit

CAMPHENE Fruit

CAPSAICIN Fruit 100–4,000 ppm

CAPSANTHIN Fruit

CAPSANTHIN-5,6-EPOXIDE Fruit

CAPSIAMIDE Fruit 20–200 ppm

CAPSIANOSIDE-A Fruit 33–250 ppm

CAPSIANOSIDE-B Fruit 2–18 ppm

CAPSIANOSIDE-C Fruit 35–103 ppm

CAPSIANOSIDE-D Fruit 21–38 ppm

CAPSIANOSIDE-E Fruit 15 ppm

CAPSIANOSIDE-F Fruit 5 ppm

CAPSIANOSIDE-I Fruit 18 ppm

CAPSIANOSIDE-II Fruit 43–138 ppm

CAPSIANOSIDE-III Fruit 15–105 ppm

CAPSIANOSIDE-IV Fruit 9 ppm

CAPSIANOSIDE-V Fruit 2 ppm

CAPSIANSIDE-A Fruit 300 ppm

CAPSICOSIDE-A-1 Root 530 ppm

CAPSICOSIDE-B-1 Root 620 ppm

CAPSICOSIDE-C-1 Root 600 ppm

CAPSIDIOL Fruit 29 ppm

CAPSOCHROME Fruit

CAPSOLUTEIN Fruit

CAPSORUBIN Fruit

CARBOHYDRATES Fruit 53,100–813,000 ppm

CARNAUBIC-ACID Seed

CARYOPHYLLENE Fruit

CHLOROGENIC-ACID Fruit

CHOLINE Pericarp 297 ppm Seed 360 ppm

CHROMIUM Fruit 0.546 ppm

CINNAMIC-ACID Tissue Culture

CIS-13'-CAPSANTHIN Fruit

CIS-9'-CAPSANTHIN Fruit

CIS-9,10-DIHYDRO-CAPSENONE Tissue Culture 1 ppm

CITRIC-ACID Fruit

CITROSTADIENOL Seed

CITROXANTHIN Fruit

CITRULLIN Fruit

COBALT Fruit 0.001–0.1 ppm

COPPER Fruit 0.5–20 ppm

CRYPTOCAPSIN Fruit

CRYPTOXANTHIN Fruit

CYCLOARTANOL Seed

CYCLOARTENOL Seed

CYCLOEUCALENOL Seed

CYCLOHEXANONE Fruit

CYCLOPENTANOL Fruit

CYSTINE Fruit 160–2,182 ppm

DECANOIC-ACID-VANILLYLAMIDE Fruit 1–68 ppm

DEHYDROASCORBIC-ACID Fruit 20,000 ppm

DELTA-3-CARENE Fruit

DIHYDROCAPSAICIN Fruit 75–1,628 ppm

DIN-N-PROPYL-AMINE Fruit 0.3 ppm

EO Fruit 16,000 ppm

ERIODICTIN Fruit

ETHYL-3-METHYLBUTYRATE Fruit

EUGENOL Fruit

FAT Fruit 2,000–144,000 ppm Seed 100,000–150,000 ppm

FIBER Fruit 12,000–351,000 ppm

FLUORINE Fruit 0.05–1 ppm

FOLACIN Fruit 3 ppm

FOLIAXANTHIN Fruit

FUNKIOSIDE Root

GALACTOSAMINE Fruit

GALACTOSE Fruit

GAMMA-TERPINENE Fruit

GLUCOSAMINE Fruit

GLUCOSE Fruit

GLUTAMIC-ACID Fruit 1,120–15,277 ppm

GLUTAMINASE Fruit

GLYCINE Fruit 310–4,228 ppm

GRAMISTEROL Seed

GROSSAMIDE Root 3 ppm

HENEICOSANE Fruit

HEPTADECANE Fruit

HESPERIDIN Fruit

HEXADECANE Fruit

HEXAN-1-AL Fruit

HEXANAL Fruit

HEXANOIC-ACID Fruit

HISTIDINE Fruit 170–2,319 ppm

HOMOCAPSAICIN Fruit 2–90 ppm

HOMODIHYDROCAPSAICIN Fruit 2–90 ppm

HYDROXY-ALPHA-CAROTENE Fruit

HYDROXY-BENZOIC-ACID-4-BETA-D-GLUCO-
SIDE Fruit

IRON Fruit 4–286 ppm

ISOHEXYL-ISOCAPROATE Fruit

ISOLEUCINE Fruit 270–3,683 ppm

L-ASPARIGINASE Fruit

LANOST-8-EN-3-BETA-OL Seed

LANOSTENOL Plant

LANOSTEROL Seed

LEAD Fruit 0.004–2 ppm

LEUCINE Fruit 440–6,002 ppm

LIMONENE Fruit

LINALOL Fruit

LINOLEIC-ACID Fruit 2,190–29,871 ppm

LITHIUM Fruit 0.284–0.4 ppm

LOPHENOL Seed

LUPEOL Seed

LUTEIN Fruit

LUTEOLIN-7-O-BETA-APIOGLUCOSIDE Leaf

LUTEOLIN-7-O-BETA-D-GLUCOSIDE Leaf

LUTEOLIN-7-O-BETA-DIGLUCOSIDE Leaf

LYSINE Fruit 380–5,183 ppm

MAGNESIUM Fruit 118–2,340 ppm

MALONIC-ACID Fruit Leaf

MANGANESE Fruit 0.7–39 ppm

MARGARIC-ACID Fruit

MERCURY Fruit 0.001–0.001 ppm

METHIONINE Fruit 100–1,364 ppm

MOLYBDENUM Fruit 15 ppm

MYRCENE Fruit

MYRISTIC-ACID Fruit 10–136 ppm

N-(13-METHYLTETRADECYL)ACETAMIDE Fruit
300–400 ppm

N-CIS-FERULOYL-TYRAMINE Root 2 ppm

N-HEXANAL Fruit

N-METHYL-ANILINE Fruit 13.1 ppm

N-NITROSO-DIMETHYLAMINE Fruit

N-NITROSO-PYRROLIDINE Fruit

N-PENTYL-AMINE Fruit 3 ppm

N-PROPYL-AMINE Fruit 2.3 ppm

N-TRANS-FERULOYL-OCTOPAMINE Root 1–2
ppm

N-TRANS-FERULOYL-TYRAMINE Root 12 ppm

N-TRANS-P-COUMAROYL-OCTOPAMINE Root
1 ppm

N-TRANS-P-COUMAROYL-TYRAMINE Root 2
ppm

NEO-BETA-CAROTENE Plant

NEOXANTHIN Fruit

NIACIN Fruit 4–172 ppm

NICKEL Fruit 0.05–5.5 ppm

NITROGEN Fruit 1,900–23,330 ppm

NONADECANE Fruit

NONANOIC-ACID-VANILLYLAMIDE Fruit 2–45
ppm

NORCAPSAICINE Fruit

NORDIHYDROCAPSAICIN Fruit 15–335 ppm

OBTUSIFOLIOL Seed

OCTANE Fruit

OCTANOIC-ACID Fruit

OLEIC-ACID Fruit 270–3,582 ppm Seed

OXALIC-ACID Fruit 257–1,171 ppm

P-AMINO-BENZALDEHYDE Root 6 ppm

P-COUMARIC-ACID Fruit 79 ppm

P-CYMENE Fruit

P-XYLENE Fruit

PALMITIC-ACID Fruit 500–6,820 ppm Seed

PALMITOLEIC-ACID Fruit 30–409 ppm

PANTOTHENIC-ACID Fruit 5 ppm

PENTADECANE Fruit

PENTADECANOIC-ACID Fruit

PHENYLALANINE Fruit 260–3,546 ppm

PHOSPHATIDYL-GLYCEROL Fruit

PHOSPHODIESTERASE Tissue Culture

PHOSPHORUS Fruit 186–3,885 ppm

PHYTOENE Fruit

PHYTOFLUENE Fruit

PIPERIDINE Fruit 5.2 ppm

PORPHOBILINOGEN-OXYGENASE Leaf

POTASSIUM Fruit 1,862–35,000 ppm

PROLINE Fruit 370–5,047 ppm

PROTEIN Fruit 8,000–184,000 ppm

PULEGONE Fruit

PYRROLIDINE Fruit 1.4 ppm

RIBOFLAVIN Fruit 19 ppm

RUBIDIUM Fruit 0.38–10 ppm

SABINENE Fruit

SCOPOLETIN Fruit

SELENIUM Fruit 0.001–0.002 ppm

SERINE Fruit 340–4,638 ppm

SILICON Fruit 1–33 ppm

SILVER Fruit 0.071–0.1 ppm
SKATOLE-PYRROLO-OXYGENASE Leaf
SODIUM Fruit 25–625 ppm
SOLANIDINE Fruit
SOLANINE Fruit Leaf 500 ppm
SOLASODINE Fruit
STEARIC-ACID Fruit 160–2,180 ppm Seed
STIGMASTEROL Fruit
STRONTIUM Fruit 2–12 ppm
SULFOQUINOVOSYL-DIACYL-GLYCEROL Fruit
SULFUR Fruit 190–2,440 ppm
TERPINEN-4-OL Fruit
TERPINOLENE Fruit
TETRADECANE Fruit
TETRAMETHYL-PYRAZINE Fruit
THIAMIN Fruit 1–15 ppm
THREONINE Fruit 310–4,228 ppm
TIN Fruit 5 ppm
TITANIUM Fruit 0.355–16 ppm
TOCOPHEROL Fruit 24 ppm
TOLUENE Fruit
TRIGONELLINE Seed 0.6 ppm
TRYPTOPHAN Fruit 110–1,500 ppm
TRYPTOPHAN-PYRROLO-OXYGENASE Leaf
TYROSINE Fruit 180–2,455 ppm
VALINE Fruit 360–4,910 ppm
VANILLOYL-GLUCOSE Fruit
VANILLYL-CAPROYLAMIDE Fruit
VANILLYL-DECANAMIDE Fruit
VANILLYL-OCTANAMIDE Fruit
VIOLAXANTHIN Fruit
VIT-B-6 Fruit 2–22 ppm
WATER Fruit 742,000–937,000 ppm
XANTHOPHYLL Plant
XANTHOPHYLL-EPOXIDE Fruit
XYLOSE Fruit
ZEAXANTHIN Fruit
ZETA-CAROTENE Fruit
ZINC Fruit 1–77 ppm
ZIRCONIUM Fruit 1.4–2 ppm

HORSERADISH

Chemicals in *Armoracia rusticana P.
GAERTN., MEYER & SCHERB.*
(*Brassicaceae*)—Horseradish

3-O-BETA-D-GLUCOSYL-BETA-D-
KAEMPFEROL-XYLOSIDE Leaf
3-O-BETA-D-GLUCOSYL-BETA-D-QUERCETIN-
XYLOSIDE Leaf
3-O-BETA-D-KAEMPFEROL-GLUCOSIDE Leaf
3-O-BETA-D-QUERCETIN-GLUCOSIDE Leaf
ALLOXURBASEN Root
ALLYL-ISOTHIOCYANATE Root 400–2,592 ppm
ALUMINUM Root 4–30 ppm
AMYLASE Root
ARGININE Root
ARSENIC Root 0.01–0.04 ppm
ASCORBIC-ACID Plant 1,220–18,200 ppm
   Root 220–3,189 ppm
ASH Plant 200,000 ppm Root 14,000–87,000
   ppm
ASPARAGINE Root
BIOSIDE Leaf
BORON Root 6–27 ppm
BROMINE Root 5–19 ppm
BUTYLISOTHIOCYANATE Plant 188–2,867
   ppm
CADMIUM Root 0.08–0.5 ppm
CALCIUM Root 240–5,512 ppm
CARBOHYDRATES Root 155,000–783,000 ppm
CHROMIUM Root 0.02–0.15 ppm
COBALT Root 0.005–0.08 ppm
COPPER Root 2–9 ppm
D-2-BUTYLISOTHIOCYANATE Seed
EO Plant 200–3,050 ppm Root 1,460–2,160
   ppm
FAT Root 2,000–12,000 ppm
FIBER Root 14,000–94,000 ppm
FLUORINE Root
FRUCTOSE Root
GENTISIC-ACID Root 15 ppm
GLUCOCOCHLEARIN Seed
GLUCOCONRINGIIN Seed
GLUCOPUTRANJIVIN Seed
GLUCOSE Root
INVERSTASE Root
IRON Root 12–106 ppm
ISOPROPYLISOTHIOCYANATE Plant
KAEMPFEROL Leaf
LEAD Root 0.02–0.15 ppm
LIMONENE Plant
LIPASE Root
MAGNESIUM Root 420–1,690 ppm
MANGANESE Root 4–19 ppm
MERCURY Root

MOLYBDENUM Root

MYROSIN Root

NIACIN Root 4–20 ppm

NICKEL Root 0.2–1.2 ppm

NITROGEN Root 8,600–38,461 ppm

P-HYDROXY-BENZOIC-ACID Root 14 ppm

PECTIN Root

PEROXIDASE Root

PHENYLETHYL-ISOTHIOCYANATE Root
    292–540 ppm

PHENYLPROPYL-ISOTHIOCYANATE Root

PHOSPHATASE Root

PHOSPHORUS Root 640–5,000 ppm

POTASSIUM Root 5,640–31,150 ppm

PROTEASE Root

PROTEIN Root 27,000–136,000 ppm

QUERCETIN Leaf

RAPHANIN Plant

RIBOFLAVIN Root 1–4 ppm

RUBIDIUM Root 0.9–4.6 ppm

RUTOSIDE Leaf

SELENIUM Root 0.001–0.01 ppm

SILICON Root 5–19 ppm

SINAPIC-ACID Plant

SINAPIN Seed

SINIGRIN Root

SODIUM Root 80–315 ppm

SULFUR Root 1,800–10,000 ppm

TANNIN Plant

THIAMIN Root 3 ppm

VANILLIC-ACID Root 45 ppm

WATER Root 740,000–802,000 ppm

ZINC Root 13–54 ppm

KALE

Chemicals in *Brassica oleracea var. acephala*
DC (*Brassicaceae*)—Kale

1-O-FERULOYL-BETA-D-GLUCOSE Leaf

1-O-SINAPOYL-BETA-D-GLUCOSE Leaf

2-HYDROXY-BUT-3-ENYL-GLUCOSINOLATE
    Leaf

3-INDOYL-METHYL-GLUCOSINOLATE Leaf

ACETYL-CHOLINE Leaf

ALANINE Leaf 1,660–10,680 ppm

ALPHA-TOCOPHEROL Leaf 359–785 ppm
    Stem 9–16 ppm

AMMONIA(NH3) Flower 15,260 ppm

ANILINE Leaf 0.7 ppm

ARACHIDONIC-ACID Leaf 20–130 ppm

ARGININE Leaf 1,840–11,840 ppm

ASCORBIC-ACID Leaf 1,200–7,720 ppm

ASH Leaf 15,000–98,500 ppm

ASPARTIC-ACID Leaf 2,950–18,985 ppm

BENZYL-AMINE Leaf 3.8 ppm

BETA-CAROTENE Leaf 50–345 ppm

CALCIUM Leaf 1,200–7,725 ppm

CARBOHYDRATES Leaf 100,000–644,000 ppm

CITRIC-ACID Leaf

COPPER Leaf 3–20 ppm

CYSTINE Leaf 440–2,830 ppm

DIMETHYL-AMINE Leaf 5.5 ppm

FAT Leaf 7,000–45,050 ppm

FIBER Leaf 15,000–96,500 ppm

FOLACIN Leaf 0.3–2 ppm

FUMARIC-ACID Leaf

GLUCOBRASSICANAPIN Leaf

GLUCOIBERIN Leaf

GLUCONAPIN Leaf

GLUTAMIC-ACID Leaf 3,740–24,065 ppm

GLYCINE Leaf 1,590–10,232 ppm

HISTIDINE Leaf 690–4,440 ppm

INDOLE-3-ACETONITRILE Shoot

INDOLE-3-CARBOXALDEHYDE Shoot

INDOLE-3-CARBOXYLIC-ACID Shoot

IRON Leaf 15–110 ppm

ISOLEUCINE Leaf 1,970–12,675 ppm

ISOPENTYL-AMINE Leaf 0.5 ppm

KAEMPFEROL Leaf 13 ppm

KILOCALORIES Leaf 500–3,220 /kg

LAURIC-ACID Leaf 20–130 ppm

LEUCINE Leaf 2,310–14,865 ppm

LINOLEIC-ACID Leaf 1,380–8,880 ppm

LINOLENIC-ACID Leaf 1,800–11,585 ppm

LYSINE Leaf 1,970–12,675 ppm

MAGNESIUM Leaf 340–2,190 ppm

MALIC-ACID Leaf

MANGANESE Leaf 8–50 ppm

METHIONINE Leaf 320–2,060 ppm

METHYL-AMINE Leaf 16.6 ppm

MUFA Leaf 520–3,345 ppm

MYRISTIC-ACID Leaf 30–190 ppm

N-BUTYL-AMINE Leaf 0.5 ppm

N-METHYL-PHENETHYLAMINE Leaf 2 ppm

N-PENTYL-AMINE Leaf 0.4 ppm

NIACIN Leaf 10–65 ppm

OLEIC-ACID Leaf 490–3,155 ppm
PALMITIC-ACID Leaf 760–4,890 ppm
PALMITOLEIC-ACID Leaf 10–65 ppm
PANTOTHENIC-ACID Leaf 1–6 ppm
PHENETHYLAMINE Leaf 3 ppm
PHOSPHORUS Leaf 560–3,600 ppm
POTASSIUM Leaf 4,270–30,000 ppm
PROGOITRIN Leaf
PROLINE Leaf 1,960–12,610 ppm
PROTEIN Leaf 33,000–212,350 ppm
PUFA Leaf 3,380–21,750 ppm
QUERCETIN Leaf 7–50 ppm
QUINIC-ACID Leaf
RIBOFLAVIN Leaf 1–8 ppm
SERINE Leaf 1,390–8,945 ppm
SFA Leaf 910–5,855 ppm
SINIGRIN Seed
SODIUM Leaf 290–3,650 ppm
STEARIC-ACID Leaf 40–260 ppm
SUCCINIC-ACID Leaf
THIAMIN Leaf 1–7 ppm
THREONINE Leaf 1,470–9,460 ppm
TOLUIDENE Leaf 1.1 ppm
TRYPTOPHAN Leaf 400–2,575 ppm
TYROSINE Leaf 1,170–7,530 ppm
VALINE Leaf 1,810–11,645 ppm
VIT-B-6 Leaf 3–17 ppm
WATER Leaf 839,000–850,000 ppm
ZINC Leaf 4–28 ppm

KELP

Chemicals in *Fucus vesiculosus L.* ( )—Bladderwrack, Kelp

4-(2",4",6" TRIHYDROXYPHENOXY)-
2,2',4',6,6'-PENTAHYDROXYBIPHENYL Plant
4-(2",4",6"-TRIHYDROXYPHENYL)-4", 6"DIHY-
DROXYPHENOXY-2,2',4',6,6'-PENTAHY
DROXYBIPHENYL Plant
ALDOBIURONIC-ACID Plant
ALGIN Plant
ALGINIC-ACID Plant
ALUMINUM Plant 631 ppm
ARACHIDONIC-ACID Plant
ARSENIC Plant 68 ppm
ASCORBIC-ACID Plant 258 ppm
BETA-CAROTENE Plant 39.6 ppm
BETA-SITOSTEROL Plant

BROMINE Plant 150 ppm
CALCIUM Plant 30,400 ppm
CARBOHYDRATES Plant 655,000 ppm
CHLOROPHYLL Plant
CHOLESTEROL Plant
CHROMIUM Plant 7 ppm
COBALT Plant 16 ppm
D-MANNITOL Plant
FAT Plant 30,000 ppm
FIBER Plant 98,000 ppm
FUCINIC-ACID Plant 1,000 ppm
FUCOIDIN Plant 600,000 ppm
FUCOL Plant
FUCOPHORETHOLS Plant
FUCOSE Plant 240,000 ppm
FUCOSTEROL Plant
GLUCURONOXYLOFUCAN Plant
HENEICOSA-1,6,9,12,15,18-HEXAEN Plant
HENEICOSA-1,6,9,12,15-PENTAEN Plant
IODINE Plant 300–5,400 ppm
IRON Plant 150 ppm
KILOCALORIES Plant 2,490 /kg
LAMINARIN Plant
LAURIC-ACID Plant
LEAD Plant 91 ppm
LUTEIN Plant
MAGNESIUM Plant 8,670 ppm
MANGANESE Plant 76 ppm
MANNITOL-DIGLUCOSIDE Plant
MANNITOL-MONOACETATE Plant
MANNITOL-MONOGLUCOSIDE Plant
MERCURY Plant 40 ppm
MUCILAGE Plant
MYRISTIC-ACID Plant
N-HENTRIACONTANE Plant
NIACIN Plant
OLEIC-ACID Plant
PALMITIC-ACID Plant
PHLOROGLUCINOL Plant
PHOSPHORUS Plant 2,490 ppm
PHYTOL Plant
PL Plant
POTASSIUM Plant 21,100 ppm
PRISTANE Plant
PROTEIN Plant 65,000 ppm
RIBOFLAVIN Plant
SELENIUM Plant
SILICON Plant 76 ppm

SODIUM Plant 56,100 ppm

SQUALENE Plant

STEARIC-ACID Plant

THIAMIN Plant

TIN Plant 24 ppm

VIOLAXANTHIN Plant

XANTHOPHYLL Plant

ZEAXANTHIN Plant

ZINC Plant 6 ppm

LETTUCE

Chemicals in *Lactuca sativa L.* (*Aster-aceae*)—Lettuce

ALANINE Leaf 560–9,333 ppm

ALPHA-LACTUCEROL Plant

ALPHA-LINOLENIC-ACID Leaf 1,130–18,833 ppm

ALPHA-TOCOPHEROL Fruit 6–139 ppm

ALUMINUM Leaf 3–126 ppm

ARGININE Leaf 710–11,833 ppm

ARSENIC Leaf 0.001–0.58 ppm

ASCORBIC-ACID Leaf 180–3,000 ppm

ASH Leaf 7,700–290,000 ppm

ASPARTIC-ACID Leaf 1,420–23,667 ppm

BARIUM Leaf 0.126–145 ppm

BETA-CAROTENE Leaf 11–190 ppm

BETA-LACTUCEROL Plant

BORON Leaf 0.9–87 ppm

BROMINE Leaf

CADMIUM Leaf 0.01–4 ppm

CAFFEIC-ACID Plant

CALCIUM Leaf 360–19,140 ppm

CAMPESTEROL Seed

CAOUTCHOUC Latex Exudate 400–1,400 ppm

CARBOHYDRATES Leaf 35,000–583,333 ppm

CERYL-ALCOHOL Leaf

CHLORINE Leaf 395 ppm

CHOLINE Leaf

CHROMIUM Leaf 0.005–20 ppm

CITRIC-ACID Leaf 500 ppm

COBALT Leaf 0.002–0.87 ppm

COPPER Leaf 0.36–29 ppm

CYSTINE Leaf 160–2,667 ppm

DELTA-5-AVENASTEROL Seed

DELTA-7-AVENASTEROL Seed

ERGOSTEROL Leaf

FAT Leaf 3,000–50,000 ppm

FERULIC-ACID Plant

FIBER Leaf 7,000–116,667 ppm

FLUORINE Leaf 0.02–8 ppm

FOLACIN Leaf

GALLIUM Stem 0.18–7 ppm

GLUTAMIC-ACID Leaf 1,820–30,333 ppm

GLYCINE Leaf 570–9,500 ppm

GUM Leaf 26,000 ppm

HISTIDINE Leaf 220–3,667 ppm

HYOSCYAMINE Plant

IRON Leaf 5–176 ppm

ISOLEUCINE Leaf 840–14,000 ppm

KAEMPFEROL Plant

LACTUCAXANTHIN Plant

LACTUCIN Plant

LACTUCOPICRIN Plant

LANTHANUM Leaf 1.26–20.3 ppm

LEAD Leaf 0.02–6 ppm

LEUCINE Leaf 790–13,167 ppm

LINOLEIC-ACID Leaf 470–7,833 ppm

LITHIUM Leaf 0.07–2.6 ppm

LUTEOLIN Plant

LYSINE Leaf 840–14,000 ppm

MAGNESIUM Leaf 110–8,700 ppm

MALIC-ACID Leaf 600 ppm

MANGANESE Leaf 1–240 ppm

MANNITOL Plant

MERCURY Leaf 0.04 ppm

METHIONINE Leaf 160–2,667 ppm

MOLYBDENUM Leaf 0.1–2 ppm

MUFA Leaf 120–2,000 ppm

N-HEXACOSYLALCOHOL Leaf

NIACIN Leaf 4–67 ppm

NICKEL Leaf 0.18–28 ppm

NITROGEN Leaf 2,200–54,000 ppm

OLEIC-ACID Leaf 90–1,500 ppm

OXALIC-ACID Leaf 110–136 ppm

P-COUMARIC-ACID Plant

PALMITIC-ACID Leaf 350–5,833 ppm

PALMITOLEIC-ACID Leaf 30–500 ppm

PANTOTHENIC-ACID Leaf 2–33 ppm

PECTINS Leaf 40,000 ppm

PHENYLALANINE Leaf 550–9,167 ppm

PHOSPHORUS Leaf 108–13,920 ppm

PHYTOSTEROLS Leaf 380–6,333 ppm

POTASSIUM Leaf 2,900–121,800 ppm

PROLINE Leaf 480–8,000 ppm

PROTEIN Leaf 13,000–216,667 ppm

PUFA Leaf 1,590–26,500 ppm
QUERCETIN Plant
SELENIUM Leaf 0.058 ppm
SERINE Leaf 390–6,500 ppm
SFA Leaf 390–6,500 ppm
SILICON Leaf 10–800 ppm
SILVER Leaf 0.018–0.58 ppm
SITOSTEROL Seed
SODIUM Leaf 28–18,560 ppm
STEARIC-ACID Leaf 40–667 ppm
STIGMAST-7-EN-3-BETA-OL Seed
STIGMASTEROL Seed
STRONTIUM Shoot 2–580 ppm
SUGAR Leaf 65,000 ppm
SULFUR Shoot 29–3,800 ppm
TARAXASTEROL Plant
THIAMIN Leaf 0.5–8.3 ppm
THREONINE Leaf 590–9,833 ppm
TITANIUM Leaf 0.09–870 ppm
TRYPTOPHAN Leaf 90–1,500 ppm
TYROSINE Leaf 320–5,333 ppm
VALINE Leaf 700–11,667 ppm
VANADIUM Leaf 0.27–20.3 ppm
VIT-B-6 Leaf 0.6–9.2 ppm
VIT-E Leaf
VIT-G Leaf
VIT-K Leaf
WATER Leaf 920,000–971,000 ppm
YTTERBIUM Leaf 0.036–0.87 ppm
YTTRIUM Leaf 0.36–8.7 ppm
ZINC Leaf 2.7–974 ppm
ZIRCONIUM Leaf 0.36–87 ppm

MUSTARD GREENS

Chemicals in *Brassica juncea* (L.) *CZERNJ.*
& *COSSON* (*Brassicaceae*)—Mustard
Greens

24-METHYLENE-25-METHYLCHOLESTEROL
  Plant
ALLYL-ISOTHIOCYANATE Seed
ASH Leaf 10,000–108,695 ppm Seed
  53,000–56,500 ppm
CALCIUM Leaf 512–5,565 ppm
COPPER Leaf 1.3–14 ppm
CROTONYL-ISOTHIOCYANATE Seed
EO Seed 4,500–30,900 ppm

FAT Leaf 12,700–138,000 ppm Seed
  300,000–380,000 ppm
FIBER Seed 80,000–85,300 ppm
GLYCOLIPIDS Plant 3,225–35,055 ppm
IRON Leaf 16–174 ppm
MAGNESIUM Leaf 353–3,837 ppm
OXALIC-ACID Leaf 1,287 ppm
PHOSPHOLIPIDS Plant 5,588–60,740 ppm
PROTEIN Leaf 28,300–307,600 ppm
WATER Leaf 908,000 ppm Seed 62,000 ppm
ZINC Leaf 6–65 ppm

OKRA

Chemicals in *Abelmoschus esculentus* (L.)
MOENCH (*Malvaceae*)—Okra

12,13-EPOXYOLEIC-ACID Seed
9-HEXADECENOIC-ACID Seed
ALANINE Fruit 730–7,300 ppm
ALPHA-TOCOPHEROL Oil 310 ppm
ARGININE Fruit 840–8,450 ppm
ASCORBIC-ACID Plant 190–2,340 ppm
ASH Fruit 7,000–70,000 ppm Seed 47,400 ppm
ASPARTIC-ACID Fruit 1,450–14,820 ppm
CALCIUM Fruit 810–8,100 ppm Seed 2,100 ppm
CARBOHYDRATES Fruit 76,300–760,000 ppm
COPPER Fruit 1–9 ppm
CYANIDIN-3-GLUCOSIDE-4'-GLUCOSIDE
  Flower
CYANIDIN-4'-GLUCOSIDE Flower
CYSTINE Fruit 180–1,900 ppm
FAT Fruit 1,000–10,000 ppm Seed
  160,000–220,000 ppm
FIBER Fruit 9,400–94,000 ppm Seed 210,200
  ppm
FOLACIN Fruit 0.7–10 ppm
GAMMA-TOCOPHEROL Oil 430 ppm
GLUTAMIC-ACID Fruit 2,710–27,100 ppm
GLYCINE Fruit 440–4,400 ppm
GOSSYPETIN Flower
GOSSYPOL Seed 70 ppm
HISTIDINE Fruit 310–3,100 ppm
IRON Fruit 8–150 ppm
ISOLEUCINE Fruit 550–6,900 ppm
KILOCALORIES Fruit 180–3,800 /kg
LEUCINE Fruit 1,050–10,500 ppm
LINOLEIC-ACID Seed 32,575–44,790 ppm
LYSINE Fruit 810–8,100 ppm

MAGNESIUM Fruit 380–6,000 ppm

MANGANESE Fruit 10–100 ppm

METHIONINE Fruit 210–2,100 ppm

MUFA Fruit 170–1,700 ppm

MYRISTIC-ACID Seed 1,120–1,540 ppm

NIACIN Fruit 10–100 ppm

OLEIC-ACID Seed 72,864–100,190 ppm

OXALIC-ACID Fruit 103 ppm

PALMITIC-ACID Seed 33,920–46,640 ppm

PANTOTHENIC-ACID Fruit 2–24 ppm

PECTIN Fruit Seed 21,500 ppm

PENTOSANS Seed 142,700 ppm

PHENYALANINE Fruit 650–6,500 ppm

PHOSPHORUS Fruit 630–6,300 ppm Seed 7,900 ppm

PHYTOSTEROLS Fruit 240–2,400 ppm

POTASSIUM Fruit 2,200–32,500 ppm Seed 8,200 ppm

PROLINE Fruit 450–14,930 ppm

PROTEIN Fruit 2,000–122,000 ppm Seed 193,800 ppm

PUFA Fruit 270–2,700 ppm

QUERCETIN Flower

RIBOFLAVIN Fruit 0.6–7 ppm

SERINE Fruit 440–4,510 ppm

SFA Fruit 260–2,600 ppm

SODIUM Fruit 10–1,000 ppm

STARCH Seed 89,200 ppm

STEARIC-ACID Seed 7,360–10,120 ppm

SUGAR Seed 40,300 ppm

SULFUR Fruit 140–1,400 ppm

THIAMIN Fruit 0.8–20 ppm

THREONINE Fruit 650–6,500 ppm

TRYPTOPHAN Fruit 170–1,710 ppm

TYROSINE Fruit 480–8,700 ppm

VALINE Fruit 910–9,100 ppm

VIT-B-6 Fruit 2–22 ppm

WATER Fruit 880,000–895,000 ppm Seed 98,900 ppm

ZINC Fruit 6–60 ppm

OLIVE

Chemicals in *Olea europaea L.* (*Oleaceae*)— Olive

(+)-CYCLO-OLIVIL Branches

1-CAFFEYL-GLUCOSE Fruit

3,4-DIHYDROXYPHENYLETHANOL-4-DIGLU-COSIDE Fruit

3,4-DIHYDROXYPHENYLETHANOL-4-MONOGLUCOSIDE Fruit

3,4-DIHYDROXYPHENYLETHYLALCOHOL Fruit

ALPHA-TOCOPHEROL Oil 119 ppm

APIGENIN Leaf

APIGENIN-7-DI-O-XYLOSIDE Leaf

APIGENIN-7-GLUCOSIDE Leaf

ARABINOSE Fruit

ARACHIDIC-ACID Fruit 300–800 ppm

ASH Fruit 64,000–294,000 ppm Leaf 61,000 ppm Twig 85,000 ppm

BETA-AMYRIN Leaf

BETA-CAROTENE Fruit 1.8–8.3 ppm

BETA-SITOSTEROL-GLUCOSIDE Leaf

BORON Fruit 1–4 ppm

CAFFEIC-ACID Fruit

CALCIUM Fruit 610–2,798 ppm Leaf 11,800 ppm

CARBOHYDRATES Fruit 13,000–60,000 ppm Leaf 735,000 ppm Twig 765,000 ppm

CATECHIN Fruit

CATECHOL-MELANIN Fruit

CHOLINE Leaf

CHRYSOERIOL-7-O-GLUCOSIDE Leaf

CINCHONIDINE Leaf

CINCHONINE Leaf

CRATAEGOLIC-ACID Fruit

CYANIDIN-3-GLUCOSIDE Fruit

CYANIDIN-3-MONOGLUCOSIDE Pericarp

CYANIDIN-3-RHAMNOSYLGLUCOSYLGLUCO-SIDE Fruit

CYANIDIN-3-RUTINOSIDE Fruit

D-1-ACETOXPINORESINOL-4″-O-METHYL-ETHER Stem

D-1-ACETOXPINORESINOL-4′-BETA-D-GLU-COSIDE Stem

D-1-HYDROXYPINORESINOL Stem

D-1-HYDROXYPINORESINOL-4″-O-METHYL-ETHER Stem

D-ACETOXPINORESINOL Stem

DEMETHYLOLEOEUROPEIN Leaf

DIHYDROCINCHONINE Leaf

DIHYDROXYPHENYLPROPANE Leaf

ELENOLIDE Fruit

ERYTHRODIOL Pericarp

ESCULETIN Stem
ESCULIN Stem
ESTRONE Seed
FAT Fruit 127,000–583,000 ppm Leaf 73,000 ppm Seed 300,000 ppm Twig 61,000 ppm
FIBER Fruit 13,000–60,000 ppm Leaf 177,000 ppm Twig 289,000 ppm
FRUCTOSE Fruit
GALACTOSE Fruit
GALACTURONIC-ACID Fruit
GAMMA-TOCOPHEROL Oil 13 ppm
GLUCOSE Fruit
IRON Fruit 16–73 ppm
KAEMPFEROL Stem
KILOCALORIES Fruit 1,160–5,320 /kg
L-OLIVIL Resin, Exudate, Sap
LIGUSTROLIDE Fruit
LINOLEIC-ACID Fruit 10,500–28,000 ppm
LUTEOLIN Leaf
LUTEOLIN-4'-O-GLUCOSIDE Leaf
LUTEOLIN-5-O-GLUCOSIDE Fruit
LUTEOLIN-7-O-GLUCOSIDE Leaf
LUTEOLINTETRAGLUCOSIDE Leaf
MANNITOL Leaf
MASLINIC-ACID Petiole
METHYL-DELTA-MASLINATE Leaf
MYRISTIC-ACID Fruit 300–800 ppm
OLEANOLIC-ACID Petiole
OLEIC-ACID Fruit 122,400–326,400 ppm
OLEOSIDE Leaf
OLEOSIDE-7-METHYL-ESTER Bark
OLEUROPEIC-ACID Root Bark
OLEUROPEIN Plant
OLIVIN Leaf
OLIVIN-4'-DIGLUCOSIDE Leaf
P-COUMARIC-ACID Fruit
PAEONIDIN-3-GLUCOSIDE Fruit
PAEONIDIN-3-RHAMNOSYLGLUCOSYLGLU-COSIDE Fruit
PALMITIC-ACID Fruit 14,250–38,000 ppm
PECTIN Fruit
PHOSPHORUS Fruit 170–780 ppm Leaf 900 ppm
POTASSIUM Fruit 550–2,523 ppm
PROTEIN Fruit 14,000–64,000 ppm Leaf 131,000 ppm Twig 89,000 ppm
PROTOCATECHUIC-ACID Fruit
QUERCETIN Stem

QUERCETIN-3-0-RUTINOSIDE Pericarp
QUERCETIN-3-O-RHAMNOSIDE Pericarp
QUINONE Fruit
RHAMNOSE Fruit
RUTIN Pericarp
SODIUM Fruit 24,000–110,092 ppm
SQUALENE Fruit
STEARIC-ACID Fruit 2,100–5,600 ppm
TANNINS Leaf
UVAOL Pericarp
VERBASCOSIDE Fruit
WATER Fruit 782,000 ppm

ONION

Chemicals in *Allium cepa L. (Liliaceae)*— Onion

1(F)-BETA-FRUCTOSYL-SUCROSE Bulb
1-(METHYLSULFINYL)-PROPYL-METHYL-DISULFIDE Bulb
1-METHYLDITHIO-PROPANE Essential Oil
1-METHYLTRITHIO-PROPANE Essential Oil
1-O-CAFFEOYL-BETA-D-GLUCOSE Leaf
1-O-FERULOYL-BETA-D-GLUCOSE Leaf
1-O-P-COUMAROYL-BETA-D-GLUCOSE Leaf
1-PROPYLTRITHIO-PROPANE Essential Oil
2,3-DIMETHYL-(DL)-BUTANE-CIS-1-CIS-DITHIAL-S,S'-DIOXIDE Bulb
2,3-DIMETHYL-5,6-DITHIA-BICYCLO(2,2,1)HEXANE-5-OXIDE Bulb
2,3-DIMETHYLTHIOPHENE Bulb
2,4-DIMETHYLTHIOPHENE Bulb
2,5-DIMETHYLTHIOPHENE Bulb
2-METHYL-BUT-2-EN-1-AL Bulb
2-METHYL-BUTYR-2-ALDEHYDE Bulb
2-METHYL-PENT-2-EN-1-AL Essential Oil
24-METHYLENE-CYCLOARTENOL Bulb
28-ISOFUCOSTEROL Bulb
3,4-DIMETHYL-2,5-DIOXO-2,5-DIHYDROTH-IOPHENE Bulb
3,4-DIMETHYLTHIOPHENE Bulb
31-NORCYCLOARTENOL Bulb
31-NORLANOSTENOL Bulb
4-ALPHA-METHYL-ZYMOSTENOL Bulb
5-DEHYDRO-AVENASTEROL Seed
5-HEXYL-CYCLOPENTA-1,3-DIONE Bulb
5-OCTYL-CYCLOPENTA-1,3-DIONE Bulb
6(G)-BETA-FRUCTOSYL-SUCROSE Bulb

9,12,13-TRIHYDROXY-OCTADEC-10-ENOIC-
ACID Bulb
9,1O,13-TRIHYDROXY-OCTADEC-11-ENOIC-
ACID Bulb
ABSCISSIC-ACID Bulb
ACETAL Bulb
ACETIC-ACID Bulb
ALANINE Bulb 330–8,597 ppm
ALLICIN Bulb
ALLIIN Bulb
ALLIOFUROSIDE-A Pericarp 220 ppm
ALLIOSPIROSIDE-A Pericarp 4,600 ppm
ALLIOSPIROSIDE-B Fruit 500 ppm
ALLIOSPIROSIDE-C Fruit 491 ppm
ALLIOSPIROSIDE-D Fruit 71 ppm
ALLYL-PROPYL-DISULFIDE Bulb
ALPHA-AMYRIN Bulb
ALPHA-SITOSTEROL Bulb
ALPHA-TOCOPHEROL Bulb 0.4–30 ppm
ALUMINUM Bulb 0.3–385 ppm
ARABINOSE Bulb
ARACHIDIC-ACID Seed
ARGININE Bulb 1,580–17,222 ppm
ARSENIC Bulb 0.002–0.076 ppm
ASCORBIC-ACID Bulb 60–2,703 ppm Leaf
390–5,000 ppm
ASH Bulb 4,000–63,000 ppm Leaf
7,000–90,000 ppm
ASPARAGINE Bulb
ASPARTIC-ACID Bulb 640–6,967 ppm
BARIUM Bulb 4–28 ppm
BENZYL-ISOTHIOCYANATE Bulb
BETA-CAROTENE Bulb 52 ppm Flower 28 ppm
Leaf 12–158 ppm
BETA-SITOSTEROL Bulb
BETA-TOCOPHEROL Seed
BORON Bulb 1–45 ppm
BRASSICASTEROL Seed
BROMINE Bulb 1–15 ppm
CADMIUM Bulb 0.005–0.38 ppm
CAFFEIC-ACID Bulb
CALCIUM Bulb 200–3,008 ppm Leaf
420–5,385 ppm
CALCIUM-OXALATE Bulb
CAMPESTEROL Bulb
CARBOHYDRATES Bulb 73,200–798,000 ppm
Leaf 47,000–603,000 ppm
CATECHOL Bulb

CEPAENES Bulb
CEPOSIDE-D Seed
CHOLEST-7-EN-3-BETA-OL Bulb
CHOLESTEROL Bulb
CHOLINE Bulb 830 ppm
CHROMIUM Bulb 0.057–4 ppm Seed 4.8 ppm
CIS-1-(PROPENYL-DITHIO)-PROPANE Essen-
tial Oil
CIS-2,3-DIMETHYL-5,6-DITHIA-
CYCLO(2,2,1)HEPTANE-5-OXIDE Bulb
CIS-3,5-DIETHYL-1,2,4-TRITHIOLANE Leaf
CIS-PROPANETHIOL-S-OXIDE Bulb
CITRIC-ACID Bulb
COBALT Bulb 0.001–0.2 ppm Seed 2.5 ppm
COPPER Bulb 0.3–11 ppm Seed 18.2 ppm
CYANIDIN-3-O-BETA-D-DIGLYCOSIDE Bulb
CYANIDIN-3-O-LAMINARIBIOSIDE Bulb
CYANIDIN-BIOSIDE Bulb
CYANIDIN-DIGLYCOSIDE Bulb
CYANIDIN-MONOGLYCOSIDE Bulb
CYCLOALLIIN Bulb
CYCLOARTENOL Bulb
CYCLOEUCALENOL Bulb
CYSTEINE Bulb
CYSTINE Bulb 210–2,289 ppm
D-MANNITOL Bulb
DIALLYL-DISULFIDE Essential Oil
DIALLYL-SULFIDE Essential Oil
DIALLYL-TRISULFIDE Essential Oil
DIHYDROALLIIN Bulb
DIMETHYL-DISULFIDE Bulb
DIMETHYL-SULFIDE Essential Oil
DIMETHYL-TRISULFIDE Essential Oil
DIPHENYLAMINE Bulb 14–11,000 ppm
DIPROPYL-DISULPHIDE Bulb
DIPROPYL-TRISULFIDE Bulb
EICOSEN-1-OL Seed
EO Bulb 50–150 ppm
ETHANOL Bulb
FAT Bulb 1,000–36,079 ppm Leaf 6,000–77,000
ppm
FERULIC-ACID Bulb
FIBER Bulb 4,400–126,000 ppm Leaf
11,000–141,000 ppm
FLUORINE Bulb 0.04–0.8 ppm
FRUCTOSAN Bulb
FRUCTOSE Bulb 65,600–162,600 ppm
FUMARIC-ACID Bulb

GAMMA-GLUTAMYL-LEUCINE Bulb
GAMMA-GLUTAMYL-PHENYLALANINE Bulb
GAMMA-GLUTAMYL-PHENYLALANINE-ETHYL-
 ESTER Bulb
GAMMA-GLUTAMYL-S-METHYL-CYSTEINE
 Plant
GAMMA-L-GLUTAMYL-ARGININE Bulb
GAMMA-L-GLUTAMYL-CYSTEINE Bulb
GAMMA-L-GLUTAMYL-ISOLEUCINE Bulb
GAMMA-L-GLUTAMYL-S(2-CARBOXY-N-
 PROPYL)L-CYSTEINE Bulb
GAMMA-L-GLUTAMYL-S-(1-PROPENYL)L-CYS-
 TEINE-SULFOXIDE Bulb
GAMMA-L-GLUTAMYL-S-(2-CARBOXY-BETA-
 METHYL-ETHYL)-CYSTEINYL-GLYCINE
 Bulb
GAMMA-L-GLUTAMYL-S-(2-CARBOXY-BETA-
 METHYL-ETHYL)-CYSTEINYL-GLYCINE-
 ETHYL
ESTER Bulb
GAMMA-L-GLUTAMYL-VALINE Bulb
GIBBERELLIN-A-4 Root
GLUCOFRUCTAN Bulb
GLUCOSE Bulb 102,000–158,600 ppm
GLUTAMINE Bulb
GLUTAN Bulb
GLYCINE Bulb 490–5,341 ppm
GLYCOLIC-ACID Bulb
GRAMISTEROL Bulb
HEXADECEN-1-OL Seed
HISTIDINE Bulb 190–2,071 ppm
IRON Bulb 2–135 ppm Leaf 34–436 ppm Seed
 235 ppm
ISOLEUCINE Bulb 420–4,578 ppm
KAEMPFEROL Bulb
KAEMPFEROL-3,4'-DI-O-BETA-D-GLUCOSIDE
 Bulb
KAEMPFEROL-4',7-DI-O-BETA-D-GLUCOSIDE
 Bulb
KAEMPFEROL-4'-O-BETA-D-GLUCOSIDE Bulb
KILOCALORIES Bulb 380–3,750 /kg Leaf
 260–3,330 /kg
LEAD Bulb 0.01–1.4 ppm
LEUCINE Bulb 410–4,469 ppm
LINOLEIC-ACID Seed Oil
LITHIUM Bulb 0.152–0.324 ppm
LOPHENOL Bulb
LYSINE Bulb 560–6,104 ppm

MAGNESIUM Bulb 76–1,230 ppm
MALIC-ACID Bulb Leaf
MANGANESE Bulb 1–38 ppm Seed 19.4 ppm
MERCURY Bulb 0.001 ppm
METHANOL Bulb
METHIONINE Bulb 100–1,090 ppm
METHIONINE-METHYLSULFONIUM Plant
METHIONINE-SULFONE Bulb
METHYL-ALLIIN Bulb
METHYL-CIS-PROPENYL-DISULFIDE Plant
METHYL-DITHIO-METHANE Essential Oil
METHYL-PROPENYL-TRISULFIDE Plant
METHYL-PROPYL-DISULFIDE Bulb
METHYLPROPYL-TRISULFIDE Bulb
MEVALONIC-ACID Bulb 0.5 ppm
MOLYBDENUM Bulb 0.1–2.3 ppm
MUFA Bulb 230–2,230 ppm
MYRISTIC-ACID Bulb 10–100 ppm
MYROSINASE Bulb
N-PROPYL-MERCAPTAN Bulb
NIACIN Bulb 1–75 ppm Leaf 7–90 ppm
NICKEL Bulb 0.05–2.5 ppm Seed 0.03–4 ppm
NITROGEN Bulb 1,700–17,690 ppm
NONADECANOIC-ACID Bulb
OLEANOLIC-ACID Bulb
OLEIC-ACID Bulb 230–2,230 ppm Seed Oil
OXALIC-ACID Bulb 10 ppm
P-COUMARIC-ACID Bulb
P-HYDROXYBANZOIC-ACID Bulb 107 ppm
PAEONIDIN-GLYCOSIDE Bulb
PALMITIC-ACID Bulb 240–2,325 ppm
PANTOTHENIC-ACID Bulb 1–16 ppm
PECTIN Bulb
PELARGONIDIN-MONOGLYCOSIDE Bulb
PENTOSAN Bulb
PEROXIDASE Bulb
PHENYLALANINE Bulb 300–3,270 ppm
PHLOROGLUCINOL Bulb 100 ppm
PHLOROGLUCINOL-CARBOXYLIC-ACID Bulb
 100 ppm
PHOSPHORUS Bulb 275–4,038 ppm Leaf
 310–5,513 ppm
PHYTOHORMONE Bulb
PHYTOSTEROLS Bulb 150–1,455 ppm
POTASSIUM Bulb 1,514–22,164 ppm
PROLINE Bulb 370–4,033 ppm
PROP-CIS-ENYL-PROPYL-DISULFIDE Bulb
PROP-CIS-ENYL-PROPYL-TRISULFIDE Bulb

PROP-TRANS-ENYL-PROPYL-DISULFIDE Bulb
PROP-TRANS-ENYL-PROPYL-TRISULFIDE Bulb
PROPAN-1-OL Bulb
PROPANE-1-THIOL Bulb
PROPIONAL Bulb
PROPIONALDEHYDE Bulb
PROSTAGLANDIN-A-1 Bulb 1 ppm
PROTEIN Bulb 10,940–162,000 ppm Leaf
  18,000–231,000 ppm
PROTOCATECHUIC-ACID Bulb 4,500–17,540
  ppm
PUFA Bulb 620–6,005 ppm
PYROCATECHOL Bulb
PYRUVIC-ACID Fruit 1,034 ppm
QUERCETIN Bulb 48,100 ppm
QUERCETIN-3,4'-DI-O-BETA-D-GLUCOSIDE
  Bulb 1,700–5,600 ppm
QUERCETIN-3-O-BETA-D-GLUCOSIDE Bulb 40
  ppm
QUERCETIN-4',7-DI-O-BETA-D-GLUCOSIDE
  Bulb 160 ppm
QUERCETIN-4-O-BETA-D-GLUCOSIDE Bulb
  100–800 ppm
QUINIC-ACID Bulb
RAFFINOSE Bulb
RHAMNOSE Bulb
RIBOFLAVIN Bulb 0.4–15 ppm
RIBOSE Bulb
RUBIDIUM Bulb 0.14–6.6 ppm
RUTIN Bulb
S-(2-CARBOXY-PROPYL)-GLUTATHIONE Bulb
  125 ppm
S-(BETA-CARBOXYBETA-METHYL-ETHER)-CYS-
  TEINE Bulb
S-ALLYL-CYSTEINE Bulb
S-METHYL-CYSTEINE Bulb
S-METHYL-CYSTEINE-SULFOXIDE Bulb
S-PROP-1-ENYL-CYSTEINE-S-OXIDE Bulb 26
  ppm
S-PROPYL-CYSTEINE-SULFOXIDE Bulb
SAPONIN Bulb
SELENIUM Bulb 0.001–0.003 ppm
SELENO-HOME-CYSTINE Plant
SELENO-METHIONINE Bulb
SELENO-METHYL-SELENOCYSTEINE Bulb
SELENO-METHYL-SELENOMETHIONINE Bulb
SELENOSIDE Plant
SERINE Bulb 350–3,815 ppm

SFA Bulb 260–2,520 ppm
SILICON Bulb 1–75 ppm
SILVER Bulb 0.038–0.054 ppm
SINAPIC-ACID Bulb
SODIUM Bulb 8–2,052 ppm
SPIRAEOSIDE Bulb 10,000–11,300 ppm
STEARIC-ACID Bulb 20–195 ppm
STIGMAST-7-EN-3-BETA-OL Seed
STIGMASTEROL Bulb
STRONTIUM Bulb 57–162 ppm
SUCCINIC-ACID Bulb
SUCROSE Bulb 82,600–145,900 ppm
SULFUR Bulb 80–4,075 ppm
TARTARIC-ACID Bulb
THIAMIN Bulb 0.3–6 ppm Leaf 0.5–6.4 ppm
THIOPROPANAL-S-OXIDE Bulb
THIOPROPIONAL-S-OXIDE Bulb
THREONINE Bulb 280–3,052 ppm
TITANIUM Bulb 0.38–11 ppm
TRANS-1-(PROPENYL-DITHIO)-PROPANE Es-
  sential Oil
TRANS-2,3-DIMETHYL-5,6-DITHIA-
  CYCLO(2,2,1)HEPTANE-5-OXIDE Bulb
TRANS-3,5-DIETHYL-1,2,4,-TRITHIOLANE Leaf
TRANS-S-(1-PROPENYL)-CYSTEINE-SULFOX-
  IDE Bulb
TRIGONELLINE Seed 13 ppm
TRYPTOPHAN Bulb 170–1,853 ppm
TSEPOSIDES Seed
TULIPOSIDE-A Root
TULIPOSIDE-B Root
TYROSINE Bulb 290–3,161 ppm
VALINE Bulb 270–2,943 ppm
VANILLIC-ACID Bulb 258 ppm
VIT-B-6 Bulb 1–18 ppm
WATER Bulb 866,000–918,000 ppm Leaf
  922,000 ppm
XYLITOL Bulb
XYLOSE Bulb
ZINC Bulb 2–53 ppm Seed 34 ppm
ZIRCONIUM Bulb 0.76–1 ppm

PAK-CHOI

Chemicals in *Brassica chinensis L.* (*Brassicaceae*)—Chinese Cabbage, Pak-Choi

ALANINE Leaf 860–18,378 ppm

ALPHA-LINOLENIC-ACID Leaf 510–10,899 ppm

ALPHA-TOCOPHEROL Leaf 2–56 ppm

ARGININE Leaf 840–17,951 ppm

ASCORBIC-ACID Leaf 450–9,713 ppm

ASH Leaf 8,000–170,960 ppm

ASPARTIC-ACID Leaf 1,080–23,080 ppm

BETA-CAROTENE Leaf 18–385 ppm

CALCIUM Leaf 1,050–22,440 ppm

CARBOHYDRATES Leaf 21,800–465,866 ppm

CYSTINE Leaf 170–3,633 ppm

FAT Leaf 2,000–42,740 ppm

FIBER Leaf 6,000–128,220 ppm

GLUTAMIC-ACID Leaf 3,600–76,932 ppm

GLYCINE Leaf 430–9,189 ppm

HISTIDINE Leaf 260–5,556 ppm

IRON Leaf 8–171 ppm

ISOLEUCINE Leaf 850–18,164 ppm

KILOCALORIES Leaf 130–2,778 /kg

LEUCINE Leaf 880–18,806 ppm

LINOLEIC-ACID Leaf 390–8,334 ppm

LYSINE Leaf 890–19,019 ppm

MAGNESIUM Leaf 106–5,844 ppm

METHIONINE Leaf 90–1,923 ppm

NIACIN Leaf 5–107 ppm

OLEIC-ACID Leaf 140–2,992 ppm

PALMITIC-ACID Leaf 220–4,701 ppm

PHENYLALANINE Leaf 440–9,402 ppm

PHOSPHORUS Leaf 370–7,907 ppm

POTASSIUM Leaf 1,804–69,143 ppm

PROLINE Leaf 310–6,625 ppm

PROTEIN Leaf 15,000–320,550 ppm

RIBOFLAVIN Leaf 0.7–15 ppm

SERINE Leaf 480–10,258 ppm

SODIUM Leaf 295–21,477 ppm

STEARIC-ACID Leaf 10–214 ppm

THIAMIN Leaf 0.4–9 ppm

THREONINE Leaf 490–10,471 ppm

TRYPTOPHAN Leaf 150–3,206 ppm

TYROSINE Leaf 290–6,197 ppm

VALINE Leaf 660–14,104 ppm

WATER Leaf 950,000–956,400 ppm

PARSLEY

Chemicals in *Petroselinum crispum* (*MILLER*) *NYMAN EX A. W. HILL* (*Apiaceae*)—Parsley

0-METHYLBENZYL-ACETATE Leaf 0.36 ppm

1,3,8-P-MENTHATRIENE Leaf 63 ppm Seed 87 ppm

1-ALLYL-2,3,4,5-TETRAMETHOXYBENZENE Seed 5–26,600 ppm

1-METHYL-4-ISOPROPENYL-BENZENE Plant

2,3-DIOXA-1-METHYL-4-(METHYL-ETHENYL)-BICYCLO-(2,2,2)-OCT-5-ENE Plant

2-(P-TOLUYL)-PROPAN-2-OL Plant

2-ALPHA-TOLYL-PROPENE Leaf

2-PENTYL-FURAN Leaf

3,8-DIOXA-4-METHYL-7-(METHYL-ETHENYL)-TRICYCLO-(5,1,0)-OCTANE Leaf

3-N-BUTYL-PHTHALIDE Seed

4-(BETA-D-GLUCOPYRANOSYLOXY)-BEN-ZOIC-ACID Seed 165 ppm

4-ISOPROPENYL-1-METHYL-BENZENE Leaf 27 ppm Seed 87 ppm

4-ISOPROPYL-CYCLOHEX-2-ENONE Leaf 0.42 ppm

4-PROPAN-1-AL-2-YL-TOLUENE Leaf

4-PROPAN-2-OL-2-YL-TOLUENE Leaf

5-METHOXY-PSORALEN Fruit 12 ppm Leaf 10 ppm

6,7-DIHYDRO-8,8-DIMETHYL-2(H),8(H)BENZO-(1,2B,5,4B'-DIPYRAN-2-6-DIONE Seed 12 ppm

6-ACETYL-7-HYDROXY-COUMARIN Seed 5 ppm

7-OCTADECANOIC-ACID Seed

8-METHOXY-PSORALEN Fruit 5 ppm

ALPHA-CADINOL Leaf 0.18 ppm

ALPHA-COPAENE Leaf 7.92 ppm

ALPHA-CUBEBENE Leaf 1.86 ppm

ALPHA-ELEMENE Leaf

ALPHA-GURJUNENE Leaf 4.92 ppm

ALPHA-NEROLIDOL Leaf 0.18 ppm

ALPHA-PHELLANDRENE Leaf 4.3 ppm Seed 0.6–210 ppm

ALPHA-PINENE Leaf 5 ppm Seed 1–31,080 ppm

ALPHA-TERPINENE Leaf 0.24 ppm

ALPHA-TERPINEOL Leaf 2.7 ppm Seed 22 ppm

ALPHA-THUJENE Leaf 0.1 ppm Seed 4–490 ppm

ALPHA-TOCOPHEROL Leaf 36–252 ppm

ALUMINUM Plant 6–390 ppm

APIGENIN Plant

APIGENIN-7-0-BETA-D-GLUCOSIDE Plant

APIGENIN-7-GLUCOAPIOSIDE Plant

APIIN Seed

APIOLE Leaf 0.36–22 ppm Seed 19,650–36,580 ppm

APIOSE Plant

ARSENIC Plant 0.01–0.21 ppm

ASCORBIC-ACID Plant 430–7,695 ppm

ASH Plant 18,000–202,464 ppm

BARIUM Plant 28–40 ppm

BENZALDEHYDE Leaf

BENZOIC-ACID-4-O-BETA-D-GLUCOSIDE Shoot 3 ppm

BERGAPTEN Root Seed Shoot 21–2,000 ppm

BETA-BISABOLENE Leaf 2.76 ppm Seed 22 ppm

BETA-CAROTENE Plant 15–267 ppm

BETA-CARYOPHYLLENE Leaf 2.46 ppm Seed 6.6–770 ppm

BETA-ELEMENE Leaf 5.4 ppm

BETA-FARNESENE Leaf 3.9 ppm Seed 25 ppm

BETA-PHELLANDRENE Leaf 60 ppm Seed 43–4,970 ppm

BETA-PHENYLETHANOL Seed

BETA-PINENE Leaf 2.4 ppm Seed 1–26,460 ppm

BETA-SELINENE Leaf 1.68 ppm

BICYCLOGERMACRENE Leaf 5.16 ppm

BIS-NORYANGONIN Tissue Culture

BORON Plant 4–54 ppm

BROMINE Plant 3–21 ppm

CADMIUM Plant 0.01–0.57 ppm

CAFFEIC-ACID Stem

CALCIUM Plant 1,000–16,850 ppm

CAMPHENE Leaf 0.24 ppm Seed 3–490 ppm

CARBOHYDRATES Plant 69,100–590,805 ppm

CARVEOL Leaf 3.9 ppm

CHALCONE-FLAVONOID-ISOMERASE Tissue Culture

CHALCONE-SYNTHASE Tissue Culture

CHLOROGENIC-ACID Stem

CHROMIUM Plant 0.06–0.7 ppm

CHRYSOERIOL-7-O-BETA-D-GLUCOSIDE Seed

CIS-3-HEXEN-1-OL Leaf 18.6 ppm Plant

CIS-BETA-OCIMENE Plant

CIS-LIGUSTILIDE Root

COBALT Plant 0.001–0.2 ppm

COPPER Plant 1–12 ppm

CRYPTONE Leaf

DELTA-3-CARENE Leaf 0.12 ppm

DELTA-CADINENE Leaf 1.38 ppm Seed 109 ppm

DELTA-CADINOL Leaf

DIMETHYL-BENZOFURAN Leaf

DIMETHYL-SULFIDE Leaf

E0 Leaf 600 ppm

ELEMICIN Leaf 18 ppm Seed 821 ppm

EO Plant 500–3,000 ppm Root 500–1,000 ppm Seed 15,000–70,000 ppm

ERIODICTYOL Plant

ESTRAGOLE Leaf 1.6 ppm

ETHANOL Plant

FALCARINONE Root

FAT Plant 3,000–53,218 ppm Seed 130,000–330,000 ppm

FIBER Plant 12,000–202,464 ppm

FLAVANONE-SYNTHASE Tissue Culture

FLUORINE Plant 0.6–7.8 ppm

FOLACIN Plant 2–17 ppm

GAMMA-CADINENE Leaf

GAMMA-ELEMENE Leaf

GAMMA-TERPINENE Leaf 0.42 ppm Seed 3–1,120 ppm

GERANIOL Leaf 1.26 ppm

GERMACRENE-D Leaf 6.9 ppm

GLYCOLIC-ACID Root Seed

GRAVEOLONE Tissue Culture

HERACLENOL Seed 3.7 ppm

HEX-3-EN-1-YL-ACETATE Plant

HEX-CIS-3-EN-1-YL-ACETATE Plant

HEXADECENOIC-ACID Leaf 0.24 ppm

HEXAN-1-AL Leaf

IMPERATORIN Fruit 1–6 ppm Leaf 0.53 ppm

INOSITOL Plant

IRON Plant 25–250 ppm

ISOIMPERATORIN Fruit 6 ppm Root

ISOPIMPINELLIN Shoot 0.3–79 ppm

JASMONIC-ACID Leaf

KAEMPFEROL Plant

LEAD Plant 0.08–4 ppm

LF Plant

LIMONENE Leaf 16 ppm Seed 6–1,470 ppm

LINALOL Leaf 0.12 ppm

LITHIUM Plant 0.76–0.792 ppm

LUTEIN Plant

LUTEOLIN-7-APIOSYL-GLUCOSIDE Seed

LUTEOLIN-7-DIGLUCOSIDE Plant

LYSINE Plant 2,190–18,724 ppm

M-XYLENE Leaf

MAGNESIUM Plant 290–5,577 ppm

MANGANESE Plant 2–375 ppm

MERCURY Plant 0.004–0.37 ppm

METHANOL Leaf

METHIONINE Plant 150–1,282 ppm

METHYL-DISULFIDE Plant

MOLYBDENUM Plant 0.1–14 ppm

MUCILAGE Root

MYRCENE Leaf 18 ppm Seed 168–1,680 ppm

MYRISTIC-ACID Seed

MYRISTICIN Leaf 131 ppm Plant 425–2,550 ppm Seed 14,785–19,800 ppm

MYRISTOLIC-ACID Seed

N-HEXANAL Leaf 0.4 ppm

N-HEXANOL Leaf 0.2 ppm

NARINGENIN Plant

NEOXANTHIN Shoot

NERAL Leaf 2.9 ppm

NIACIN Plant 5–87 ppm

NICKEL Plant 0.1–8.5 ppm

NICOTINAMIDE Plant

NICOTINIC-ACID Sprout Seedling

NICOTINIC-ACID-BETA-D-GLUCOSIDE Tissue Culture

NICOTINIC-ACID-N-ALPHA-L-ARABINOSIDE Tissue Culture

NITROGEN Leaf 4,900–40,700 ppm

OLEIC-ACID Seed 53,000 ppm

OSTHOLE Plant 840–3,975 ppm

OXYPEUCEDANIN Fruit 7–26 ppm Leaf 100 ppm

P-COUMARIC-ACID Stem

P-CYMENE Leaf 1.44 ppm Seed 34 ppm

P-CYMENE-8-OL Leaf 4.38 ppm Seed 28 ppm

P-MENTHATRIENE Leaf 0.36 ppm

P-MENTHATRIENOLE Leaf 0.84–18.3 ppm

P-MENTHYL-ACETOPHENONE Leaf 3.66 ppm Seed 31 ppm

P-XYLENE Leaf

PALMITIC-ACID Seed 5,000 ppm

PANTOTHENIC-ACID Plant 3–26 ppm

PENTATRIACONTANE Leaf 0.18 ppm

PETROSELINIC-ACID Seed 715,000 ppm

PHENYALANINE-AMMONIA-LYASE Tissue Culture

PHENYL-ACETALDEHYDE Leaf

PHOSPHORUS Plant 405–6,425 ppm

POTASSIUM Plant 4,425–53,833 ppm

PROTEIN Plant 20,000–254,096 ppm Seed 191,000 ppm

PROTOCATECHUIC-ACID Stem

PSORALEN Fruit 1–10 ppm Leaf 2.5 ppm

QUERCETIN Plant

RIBOFLAVIN Plant 2–14 ppm

ROSMARINIC-ACID Plant

RUBIDIUM Leaf 2.2–65 ppm

RUTIN Leaf 30,000 ppm

SABINENE Leaf 0.54 ppm Seed 1–1,190 ppm

SANTENE Seed 1–140 ppm

SEDANENOLIDE Seed

SELENIUM Plant 0.001–0.021 ppm

SENKYUNOLIDE Root 5 ppm

SESQUIPHELLANDRENE Leaf

SILICON Leaf 60–1,425 ppm

SILVER Plant 0.19–0.2 ppm

SODIUM Plant 213–5,569 ppm

STEARIC-ACID Seed

STRONTIUM Plant 285–396 ppm

SUCCINIC-ACID Plant

SULFUR Plant 380–4,700 ppm

TAURINE Plant

TERPINEN-4-OL Leaf 0.72 ppm

TERPINOLENE Leaf 33 ppm Seed 6–700 ppm

TETRADECANAL Leaf 3.84 ppm

THIAMIN Plant 7 ppm

TITANIUM Plant 1–2 ppm

TOLUENE Leaf

TRANS-2-HEXENAL Leaf 12.5 ppm

TRANS-2-HEXENOL Leaf 0.2 ppm

TRANS-BETA-OCIMENE Plant

TRIGONELLINE Tissue Culture

VIT-B-6 Plant 2–14 ppm

WATER Plant 73,000–889,450 ppm

XANTHOTOXIN Shoot 3–289 ppm

ZINC Plant 7–164 ppm

ZIRCONIUM Plant 3.8–4 ppm

PARSNIP

Chemicals in *Pastinaca sativa* L. (*Apiaceae*)—Parsnip

5-ALPHA-ANDROST-16-EN-3-ONE Root

5-METHOXY-PSORALEN Root 7.3 ppm

ALPHA-LINOLENIC-ACID Root 30–145 ppm

ALPHA-PHELLANDRENE Root

ALPHA-TERPINENE Root

ALPHA-THUJENE Root

ALUMINUM Root 1–35 ppm

ANGELICIN Root 34 ppm

APTERIN Root

ARSENIC Root 0.01 ppm

ASCORBIC-ACID Root 160–830 ppm

ASH Root 9,800–90,000 ppm Seed 12,000 ppm

BERGAPTEN Root 3.2–3,800 ppm Seed

BETA-BISABOLENE Root

BETA-CAROTENE Root 0.2–1 ppm

BETA-PHELLANDRENE Root

BETA-PINENE Root

BETA-TRANS-FARNESENE Root

BORON Root 4–25 ppm

BROMINE Root

CADMIUM Root 0.01–0.4 ppm

CALCIUM Root 315–3,525 ppm

CAMPHENE Root

CARBOHYDRATES Root 17,500–902,000 ppm

CHROMIUM Root 0.01–0.1 ppm

CIS-ALLO-OCIMENE Root

CIS-BETA-OCIMENE Root

COBALT Root

COPPER Root 0.8–12 ppm

FAT Root 3,000–24,000 ppm Seed
173,000–288,000 ppm

FIBER Root 15,000–97,700 ppm

FLUORINE Root 0.1 ppm

FOLACIN Root 0.6–3.6 ppm

GAMMA-TERPINENE Root

IMPERATORIN Leaf Root 1,700 ppm Seed

IRON Root 4–112 ppm

ISOBERGAPTEN Plant

ISOIMPERATORIN Seed

ISOPIMPINELLIN Seed

ISORHAMNETIN Leaf

ISORHAMNETIN-3-GLUCOSIDE-4-RHAMNO-
SIDE Plant

KAEMPFEROL Seed

KILOCALORIES Root 650–3,664 ppm

LEAD Root 0.01–0.1 ppm

LIMONENE Root

LINOLEIC-ACID Root 410–2,000 ppm Seed
36,330 ppm

MAGNESIUM Root 230–2,100 ppm

MANGANESE Root 2–33 ppm

MERCURY Root 0.001–0.002 ppm

MOLYBDENUM Root 0.1–0.5 ppm

MUFA Root 1,120–5,470 ppm

MYRCENE Root

MYRISTIC-ACID Root 30–145 ppm

MYRISTICIN Root Essent. Oil 183,000–662,000
ppm

N-HEPTACOSANE Seed

N-HEXACOSANE Seed

N-NONACOSANE Seed

N-NONADECANE Seed

N-OCTACOSANE Seed

N-OCTADECANE Seed

N-OCTYL-ALCOHOL Seed

N-TRIACONTANE Seed

NIACIN Root 2–34 ppm

NICKEL Root 0.04–1.6 ppm

NITROGEN Root 3,000–33,160 ppm

OCTYL-BUTYRATE Plant

OCTYL-PROPIONATE Plant

OLEIC-ACID Seed 1,020–158,000 ppm

OXALIC-ACID Root 205 ppm

P-CYMENE Root

PALMITIC-ACID Root 300–1,730 ppm Seed
1,730–2,880 ppm

PALMITOLEIC-ACID Root 30–145 ppm

PANTOTHENIC-ACID Root 6–29 ppm

PASTINACIN Seed

PETROSELINDIOLEIN Seed

PETROSELINIC-ACID Seed 79,580–132,500
ppm

PETROSELINOLEIN Seed

PHOSPHORUS Root 400–7,365 ppm

PIMPINELLIN Plant

POTASSIUM Root 3,300–40,000 ppm

PROTEIN Root 12,000–85,000 ppm Seed
150,000–155,000 ppm

PSORALEN Root 7.1–10.5 ppm

PUFA Root 470–2,300 ppm

PYRUVIC-CARBOXYLASE Root

QUERCETIN Leaf

QUERCETIN-3-O-BETA-D-GLUCOSIDE Leaf

QUERCETIN-3-RHAMNOGLUCOSIDE Leaf

RIBOFLAVIN Root 0.5–4 ppm

RUBIDIUM Root 0.6–10 ppm

RUTIN Plant

SABINENE Root

SELINIUM Root 0.001–0.002 ppm

SFA Root 500–2,445 ppm

SILICON Root 2–50 ppm

SODIUM Root 100–575 ppm

SPHONDIN Root

STEARIC-ACID Root 140–685 ppm

SUBERIN Root

SULFUR Root 270–11,050 ppm

TERPINOLENE Root Essent. Oil
253,000–666,000 ppm

THIAMIN Root 0.8–11.4 ppm

TRANS-BETA-OCIMENE Root

TRIPETROSELINENE Seed

UMBELLIFERONE Plant

VIT-B-6 Root 0.9–4.4 ppm

WATER Root 724,000–812,000 ppm

XANTHOTOXIN Leaf 800 ppm Root 26–1,000
ppm

XANTHOTOXOL Plant

ZINC Root 5–70 ppm

PLANTAIN

Chemicals in *Musa x paradisiaca L.*
(*Musaceae*)—Banana, Plantain

(24R)-4ALPHA,14ALPHA,24-TRIMETHYL-
5ALPHA-CHOLESTA-8,25(27)-3BETA-OL
Plant

(24S)-24-METHYL-25-DEHYDROCHOLES-
TEROL Fruit

2,4-METHYLENE-CHOLESTEROL Fruit

24-METHYL-CHOLESTEROL Fruit

24-METHYLENE-31-NOR-5ALPHA-CYCLOAR-
TAN-3-ONE Fruit

24-METHYLENE-31-NOR-5ALPHA-LANOST-
9(11)-3BETA-OL Fruit

24-METHYLENE-CYCLOARTENOL Fruit Plant

24-METHYLENE-CYCLOARTENOL-PALMITATE
Fruit

24-METHYLENEPOLLINASTANOL Fruit

31-NOR-24BETA-METHYL-9,19-CY-
CLOLANOST-25-EN-3ALPHA-OL Flower

31-NORCYCLOLAUDENOL Fruit

31-NORCYCLOLAUDENONE Fruit

5-HYDROXYTRYPTAMINE Plant

6G-BETA-D-FRUCTOFURANOSYLSUCROSE
Fruit

ACETIC-ACID Fruit

ALANINE Fruit 390–1,515 ppm

ALPHA-CAROTENE Fruit 0.12–0.36 ppm

ALPHA-KETO-GLUTARIC-ACID Leaf

ALPHA-LINOLENIC-ACID Fruit 330–1,282 ppm

ALPHA-TOCOPHEROL Hull Husk 30 ppm

ALUMINUM Fruit 1–35 ppm

AMYLASE Fruit

AMYLOSE Fruit 205,000 ppm

ANHYDROGALACTURONIC-ACID Fruit

ARABINOSE Fruit

ARGININE Fruit 470–1,826 ppm

ARSENIC Fruit 0.04–0.35 ppm

ASCORBIC-ACID Fruit 88–367 ppm Hull Husk
1,380 ppm

ASCORBIC-ACID-OXIDASE Fruit

ASH Flower 12,000 ppm Fruit 7,100–31,900
ppm Hull Husk 121,000 ppm
Leaf 88,000 ppm Pith 6,000 ppm Shoot
11,710–158,300 ppm Sprout Seedling 143,000
ppm

ASPARTIC-ACID Fruit 1,130–4,390 ppm

BETA-CAROTENE Fruit 0.4–2.1 ppm Hull Husk
0.6–16.6 ppm

BETA-SITOSTEROL Fruit Leaf

BIOTIN Fruit

BORIC-ACID Fruit

BORON Fruit 1–17.7 ppm

BROMINE Fruit 0.3–27 ppm

BUTYRIC-ACID Fruit Plant

CADMIUM Fruit

CALCIUM Flower 300 ppm Fruit 40–460 ppm
Leaf 7,500 ppm Pith 100 ppm
Sprout Seedling 11,600 ppm

CALCIUM-PECTATE Fruit 42,000 ppm

CAMPESTEROL Fruit

CAPRIC-ACID Fruit 10–39 ppm

CAPROLIC-ACID Plant

CAPRYLIC-ACID Plant

CARBOHYDRATES Flower 50,000 ppm Fruit
234,300–910,256 ppm Hull Husk 631,000
ppm Leaf 695,000 ppm Pith 97,000 ppm
Shoot 39,000–527,000 ppm Sprout Seedling
810,000 ppm

CATALASE Fruit

CELLULOSE Fruit

CHLORINE Fruit 1,250 ppm

CHLOROPHYLL Hull Husk 52–103 ppm

CHOLESTEROL Fruit

CHROMIUM Fruit 0.02–0.15 ppm

CITRIC-ACID Fruit

COBALT Fruit

COPPER Fruit 1–7 ppm

CYANIDIN Inflorescence

CYCLOARTENOL Fruit

CYCLOEUCALENOL Fruit

CYCLOEUCALENONE Fruit

CYCLOLAUDENOL Fruit

CYSTINE Fruit 170–660 ppm

DEHYDROASCORBIC-ACID Fruit 10–51 ppm

DELPHINIDIN Inflorescence Plant

DOPA Fruit

DOPAMINE Fruit Hull Husk 700 ppm

ERUCIC-ACID Plant

FAT Flower 2,000 ppm Fruit 3,450–23,693 ppm Hull Husk 87,000 ppm

Leaf 118,000 ppm Pith 1,000 ppm Shoot 8,480–115,000 ppm Sprout Seedling 23,000 ppm

FIBER Flower 19,000 ppm Fruit 5,000–19,425 ppm Hull Husk 100,000 ppm

Leaf 240,000 ppm Pith 8,000 ppm Shoot 13,210–178,600 ppm Sprout Seedling 205,000 ppm

FLUORINE Fruit 0.1–0.4 ppm

FOLACIN Fruit 0.2–0.9 ppm

FORMIC-ACID Fruit

FRUCTOSE Fruit 35,000 ppm

GABA Fruit

GADOLEIC-ACID Plant

GALACTOSE Fruit

GAMMA-GUANIDINO-N-BUTYRIC-ACID Fruit

GAMMA-GUANIDINOBUTYRIC-ACID Fruit

GLUCOSE Fruit 45,000 ppm

GLUTAMIC-ACID Fruit 1,110–4,312 ppm

GLUTARIC-ACID Leaf

GLYCERIC-ACID Leaf

GLYCINE Fruit 370–1,437 ppm

GLYCOLIC-ACID Leaf

GLYOXALIC-ACID Leaf

HEMICELLULOSE Fruit

HISTIDINE Fruit 810–3,147 ppm

INDOLE-3-ACETIC-ACID Fruit

INOSITOL Fruit 340 ppm

INVERTASE Fruit

IRON Flower 1 ppm Fruit 3–25 ppm Pith 11 ppm

ISOFUCISTEROL Fruit

ISOLEUCINE Fruit 330–1,282 ppm

ISOVALERIANIC-ACID Plant

KAEMPFEROL Fruit Plant

KILOCALORIES Fruit 920–3,574 /kg

L-OCTACOSANOL Plant

L-TRIACONTAOL Plant

LATEX Hull Husk 20,000 ppm

LAURIC-ACID Fruit 20–78 ppm

LEAD Fruit 0.02–0.2 ppm

LEUCINE Fruit 710–2,758 ppm

LEUCOCYANIDIN Fruit

LEUCODELPHINIDIN Fruit

LIGNIN Fruit

LINOLEIC-ACID Fruit 560–2,176 ppm

LIPASE Fruit

LUTEIN Fruit 0.033–0.1 ppm

LYSINE Fruit 480–1,865 ppm

MAGNESIUM Fruit 277–1,465 ppm

MALIC-ACID Fruit 530–3,730 ppm

MALONIC-ACID Leaf

MALTOSE Fruit

MALVIDIN Inflorescence

MANGANESE Fruit 1.4–18 ppm

MERCURY Fruit 0.001–0.007 ppm

METHIONINE Fruit 110–427 ppm

MFA Fruit 410–1,593 ppm

MOLYBDENUM Fruit

MUFA Fruit 410–1,593 ppm

MYRISTIC-ACID Fruit 30–117 ppm

NEO-BETA-CAROTENE-U Hull Husk 0.1–0.3 ppm

NIACIN Flower 6 ppm Fruit 5–23 ppm Hull Husk 50 ppm Pith 2 ppm

NICKEL Fruit 0.01–0.1 ppm

NITROGEN Fruit 1,600–15,000 ppm

NONACOSANE Plant

NOREPINEPHRINE Fruit Hull Husk 122 ppm

OBTUSIFOLIOL Fruit

OLEIC-ACID Fruit 270–1,049 ppm

OXALIC-ACID Fruit 22–5,240 ppm Leaf

OXYGENASE Fruit

PALMITIC-ACID Fruit 1,250–4,856 ppm

PALMITOLEIC-ACID Fruit 120–466 ppm

PANTOTHENIC-ACID Fruit 2.6–10.1 ppm

PECTIN Fruit 7,000–40,000 ppm Hull Husk 3,800–12,800 ppm

PELARGONIDIN Inflorescence

PEONIDIN Inflorescence

PEROXIDASE Fruit

PETUNIDIN Inflorescence

PHENYLALANINE Fruit 380–1,476 ppm

PHOSPHATASE Fruit

PHOSPHORIC-ACID Fruit

PHOSPHORUS Flower 500 ppm Fruit 200–1,190 ppm Leaf 2,400 ppm Pith 100 ppm

PHYTOSTEROLS Fruit 160–622 ppm

PIPECOLIC-ACID Fruit

POTASSIUM Fruit 3,100–16,150 ppm

PROLINE Fruit 400–1,554 ppm

PROTEASE Fruit

PROTEIN Flower 61,000 ppm Fruit 10,040–41,026 ppm Leaf 99,000 ppm Pith 5,000 ppm Shoot 18,930–255,900 ppm Sprout Seedling 24,000 ppm

PUFA Fruit 890–3,458 ppm

PYRUVIC-ACID Leaf

QUERCETIN Fruit Plant

QUINIC-ACID Fruit

RHAMNOSE Fruit

RIBOFLAVIN Fruit 1–3.9 ppm

RUBIDIUM Fruit 2.5–20 ppm

RUTIN Fruit

SELENIUM Fruit 0.001–0.04 ppm

SERINE Fruit 470–1,826 ppm

SEROTONIN Fruit Hull Husk 47–93 ppm

SFA Fruit 1,850–7,187 ppm

SHIKIMIC-ACID Leaf

SILICA Fruit 238 ppm

SILICON Fruit 70–350 ppm

SITOINDOSIDE Fruit

SITOSATEROL Fruit

SODIUM Fruit 6–44 ppm

STARCH Fruit 7,000–17,500 ppm Stem 50,000 ppm

STEARIC-ACID Fruit 60–233 ppm

STIGMASTEROL Fruit

SUCCINIC-ACID Fruit Leaf

SUCROSE Fruit 119,000 ppm

SULFUR Fruit 78–500 ppm

TARTARIC-ACID Fruit

THIAMIN Fruit 0.45–1.7 ppm

THREONINE Fruit 340–1,321 ppm

TOCOPHEROL Fruit 2–11 ppm

TRYPTOPHAN Fruit 120–466 ppm

TYROSINE Fruit 240–932 ppm

VALINE Fruit 470–1,826 ppm

VANILLIC-ACID Plant

VIT-B-6 Fruit 6–22.5 ppm

WATER Bulb 902,000 ppm Flower 902,000 ppm Fruit 738,790–746,410 ppm Latex Exudate 114,600 ppm Pith 883,000 ppm Shoot 926,000 ppm

XANTHOPHYLLS Hull Husk 1–7.3 ppm

XYLOSE Fruit

ZINC Fruit 1.5–10 ppm

POTATO

Chemicals in *Solanum tuberosum L.* (*Solanaceae*)—Potato

(25S)-BAROGENIN Tuber 9.5 ppm

1,4-DIMETHYLNAPTHALENE Plant

1,6-DIMETHYLNAPTHALENE Plant

11-HYDROXY-11-METHYL-ETHYL-6,10-DI-METHYL-SPIRO-(4,5)-DEC-6-EN-8-ONE Tuber 81 ppm

16-HYDROXY-HEXADECANOIC-ACID Leaf

18-HYDROXY-OCTADECANOIC-ACID Leaf

18-HYDROXY-OCTADECENOIC-ACID Leaf

2'-CHLORO-DIAZEPAM Tuber

2'-CHLORO-N-DEMETHYL-DIAZEPAM Tuber

2-(1',2'DIHYDROXY-1'-METHYL-ETHYL)-6,10-DIMETHYL-9-HYDROXY-SPIRO-(4,5)-DEC-6-EN-8-ONE Tuber

2-(12-O-BETA-D-GLUCOSYL-11-HYDROXY-11-METHYL-ETHYL)-6,10-DIMETHYL-SPIRO-4,5)-DEC-6-EN-8-ONE Tuber 262 ppm

2-ALPHA-ETHOXY-DIHYDRO-PHYTUBERIN Tuber

2-BETA-ETHOXY-DIHYDRO-PHYTUBERIN Tuber

2-PENTYL-FURAN Plant

22-HYDROXY-DOCOSANOIC-ACID Leaf

24-HYDROXY-TETRACOSANOIC-ACID Leaf

24-METHYLENE-CYCLOARTENOL Fruit

24-METHYLENE-LOPHENOL Plant

26-HYDROXY-HEXACOSANOIC-ACID Leaf

28-HYDROXY-OCTACOSANOIC-ACID Leaf

3,4-DICAFFEOYL-QUINIC-ACID Tuber 3 ppm

3,5-DICAFFEOYL-QUINIC-ACID Tuber

3-HYDROXY-2'CHLORO-N-DEMETHYL-DI-AZEPAM Tuber

4-ALPHA,14-ALPHA-DIMETHYLCHOLESTA-
8,24-DIEN-3-BETA-OL Plant

5-ALPHA-CHOLESTANE Tuber

6,10-DIMETHYL-SPIRO-(4,5)-DEC-6-EN-2,8-
DIONE Tuber

6-(3-METHYL-2-BUTANYL-AMINO)PURINE-9-
BETA-D-RIBOFURANOSIDE Tuber

6-(3-METHYL-2-BUTENYL-AMINO)PURINE
Tuber

9,10,18-TRIHYDROXY-OCTADECANOIC-ACID
Leaf

9,10,18-TRIHYDROXY-OCTADECENOIC-ACID
Leaf

9-DIHYDRO-OCTADECADIENOIC-ACID Leaf

9-HYDROXYNONANOIC-ACID Leaf

ACETALDEHYDE Plant

ACETONE Plant

ACETYL-CHOLINE Plant

ACETYL-DEHYDRO-RISHITINOL Tuber

ACONITIC-ACID Plant

ACROLEIN Essential Oil

ADENINE Plant

ALANINE Tuber 1,140–5,700 ppm

ALLANTOIN Plant

ALLOCYANIDOL Plant

ALPHA-AMINO-BUTYRIC-ACID Plant

ALPHA-AMYLASE Plant

ALPHA-CHACONINE Tuber 0.5–635 ppm

ALPHA-GLUCOSIDASE Tuber

ALPHA-KETO-GLUTARIC-ACID Plant

ALPHA-SOLAMARINE Plant

ALPHA-SOLANINE Tuber 5–125,100 ppm

ALPHA-TOCOPHEROL Tuber 0.5–2.8 ppm

ALUMINUM Tuber 3.9–255 ppm

ANHYDROGALACTURONIC-ACID Plant

ARABINOSE Plant

ARABINOSYL-GLUCOSE Plant

ARGININE Tuber 950–6,850 ppm

ARSENIC Tuber 0.001–0.6 ppm

ASCORBIC-ACID Tuber 170–990 ppm

ASH Tuber 8,100–85,000 ppm

ASPARTIC-ACID Tuber 4,340–24,050 ppm

BARIUM Tuber 0.078–60 ppm

BEHENIC-ACID Leaf

BEHENYL-FERULATE Tuber

BENZOTHIAZOL Plant

BETA-2-CHACONINE Tuber

BETA-AMYLASE Plant

BETA-ANHYDROROTUNDOL Tuber

BETA-CAROTENE Tuber 1 ppm

BETA-CAROTENE-5,6-MONOEPOXIDE Plant

BETA-CHACONINE Tuber

BETA-SITOSTEROL Plant

BETA-SOLAMARINE Plant

BORON Tuber 1–8 ppm

BROMINE Tuber 0.2–30 ppm

CADAVERINE Plant

CADMIUM Tuber 0.004–0.455 ppm

CAFFEIC-ACID Tuber 280 ppm

CALCIUM Tuber 34–2,550 ppm

CAMPESTEROL Plant

CAPRIC-ACID Tuber 10–48 ppm

CAPROIC-ACID Leaf

CARBOHYDRATES Tuber 171,000–862,000
ppm

CAROTENOIDS Tuber 3 ppm

CATECHOLASE Plant

CELLULOSE Plant

CHLORINE Tuber 16 ppm

CHLOROGENIC-ACID Tuber 22–71 ppm

CHOLESTEROL Plant

CHOLINE Tuber 330–1,000 ppm

CHROMIUM Tuber 0.002–1.4 ppm

CIS-ANTHERAXANTHIN-5,6-MONOEPOXIDE
Plant

CIS-NEOXANTHIN Plant

CIS-VIOLAXANTHIN Plant

CITRIC-ACID Tuber 2,000 ppm

CITROSTADIENOL Plant

COBALT Tuber 0.002–0.3 ppm

COPPER Tuber 0.48–14 ppm

CROTONALDEHYDE Plant

CRYPTOCHLOROGENIC-ACID Tuber 11 ppm

CRYPTOXANTHIN Plant

CRYPTOXANTHIN-5,6-DIEPOXIDE Plant

CUSCOHYGRINE Root

CYANIN Flower

CYANOSIDE Plant

CYCLOARTENOL Tuber

CYCLODEHYDROISOLUBIMIN Tuber 0.7 ppm

CYCLOLAUDENOL Fruit

CYNAROSIDE Flower

CYSTINE Tuber 230–1,235 ppm

DEACETYL-PHYTUBERIN Tuber 36 ppm

DELPHINIDIN-3-RUTINOSIDE Plant

DELPHININ Flower

DEMISSIDINE Tuber

DEMISSINE Tuber

DI-GALACTOSYL-GLYCEROL Plant

DIAZEPAM Tuber

DIHYDROXY-HEXADECANOIC-ACID Leaf

DIMETHYL-SULFIDE Plant

DOCOSAN-1-OL Leaf

EICOSAN-1-OL Leaf

EICOSANOIC-ACID Leaf

EICOSYL-FERULATE Tuber

EO Plant 2 ppm

EPILUBIMIN Tuber

ETHANETHIOL Plant

FAT Tuber 1,000–9,000 ppm

FERULIC-ACID Tuber 28 ppm

FIBER Tuber 3,000–27,000 ppm

FLUROINE Tuber 0.06–1 ppm

FOLACIN Tuber 0.074 ppm

FRUCTOSE Plant

FUCOSE Plant

FUMARIC-ACID Tuber

FURFUROL Plant

GALACTINOL Plant

GALACTOSE Plant

GAMMA-AMINOBUTYRIC-ACID Plant

GAMMA-CHACONINE Tuber

GERANIOL Plant

GIBBERELLINS Tuber

GLUCINOL Tuber

GLUCOSE Plant

GLUCOSYL-MYOINOSITOL Plant

GLUTAMIC-ACID Tuber 3,470–24,150 ppm

GLUTAMINE Plant

GLUTATHIONE Plant

GLYCINE Tuber 620–5,700 ppm

GLYOXALIC-ACID Plant

HEMICELLULOSE Plant

HEPTADECAN-1-OL Leaf

HEPTADECANOIC-ACID Leaf

HEPTADECENEDOIC-ACID Leaf

HEXACOSAN-1-OL Leaf

HEXACOSANOIC-ACID Leaf

HEXACOSYL-FERULATE Tuber

HEXADECAN-1-OL Leaf

HEXADECANEDIOIC-ACID Leaf

HEXADECANOIC-ACID Leaf

HEXADECYL-FERULATE Tuber

HISTIDINE Tuber 450–2,140 ppm

HYDROGEN-SULFIDE Plant

HYDROXYMALONIC-ACID Plant

HYPOXANTHINE Plant

INVERTASE Plant

IODINE Plant 0.011 ppm

IRON Tuber 5–128 ppm

ISOBUTYRALDEHYDE Essential Oil

ISODITYROSINE Tissue Culture

ISOFRAXIDIN-7-O-BETA-D-GLUCOSIDE Tuber 19 ppm

ISOLEUCINE Tuber 840–5,700 ppm

ISOLUBIMIN Tuber

ISOQUERCITRIN Plant

ISOVALERALDEHYDE Essential Oil

JASMONIC-ACID Tuber

KAEMPFEROL Flower

KAEMPFEROL-3-0-SOPHOROSIDE Seed

KAEMPFEROL-3-DIGLUCOSIDE-7-RHAMNO-SIDE Plant

KAEMPFEROL-3-SOPHOROSIDE-RHAMNO-SIDE Seed

KAEMPFEROL-3-TRIGLUCOSIDE-7-RHAMNO-SIDE Plant

KILOCALORIES Tuber 780–3,755 /kg

LACTIC-ACID Plant

LAURIC-ACID Tuber 30–143 ppm

LEAD Tuber 0.01–4.2 ppm

LECITHINASE Plant

LEPTINE Plant

LEUCINE Tuber 1,240–7,100 ppm

LIGNOCERYL-FERULATE Tuber

LINOLEIC-ACID Tuber 320–1,520 ppm

LINOLENIC-ACID Tuber 100–475 ppm

LITHIUM Tuber 0.104–0.28 ppm

LORMETAZEPAM Tuber

LUBIMIN Tuber

LUBIMINOL Tuber

LUTEIN Plant

LUTEOLIN Flower

LYCOPHENOL Fruit

LYSINE Tuber 1,260–6,800 ppm

MAGNESIUM Tuber 190–4,250 ppm

MALIC-ACID Tuber 1,120 ppm

MALTOTRIOSE Plant

MANGANESE Tuber 1.3–22 ppm

MANNINOTRIOSE Plant

MANNOSE Plant

MELIBIOSE Plant

MERCURY Tuber 0.05 ppm

METHANETHIOL Plant

METHIONINE Tuber 310–1,568 ppm

METHIONINE-SULFOXIDE Plant

METHYL-ISOPROPYLKETONE Plant

MEVALONIC-ACID Tuber

MOLYBDENUM Tuber 0.1–2.1 ppm

MONOHYDROXY-HEXADECANDIOIC-ACID
Leaf

MONOHYDROXY-PENTADECANEDIOIC-ACID
Leaf

MUCILAGE Plant

MUFA Tuber 20–95 ppm

MYO-INOSITOL Plant

MYRICETIN Flower

MYRISTIC-ACID Tuber 10–48 ppm

N-AMYL-ALCOHOL Plant

N-BUTYRALDEHYDE Essential Oil

N-DEMETHYL-DIAZEPAM Tuber

N-HEPTANOL Plant

N-HEXANAL Plant

N-OCTANAL Plant

N-PENTANAL Plant

NEGRETINE Plant

NEO-CHLOROGENIC-ACID Tuber 7 ppm

NIACIN Tuber 148–74 ppm

NICKEL Tuber 0.02–2.6 ppm

NICOTINE Plant

NICOTINIC-ACID Tuber 12 ppm

NITROGEN Tuber 2,200–17,000 ppm

NONACOSANOIC-ACID Leaf

NONADECAN-1-OL Leaf

NONANEDIOIC-ACID Leaf

NORADRENALIN Fruit

NOREPINEPHRINE Tuber

O-ALPHA-D-GLUCOPYRANOSYL-(1-{4-O-
ALPHA-D-GLUCOPYRANOSYL . . . TU Plant

OCTACOSAN-1-OL Leaf

OCTACOSANOIC-ACID Leaf

OCTACOSYL-FERULATE Tuber

OCTADECADIENOIC-ACID Leaf

OCTADECAN-1-OL Leaf

OCTADECANOIC-ACID Leaf

OCTADECENDIOIC-ACID Leaf

OCTADECENOIC-ACID Leaf

OCTADECYL-FERULATE Tuber

OCTEN-1-OL Plant

OLEIC-ACID Tuber 10–48 ppm

OXALIC-ACID Tuber 150 ppm

OXYEPILUBIMIN Tuber

OXYGLUTINOSONE Tuber

OXYLUBIMIN Tuber

P-COUMARIC-ACID Tuber 4 ppm

P-COUMAROYL-GLUCOSE Fruit

PAEONANIN Plant

PALMITIC-ACID Tuber 160–760 ppm

PALMITOLEIC-ACID Tuber 10–48 ppm

PANTOTHENIC-ACID Tuber 3–18 ppm

PATATIN Tuber

PECTIN Leaf 21,000–73,000 ppm Tuber
18,000–33,000 ppm

PENTADECANOIC-ACID Leaf

PETANIN Plant

PETUNIDIN-3-RUTINOSIDE Plant

PHELLOGENIC-ACID Leaf

PHENOL-OXIDASE Plant

PHENYL-ACETALDEHYDE Plant

PHENYLALANINE Tuber 920–5,550 ppm

PHOSPHOLIPASE Plant

PHOSPHORUS Tuber 320–4,200 ppm

PHOSPHORYLASE Plant

PHYTIC-ACID Plant

PHYTIN Plant

PHYTOSTEROLS Tuber 50–240 ppm

PHYTUBERIN Tuber

PLANTEOSE Plant

POLYPHENOL-OXIDASE Plant

POTASSIUM Tuber 2,470–30,000 ppm

PROLINE Tuber 740–6,700 ppm

PROTEIN Tuber 10,000–127,000 ppm

PUFA Tuber 430–2,043 ppm

PYRIDINE Plant

QUERCETIN Flower

QUERCITIN-3-GLUCOSIDE Plant

QUERCITIN-3-GLUCOSYL-RHAMNOSIDE
Flower

QUERCITIN-3-RUTINOSIDE Plant

QUINIC-ACID Tuber

RAFFINOSE Plant

RHAMNOSE Plant

RIBOFLAVIN Tuber 0.4–1.9 ppm

RIBOFURANOSYL-CIS-ZEATIN Tuber

RIBOFURANOSYL-TRANS-ZEATIN Tuber

RIBOSYL-GLUCOSE Plant

RISBITIN Plant

RISHITIN Tuber 11 ppm

RISHITINOL Tuber 9 ppm
RISHITINONE Tuber 0.4 ppm
RUBIDIUM Tuber 0.64–23 ppm
RUTIN Shoot
SCOPOLETIN Tuber Epidermis
SCOPOLIN Tuber 98 ppm
SELENIUM Tuber 0.01 ppm
SERINE Tuber 90–5,250 ppm
SFA Tuber 260–1,235 ppm
SILICON Tuber 1–10 ppm
SILVER Tuber 0.026–0.07 ppm
SINAPIC-ACID Tuber 3 ppm
SODIUM Tuber 2.6–323 ppm
SOLAMINE Sprout Seedling
SOLANESOL Leaf
SOLANIDINE Tuber
SOLANIDINE-T Plant
SOLANINE Fruit 10,000 ppm Leaf 6,000–7,000 ppm Tissue Culture 600 ppm
SOLANINES Tuber 20–100 ppm
SOLANOLONE Tuber 2.2 ppm
SOLANTHRENE Tuber
SOLASODINE Tuber
SOLAVETIVONE Tuber 6–83 ppm
SPIROVETIVA-1(10),11,DIEN-2-ONE Tuber
SPIROVETIVA-1(10),3,11,TRIEN-2-ONE Tuber
STACHYOSE Plant
STARCH Tuber 150,000–800,000 ppm
STEARIC-ACID Tuber 40–190 ppm
STIGMASTEROL Plant
STRONTIUM Tuber 0.39–60 ppm
SUBERIN Tuber
SUCCINIC-ACID Plant
SULFUR Tuber 16–1,900 ppm
TANNIN Leaf 32,000 ppm
TARTARIC-ACID Plant
TETRACOSAN-1-OL Leaf
TETRACOSANEDIOIC-ACID Leaf
TETRACOSANOIC-ACID Leaf
TETRADECANOIC-ACID Leaf
THIAMIN Tuber 1–5 ppm
THREONINE Tuber 750–4,300 ppm
TITANIUM Tuber 0.13–17 ppm
TOLATID-5-EN-3BETA-OL Plant
TOMATIDINE Tuber
TOMATINE Tuber
TRANS-N-FEROLOYL-PUTRESCINE Tuber
TRANS-NONEN-2-OL Plant

TRANS-OCTEN-2-AL Plant
TRANS-OCTEN-2-OL Plant
TRANS-ZEATIN Tissue Culture
TRIACONTAN-1-OL Leaf
TRIACONTANOIC-ACID Leaf
TRIGALACTOSYL-GLYCEROL Plant
TRIGONELLINE Plant
TRITRIACONTANONE Plant
TRYPTOPHAN Tuber 320–2,250 ppm
TUBERONIC-ACID-5'-O-BETA-D-GLUCOSIDE Leaf 0.027 ppm
TUBEROSIN Plant
TYRAMINE Fruit
TYROSINASE Plant
TYROSINE Tuber 770–3,900 ppm
UMBELLIFERONE Tuber
VALINE Tuber 117–6,450 ppm
VIT-B-6 Tuber 2.5–12.5 ppm
WATER Tuber 700,000–800,000 ppm
XYLOSYL-GLUCOSE Plant
YAMOGENIN Plant
ZINC Tuber 1.9–44.1 ppm
ZIRCONIUM Plant 0.52–1.4 ppm

POTATO YAM

Chemicals in *Dioscorea bulbifera L.* (*Dioscoreaceae*)—Air Potato, Potato Yam

2,4,5,6-TETRAHYDROXYPHENANTHRENE Tuber
2,4,6,7-TETRAHYDROXY-9,10-DIHYDROPHENANTHRENE Tuber
ARSENIC Rhizome 0.37 ppm
ASH Tuber 9,000–31,000 ppm
CALCIUM Rhizome 690–2,379 ppm
CALCIUM-OXALATE Tuber
CARBOHYDRATES Tuber 265,000–914,900 ppm
COPPER Rhizome 8 ppm
D-SORBITOL Rhizome
DIOSBULBIN-A Tuber
DIOSBULBIN-B Tuber
DIOSBULBIN-C Tuber
DIOSBULBIN-D Tuber
DIOSBULBIN-E Tuber
DIOSBULBIN-F Tuber
DIOSBULBIN-G Tuber
DIOSBULBIN-H Tuber

DIOSBULBINOSIDE-D Tuber

DIOSBULBINOSIDE-F Tuber

DIOSGENIN Tuber 4,500 ppm

FAT Tuber 1,000–12,800 ppm

FIBER Tuber 9,000–96,400 ppm

GUM Tuber 900 ppm

IRON Rhizome 40 ppm

KILOCALORIES Tuber 1,120–3,860 /kg

MAGNESIUM Rhizome 370 ppm

MANGANESE Rhizome 4 ppm

MERCURY Rhizome 0.02 ppm

PHOSPHORUS Tuber 290–1,000 ppm

PHOSPHORUS-OXIDE-(P2O5) Tuber
4,500–7,700 ppm

POTASSIUM Rhizome 3,570 ppm

PROTEIN Tuber 15,000–133,100 ppm

SAPONIN Tuber 57,000 ppm

SODIUM Rhizome 378 ppm

STARCH Tuber 800,000 ppm

TANNIN Tuber

WATER Tuber 710,000 ppm

ZINC Rhizome 12 ppm

PUMPKIN

Chemicals in *Cucurbita pepo L.* (*Cucurbitaceae*)—Pumpkin

(+)-CIS-ABSCISIC-ACID Plant

(+)-DEHYDROVOMIFOLIOL Plant

(+)-TRANS-ABSCISIC-ACID Plant

(+)-VOMIFOLIOL Plant

24-ETHYL-5-ALPHA-CHOLESTA-7,22,25-TRIEN-
3-BETA-OL Seed

24-ETHYL-5-ALPHA-CHOLESTA-7,25-DIEN-3-
BETA-OL Seed

24-ALPHA-ETHYLLATHOSTEROL Plant

5-ALPHA-STIGMASTA-7,25-DIEN-3-BETA-OL
Plant

ADENINE Flower

ADENOSINE Flower

ALANINE Fruit 280–3,333 ppm Seed
11,580–12,441 ppm

ALPHA-AMINO-ADIPIC-ACID Flower

ALPHA-AMINO-BUTYRIC-ACID Flower

ALPHA-KETO-BETA-METHYL-BUTYRIC-ACID
Juice 100 ppm

ALPHA-KETO-BETA-METHYL-VALERAINIC-
ACID Juice 180 ppm

ALPHA-LINOLENIC-ACID Flower 20–410 ppm
Fruit 30–357 ppm Seed 1,810–1,945 ppm

ALPHA-SPINASTEROL Flower Seed

ALPHA-SPINASTERYL-BETA-D-GLUCOSIDE
Flower

ALPHA-TOCOPHEROL Fruit 10–119 ppm

ALUMINUM Seed 11 ppm

ARACHIDIC-ACID Seed 200 ppm

ARGININE Fruit 370–6,429 ppm Seed
40,330–43,328 ppm

ASCORBIC-ACID Flower 280–5,773 ppm Fruit
90–1,071 ppm

ASH Flower 4,800–98,970 ppm Fruit
7,500–95,238 ppm Seed 47,530–70,000 ppm

ASPARTIC-ACID Fruit 1,020–12,143 ppm Seed
24,770–26,612 ppm

BETA-AMINO-ISOBUTYRIC-ACID Flower

BETA-CAROTENE Flower 12–240 ppm Fruit
9.6–114 ppm Seed 2–2.5 ppm

BETA-HYDROXYBUTYRIC-ACID Fruit

BETA-SITOSTEROL Seed

BORON Fruit 1 ppm

CAFFEIC-ACID Leaf

CALCIUM Flower 390–8,041 ppm Fruit
210–2,500 ppm Seed 418–474 ppm

CARBOHYDRATES Flower 32,800–676,290
ppm Fruit 65,000–773,809 ppm Seed
178,100–191,341 ppm

CHOLESTEROL Plant

CHROMIUM Seed 17 ppm

COBALT Seed 143 ppm

CODECARBOXYLASE Plant

COPPER Seed 14–15 ppm

CRYPTOXANTHIN Flower

CUCURBIC-ACID Plant

CUCURBIC-ACID-GLUCOSIDE Plant

CUCURBIC-ACID-METHYL-ESTER Plant

CUCURBITAXANTHIN Fruit

CUCURBITIN Seed 16,600–66,300 ppm

CUCURBITOL Seed

CYSTINE Fruit 30–700 ppm Seed 3,010–3,234
ppm

DEHYDROASCORBIC-ACID Seed

DELTA-HYDROXYLYSINE Flower

DL-CITRULLIN Seed

EDESTINE Seed

FAT Flower 700–14,430 ppm Fruit 1,000–11,905
ppm Seed 384,500–520,000 ppm

FERULIC-ACID Plant

FIBER Flower 6,300–130,000 ppm Fruit 11,000–130,952 ppm Seed 19,690–26,538 ppm

FLAVOXANTHIN Juice

GABA Seed

GIBBERELLIN-A39 Plant

GIBBERELLIN-A48 Plant

GIBBERELLIN-A49 Plant

GLUTAMIC-ACID Fruit 1,840–35,000 ppm Seed 43,150–46,358 ppm

GLUTINOL Flower

GLYCINE Fruit 270–8,000 ppm Seed 17,960–19,295 ppm

GLYOXALIC-ACID Juice 200 ppm

GUANOSINE Sprout Seedling

HISTIDINE Fruit 140–1,905 ppm Seed 6,810–7,316 ppm

HYDROXYBRENZTRAUBEN-ACID Fruit

IRON Flower 7–144 ppm Seed 86–172 ppm

ISOLEUCINE Fruit 310–3,690 ppm Seed 12,640–13,580 ppm

ISORHAMNETIN-3-O-RUTINOSIDE-4'-O-RHAMNOSIDE Flower

KAEMPFEROL Leaf

KILOCALORIES Flower 150–3,092 /kg Fruit 220–3,095 /kg Seed 2,730–5,812 /kg

LAURIC-ACID Flower 10–205 ppm Fruit 10–119 ppm Seed 440–472 ppm

LECITHIN Seed 4,000 ppm

LEUCINE Fruit 460–5,476 ppm Seed 20,790–22,336 ppm

LINOLEIC-ACID Flower 20–410 ppm Fruit 20–238 ppm Seed 209,040–222,411 ppm

LUPEOL Flower

LUTEIN Flower

LYSINE Fruit 470–6,429 ppm Seed 18,330–19,693 ppm

M-CARBOXYPHENYLALANINE Seed

MAGNESIUM Flower 240–4,950 ppm Fruit 120–1,429 ppm Seed 5,140–5,748 ppm

MANGANESE Seed 40 ppm

MANNITOL Fruit 150,000–200,000 ppm

METHIONINE Fruit 110–1,310 ppm Seed 5,510–5,920 ppm

MUFA Flower 90–1,855 ppm Fruit 130–1,548 ppm Seed 142,580–153,180 ppm

MYRISTIC-ACID Flower 50–1,030 ppm Fruit 60–714 ppm Seed 200–559 ppm

NEOXANTHIN Flower

NIACIN Flower 7–142 ppm Fruit 7–16 ppm Seed 14–22 ppm

OLEIC-ACID Flower 40–825 ppm Fruit 60–714 ppm Seed 141,460–151,977 ppm

ORNITHINE Flower

OXALIC-ACID Juice 400 ppm

OXYCEROTINIC-ACID Seed

PALMITIC-ACID Flower 260–5,360 ppm Fruit 370–4,405 ppm Seed 56,120–60,292 ppm

PALMITOLEIC-ACID Flower 50–1,030 ppm Fruit 60–714 ppm Seed 990–1,064 ppm

PHENYLALANINE Fruit 300–3,810 ppm Seed 12,220–13,128 ppm

PHOSPHOLIPIDS Seed

PHOSPHORUS Flower 490–10,100 ppm Fruit 440–5,238 ppm Seed 10,600–12,982 ppm

PHYTIC-ACID Seed 15,000–22,000 ppm

PHYTOSTEROLS Fruit 120–1,428 ppm

POTASSIUM Flower 1,730–35,670 ppm Fruit 3,400–40,476 ppm Seed 5,540–8,670 ppm

PROLINE Fruit 260–17,100 ppm Seed 10,000–10,743 ppm

PROTEIN Fruit 10,000–140,000 ppm Seed 86,000–271,797 ppm

PUFA Flower 40–825 ppm Fruit 50–595 ppm Seed 209,040–224,581 ppm

QUERCETIN Leaf

RHAMNAZIN-3-RUTINOSIDE Flower

RIBOFLAVIN Flower 0.7–15 ppm Fruit 1.1–13.1 ppm Seed 2.7–4.9 ppm

SALICYLIC-ACID Seed

SELENIUM Seed

SERINE Fruit 440–6,100 ppm Seed 11,480–12,333 ppm

SFA Flower 360–7,425 ppm Fruit 520–6,190 ppm Seed 86,740–93,180 ppm

SILICON Seed

SODIUM Flower 50–1,030 ppm Fruit 10–119 ppm Seed 180–193 ppm

STEARIC-ACID Flower 20–410 ppm Fruit 30–357 ppm Seed 28,110–30,200 ppm

STIGMAST-7-ENOL Flower

STIGMAST-7-ENYL-D-GLUCOSIDE Flower

SUCROSE Seed 14,000 ppm

THIAMIN Flower 0.4–8.6 ppm Fruit 0.5–5.9
ppm Seed 1.9–3.7 ppm
THREONINE Fruit 250–3,452 ppm Seed
9,030–9,701 ppm
TIN Seed 23 ppm
TRIGONELLINE Sprout Seedling
TRYPTOPHAN Fruit 120–1,800 ppm Seed
4,310–4,630 ppm
TYROSINE Fruit 130–5,000 ppm Seed
10,190–10,948 ppm
UREASE Seed
VALINE Fruit 350–4,167 ppm Seed
19,720–21,186 ppm
VIOLAXANTHIN Flower
WATER Fruit 916,000 ppm Seed 65,200–73,110
ppm
XANTHOPHYLL Flower
ZEAXANTHIN Flower
ZINC Seed 74–83 ppm

RADISH

Chemicals in *Raphanus sativus L.* (*Brassicaceae*)—Radish

4-METHYLSULFOXIDEBUTEN-(3)-YL-CYANIDE
Seed 200 ppm
ALANINE Root 220–4,265 ppm
ALUMINUM Root 6–185 ppm
ARGININE Plant
ARSENIC Root
ASCORBIC-ACID Fruit 690–7,822 ppm Leaf
810–7,043 ppm Root 226–6,216 ppm
ASH Root 10,000–185,700 ppm
ASPARTIC-ACID Root 480–9,300 ppm
BETA-CAROTENE Fruit 0.3–26.2 ppm Leaf
24.7–214 ppm Root 1 ppm
BETA-HEXYLALDEHYDE Seed
BORON Root 0.6–64 ppm
BROMINE Root
CADMIUM Root 0.005–0.57 ppm
CAFFEIC-ACID Root 91 ppm
CALCIUM Fruit 260–10,130 ppm Leaf
2,380–19,130 ppm Root 190–8,570 ppm
Seed 3,670 ppm
CARBOHYDRATES Fruit 54,000–701,000 ppm
Leaf 57,000–496,000 ppm Root
36,000–757,000 ppm
CHROMIUM Root 0.01–0.14 ppm

COBALT Root
COPPER Root 0.3–8 ppm Seed 6 ppm
CYSTINE Root 50–970 ppm
DIALLYL-SULFIDE Root
ERUCIC-ACID Seed
FAT Fruit 3,000–50,000 ppm Leaf 6,000–52,000
ppm Root 1,000–187,000 ppm Seed
298,000–410,000 ppm
FERULIC-ACID Root 16 ppm
FIBER Fruit 11,000–147,000 ppm Leaf
11,000–96,000 ppm Root 5,200–176,000
ppm
FLUORINE Root
FOLACIN Root 0.3–5.8 ppm
GLUCOBRASSICIN Plant
GLUCOCAPPARIN Seed
GLUCOLEPIDIIN Seed
GLUCOPUTRANJIVIN Root
GLUCORAPHANIN Root
GLUTAMIC-ACID Root 1,320–25,580 ppm
GLYCEROL-SINAPATE Seed
GLYCINE Root 220–4,265 ppm
HISTIDINE Root 130–2,520 ppm
INDOLE-ACETIC-ACID Root
INDOLEACETONITRILE Root
IRON Fruit 4–295 ppm Leaf 41–357 ppm Root
2–189 ppm Seed 120 ppm
ISOBUTYRALDEHYDE Leaf
ISOLEUCINE Root 300–5,815 ppm
KILOCALORIES Fruit 340–3,370 /kg Leaf
330–2,870 /kg Root 170–3,510 /kg
L-SULFORAPHENE Root
LEAD Root 0.01–0.57 ppm
LEUCINE Root 370–7,170 ppm
LINOLEIC-ACID Root 160–3,100 ppm
LINOLENIC-ACID Root 290–5,620 ppm
LYSINE Root 350–6,785 ppm
MAGNESIUM Root 85–3,570 ppm Seed 3,960
ppm
MANGANESE Root 0.5–20 ppm Seed 40 ppm
MERCURY Root 0.014 ppm
METHIONINE Root 70–1,355 ppm
METHYL-MERCAPTAN Seed
MOLYBDENUM Root
MUFA Root 170–3,295 ppm
MYRISTIC-ACID Root
N-BUTYRALDEHYDE Leaf

NIACIN Fruit 2-59 ppm Leaf 40-348 ppm
Root 3-68 ppm
NICKEL Root 0.01-0.71 ppm
NITROGEN Root 2,000-38,570 ppm
OLEIC-ACID Root 160-3,100 ppm
OXALIC-ACID Root 92 ppm
P-COUMARIC-ACID Root 91 ppm
PALMITIC-ACID Root 260-5,040 ppm
PANTOTHENIC-ACID Root 0.8-18 ppm
PHENYLALANINE Root 230-4,455 ppm
PHOSPHORUS Fruit 240-10,526 ppm Leaf
300-2,609 ppm Root 160-5,850 ppm
PHYTOSTEROLS Root 70-1,355 ppm
POTASSIUM Fruit 2,070-20,495 ppm Leaf
5,000-43,478 ppm Root 2,215-85,700 ppm
Seed 11,900 ppm
PROLINE Root 180-3,490 ppm
PROTEIN Fruit 13,000-257,000 ppm Leaf
33,000-287,000 ppm Root 5,260-182,000
ppm Seed 236,000-336,000 ppm
PUFA Root 450-8,720 ppm
PUTRESCINE Leaf
RAPHANIN Seed
RAPHANUSIN-A Root
RAPHANUSIN-B Root
RAPHANUSIN-C Root
RAPHANUSIN-D Root
RIBOFLAVIN Fruit 0.3-5.3 ppm Leaf 2.6-24
ppm Root 0.3-9.3 ppm
RUBIDIUM Root 0.44-15.7 ppm
S-METHYL-L-CYSTEINSULFOXIDE Root
SELENIUM Root
SERINE Root 210-4,070 ppm
SILICON Root 10-425 ppm
SINAPIC-ACID Root
SINIGRIN Seed
SODIUM Fruit 50-495 ppm Leaf 1,100-9,565
ppm Root 100-5,020 ppm Seed 134 ppm
SPERMINE Leaf
SPERMINIDINE Leaf
STEARIC-ACID Root 40-775 ppm
SULFUR Root 350-6,140 ppm
THIAMIN Fruit 0.3-7.9 ppm Leaf 1.4-7 ppm
Root 0.3-9.7 ppm
THREONINE Root 290-5,620 ppm
TRIACONTANE Seed
TRYPTOPHAN Root 40-775 ppm
TYROSINE Root 130-2,520 ppm

VALINE Root 320-6,200 ppm
VIT-B-6 Root 0.7-14.5 ppm
WATER Fruit 899,000-923,000 ppm Leaf
856,000 ppm Root 926,000-945,000 ppm
ZINC Root 2-72 ppm Seed 29 ppm

RHUBARB

Chemicals in *Rheum rhabarbarum L.* (*Polygonaceae*)—Rhubarb

(+)-CATECHIN Root
(+)-CATECHIN-5-O-GLUCOSIDE Root
1,2,6-TRI-O-GALLOYL-GLUCOSE Root
1,6-DI-O-GALLOYL-GLUCOSE Root
1-O-GALLOYL-GLYCEROL Root
2-O-CINNAMOYLGLUCOGALLIN Root
3,3',5-TRIHYDROXY-4'-METHOXYSTILBEN-3-
BETA-D-GLUCOPYRANOSIDE Plant
3,5,4'-TRIHYDROXYSTILBENE-4'-O-(6''-O-GAL-
LOYL)-GLUCOSIDE Root
3,5,4'-TRIHYDROXYSTILBENE-4'-O-GLUCO-
SIDE Root
4-(P-HYDROXYPHENYL)BUTANONE-O-GLU-
COSIDE Root
6-HYDROXYMUSIZIN-8-O-GLUCOSIDE Root
6-O-GALLOYL-GLUCOSE Root
ACETIC-ACID Pt
ALOE-EMODIN-8-O-GLUCOSIDE Root
ALPHA-TOCOPHEROL Leaf 1,197-1,238 ppm
Pt 2-48 ppm
ALUMINUM Pt 1-80 ppm
ANHYDRORHAPONTIGENIN Root
ANTHRAQUINONE-GLYCOSIDES Leaf
ANTHRONES Leaf 10,000-15,000 ppm
ARSENIC Pt 0.01 ppm
ASCORBIC-ACID Leaf 110-1,833 ppm Pt
80-2,581 ppm
ASH Leaf 10,000-194,000 ppm Pt
8,000-160,000 ppm
BETA-CAROTENE Leaf 0.3-5 ppm Pt 0.6-12
ppm
BORON Pt 0.1-36 ppm
BROMINE Pt 1-20 ppm
CADMIUM Pt 0.005-0.6 ppm
CAFFEIC-ACID Pt 8 ppm
CALCIUM Leaf 470-14,400 ppm Pt 600-18,462
ppm
CALCIUM-OXALATE Leaf

CARBOHYDRATES Leaf 41,000–683,000 ppm Pt 37,000–774,000 ppm

CHROMIUM Pt 0.005–0.1 ppm

CHRYSARONE Root

CHRYSARONE-METHYL-ETHER Root

CHRYSOPHANIC-ACID Root Essent. Oil

CHRYSOPHANIN Root

CHRYSOPHANOL Root

CHRYSOPHANOL-1-O-GLUCOSIDE Root

CHRYSOPHANOL-8-O-GLUCOSIDE Root

CHRYSOPONTIN Root

CHRYSORHAPONTIN Root

CITRIC-ACID Pt

COBALT Pt 0.005–0.1 ppm

COPPER Pt 0.2–5.2 ppm

CYANIDIN-3-GLUCOSIDE Leaf

CYANIDIN-3-RUTINOSIDE Leaf

DESOXYRHAPONTICIN Root

DIHYDROXYGLUTAMIC-ACID Leaf

EMODIN Root

EMODIN-8-O-GLUCOSIDE Root

EMODIN-METHYL-ETHER Root

EO Root

EPICATECHIN Root

EPICATECHIN-3-O-GALLATE Root

FAT Leaf 1,000–65,000 ppm Pt 1,000–32,000 ppm

FERULIC-ACID Pt 8 ppm Root

FIBER Leaf 7,000–125,000 ppm Pt 3,000–135,000 ppm

FLUORINE Pt 0.1–4 ppm

FOLACIN Pt 0.06–0.1 ppm

FRANGULA-EMODIN-ANTHRONE Leaf

FUMARIC-ACID Pt

GALLIC-ACID Pt 53 ppm Root

GALLIC-ACID-3-O-(6'-O-GALLOYL)-GLUCO-SIDE Root

GALLIC-ACID-4-O-(6'-O-GALLOYL)-GLUCO-SIDE Root

GLUCOCHRYSARONE Root

GLYCOCHRYSARONE Root

GLYCOGALLIN Root

IRON Leaf 3–250 ppm Pt 1–154 ppm

ISOEMODIN Root

ISOLINDLEYIN Root

ISOQUERCITRIN Leaf

ISORHAPONTIGENIN Root

LACTIC-ACID Pt

LEAD Pt 0.02–1 ppm

LINDLEYIN Root

LUTEIN Pt 1.7–34 ppm

MAGNESIUM Pt 90–1,975 ppm

MAGNESIUM-OXALATE Pt

MALIC-ACID Pt

MANGANESE Pt 2–35 ppm

MERCURY Pt 0.002–0.14 ppm

METHYL-CHRYSOPHANIC-ACID Root

MOLYBDENUM Pt 0.1 ppm

NIACIN Leaf 1–33 ppm Pt 2–57 ppm

NICKEL Pt 0.1–4 ppm

NITROGEN Pt 1,100–22,000 ppm

OXALIC-ACID Leaf 3,000–11,000 ppm Pt 4,400–13,360 ppm

P-COUMARIC-ACID Pt 44 ppm Root

PANTOTHENIC-ACID Pt 0.8–13.3 ppm

PECTINS Pt 1,020 ppm

PHOSPHORUS Leaf 160–3,472 ppm Pt 100–3,462 ppm

PHYSCION Root

PHYSCION-8-O-GLUCOSIDE Root

PICEATANNOL-3'-O-GLUCOSIDE Plant

POTASSIUM Pt 2,510–66,400 ppm

PROCYANIDIN-B-2-3,3'-DI-O-GALLATE Root

PROCYANIDIN-B1,3'-O-GALLATE Root

PROTEIN Leaf 7,000–276,000 ppm Pt 4,000–115,000 ppm

PROTOCATECHUIC-ACID Pt

QUERCETIN-3'-GLUCOSIDE Pt

QUERCETIN-3-0-RHAMNOSIDE Pt

QUERCETIN-3-0-RUTINOSIDE Pt

RHAPONTIC-ACID Root

RHAPONTICIN Root 14,200 ppm

RHAPONTIGENIN Root

RHEIN Root

RHEINOSIDES Root 12,900 ppm

RIBOFLAVIN Leaf 0.2–3 ppm Pt 0.3–14 ppm

RUBIDIUM Pt 1.1–58 ppm

RUTIN Leaf 6,000 ppm

SELENIUM Pt

SENNOSIDE-A Root

SENNOSIDE-B Root

SILICON Pt 3–200 ppm

SINAPIC-ACID Pt 6 ppm Root

SODIUM Pt 20–855 ppm

SUCCINIC-ACID Pt

SULFUR Pt 62–1,240 ppm

THIAMIN Leaf 0.2–3.3 ppm Pt 0.2–6.5 ppm

TORACHRYSONE-8-O-GLUCOSIDE Root

VANILLIC-ACID Pt 4 ppm

WATER Leaf 927,000–950,000 ppm Stem
  927,000–950,000 ppm

ZINC Pt 1–46 ppm

SOYBEAN

Chemicals in *Glycine max* (*L.*) *MERR.*
(*Fabaceae*)—Soybean

(+)-CATECHIN Leaf

(6AR,11AR)-3-6(A)-9-TRIHYDROXYPTERO-
  CARPAN Cotyledon

1-DODECENE Plant

1-HEXANOL Plant

1-O-FERULOYL-BETA-D-GLUCOSE Sprout
  Seedling

1-O-PARA-COUMAROYL-BETA-D-GLUCOSE
  Sprout Seedling

2,2-DIMETHYL-HEXANAL Leaf

2,4-HEXADIEN-1-OL Plant

2-HEXENAL Plant

24-METHYLENE-CYCLOARTENOL Seed

3,5,5,TRIMETHYL-2-HEXENE Seed

3-HEXENAL-1-OL Plant

3-HYDROXY-LINOLEIC-ACID Tissue Culture

3-HYDROXY-OLEIC-ACID Tissue Culture

3-OCTANOL Leaf

3-OCTANONE Leaf

3-TETRADECENE Leaf

4'-5-7-TRIACETOXYISOFLAVONE Shoot

4'-5-7-TRIMETHOXYISOFLAVONE Shoot

4'-7-DIACETOXYISOFLAVONE Shoot

4'7-DIMETHOXYISOFLAVONE Shoot

4-HEXENYLOL-ACETATE Plant

4-HYDROXY-BENZOIC-ACID Leaf Root

4-HYDROXYCINNAMIC-ACID Leaf

5"-O-ACETYL-DAIDZIN Seed 145 ppm

6"-O-ACETYL-DAIDZIN Seed 80 ppm

6"-O-ACETYL-GENISTIN Seed 17–145 ppm

6,8-DI-HEXOSYL-GENKWANIN Root

6-CARBOXY-PTERIN Seed 0.087 ppm

6-HYDROXY-METHYL-PTERIN Plant

7-DEHYDRO-AVENASTEROL Seed

7-OCTEN-4-OL Leaf

ABSCISIC-ACID Seed

ACETALDEHYDE Plant

ACETIC-ACID Seed

ACETIC-ACID-CYCLOHEXYL-ESTER Leaf

ACETIC-ACID-HEXYL-ESTER Leaf

ACETONE Plant

ACETYL-SOYASAPONIN-A-1 Seed 410 ppm

ACETYL-SOYASAPONIN-A-2 Seed 110 ppm

ACETYL-SOYASAPONIN-A-3 Seed 30 ppm

ACETYL-SOYASAPONIN-A-4 Seed 378 ppm

ACETYL-SOYASAPONIN-A-5 Seed 89 ppm

ACETYL-SOYASAPONIN-A-6 Seed 50 ppm

ACID-PHOSPHATASE Plant

ADENINE Seed 210–500 ppm Sprout Seedling

ADENOSINE Sprout Seedling

ADENYLIC-ACID Sprout Seedling

AFROMOSIN Leaf

ALANINE Seed 17,190–18,795 ppm

ALCOHOL-DEHYDROGENASE Plant

ALLANTOIC-ACID Leaf

ALLANTOIN Seed

ALLANTOINASE Seed

ALPHA-AMYLASE Seed

ALPHA-AMYRIN Sprout Seedling

ALPHA-KETO-GLUTARIC-ACID Seed

ALPHA-LINOLENIC-ACID Seed 13,300–14,540
  ppm

ALPHA-TOCOPHEROL Leaf 29–280 ppm Oil
  95 ppm Seed 8–19 ppm

ALUMINUM Seed 2–60 ppm

AMMONIA Seed 8,600 ppm

AMYLASE Seed

ANTHEROXANTHIN Leaf

ANTHOCYANIN Seed

ARABINOGALACTAN Seed

ARABINOSE Seed

ARACHIDONIC-ACID Seed

ARGININE Seed 28,310–30,950 ppm

ASCORBIC-ACID Fruit 290–942 ppm Seed 849
  ppm Sprout Seedling 100–949 ppm

ASCORBICASE Seed

ASH Fruit 16,000–52,000 ppm Plant
  55,000–119,000 ppm Seed 17,000–61,000
  ppm Sprout Seedling 8,000–58,000 ppm

ASPARAGIC-ACID Seed

ASPARTATE-AMINO-TRANSFERASE Plant

ASPARTIC-ACID Seed 45,890–50,175 ppm

ASTRAGALIN Leaf

BARIUM Seed 1–90 ppm

BETA-AMYLASE Seed

BETA-AMYRIN Sprout Seedling

BETA-CAROTENE Fruit 4.1–13.4 ppm Plant 0.3 ppm Seed 11.3 ppm Sprout Seedling 0.2–3.5 ppm

BETA-CONGLYCIN Seed

BETA-INDOLACETIC-ACID Shoot

BETA-NEOCAROTENE Seed

BETA-SITOSTEROL Seed 900 ppm

BETA-TOCOPHEROL Seed

BETAINE Seed

BIOCHANIN-C Seed

BIOTIN Seed 750 ppm

BORNESITOL Leaf

BORON Seed 4–18 ppm

BOWMAN-BIRK-INHIBITOR Seed 500–3,000 ppm

BUTANOIC-ACID-3-HEXENYL-ESTER Leaf

BUTYROSPERMOL Seed

CADAVERINE Seed

CAFFEIC-ACID Seed 1–4 ppm

CALCIUM Fruit 670–2,200 ppm Plant 9,400–13,000 ppm Seed 780–4,440 ppm Sprout Seedling 480–3,504 ppm

CAMPESTEROL Seed

CANAVANINE Seed

CARBOHYDRATES Fruit 132,000–429,000 ppm Plant 658,000–781,000 ppm Seed 53,000–432,000 ppm

CARBOXYLASE Seed

CARLINOSIDE Root

CATALASE Seed

CEPHALIN Seed 4,650–7,750 ppm

CHIRO-INOSITOL Root 620 ppm

CHLORINE Seed 200 ppm

CHLOROGENIC-ACID Shoot

CHLOROPHYLL Seed

CHOLESTEROL Seed

CHOLINE Seed 2,490 ppm

CICERITOL Seed 230–800 ppm

CINNAMIC-ACID-4-HYDROXYLASE Tissue Culture

CIS-ACONITIC-ACID Root

CITRIC-ACID Seed 8,000–13,000 ppm

COBALT Seed 0.78 ppm

COPPER Seed 4.3–18 ppm

COPROPORPHYRIN Tissue Culture

COUMESTRIN Root

COUMESTROL Seed 1.2 ppm Shoot

CROCETIN Leaf

CYANIDIN-3-GLUCOSIDE Seed

CYANIDIN-3-MONOGLUCOSIDE Seed

CYCLOARTENOL Sprout Seedling

CYCLOLAUDENOL Sprout Seedling

CYSTEINE Seed 5,880–6,430 ppm

D-GALACTOSE Seed

D-ONITOL Leaf

D-PINITOL Seed Stem

DAIDZEIN Cotyledon 14–28 ppm Hypocotyl 140–190 ppm Seed 8–328 ppm Testa 7–10 ppm

DAIDZIN Cotyledon 375–1,028 ppm Hypocotyl 7,599–10,315 ppm Seed 129–8,100 ppm Testa 66–86 ppm

DELPHINIDIN-3-MONOGLUCOSIDE Seed

DELTA-TOCOPHEROL Seed

DI-GALACTOSYL-GLYCEROL Seed 100–170 ppm

DIAPHORASE Plant

DIHYDRO-BETA-SITOSTEROL Seed

DIMETHYL-AMINE Seed 8 ppm

ERGOST-4-EN-3-6-DION Tissue Culture

ERGOST-4-EN-3-ONE Tissue Culture

ERGOSTEROL Seed

ERUCIC-ACID Seed

ERYTHRO-NEOPTERIN Seed 0.014 ppm

ESTERASE Plant

ETHANOL Plant

ETHYL-AMINE Seed 0.5 ppm

ETHYLENE Tissue Culture

ETHYLVINYLKETONE Seed

FAT Fruit 51,000–160,000 ppm Plant 25,000–62,000 ppm Seed 45,000–218,000 ppm Sprout Seedling 14,000–102,000 ppm

FERULIC-ACID Plant 1–4 ppm Seed 1–4 ppm

FIBER Fruit 14,000–45,000 ppm Plant 281,000–355,000 ppm Seed 19,000–63,000 ppm Sprout Seedling 7,000–58,000 ppm

FICAPRENOL-10 Leaf

FICAPRENOL-11 Leaf

FICAPRENOL-12 Leaf

FISETIN Leaf

FLAVONOL-3-O-BETA-D-GLUCOSIDE Leaf

FLAZIN Seed 10 ppm

FLUORINE Seed 0.06 ppm

FOLACIN Seed 0.3–4 ppm

FORMIC-ACID Root

FORMOMONETIN Plant

FRUCTOSE Stem

FUMARIC-ACID Seed

GALACTOPINITOL-A Seed 1,520–4,280 ppm

GALACTOPINITOL-B Seed 500–1,800 ppm

GALACTINOL Seed 120–230 ppm

GALACTOMANNAN Seed

GALLIC-ACID Leaf 0.1–2.9 ppm

GAMMA-CONGLYCIN Seed

GAMMA-COUMARIC-ACID Seed

GAMMA-SITOSTEROL Seed

GAMMA-TOCOPHEROL Oil 699 ppm Seed 140 ppm

GENISTEIN Cotyledon 28–59 ppm Endosperm 267 ppm Hypocotyl 242–247 ppm Seed 20–46 ppm Testa 5–15 ppm

GENISTIN Cotyledon 1,139–2,058 ppm Hypocotyl 53–91 ppm Seed 522–13,400 ppm Testa 28–74 ppm

GENTISIC-ACID Seed

GLUCOSAMINE Seed

GLUCOSE Seed 300–570 ppm

GLUCOSE-6-PHOSPHATE-DEHYDROGENASE Plant

GLUCOSIDASE Seed

GLUCURONIC-ACID Seed

GLUTAMATE-OXALOACETIC-TRANSAMINASE Plant

GLUTAMIC-ACID Seed 70,680–77,280 ppm

GLUTAMYL-ALANINE Seed

GLUTAMYL-TYROSINE Seed

GLUTARIC-ACID Root

GLYCEOLLIN-I Sprout Seedling

GLYCEOLLIN-II Sprout Seedling

GLYCEOLLIN-III Sprout Seedling

GLYCEOLLIN-IV Cotyledon

GLYCINE Seed 16,870–18,445 ppm

GLYCININE Seed 345,000–388,880 ppm

GLYCINOPRENOL-10 Leaf

GLYCINOPRENOL-11 Leaf

GLYCINOPRENOL-9 Leaf

GLYCITEIN Hypocotyl 93–118 ppm Seed 13–30 ppm Testa 15 ppm

GLYCITEIN-7-O-BETA-D-GLUCOSIDE Seed 129 ppm

GLYCITIN Seed

GLYCITIN-7-BETA-GLUCOSIDE Cotyledon

16–17 ppm Hypocotyl 5,888–6,641 ppm Seed 95–159 ppm

GLYCOLIC-ACID Root Seed Sprout Seedling

GOSSYPOL Seed 60 ppm

GUANIDINE Seed

HEXAN-1-AL Plant

HISPIDINIC-ACID Sprout Seedling

HISPIDOL Seed

HISTIDINE Seed 9,840–10,770 ppm Sprout Seedling

HYDROXYPHASEOLIN Seed

HYPOGEIC-ACID Sprout Seedling

HYPOXANTHINE Sprout Seedling

INDOLE-3-ACETIC-ACID Root

INOSITOL Sprout Seedling

INOSITOL-HEXAPHOSPHATE Seed 14,000 ppm

INVERTASE Tissue Culture

IODINE Seed 0.5–16 ppm

IRON Fruit 28–91 ppm Plant 210 ppm Seed 38–180 ppm Sprout Seedling 10–73 ppm

ISOCAPRIC-ACID Seed

ISOCITRATE-DEHYDROGENASE Plant

ISOCOUMARIC-ACID Plant

ISOFERULIC-ACID Seed

ISOFLAVONES Seed 3,010–10,000 ppm

ISOFUCOSTEROL Seed

ISOLEUCINE Seed 19,353 ppm

ISOLIQUIRITIGENIN Seed

ISOPROPYL-AMINE Seed

ISOQUERCITRIN Leaf

ISOSCHAFTOSIDE Root 278 ppm

ISOVALERIANIC-ACID Seed

ISOXANTHOPTERIN Seed 0.062 ppm

JASMONIC-ACID Petiole

KAEMPFEROL Plant

KAEMPFEROL-3-0-BETA-D-RUTINOSIDE Plant

KAEMPFEROL-3-0-SOPHOROSIDE Leaf

KAEMPFEROL-3-O-BETA-D-NEOHESPERIDO-SIDE Leaf

KAEMPFEROL-3-O-BETA-D-O-2-RHAMNOSYL-GENTIOBIOSIDE Leaf

KAEMPFEROL-3-O-BETA-D-O-2-RHAMNOSYL-RUTINOSIDE Leaf

KAEMPFEROL-3-O-BETA-O-2-GENTIOBIOSIDE Leaf

KAEMPFEROL-3-O-BETA-O-2-GLUCOSYL-GEN-TIOBIOSIDE Leaf

KAEMPFEROL-3-O-BETA-O-2-GLUCOSYL-RUTI-
NOSIDE Leaf
KILOCALORIES Fruit 1,340–4,350 /kg Seed
1,390–4,548 /kg Sprout Seedling 460–3,360 /kg
KUNITZ-TRYPSIN-INHIBITOR Seed 500 ppm
LECITHIN Seed 15,000–25,000 ppm
LECTIN,SOYBEAN(SBL) Seed 9,760 ppm
LEGUMELIN Seed
LEUCINE Seed 29,720–32,500 ppm
LEUCINE-AMINO-PEPTIDASE Plant
LIGNIN Tissue Culture
LIGNOCERIC-ACID Seed
LINOLEIC-ACID Seed 70,335–126,082 ppm
LINOLENIC-ACID Seed 6,666–9,027 ppm
LIPASE Seed
LIPOXIDASE Seed
LIPOXIYGENASE Sprout Seedling
LIPOXYGENASE Plant
LUMAZINE Seed
LUPEOL Seed
LUTEIN Leaf
LYSINE Seed 24,290–26,560 ppm
MAGNESIUM Seed 430–3,160 ppm
MALATE-DEHYDROGENASE Plant
MALIC-ACID Seed 700–1,000 ppm
MALTOSE Sprout Seedling
MANGANESE Seed 8–60 ppm
MANNOSE-6-PHOSPHATE-ISOMERASE Plant
METHANOL Plant
METHIONINE Seed 4,920–5,380 ppm
METHYL-AMINE Seed 0.5–50 ppm
METHYLGENISTEIN Seed
MOLYBDENUM Seed 4 ppm
MUFA Seed 44,040–48,150 ppm
MYO-INOSITOL Root 900 ppm
MYRISTIC-ACID Seed 550–600 ppm
N-ACYL-PHOSPHATIDYL-ETHANOLAMINE
Sprout Seedling
N-BUTYL-AMINE Seed 1 ppm
N-CAPRIC-ACID Seed
N-CAPRYLIC-ACID Seed
N-METHYL-PHENETHYLAMINE Seed 50 ppm
N-NONANOIC-ACID Seed
N-VALERIANIC-ACID Seed
NADP-ACTIVE-ISOCITRATE-DEHYDROGENASE
Plant
NARINGENIN Leaf
NEO-CHLOROGENIC-ACID Plant

NEOXANTHIN Leaf
NEURAMINIC-ACID Seed
NH3 Seed 8,600 ppm
NIACIN Fruit 14–46 ppm Seed 13–32 ppm
Sprout Seedling 8–58 ppm
NICKEL Seed 1–30 ppm
NICOTIFLORIN Leaf
NITROGENASE Tissue Culture
O-BETA-D-GLUCOSYL-DIHYDROZEATIN Leaf
O-BETA-D-GLUCOSYL-DIHYDROZEATIN-RI-
BOSIDE Leaf
O-BETA-D-GLUCOSYL-ZEATIN Leaf
O-BETA-D-GLUCOSYL-ZEATIN-RIBOSIDE Leaf
O-COUMARIC-ACID Seed
OCTADECA-2,9,12-TRIENOIC-ACID Tissue Culture
OCTADECA-2,9-DIENOIC-ACID Tissue Culture
OCTADECA-9,12-DIENOIC-ACID Tissue Culture
OLEIC-ACID Seed 40,230–72,116 ppm
ONONIN Plant
ONONITOL Root 190 ppm
OXALIC-ACID Root Seed 770 ppm
P-COUMARIC-ACID Seed 1–4 ppm
P-HYDROXY-BENZOIC-ACID Seed 0.7–2.7
ppm
PALMITIC-ACID Seed 14,895–26,862 ppm
PALMITOLEIC-ACID Seed 550–600 ppm
PANTOTHENIC-ACID Seed 6–12 ppm
PENTANAL Plant
PENTANE Plant
PERLOLIDIN Seed
PEROXIDASE Seed
PHASEOL Leaf
PHASEOLIN Seed
PHASIN Seed
PHENYLALANINE Seed 19,050–20,830 ppm
PHENYLALANINE-AMMONIA-LYASE Tissue
Culture
PHOSPHATIDES Seed 1,350–7,260 ppm
PHOSPHATIDIC-ACID Sprout Seedling
PHOSPHATIDYL-CHOLINE Seed
PHOSPHATIDYL-ETHANOLAMINE Sprout
Seedling
PHOSPHATIDYL-GLYCEROLE Sprout Seedling
PHOSPHATIDYL-INOSITOL Sprout Seedling
PHOSPHOGLUCOMUTASE Plant
PHOSPHOGLUCOSE-ISOMERASE Plant
PHOSPHORUS Fruit 2,250–7,305 ppm Plant

2,400–5,410 ppm Seed 1,580–8,040 ppm
Sprout Seedling 580–4,891 ppm
PHYSETOLIC-ACID Seed
PHYTASE Seed
PHYTIC-ACID Seed
PHYTOHEMAGGLUTININ Seed
PHYTOSTEROLS Seed 1,610–1,760 ppm
PINITOL Leaf 10,000 ppm Root 550 ppm Seed
2,000–2,980 ppm
PIPERIDINE Seed
POLYSACCHARIDES Seed 120,000 ppm
POTASSIUM Plant 10,600 ppm Seed
4,100–27,600 ppm Sprout Seedling
2,790–15,081 ppm
PROLINE Seed 21,350–23,344 ppm
PROPANAL Plant
PROPIONIC-ACID Seed
PROTEASE Seed
PROTEIN Fruit 109,000–354,000 ppm Plant
139,000–166,000 ppm Seed
130,000–409,000 ppm Sprout Seedling
62,000–453,000 ppm
PROTOCATECHUIC-ACID Plant 0.2–0.5 ppm
PTERIN Seed 0.052 ppm
PUFA Seed 112,550–123,060 ppm
PYRIDOXINE Seed 6.4 ppm
PYROGLUTAMIC-ACID Seed 1,000–3,000 ppm
QUERCETIN Plant
QUERCETIN-3-O-BETA-D-2-GLUCOSYL-RUTI-
NOSIDE Leaf
QUERCETIN-3-O-BETA-O-SOPHOROSIDE Leaf
QUERCITRIN Leaf
RAFFINOSE Seed 5,000–15,000 ppm
RIBOFLAVIN Fruit 1.6–5 ppm Seed 1.7–13 ppm
Sprout Seedling 1.5–15 ppm
RIBOSE-1,5-DIPHOSPHATE-CARBOXYLASE Tis-
sue Culture
ROTENOIDS Seed 1,000 ppm
RUTIN Shoot
SALICYLIC-ACID Seed
SAPOGENOL-C Sprout Seedling
SAPONINS Seed 50,000 ppm
SELENIUM Seed 0.04–1.25 ppm
SEQUOYITOL Leaf
SERINE Plant Seed 21,150–23,125 ppm
SFA Seed 14,850–32,670 ppm
SILICON Seed
SINAPIC-ACID Leaf Seed

SODIUM Seed 9–3,800 ppm Sprout Seedling
300–1,622 ppm
SOJAGOL Plant
SOPHORAFLAVANOLOSIDE Leaf
SOYASAPOGENOL-A Seed
SOYASAPOGENOL-B Seed
SOYASAPOGENOL-B-1 Seed
SOYASAPOGENOL-C Seed
SOYASAPONIN-A Seed
SOYASAPONIN-A-1 Seed 239–400 ppm
SOYASAPONIN-A-2 Embryo
SOYASAPONIN-A-3 Seed 100 ppm
SOYASAPONIN-A-4 Seed
SOYASAPONIN-A-5 Seed
SOYASAPONIN-A-6 Seed
SOYASAPONIN-B Seed
SOYASAPONIN-C Seed
SOYASAPONIN-D Seed
SOYASAPONIN-E Seed
SOYASAPONIN-I Cotyledon 300–3,000 ppm
Hypocotyl 5,000–19,000 ppm Leaf
1,500–11,100 ppm Pericarp 100–2,500 ppm
Root 600–3,300 ppm Seed 139–1,200 ppm
Stem 300–1,300 ppm
SOYASAPONIN-II Seed 47–150 ppm
SOYASAPONIN-III Seed 10–22 ppm
SOYASAPONIN-IV Seed 140–160 ppm
SOYASAPONIN-V Seed
SQUALENE Seed
STACHYOSE Seed 22,300–51,050 ppm
STARCH Seed 10,000 ppm
STEARIC-ACID Seed 4,320–7,785 ppm
STIGMAST-4-EN-3-6-DIONE Tissue Culture
STIGMAST-4-EN-3-ONE Tissue Culture
STIGMASTA-4-22-DIEN-3-6-DIONE Tissue Cul-
ture
STIGMASTA-4-22-DIEN-3-ONE Tissue Culture
STIGMASTEROL Seed
STRONTIUM Seed 3–42 ppm
SUCCINIC-ACID Root Seed Sprout Seedling
SUCROSE Seed 27,950–71,700 ppm
SUGARS Seed 125,000 ppm
SULFUR Seed 4,066 ppm
SYRINGIC-ACID Root 4.1–4.7 ppm Seed
TATOIN Seed
TETRAMETHYL-PYRAZINE Seed
THIAMIN Fruit 4.4–14 ppm Seed 4–10 ppm
Sprout Seedling 1.9–17 ppm

THREONEOPTERIN Seed 0.017 ppm
THREONINE Seed 15,850–17,330 ppm
TITANIUM Seed 12 ppm
TRANS-ACONITIC-ACID Root
TRANS-OCIMENE Plant
TRIGONELLINE Fruit 3.7–16.2 ppm Leaf
  10.5–63.2 ppm Root 1.1 ppm
Seed 19.7–71.8 ppm Stem 1.5–7.6 ppm
TRYPOTPHAN Seed 5,300–5,795 ppm
TYROSINE Seed 13,800–15,090 ppm
UNDYLIC-ACID Sprout Seedling
UREASE Seed
URICASE Seed
UROPORPHYRIN Tissue Culture
VALINE Seed 18,210–19,910 ppm
VANILLIC-ACID Root 1–4 ppm Seed
VERBACOSE Seed 280–410 ppm
VERBASCOSE Seed 3,000 ppm
VIOLAXANTHIN Leaf
VIT-B-6 Seed 3–6 ppm
VIT-D Seed
VIT-E Seed
VIT-K Seed
VITEXIN Root
VITEXIN-2"-O-RHAMNOSIDE Root
WATER Fruit 692,000 ppm Seed
  83,980–682,000 ppm Sprout Seedling
  815,000–863,000 ppm
XANTHINE Sprout Seedling
XYLOGALACTOMANNAN Seed
XYLOSE Seed
ZINC Seed 22–90 ppm
ZIRCONIUM Seed 0.8–2.4 ppm

SPINACH

Chemicals in *Spinacia oleracea L.* (*Chenopodiaceae*)—Spinach

3-HYDROXYTYRAMINE Leaf
6-(HYDROXYMETHYL)-LUMAZINE Leaf
7-STIGMASTEROL Leaf
ACETYL-CHOLINE Leaf
ALANINE Plant 1,420–16,864 ppm
ALPHA-LINOLENIC-ACID Plant 480–13,657
  ppm
ALPHA-TOCOPHEROL Leaf 12–419 ppm
ALUMINUM Leaf 5–270 ppm
ARGININE Plant 1,620–19,239 ppm

ARSENIC Leaf 0.02–0.29 ppm
ASCORBATE Plant 212–4,450 ppm
ASCORBIC-ACID Plant 239–7,595 ppm
ASH Plant 16,850–285,700 ppm
ASPARTIC-ACID Plant 2,400–28,502 ppm
BETA-CAROTENE Plant 4–690 ppm
BORON Leaf 2.4–40 ppm
BROMINE Leaf 4 ppm
CADMIUM Leaf 0.05–5 ppm
CALCIUM Plant 730–15,700 ppm
CARBOHYDRATES Plant 35,000–415,660 ppm
CEPHALIN Leaf
CHLORINE Plant 540–6,835 ppm
CHOLESTEROL Leaf
CHROMIUM Flower 0.01–0.42 ppm
COBALT Plant 0.001–1.2 ppm
COLAMINE Leaf
COPPER Plant 0.1–24 ppm
CYSTINE Plant 350–4,157 ppm
DIGALACTOSYLDIACYLGLYCEROL Plant
FAT Plant 3,070–46,672 ppm
FERULIC-ACID Leaf 16 ppm
FIBER Plant 6,000–111,634 ppm
FLUORINE Leaf 0.3–5.7 ppm
FOLACIN Plant 1.2–27.13 ppm
GLUTAMIC-ACID Plant 3,430–40,735 ppm
GLUTATHIONE Plant 90–1,065 ppm
GLYCINE Plant 1,340–15,914 ppm
HEXADECA-7,10,13-TRIENOIC-ACID Leaf
HEXOSAMINE Seed 380 ppm
HISTIDINE Plant 640–7,601 ppm
IODINE Plant 0.2 ppm
IRON Plant 8–384 ppm
ISOLEUCINE Plant 1,470–17,458 ppm
KAEMPFEROL Plant
KILOCALORIES Plant 220–2,613 /kg
LEAD Leaf 0.03–3 ppm
LECITHIN Leaf
LEUCINE Plant 2,230–26,483 ppm
LINOLEIC-ACID Plant 104–2,613 ppm
LYSINE Plant 1,740–20,664 ppm
MAGNESIUM Plant 420–11,000 ppm
MANGANESE Plant 3–485 ppm
MERCURY Leaf 0.003–0.11 ppm
METHIONINE Plant 530–6,294 ppm
MOLYBDENUM Plant 0.06–0.8 ppm
MONOGALACTOSYLDIACYLGLYCEROL Plant
MYRISTIC-ACID Plant 1–950 ppm

N,N-DIMETHYLHISTAMINE Leaf
N-ACETYLHISTAMINE Leaf
NIACIN Plant 6.9–89.8 ppm
NICKEL Plant
NITROGEN Leaf 3,200–45,700 ppm
OLEIC-ACID Plant 18–475 ppm
OXALIC-ACID Leaf 6,580 ppm
P-COUMARIC-ACID Leaf 133 ppm
PALMITIC-ACID Plant 106–4,869 ppm
PALMITOLEIC-ACID Plant 21–475 ppm
PANTOTHENIC-ACID Plant 0.57–8.7 ppm
PATULETIN Leaf
PHENYLALANINE Plant 1,290–15,320 ppm
PHOSPHATIDYL-CHOLINE Plant
PHOSPHATIDYL-ETHANOLAMINE Plant
PHOSPHATIDYL-GLYCEROL Leaf
PHOSPHATIDYL-INOSITOL Leaf
PHOSPHATIDYL-SERINE Leaf
PHOSPHORUS Plant 250–6,232 ppm
PHYTOSTEROLS Plant 90–1,800 ppm
POLYPHENOL-OXIDASE Leaf
POTASSIUM Plant 2,060–69,077 ppm
PROLINE Plant 1,120–13,301 ppm
PROTEIN Plant 27,480–352,954 ppm
QUERCETIN Leaf 19 ppm
RIBOFLAVIN Plant 1.8–23.4 ppm
RUBIDIUM Leaf 0.9–90 ppm
RUTIN Leaf 170 ppm
SELENIUM Leaf 0.057 ppm
SERINE Plant 1,040–12,351 ppm
SILICON Leaf 1–855 ppm
SODIUM Plant 585–10,669 ppm
SPINASAPONINS Plant
SPINASTEROL Leaf
STEARIC-ACID Plant 7–356 ppm
STRONTIUM Plant 0.06–0.77 ppm
SULFOLIPIDS Plant
SULFUR Plant 270–5,700 ppm
THIAMIN Plant 0.7–10.2 ppm
THREONINE Plant 1,220–14,489 ppm
TRIMETHYLHISTAMINE Leaf
TRYPTOPHAN Plant 390–4,632 ppm
TYROSINE Plant 1,080–12,826 ppm
VALINE Plant 1,610–19,120 ppm
VIT-B-6 Plant 1.9–24 ppm
WATER Plant 913,120–930,000 ppm
ZINC Plant 4–185 ppm

SPIRULINA

Chemicals in *Spirulina pratensis*—Spirulina

ASCORBIC-ACID Plant
ASH Plant 182,000 ppm
BETA-CAROTENE Plant 478 ppm
CALCIUM Plant 280 ppm
CARBOHYDRATES Plant 245,000 ppm
FAT Plant 21,000 ppm
FIBER Plant 2,000 ppm
IRON Plant 713 ppm
KILOCALORIES Plant 3,800 /kg
MAGNESIUM Plant 2,550 ppm
NIACIN Plant
PHOSPHORUS Plant 3,190 ppm
POTASSIUM Plant 1,600 ppm
PROTEIN Plant 713,000 ppm
RIBOFLAVIN Plant 46 ppm
SODIUM Plant 128 ppm
THIAMIN Plant 51 ppm

STRING BEAN

Chemicals in *Phaseolus vulgaris L.*
(*Fabaceae*)—Black Bean, Garden Bean,
Green Bean, Haricot, String Bean

12-DICARBONIC-ACID Hull Husk
17-BETA-ESTRADIOL Flower
2'-HYDROXYGENISTEIN Fruit
2-METHOXYPHASEOLINISOFLAVAN Sprout
  Seedling
ALANINE Fruit 840–8,633 ppm Seed
  9,050–10,171 ppm Sprout Seedling
  1,740–18,710 ppm
ALLANTOIC-ACID Fruit
ALPHA-LINOLENIC-ACID Fruit 360–3,700 ppm
  Seed 2,780–3,124 ppm Sprout Seedling
  1,690–18,172 ppm
ALPHA-TOCOPHEROL Fruit 0.2–14 ppm Leaf
  698–719 ppm
ALUMINUM Fruit 1–1,050 ppm Seed 5–73 ppm
APIGENIN Plant
ARGININE Fruit 730–7,503 ppm Seed
  13,370–15,026 ppm Sprout Seedling
  2,280–24,516 ppm
ARSENIC Fruit 0.003–0.01 ppm Seed
  0.002–0.002 ppm
ASCORBIC-ACID Fruit 10–2,389 ppm Leaf

1,100–8,333 ppm Seed 177 ppm Sprout
Seedling 387–4,161 ppm

ASH Fruit 6,000–156,000 ppm Leaf
26,000–177,000 ppm Seed 17,000–62,000
ppm Sprout Seedling 5,000–53,763 ppm

ASPARAGINE Fruit

ASPARTIC-ACID Fruit 2,550–26,208 ppm Seed
26,130–29,366 ppm Sprout Seedling
5,460–58,710 ppm

BARIUM Fruit 0.4–45 ppm Seed 0.1–7.3 ppm

BETA-CAROTENE Fruit 2.2–66 ppm Leaf
32.4–245.5 ppm Seed 0.1–9.8 ppm Sprout
Seedling

BIOTIN Root

BORON Fruit 0.1–45 ppm Seed 2–43 ppm

BROMINE Fruit 2–20 ppm

CADMIUM Fruit 0.002–0.2 ppm Seed
0.007–0.039 ppm

CALCIUM Fruit 356–18,000 ppm Leaf
2,740–20,758 ppm Seed 510–3,295 ppm
Sprout Seedling 170–1,828 ppm

CARBOHYDRATES Fruit 56,000–733,778 ppm
Leaf 66,000–500,000 ppm Seed
278,000–701,039 ppm Sprout Seedling
41,000–440,860 ppm

CEREBROSIDE Fruit

CHOLINE Fruit

CHROMIUM Fruit 0.005–1.5 ppm Seed
0.051–4.9 ppm

COBALAMINE Root

COBALT Fruit 10.5 ppm Seed 0.034–1.05 ppm

COPPER Fruit 0.62–45 ppm Seed 2–15 ppm

CYSTINE Fruit 180–1,850 ppm Seed
2,350–2,641 ppm Sprout Seedling 480–5,161
ppm

DEC-2-EN Hull Husk

ESTROL Flower

ESTRONE Flower

FAT Fruit 2,000–47,000 ppm Leaf 4,000–54,000
ppm Seed 3,000–24,000 ppm Sprout
Seedling 5,000–53,763 ppm

FERRITINE Flower

FERULIC-ACID Plant

FIBER Fruit 10,000–159,000 ppm Leaf
28,000–212,000 ppm Seed 37,000–88,700
ppm

FLUORINE Fruit 0.1–2 ppm

FOLACIN Seed 4.1–5.3 ppm Sprout Seedling
0.3–4.1 ppm

GENISTEIN Fruit

GIBBERELIN-A-37 Plant

GIBBERELIN-A-38 Plant

GLUCOKININ Fruit

GLUTAMIC-ACID Fruit 1,870–19,219 ppm Seed
32,940–37,019 ppm Sprout Seedling
5,120–55,054 ppm

GLUTATHIONE Root

GLYCINE Fruit 650–6,680 ppm Seed
8,430–9,474 ppm Sprout Seedling
1,440–15,484 ppm

HISTIDINE Fruit 340–3,494 ppm Seed
6,010–6,754 ppm Sprout Seedling
1,180–12,688 ppm

INOSITOL Fruit

IRON Fruit 6–1,050 ppm Leaf 92–697 ppm
Seed 24–147 ppm Sprout Seedling 8–87 ppm

ISOLEUCINE Fruit 660–6,783 ppm Seed
9,540–10,722 ppm Sprout Seedling
1,860–20,000 ppm

KAEMPFEROL-3-GLUCURONIDE Leaf

KILOCALORIES Fruit 280–3,830 /kg Leaf
360–2,730 /kg Seed 3,230–3,832 /kg Sprout
Seedling 290–3,118 /kg

LEAD Fruit 0.01–10.5 ppm Seed 0.7–1 ppm

LEUCINE Fruit 1,120–11,511 ppm Seed
17,250–19,386 ppm Sprout Seedling
3,020–32,473 ppm

LIGNIN Seed 4,100–10,800 ppm

LINOLEIC-ACID Fruit 230–2,364 ppm Seed
3,320–3,731 ppm Sprout Seedling
1,070–11,505 ppm

LITHIUM Fruit 0.216–2.7 ppm Seed 0.136–2.45
ppm

LUTEOLIN Plant

LYSINE Fruit 880–9,044 ppm Seed
14,830–16,667 ppm Sprout Seedling
2,390–25,700 ppm

MAGNESIUM Fruit 210–18,000 ppm Seed
510–3,430 ppm Sprout Seedling 210–2,258
ppm

MALONIC-ACID Fruit

MANGANESE Fruit 1–150 ppm Seed 2–24 ppm

MERCURY Fruit 0.02 ppm

METHIONINE Fruit 220–2,261 ppm Seed

3,250–3,653 ppm Sprout Seedling 440–4,731 ppm

MOLYBDENUM Fruit 20 ppm Seed 0.5–14 ppm

MUFA Fruit 50–514 ppm Seed 1,230–1,382 ppm Sprout Seedling 390–4,194 ppm

NIACIN Fruit 5–77 ppm Leaf 13–98 ppm Seed 15–38 ppm Sprout Seedling 29–312 ppm

NICKEL Fruit 15 ppm Seed 0.5–7 ppm

NITROGEN Fruit 3,600–41,000 ppm

OLEIC-ACID Fruit 40–411 ppm Seed 1,230–1,382 ppm Sprout Seedling 390–4,194 ppm

OXALIC-ACID Fruit 312 ppm

P-COUMARIC-ACID Plant

PALMITIC-ACID Fruit 220–2,261 ppm Seed 3,430–3,855 ppm Sprout Seedling 640–6,882 ppm

PANTOTHENIC-ACID Fruit 0.9–10 ppm Seed 9–10 ppm

PHASELIC-ACID Plant

PHASEOLIDES Plant

PHASEOLLIDIN Plant

PHASEOLLIN Plant

PHASEOLLIN-ISOFLAVONE Plant

PHENYLALANINE Fruit 670–6,886 ppm Seed 11,680–13,127 ppm Sprout Seedling 2,120–22,796 ppm

PHOSPHORUS Fruit 370–13,500 ppm Leaf 750–5,682 ppm Seed 2,130–5,880 ppm Sprout Seedling 370–3,978 ppm

PHYTIC-ACID Seed 4,800 ppm

PHYTOSTEROLS Seed

PIPECOLIC-ACID Fruit

POTASSIUM Fruit 1,960–58,500 ppm Seed 9,840–21,070 ppm Sprout Seedling 1,870–20,108 ppm

PROLINE Fruit 680–6,989 ppm Seed 9,160–10,294 ppm Sprout Seedling 1,690–18,172 ppm

PROTEIN Fruit 17,700–224,000 ppm Leaf 36,000–297,000 ppm Seed 98,000–394,000 ppm Sprout Seedling 42,000–451,613 ppm

PUFA Fruit 590–6,064 ppm Seed 6,100–6,855 ppm Sprout Seedling 2,760–29,677 ppm

PYRROLIDINONCARBONIC-ACID Fruit

QUERCETIN-3-GLUCURONIDE Leaf

RIBOFLAVIN Fruit 1–12 ppm Leaf 0.6–4.5 ppm Seed 1.2–3 ppm Sprout Seedling 2.5–27 ppm

RUBIDIUM Fruit 0.47–7 ppm

SELENIUM Fruit 0.001–0.008 ppm Seed 0.01 ppm

SERINE Fruit 990–10,175 ppm Seed 11,750–13,205 ppm Sprout Seedling 2,240–24,086 ppm

SFA Fruit 260–2,672 ppm Seed 3,660–4,113 ppm Sprout Seedling 720–7,742 ppm

SILICON Fruit 80–1,200 ppm

SILVER Fruit 0.3 ppm Seed 0.034–0.147 ppm

SODIUM Fruit 5.4–707 ppm Seed 0.85–112 ppm

STEARIC-ACID Fruit 40–411 ppm Seed 220–247 ppm Sprout Seedling 90–968 ppm

STRONTIUM Fruit 2–105 ppm Seed 0.7–34 ppm

SUCCINIC-ACID Fruit

SULFUR Fruit 54–875 ppm Seed 54–137 ppm

THIAMIN Fruit 0.5–8.8 ppm Leaf 1.8–13.6 ppm Seed 3.7–10 ppm Sprout Seedling 3.7–40 ppm

THREONINE Fruit 790–8,119 ppm Seed 9,090–10,216 ppm Sprout Seedling 1,760–18,925 ppm

TITANIUM Fruit 0.1–105 ppm Seed 0.17–7.4 ppm

TRAUMATINIC-ACID Hull Husk

TRIGONELLINE Fruit

TRYPTOPHAN Fruit 190–1,953 ppm Seed 2,560–2,877 ppm Sprout Seedling 440–4,731 ppm

TYROSINE Fruit 420–4,317 ppm Seed 6,080–6,833 ppm Sprout Seedling 1,440–15,484 ppm

VALINE Fruit 900–9,250 ppm Seed 11,300–12,699 ppm Sprout Seedling 2,160–23,226 ppm

VANADIUM Fruit 0.24–105 ppm

VIT-B-6 Fruit 0.74–7.6 ppm Seed 2.8–3.3 ppm

WATER Fruit 688,000–942,000 ppm Leaf 868,000 ppm Seed 63,000–604,000 ppm Sprout Seedling 907,000 ppm

ZINC Fruit 2–150 ppm Seed 19–50 ppm

ZIRCONIUM Fruit 1–22 ppm Seed 0.68–1.47 ppm

SUMMER SQUASH

Chemicals in *Cucurbita spp* (*Cucurbitaceae*)—Summer Squash

ALANINE Fruit 620–9,810 ppm

ARGININE Fruit 500–7,910 ppm

ASCORBIC-ACID Fruit 148–2,340 ppm

ASH Fruit 5,550–96,045 ppm

ASPARTIC-ACID Fruit 1,440–22,785 ppm

BETA-CAROTENE Fruit 0.12–1.9 ppm

CALCIUM Fruit 200–3,165 ppm

CARBOHYDRATES Fruit 43,500–688,300 ppm

COPPER Fruit 0.7–12 ppm

CYSTINE Fruit 120–1,900 ppm

FAT Fruit 2,100–33,230 ppm

FIBER Fruit 6,000–94,935 ppm

FOLACIN Fruit 0.2–4.6 ppm

GLUTAMIC-ACID Fruit 1,260–19,935 ppm

GLYCINE Fruit 440–6,962 ppm

HISTIDINE Fruit 250–3,955 ppm

IRON Fruit 4–73 ppm

ISOLEUCINE Fruit 420–6,645 ppm

KILOCALORIES Fruit 200–3,165 /kg

LAURIC-ACID Fruit 10–160 ppm

LEUCINE Fruit 690–10,920 ppm

LINOLEIC-ACID Fruit 330–5,220 ppm

LINOLENIC-ACID Fruit 560–8,860 ppm

LYSINE Fruit 650–10,285 ppm

MAGNESIUM Fruit 230–3,640 ppm

MANGANESE Fruit 1–27 ppm

METHIONINE Fruit 170–2,690 ppm

MUFA Fruit 160–2,530 ppm

MYRISTIC-ACID Fruit 10–160 ppm

NIACIN Fruit 5–85 ppm

OLEIC-ACID Fruit 140–2,215 ppm

PALMITIC-ACID Fruit 380–6,015 ppm

PALMITOLEIC-ACID Fruit 10–169 ppm

PANTOTHENIC-ACID Fruit 1–18 ppm

PECTIN Fruit 6,000–94,935 ppm

PHENYLALANINE Fruit 410–6,485 ppm

PHOSPHORUS Fruit 350–5,540 ppm

POTASSIUM Fruit 1,950–30,855 ppm

PROLINE Fruit 370–5,855 ppm

PROTEIN Fruit 11,800–186,700 ppm

PUFA Fruit 890–14,080 ppm

RIBOFLAVIN Fruit 0.4–6 ppm

SERINE Fruit 480–7,595 ppm

SFA Fruit 440–6,960 ppm

SODIUM Fruit 20–315 ppm

STEARIC-ACID Fruit 40–635 ppm

THIAMIN Fruit 0.6–10 ppm

THREONINE Fruit 280–4,430 ppm

TRYPTOPHAN Fruit 110–1,740 ppm

TYROSINE Fruit 310–4,905 ppm

VALINE Fruit 530–8,385 ppm

VIT-B-6 Fruit 1–18 ppm

WATER Fruit 936,800 ppm

ZINC Fruit 2–41 ppm

TOMATO

Chemicals in *Lycopersicon esculentum
MILLER (Solanaceae)*—Tomato

1',2'-EPOXY-1',2'-DIHYDRO-BETA-EPSILON-
PSEUDOCAROTENE Fruit

1',2'-EPOXY-1',2'-DIHYDRO-BETA-PSI-
CAROTENE Fruit

1,2-EPOXY-1,2-DIHYDRO-PSI,PSI-CAROTENE
Fruit

1-BUTYL-2-THIAZOL Fruit

1-O-FERULOYL-BETA-D-GLUCOSE Fruit

1-O-P-COUMAROYL-BETA-D-GLUCOSE Fruit

10,16-DIHYDROXY-DECANOIC-ACID Fruit

10,16-DIHYDROXY-HEXADECANOIC-ACID
Fruit

16-HYDROXY-HEXADECANOIC-ACID Fruit

2,7-DIMETHYL-OCT-4-ENEDIOIC-ACID Shoot
1.2 ppm

2,7-DIMETHYL-OCTA-2,4-DIENOIC-ACID
Shoot 1.8 ppm

2-BUTANONE Fruit

2-PENTANONE Fruit

2-PROPANONE Fruit

24-®-ETHYL-LOPHENOL Seed

24-METHYL-31-NOR-LANOST-9(11)-EN-3-
BETA-OL Seed

24-METHYL-LOPHENOL Seed

24-METHYLENE-CYCLOARTANAL Seed

24-METHYLENE-CYCLOARTENAL Plant

3-BETA-HYDROXY-5-ALPHA-PREG-16-EN-20-
ONE Shoot

3-O-FERULOYL-QUINIC-ACID Leaf

31-NOR-LANOST-8-EN-3-BETA-OL Seed

31-NOR-LANOST-9(11)-EN-3-BETA-OL Seed

31-NORCYCLOARTENAL Seed

4-ALPHA-24-DIMETHYL-CHOLESTA-7,24-
DIEN-3-BETA-OL Seed

4-ALPHA-METHYL-24-ETHYL-CHOLESTA-7,24-
DIEN-3-BETA-OL Seed

4-VINYL-GUAIACOL Leaf Seed

5,6-EPOXY-5,6-DIHYDRO-PSEUDO-PSEUDO-
 CAROTENE Fruit
5-HYDROXYTRYPTAMINE Fruit
5ALPHA-FUROSTANE-3BETA,22,26TRIOL-3-O-
 BETA-D-GLUCOPYRANOSYL . . . Plant
9,10,16-TRIHYDROXYHEXADECANOIC-ACID
 Fruit
9,10,18-TRIHYDROXY-OCTADECANOIC-ACID
 Fruit
ABSCISIC-ACID Leaf
ABSCISIC-ACID-1',4'-TRANS-DIOL Fruit Leaf
ABSCISIC-ACID-1'O-BETA-D-GLUCOPYRA-
 NOSIDE Stem
ACETALDEHYDE Fruit
ACETIC-ACID Fruit
ACETONE Fruit
ADENOSINE Flower
ALANINE Fruit 30–4,132 ppm
ALPHA-AMYRIN Fruit
ALPHA-CAPROLACTONE Fruit
ALPHA-IONENE Fruit
ALPHA-KETO-GLUTARIC-ACID Fruit
ALPHA-LINOLENIC-ACID Fruit 30–496 ppm
ALPHA-NONALACTONE Fruit
ALPHA-OCTALACTONE Fruit
ALPHA-OXOGLUTARIC-ACID Fruit
ALPHA-PINENE Fruit
ALPHA-TOCOPHEROL Fruit 7–143 ppm
ALUMINUM Fruit 0.3–1,700 ppm
ARABIC-ACID Fruit
ARGININE Fruit 1–3,637 ppm
ARSENIC Fruit 0.003–0.043 ppm
ASCORBIC-ACID Fruit 50–2,952 ppm
ASH Fruit 5,700–105,461 ppm
ASPARAGINE Fruit 300 ppm
ASPARTIC-ACID Fruit 1,230–20,332 ppm
AUROXANTHIN Fruit
BARIUM Fruit 60 ppm
BENZALDEHYDE Fruit
BENZYL-ALCOHOL Fruit
BETA-ALANINE Fruit 6 ppm
BETA-AMYRIN Fruit
BETA-CAROTENE Fruit 7–113 ppm
BETA-D-GLUCOPYRANOSYL-PHASEIC-ACID
 Plant
BETA-IONENE Fruit
BETA-SITOSTEROL Fruit
BETAINE Root 23 ppm Shoot 69 ppm

BIOTIN Fruit
BORON Fruit 96 ppm
BUTANOL-2-ON-3 Fruit
BUTANOLS Fruit
BUTYROLACTONE Fruit
CADMIUM Fruit 0.005–1.7 ppm
CAFFEIC-ACID Fruit 6 ppm
CAFFEIC-ACID-4-O-BETA-D-GLUCOSIDE Fruit
CALCIUM Fruit 60–2,400 ppm Leaf 60,800
 ppm
CAMPESTEROL Fruit
CAPRYLIC-ACID Fruit
CARBOHYDRATES Fruit 43,400–717,400 ppm
CARBOXYLIC-ACID Leaf
CELLULASE Fruit
CELLULOSE Fruit
CERIUM Fruit 7–60 ppm
CHLORINE Fruit 510 ppm
CHLOROGENIC-ACID Fruit 18 ppm
CHLOROPHYLL Fruit 3–30 ppm
CHLOROPHYLL-A Fruit
CHLOROPHYLL-B Fruit
CHOLINE Root 36 ppm Shoot 48 ppm
CHROMIUM Fruit 3 ppm
CINNAMALDEHYDE Fruit
CIS-3-HEXENOL-1 Fruit 4–40 ppm
CIS-5'-BETA-PSEUDOCAROTENE Fruit
CIS-5'-EPSILON-PSEUDOCAROTENE Fruit
CIS-5'-NEUROSPORENE Fruit
CIS-5,CIS-5'-LYCOPENE Fruit 1–20 ppm
CIS-5-LYCOPENE Fruit 1–20 ppm
CIS-HEXEN-3-AL Fruit
CITRAL Fruit
CITRIC-ACID Fruit
CITROSTADIENOL Seed
COBALT Fruit 1.4 ppm
COPPER Fruit 0.4–100 ppm
CUTIN Fruit
CYCLOARTANOL Seed
CYCLOARTENOL Seed
CYCLOEUCALENOL Seed
CYCLOHEXANOL Fruit
CYSTINE Fruit 120–1,984 ppm
DAMASCENONE Fruit
DECADIEN-TRANS-2,TRANS-4-AL Fruit
DIACETYL Fruit
DIHYDROXYTARTARIC-ACID Fruit
DIHYDROZEATIN Flower

EPOXY-5,6-IONENE Fruit

EPOXY-LUTEIN Fruit

ETHANOL Fruit

ETHYL-PHENOL Fruit

ETHYLENE Fruit

EUGENOL Fruit

FALCARINDIOL Seed

FALCARINOL Seed

FARNESAL Fruit

FARNESYL-ACETONE Fruit

FAT Fruit 1,330–47,441 ppm Seed
150,000–250,000 ppm

FERULIC-ACID Fruit

FERULIC-ACID-O-BETA-D-GLUCOSIDE Fruit

FIBER Fruit 4,700–77,691 ppm

FLUORINE Fruit 0.02–1.7 ppm

FOLACIN Fruit 2 ppm

FORMIC-ACID Fruit

FRUCTOSE Fruit 11,700 ppm

FUMARIC-ACID Fruit

FURFURAL Fruit

GABA Fruit 220–480 ppm

GAMMA-CAROTENE Fruit

GENTISIC-ACID Leaf

GERANYL-ACETONE Fruit

GIBBERELLINS Fruit

GLUCOSE Fruit 16,300 ppm

GLUTAMIC-ACID Fruit 90–54,053 ppm

GLYCERIC-ACID Fruit

GLYCINE Fruit 23–3,637 ppm

GLYCOLIC-ACID Fruit

GLYOXAL Fruit

GRAMISTEROL Seed

GUAIACOL Fruit

HEMICELLULOSE Fruit

HEPTADIEN-TRANS-2,CIS-4-AL Fruit

HEPTADIEN-TRANS-2,TRANS-4-AL Fruit

HEPTULOSE Fruit

HEXADIEN-TRANS-2-,TRANS-4-AL Fruit

HEXANOLS Fruit

HISTIDINE Fruit 30–2,149 ppm

HYDROCINNAMALDEHYDE Fruit

I-VALERALDEHYDE Fruit

I-VALERIC-ACID Fruit

INDOLE-3-ACETIC-ACID Root

IODINE Fruit

IRON Fruit 1–800 ppm

ISOAMYLOL Fruit 7–40 ppm

ISOLEUCINE Fruit 210–3,471 ppm

ISOPENTENYL-ADENINE Root

ISOPENTENYL-ADENOSINE Root

ISOVALERALDEHYDE Fruit 0.006 ppm

JSGGALACTURONIC-ACID Fruit

KAEMPFEROL Seed

KETOHEPTOSE Fruit

LACTIC-ACID Fruit

LANOSTEROL Seed

LEAD Fruit 0.003–60 ppm

LEUCINE Fruit 330–5,455 ppm

LEUCINES Fruit 1–90 ppm

LEUCIONPINE Tissue Culture

LEUCIONPINE-LACTAM Tissue Culture

LINALOL Fruit

LINOLEIC-ACID Fruit 830–13,720 ppm

LINOLENIC-ACID Fruit

LITHIUM Fruit 0.28–0.68 ppm

LOPHENOL Seed

LUPEOL Plant

LUTEIN Fruit

LUTEIN-5,6-EPOXIDE Fruit

LUTEIN-EPOXIDE Fruit

LYCOPENE Fruit 1–20 ppm

LYCOPERSICONOL Root

LYCOPERSICONOLIDE Root 6.7 ppm

LYCOPHYLL Fruit

LYCOXANTHIN Fruit

LYSINE Fruit 20–5,455 ppm

MAGNESIUM Fruit 70–6,000 ppm Leaf 4,300
ppm

MALIC-ACID Fruit

MANGANESE Fruit 0.6–100 ppm

MERCURY Fruit 0.001–0.002 ppm

METHANOL Fruit

METHIONINE Fruit 16–1,322 ppm

METHYL-2-BUTYRIC-ACID Fruit

METHYL-6-HEPTEN-5-ON-2 Fruit

METHYL-GLYOXAL Fruit

METHYL-SALICYLATE Fruit

MEVALONIC-ACID Fruit 3–4 ppm

MOLYBDENUM Fruit 6 ppm

MYRISTIC-ACID Fruit

N(6)-ISOPENT-2-ENYL-ADENINE Flower

N-DOTRIACONTANE Fruit

N-HENTRIACONTANE Fruit

N-HEXANOL Fruit

N-PENTANOL Fruit 7–40 ppm

N-TETRATRIACONTANE Fruit
N-TRITRIACONTANE Fruit
NARCOTINE Fruit
NARINGENIN Fruit
NEO-BETA-CAROTENE-B Fruit
NEO-BETA-CAROTENE-U Fruit
NEO-CHLOROGENIC-ACID Leaf
NEODYMIUM Fruit 2–30 ppm
NEOLYCOPENE-A Fruit
NEOLYCOPENE-B Fruit
NEOTIGOGENIN Tissue Culture 300–1,500 ppm
NEOXANTHIN Fruit
NESTIGOGENIN Fruit
NEUROSPORINE Fruit
NIACIN Fruit 6–99 ppm
NICKEL Fruit 0.01–5 ppm
NICOTIANAMINE Leaf
NITROGEN Fruit 1,300–23,330 ppm Leaf 26,000 ppm
NONACOSANE Fruit
O-CRESOL Fruit
O-HYDROXY-ACETOPHENONE Fruit
OBTUSIFOLIOL Seed
OLEIC-ACID Fruit 310–5,124 ppm
OXALIC-ACID Fruit 36–263 ppm
P-COUMARIC-ACID Fruit
P-COUMARIC-ACID-O-BETA-D-GLUCOSIDE Fruit
P-HYDROXYBENZALDEHYDE Plant
PALMITIC-ACID Fruit 210–3,471 ppm
PALMITOLEIC-ACID Fruit 10–165 ppm
PANTOTHENIC-ACID Fruit 1–61 ppm
PECTIN Fruit 100–31,000 ppm
PECTINESTERASE Fruit
PENTANOLS Fruit
PENTEN-1-OL-3 Fruit
PHENOL Fruit
PHENOLICS Fruit 27–570 ppm
PHENYL-2-ETHANOL Fruit
PHENYL-ACETALDEHYDE Fruit
PHENYLACETONITRILE Fruit
PHENYLALANINE Fruit 72–3,801 ppm
PHOSPHATIDYL-GLYCEROL Leaf
PHOSPHORUS Fruit 110–8,400 ppm Leaf 5,500 ppm
PHYTOENE Fruit
PHYTOENE-1,2-OXIDE Fruit

PHYTOFLUENE Fruit
PHYTOSTEROLS Fruit 70–1,157 ppm
PIPECOLIC-ACID Fruit
POLYGALACTURONASE Fruit
POTASSIUM Fruit 780–58,800 ppm Leaf 47,000 ppm
PROLINE Fruit 170–2,810 ppm Root 725 ppm
PROLYCOPENE Fruit
PROPANOLS Fruit
PROPIONIC-ACID Fruit
PROTEIN Fruit 8,790–148,935 ppm
PROTOPECTIN Fruit 11,700–24,200 ppm
PYRUVIC-ACID Fruit
QUERCETIN Fruit
QUERCETIN-3-0-RHAMNOSIDE Fruit
QUERCITRIN Fruit
RIBOFLAVIN Fruit 1–8 ppm
RISHITIN Plant
RUBIDIUM Fruit 0.3–22 ppm
RUTIN Fruit Leaf 24,000 ppm
RUTINOSIDE Fruit
S-METHYL-METHIONINE Fruit 16–35 ppm
SALICYLALDEHYDE Fruit
SELENIUM Fruit 0.001–0.034 ppm
SERINE Fruit 57–3,967 ppm
SILICON Fruit
SILVER Fruit 1.4 ppm
SODIUM Fruit 10–6,600 ppm
SOLADULCIDINE Shoot
SOLANINE Fruit
SQUALENE Fruit
STARCH Fruit 120–10,000 ppm
STEARIC-ACID Fruit 80–1,322 ppm
STIGMASTEROL Fruit
STRONTIUM Fruit 140 ppm
SUCCINIC-ACID Fruit
SUCROSE Fruit
SUGARS Fruit 15,000–45,000 ppm
SULFOQUINOVOSYL-DIACYL-GLYCEROL Leaf
SULFUR Fruit 107–2,330 ppm
SYRINGALDEHYDE Plant
TARTARIC-ACID Fruit
TETRA-DECA-CIS-6-ENE-1,3-DIYNE-5,8-DIOL Stem
THIAMIN Fruit 1–10 ppm
THREONINE Fruit 65–3,637 ppm
TITANIUM Fruit 140 ppm
TOMATIDA-3,5-DIENE Shoot

TOMATIDINE Plant
TOMATINE Flower Leaf 6–8 ppm
TOMATOSIDE-A Seed
TRANS-ACONITIC-ACID Fruit
TRANS-METHYL-6-HEPTADIENE-3,5-ON-2
  Plant
TRIACONTANE Fruit
TRICODECAN-3-ONE Leaf
TRIDECAN-2-ONE Leaf
TRIDECAN-3-ONE Leaf
TRIGONELLINE Root 69 ppm
TRIMETHYL-2,6,6-HYDROXY-2-CYCLOHEXA-
  NONE Fruit
TRYPTAMINE Fruit
TRYPTOPHAN Fruit 1–1,157 ppm
TYRAMINE Fruit
TYROSINE Fruit 38–2,479 ppm
UBIQUINONE-10 Tissue Culture 60 ppm
VALINE Fruit 1–3,801 ppm
VANADIUM Fruit 6 ppm
VANILLIN Plant
VIOLAXANTHIN Fruit
VIT-B-6 Fruit 9 ppm
WATER Fruit 910,000–982,000 ppm
XANTHOPHYLL Fruit
YTTRIUM Fruit 6 ppm
ZEATIN Fruit
ZEATIN-GLUCOSIDE Flower
ZEATIN-RIBOSIDE Flower
ZEAXANTHIN Fruit
ZETA-CAROTENE Fruit
ZINC Fruit 1–120 ppm
ZIRCONIUM Fruit 4 ppm

TURNIP

Chemicals in *Brassica rapa var. rapa* (*Brassicaceae*)—Turnip

(+)-CYSTEINE Root
(+)-S-METHYL-L-CYSTEINE-SULFOXIDE Root
4ALPHA,7ALPHA,24-TRIMETHYL-5ALPHA-
  CHOLESTA-8,24-DIEN-3BETA-OL Plant
ALANINE Root 350–4,305 ppm
ALLANTOIC-ACID Root
ALLANTOIN Root
ALUMINUM Root 2–10 ppm
ARGININE Root 240–2,950 ppm
ARSENIC Root

ASCORBIC-ACID Root 210–2,580 ppm
ASH Root 7,000–86,000 ppm
ASPARTIC-ACID Root 630–7,750 ppm
BETA-CAROTENE Root
BORON Root 2–20 ppm
BRASSICASTEROL Plant
BROMINE Root
CADMIUM Root 0.01–0.1 ppm
CALCIUM Root 300–3,690 ppm
CAMPESTEROL Plant
CARBOHYDRATES Root 62,300–766,290 ppm
CHROMIUM Root 0.005–0.05 ppm
COBALT Root
COPPER Root 0.4–4 ppm
CYSTINE Root 50–615 ppm
FAT Root 1,000–12,300 ppm
FIBER Root 9,000–110,700 ppm
FLUORINE Root
FOLACIN Root 0.14–2 ppm
GLUTAMIC-ACID Root 1,300–15,990 ppm
GLYCINE Root 250–3,075 ppm
HISTIDINE Root 140–1,720 ppm
IRON Root 2–37 ppm
ISOLEUCINE Root 360–4,425 ppm
KILOCALORIES Root 270–3,321 /kg
LEAD Root 0.02–0.2 ppm
LEUCINE Root 330–4,060 ppm
LINOLEIC-ACID Root 120–1,475 ppm
LINOLENIC-ACID Root 400–4,920 ppm
LYCOPENE Root
LYSINE Root 360–4,425 ppm
MAGNESIUM Root 110–2,000 ppm
MANGANESE Root 0.6–7 ppm
MERCURY Root 0.001–0.01 ppm
METHIONINE Root 110–1,350 ppm
MOLYBDENUM Root 0.1–1 ppm
MUFA Root 60–740 ppm
NIACIN Root 4–49 ppm
NICKEL Root 0.01–0.1 ppm
NITROGEN Root 1,800–18,000 ppm
OLEIC-ACID Root 60–740 ppm
PALMITIC-ACID Root 100–1,230 ppm
PALMITOLEIC-ACID Root 10–120 ppm
PANTOTHENIC-ACID Root 2–25 ppm
PHENYLALANINE Root 170–2,090 ppm
PHOSPHORUS Root 270–5,000 ppm
POTASSIUM Root 1,700–30,000 ppm
PROTEIN Root 9,000–110,700 ppm

PUFA Root 530–6,520 ppm

RAPIN Root

RIBOFLAVIN Root 0.3–4 ppm

RUBIDIUM Root 1–10 ppm

SELENIUM Root

SERINE Root 290–3,565 ppm

SFA Root 110–1,350 ppm

SILICON Root 120–1,200 ppm

SODIUM Root 400–11,600 ppm

STEARIC-ACID Root 10–120 ppm

SULFUR Root 510–5,100 ppm

THIAMIN Root 0.4–5 ppm

THREONINE Root 250–3,075 ppm

TRYPTOPHAN Root 90–1,100 ppm

TYROSINE Root 130–1,600 ppm

VALINE Root 300–3,690 ppm

VIT-B-6 Root 1–11 ppm

WATER Root 900,000–921,120 ppm

ZINC Root 2–23 ppm

WATER CHESTNUT

Chemicals in *Eleocharis dulcis* (*BURM. F*)
TRIN. (*Cyperaceae*)—Water chestnut

ASCORBIC-ACID Tuber 40–317 ppm

ASH Tuber 11,000–60,000 ppm

BETA-CAROTENE Tuber

CALCIUM Tuber 40–265 ppm

CARBOHYDRATES Tuber 161,000–876,000 ppm

FAT Tuber 2,000–16,000 ppm

FIBER Tuber 6,000–39,000 ppm

IRON Tuber 6–37 ppm

KILOCALORIES Tuber 680–3,640 /kg

NIACIN Tuber 10–53 ppm

PHOSPHORUS Tuber 650–4,075 ppm

POTASSIUM Tuber 4,810–25,450 ppm

PROTEIN Tuber 14,000–85,000 ppm

PUCHIIN Tuber

RIBOFLAVIN Tuber 0.2–9 ppm

SODIUM Tuber 100–920 ppm

STARCH Tuber 70,000–400,000 ppm

SUCROSE Tuber 63,500–317,500 ppm

THIAMIN Tuber 0.3–6 ppm

WATER Tuber 773,000–811,000 ppm

WATERCRESS

Chemicals in *Nasturtium officinale R. BR.*
(*Brassicaceae*)—Berro, Watercress

ALANINE Herb 1,370–27,400 ppm

ARGININE Herb 1,500–30,000 ppm

ASCORBIC-ACID Herb 430–13,690 ppm

ASH Herb 13,000–179,000 ppm

ASPARTIC-ACID Herb 1,870–37,400 ppm

BETA-CAROTENE Herb 28–560 ppm

BIOTIN Plant

CALCIUM Herb 1,200–24,000 ppm

CARBOHYDRATES Herb 12,900–25,800 ppm

COPPER Plant

CYSTINE Herb 70–1,400 ppm

DIASTASE Plant

EO Plant 600–660 ppm

FAT Herb 1,000–20,000 ppm

FIBER Herb 700–77,670 ppm

FOLACIN Plant

GLUCONASTURTIN Plant

GLUTAMIC-ACID Herb 1,900–38,000 ppm

GLYCINE Herb 1,120–22,400 ppm

HISTIDINE Herb 400–8,000 ppm

IRON Herb 2–262 ppm

ISOLEUCINE Herb 530–10,600 ppm

KILOCALORIES Herb 300–2,915 /kg

LEUCINE Herb 1,660–33,200 ppm

LYSINE Herb 1,340–26,800 ppm

MAGNESIUM Herb 210–4,200 ppm

MANGANESE Plant

METHIONINE Herb 200–4,000 ppm

NIACIN Herb 2–113 ppm

PANTOTHENIC-ACID Plant 3–62 ppm

PHENYLALANINE Herb 1,140–22,800 ppm

PHENYLETHYL-ISOTHIOCYANATE Plant

PHOSPHORUS Herb 600–12,000 ppm

POTASSIUM Herb 3,300–66,000 ppm

PROLINE Herb 960–19,200 ppm

PROTEIN Herb 23,000–460,000 ppm

RIBOFLAVIN Herb 1–25 ppm

SERINE Herb 600–12,000 ppm

SODIUM Herb 410–8,200 ppm

THIAMIN Herb 1–18 ppm

THREONINE Herb 1,330–26,600 ppm

TRYPTOPHAN Herb 300–6,000 ppm

TYROSINE Herb 630–12,600 ppm

VALINE Herb 1,370–27,400 ppm
VIT-B-6 Herb 1–26 ppm
WATER Herb 897,000–951,000 ppm
ZINC Plant

WHEATGRASS

Chemicals in *Elytrigia repens* (*L.*) *DESV. EX NEVSKI* (*Poaceae*)—Couchgrass, Doggrass, Quackgrass, Twitchgrass, Wheatgrass

AGROPYRENE Rhizome 494 ppm
ALUMINUM Plant 331 ppm
ASH Plant 61,000–78,000 ppm
BETA-ALANINE Rhizome
CALCIUM Plant 3,000–9,280 ppm
CARBOHYDRATES Plant 772,000–797,000 ppm
CHROMIUM Plant 37 ppm
COBALT Plant 18 ppm
EO Rhizome 500–520 ppm
FAT Plant 28,000–38,000 ppm Rhizome 15,000 ppm Seed 18,000–121,000 ppm
FIBER Plant 317,000–339,000 ppm
INFUSION Plant
INOSITOL Rhizome 10,000–15,000 ppm
IRON Plant 311 ppm
MAGNESIUM Plant 7,570 ppm
MALIC-ACID Rhizome
MANGANESE Plant 188 ppm
MANNITOL Rhizome 10,000–15,000 ppm
MUCILAGE Rhizome 110,000 ppm
PHOSPHORUS Plant 2,800–9,510 ppm
POTASSIUM Plant 9,780 ppm
PROTEIN Plant 106,000–112,000 ppm Seed 168,000–212,000 ppm
SAPONIN Rhizome
SELENIUM Plant
SILICON Plant 253 ppm
SODIUM Plant
TIN Plant 67 ppm
TRITICIN Rhizome 50,000–80,000 ppm
VANILLIN Rhizome
VANILLIN-GLYCOSIDE Rhizome
WATER Plant 789,000 ppm
ZINC Plant

YARROW

Chemicals in *Achillea millefolium L.* (*Asteraceae*)—Yarrow

1,8-CINEOLE Leaf 24–960 ppm
2,3-DIHYDROACETOXYMATRICIN Plant
5-HYDROXY-3,6,7,4'-TETRAM-ETHOXYFLAVONE Plant
8-ACETOCYARTABSIN Plant
8-ANELOOXYARTABSIN Plant
ACETYLBALCHANOLIDE Plant
ACHICEINE Plant
ACHILLEINE Plant
ACHILLETINE Plant
ACHILLICIN Plant
ACHILLIN Plant
ACONITIC-ACID Plant
ALLO-OCIMENE Leaf 4–140 ppm
ALPHA-PINENE Leaf 25–1,000 ppm
ALPHA-TERPINENE Leaf 3–130 ppm
ALPHA-THUJONE Plant
ALUMINUM Plant 34 ppm
APIGENIN Plant
APIGENIN-GLUCOSIDE Plant
ARABINOSE Plant
ARTEMITIN Plant
ASCORBIC-ACID Leaf 580–3,100 ppm
ASH Plant 100,000–125,000 ppm
ASPARAGINE Plant
AUSTRICIN Plant
AZULENE Leaf 7,140 ppm
BALCHANOLIDE Plant
BENZALDEHYDECYANHYDRINGLYCOSIDE Plant
BETA-CAROTENE Plant
BETA-PINENE Leaf 18–720 ppm
BETA-SITOSTEROL Plant
BETA-SITOSTEROL-ACETATE Plant
BETAINE Plant
BETONICINE Plant
BORNEOL Leaf 6–275 ppm
BORNYL-ACETATE Plant
BUTYRIC-ACID Plant
CAFFEIC-ACID Plant
CALCIUM Plant 8,670 ppm
CAMPHENE Leaf 15–600 ppm
CAMPHOR Leaf 45–1,780 ppm

CARBOHYDRATES Plant 713,000–752,000 ppm
CARYOPHYLLENE Leaf 4–160 ppm
CASTICIN Plant
CEROTINIC-ACID Plant
CHAMAZULENE Plant 50–2,800 ppm
CHAMAZULENE-CARBOXYLIC-ACID Plant
CHOLINE Plant
CHROMIUM Plant 25 ppm
CINEOLE Plant
CIS-DEHYDROMATRICARIA-ESTER Leaf
COBALT Plant 31 ppm
COPAENE Leaf 1.5–60 ppm
COUMARINS Plant
CUMINALDEHYDE Leaf 0.3–11 ppm
DEACETYLMATRICARIN Plant
DELTA-CADINENE Leaf 0.2–8 ppm
DULCITOL Plant
EO Flower 700–5,000 ppm Leaf 250–14,000 ppm
EUGENOL Plant
FARNESENE Plant
FAT Plant 18,000–40,000 ppm Seed 223,000–334,000 ppm
FIBER Plant 69,000–201,000 ppm
FOLACIN Plant
FORMIC-ACID Plant
FURFURAL Plant
FURFURYL-ALCOHOL Plant
GALACTOSE Plant
GAMMA-TERPINENE Leaf 9–370 ppm
GLUCOSE Plant
GUAIAZULENE Plant
HEPTADECANE Plant
HOMOSTACHYDRINE Plant
HUMULENE Leaf 0.5–22 ppm
HYDROXYACHILLIN Plant
INOSITOL Plant
INULIN Plant
IRON Plant
ISOARTEMISIA-KETONE Plant
ISOBUTYL-ACETATE Plant
ISORHAMNETIN Plant
ISOVALERIC-ACID Plant
KILOCALORIES Plant 2,900 /kg
LEUCODIN Plant
LIMONENE Leaf 4–170 ppm
LUTEOLIN Plant
LUTEOLIN-7-GLUCOSIDE Plant

MAGNESIUM Plant 1,920 ppm
MANGANESE Plant 50 ppm
MANNITOL Plant
MENTHOL Plant
MILLEFIN Plant
MILLEFOLIDE Plant
MOSCHATINE Plant
MYRCENE Leaf 0.5–20 ppm
MYRISTIC-ACID Plant
NIACIN Plant
OLEIC-ACID Plant
P-CYMENE Leaf 9–370 ppm
PALMITIC-ACID Plant
PENTACOSANE Plant
PHOSPHORUS Plant 2,950 ppm
PONTICAEPOXIDE Plant
POTASSIUM Plant 17,800 ppm
PROAZULENE Plant
PROTEIN Plant 108,000–144,000 ppm Seed 286,000–369,000 ppm
QUERCETIN Plant
QUERCETIN-GLYCOSIDE Plant
QUERCITRIN Plant
RESIN Plant 6,000 ppm
RIBOFLAVIN Plant 5–6 ppm
RUTIN Plant
SABINENE Leaf 30–1,225 ppm
SALICYLIC-ACID Plant
SELENIUM Plant
SILICON Plant 45 ppm
SODIUM Plant 82 ppm
STACHYDRINE Plant
STIGMASTEROL Plant
SUCCINIC-ACID Plant
TANNIN Plant 28,000 ppm
TERPINEN-4-OL Leaf 10–430 ppm
TERPINEOL Plant
THIAMIN Plant
THIOPHENES Flower 167 ppm Leaf 167 ppm
THUJONE Plant
TIN Plant 26 ppm
TRANS-DEHYDROMATRICARIA-ESTER Leaf
TRICOSANE Plant
TRICYCLENE Leaf 0.6–27 ppm
TRIGONELLINE Plant
VIBURNITOL Plant
WATER Plant 823,000 ppm
ZINC Plant

Appendix D

Scientific Article Abstracts

Throughout this book you've learned about the happy coincidence that foods that help you lose weight—such as vegetables, fruits, and whole grains—tend to be the foods that are better for you healthwise and longevity-wise. You've also learned that, conversely, the more fattening foods—such as meat and dairy products—are the less healthful dietary choices. If you make the dietary choices I've recommended and combine that with an aerobics-based exercise program, you'll have no problem seeing the pounds come off. You'll also feel more energized.

The problem is that you may not initially perceive the long-term health benefits of these choices because long term, by definition, involves waiting decades, and society is still filled with inaccurate and misleading information about our food choices. This appendix attempts to set the record straight once and for all. The idea is that if you can get the facts—not from me this time, but from the latest unversity and medical school research—your motivation to continue making weight-busting and health-boosting dietary choices will be reinforced.

Here I review the current peer-reviewed scientific literature on many of the dietary choices discussed in this book and evaluate the evidence for or against inclusion of these items in any given diet. The information here comes directly from prestigious "establishment" medical and scientific journals; all I've done is summarize the article abstracts in lay language so that readers without scientific training can understand the conclusions easily. I've looked at high-protein diets, meat, milk, saturated fat, alcohol, dietary-disease connections, and vegetarian diets. Other subjects of interest include pesticides, exercise, and fiber. The nearly one thousand articles summarized here represent only a small sampling of what could have been included; this section could have been expanded tenfold. But I hope this will be enough to get you to understand that the advice given in this book, "alternative" as it may sound, is actually

600

based on hard, mainstream-derived, scientific evidence. And if you like, you can read more about each of these topics on your own.

Here's a scenario I envision. When you're starting to make beneficial dietary changes, many times other people will try to get you off course by saying things like "You know, you really should use a high-protein diet to lose weight," or "Don't give up meat; it's good for you." These people aren't trying to sabotage your plans; they're just misinformed. But with this appendix, *you're* informed. I envision you countering critics by saying "I'm not going the high-protein route because research shows that it's bad for the kidneys and can increase the risk of osteoporosis," or "A meatless diet reduces breast cancer rates, and that's important to me." You also can counter any self-doubt you may have about eating in a new way that may, admittedly, feel strange at first.

By the way, sometimes doctors or others will say "You can eat anything you want, as long as you eat it in a moderate amount." As you know by now, I don't subscribe to this view. If something is toxic, it is still toxic in a moderate amount. It may take awhile for that substance to make you sick, but why risk it? Besides, how many other toxic things are you consuming in "moderate amounts" beyond that one item? That's an important question, because the health-destroying effects of these various items are going to build up without your being aware of it. Remember that we swim in a proverbial sea of 100,000 man-made chemicals, many of dubious effect, and many of which we can do nothing about. As I see it, the purer we can keep our diets, which we *can* do something about, the better.

You may want to skim through this section, read it in depth, or read parts that pique your interest. Think of it, along with your stove, pots, pans, and juicer, as something that will get you further on your way to producing healthful, slimming meals and shedding those unwanted pounds.

OBESITY STATISTICS TODAY

"Increasing Pediatric Obesity in the United States"

Gortmaker SL; Dietz WH Jr; Sobol AM; Wehler CA
Am J Dis Child 1987 May; 141(5):535–40
This study shows that in the four-year period from 1976 to 1980, the prevalence of obesity, compared to data from 1963 through 1965, increased by 45 percent in children six to eleven years old and by 39 percent in children twelve to seventeen years old. In the same time period, the prevalence of superobesity increased by 98 percent in children six to eleven years old and by 64 percent in children twelve to seventeen years old.

"Prevalence of Overweight among Preschool Children in the United States, 1971 through 1994"

Ogden CL; Troiano RP; Briefel RR; Kuczmarski RJ; Flegal KM; Johnson CL
Pediatrics 1997 Apr; 99(4):E1

This article shows that in the period from 1988 through 1994, more than 10 percent of four- and five-year-old girls were overweight. In the period from 1971 through 1974, 5.8 percent of girls of the same age were overweight.

"Overweight School Children in New York City: Prevalence Estimates and Characteristics"

Melnik TA; Rhoades SJ; Wales KR; Cowell C; Wolfe WS

Int J Obes Relat Metab Disord 1998 Jan; 22(1):7–13

This study shows that, in a sample of children from New York City schools, 37.5 percent of second-grade children and about a third of fifth-grade children were overweight based on the 85th percentile of body index mass, whereas almost 20 percent of them were overweight based on the 95th percentile of body index mass.

"Obesity as a Chronic Disease: Modern Medical and Lifestyle Management"

Rippe JM; Crossley S; Ringer R

J Am Diet Assoc 1998 Oct; 98(10 Suppl 2):S9–15

This article shows that the prevalence of obesity in the United States has increased by 40 percent between 1980 and 1990, affecting more than one third of the adult population. It also emphasizes that obesity is associated with coronary heart disease, type 2 diabetes, hypertension, and dyslipidemia.

"Long-term Morbidity and Mortality of Overweight Adolescents. A Follow-up of the Harvard Growth Study of 1922 to 1935"

Must A; Jacques PF; Dallal GE; Bajema CJ; Dietz WH

N Engl J Med 1992 Nov 5; 327(19):1350–55

This study shows that overweight adolescent males have an 80 percent increased risk of mortality from all causes and an over twofold increased risk of mortality from coronary heart disease. Overweight in adolescence was also positively associated with increased morbidity from coronary heart disease and atherosclerosis in men and women, and with increased risk of colorectal cancer and gout in men and of arthritis in women.

"Divergent Trends in Obesity and Fat Intake Patterns: The American Paradox"

Heini AF; Weinsier RL

Am J Med 1997 Mar; 102(3):259–64

This article shows that in 1991, 33.3 percent of the U.S. population was estimated to be overweight, a 31 percent increase compared to 1980. At the same time, consumption of fat and of total calories decreased, and the percentage of people eating low-fat products increased from 19 percent of the population in 1978 to 76 percent in 1991.

"The 25–year Health Care Costs of Women Who Remain Overweight after 40 Years of Age"

Gorsky RD; Pamuk E; Williamson DF; Shaffer PA; Koplan JP

Am J Prev Med 1996 Sep-Oct; 12(5):388–94

This study estimates that, over twenty-five years, the treatment of conditions in middle-age women associated with overweight cost $16 billion.

"Overweight and Chronic Illness—A Retrospective Cohort Study, with a Follow-up of 6–17 Years, in Men and Women of Initially 20–50 Years of Age"
Seidell JC; Bakx KC; Deurenberg P; van den Hoogen HJ; Hautvast JG; Stijnen T
J Chronic Dis 1986; 39(8):585–93

This study shows that the incidence of diabetes, gout, arteriosclerotic disease, and arthrosis in men and women, and of varicose veins in women, is higher in overweight individuals.

"Adolescent Overweight Is Associated with Adult Overweight and Related Multiple Cardiovascular Risk Factors: The Bogalusa Heart Study"
Srinivasan SR; Bao W; Wattigney WA; Berenson GS
Metabolism 1996 Feb; 45(2):235–40

This study shows that 52 percent of overweight adolescent black males and 62 percent of females are at risk of remaining overweight as adults. Overweight individuals have 8.5 and 3 to 8 times higher risk of hypertension and dyslipidemia compared to lean controls.

"Body Weight and Mortality: A Prospective Evaluation in a Cohort of Middle-aged Men in Shanghai, China"
Yuan JM; Ross RK; Gao YT; Yu MC
Int J Epidemiol 1998 Oct; 27(5):824–32

This study, performed on a cohort of 18,244 Chinese men aged forty-five to sixty-four years, shows that overweight nonsmokers individuals have a twofold excess risk of death from cardiovascular and cerebrovascular diseases compared to lean controls.

"Predictors of Overweight and Overfatness in a Multiethnic Pediatric Population. Child and Adolescent Trial for Cardiovascular Health Collaborative Research Group"
Dwyer JT; Stone EJ; Yang M; Feldman H; Webber LS; Must A; Perry CL; Nader PR; Parcel GS
Am J Clin Nutr 1998 Apr; 67(4):602–10

This study shows that overweight children have significantly higher plasma levels of total blood cholesterol, lower HDL cholesterol, and lower running performances compared to lean controls, and are at higher risk of cardiovascular disease.

THE BENEFITS OF EXERCISE

"Dietary and Lifestyle Determinants of Mortality among German Vegetarians"
Chang-Claude J; Frentzel-Beyme R
Int J Epidemiol 1993 Apr; 22(2):228–36

This study found that, in a cohort of 1,904 vegetarians, those who reported a medium or high level of physical activity had only half the total mortality of those who reported low level of exercise. Reduction risk was also associated with duration of vegetarianism and vegetarian status (strict versus moderate).

"Effect of Diet and Moderate Exercise on Central Obesity and Associated Disturbances, Myocardial Infarction and Mortality in Patients with and without Coronary Artery Disease"

Singh RB; Rastogi V; Rastogi SS; Niaz MA; Beegom R
J Am Coll Nutr 1996 Dec; 15(6):592–601

In this study, performed on a sample population of 463 patients with coronary artery disease or risk factors, 231 patients were advised to follow a low-fat diet rich in fruits, vegetables, and legumes, and perform moderate physical activity (group A), while 232 patients were advised to follow a low-fat diet only (group B). Abdominal obesity decreased by 6.2 percent in group A versus 1.2 percent in group B; 29 patients experienced cardiac events in group A versus 43 in group B; 16 patients died in group A versus 24 in group B. Within group A, patients with better adherence to the program experienced even greater reduction of abdominal obesity and lower morbidity and mortality rates.

"Physical Activity and 10-year Mortality from Cardiovascular Diseases and All Causes: The Zutphen Elderly Study"

Bijnen FC; Caspersen CJ; Feskens EJ; Saris WH; Mosterd WL; Kromhout D
Arch Intern Med 1998 Jul 27; 158(14):1499–505

This study, conducted on a population of 802 Dutch men sixty-four to eighty-four years of age, shows that physical activity like walking or biking performed at least three times per week for twenty minutes reduced mortality from cardiovascular disease by 31 percent and total mortality by 29 percent.

"Lifelong Exposures and the Potential for Stroke Prevention: The Contribution of Cigarette Smoking, Exercise, and Body Fat"

Shinton R
J Epidemiol Community Health 1997 Apr; 51(2):138–43

This study, performed on a sample population of 125 individuals with history of stroke and 188 matched controls, estimates that 49 percent of the strokes were caused by cigarette smoking, while the combination of cigarette smoking, lack of physical exercise, and obesity was estimated to have caused 80 percent of the strokes in this population.

"Comparison of 2-year Weight Loss Trends in Behavioral Treatments of Obesity: Diet, Exercise, and Combination Interventions"

Skender ML; Goodrick GK; Del Junco DJ; Reeves RS; Darnell L; Gotto AM; Foreyt JP
J Am Diet Assoc 1996 Apr; 96(4):342–46

In this study 127 individuals were randomly counseled to follow one of three weight-loss approaches: diet only, exercise only, or a combination of diet and exercise. After one year, the most weight loss was noted in the combination group, while the exercise-only group had the least weight loss. After two years, the diet-only group regained weight above baseline, while the exercise-only group retained the most weight loss, followed by the combination group.

"A Meta-Analysis of the Past 25 Years of Weight Loss Research Using Diet, Exercise or Diet Plus Exercise Intervention"

Miller WC; Koceja DM; Hamilton EJ

Int J Obes Relat Metab Disord 1997 Oct; 21(10):941–47

This study reviews all the literature published in peer-reviewed journals on weight loss through diet, exercise, or diet plus exercise, and concluded that the most effective approach to maintain the weight loss is through a combination of nutritional changes and physical activity.

"Physical Activity and Physical Fitness in African-American girls with and without Obesity"

Ward DS; Trost SG; Felton G; Saunders R; Parsons MA; Dowda M; Pate RR

Obes Res 1997 Nov; 5(6):572–75

This study, performed on a sample population of 150 African American girls, 54 of whom were obese and 96 of whom were lean, shows that moderate and vigorous exercise was inversely related to body mass index and was performed significantly more by the girls in the lean group, thus suggesting that lack of physical activity is a contributing factor to obesity.

"The Role of Physical Activity in the Prevention and Management of Obesity"

Rippe JM; Hess S

J Am Diet Assoc 1998 Oct; 98(10 Suppl 2):S31–38

This review presents the studies showing that a combination of physical activity and proper nutrition is the most effective way to induce and maintain weight loss. Physical activity increases energy expenditure and resting metabolic rate and is beneficial to health even when it is not associated with weight loss.

"Preliminary Results of Triple Therapy for Obesity"

Huang MH; Yang RC; Hu SH

Int J Obes Relat Metab Disord 1996 Sep; 20(9):830–36

In this study, forty-five individuals with simple obesity entered an eight-week weight-loss program consisting of acupuncture, diet, and aerobic exercise. This approach resulted in 87 percent rate of effectiveness with a 4.4 +/-2.9 kg reduction in body weight and a 5.6 +/-3.0 percent reduction in body fat. At one year follow-up, weight rebound of more than 1.5 kg occurred in 19 percent of the individuals. There was a direct correlation between frequency of aerobic exercise and weight loss and maintenance.

"Effect of Exercise Training on Long-term Weight Maintenance in Weight-reduced Men"

Pasman WJ; Saris WH; Muls E; Vansant G; Westerterp-Plantenga MS

Metabolism 1999 Jan; 48(1):15–21

In this study two groups of obese individuals underwent a four-month program consisting of diet and exercise. At the end of the program one group interrupted physical activity while the other maintained it. Follow-up at sixteen months showed that body-weight regain was similar in both groups while fat-mass regain was significantly lower in the trained group.

"The Relation of Physical Activity to Risk for Symptomatic Gallstone Disease in Men"
Leitzmann MF; Giovannucci EL; Rimm EB; Stampfer MJ; Spiegelman D; Wing AL; Willett WC
Ann Intern Med 1998 Mar 15; 128(6):417–25

This study, performed on a cohort of 45,813 U.S. men, shows that those aged forty to sixty-four in the highest versus the lowest quintile of physical activity had a 42 percent lower risk of symptomatic gallstone disease. For men sixty-five years or older in the highest versus the lowest quintile of exercise, the risk decreased by 25 percent. It was estimated that thirty minutes of endurance training five times per week would prevent 34 percent of symptomatic gallstone disease in this population.

"Randomised Comparison of Diets for Maintaining Obese Subjects' Weight after Major Weight Loss: Ad Lib, Low Fat, High Carbohydrate Diet vs. Fixed Energy Intake"
Toubro S; Astrup A
BMJ 1997 Jan 4; 314(7073):29–34

In this study, forty-three patients, after a period of slow or rapid weight loss, were randomized to a one-year program of ad lib diet or fixed energy intake diet. At the end of the study period, the group on a fixed energy diet regained more than twice as much weight as the ad lib group, while weight loss of more than 5 kg was kept in 40 percent of the energy intake group and in 65 percent of the ad lib group.

THE BENEFITS OF CERTAIN FATS

"Polyunsaturated Fats Enhance Peripheral Glucose Utilization in Rats"
Lardinois CK; Starich GH
J Am Coll Nutr 1991 Aug; 10(4):340–45

This study shows that rats consuming a diet rich in polyunsaturated fatty acids (PUFA) from fish sources have significantly lower plasma insulin concentration, and therefore likely better peripheral glucose utilization, compared to rats fed a diet rich in saturated fatty acids from cocoa butter or monounsaturated fatty acid from olive oil.

"Ectopic Calcification of Rat Aortas and Kidneys Is Reduced with n-3 Fatty Acid Supplementation"
Schlemmer CK; Coetzer H; Claassen N; Kruger MC; Rademeyer C; van Jaarsveld L; Smuts CM

Prostaglandins Leukot Essent Fatty Acids 1998 Sep; 59(3):221–27

This study shows that the calcium glubionate–experimentally induced calcification of the aorta and kidneys is reduced in rats fed a diet supplementation with essential fatty acids toward values similar to those found in saline-injected controls.

"Dietary Factors Determining Diabetes and Impared Glucose Tolerance. A 20-year Follow-up of the Finnish and Dutch Cohorts of the Seven Countries Study"

Feskens EJ; Virtanen SM; Rasanen L; Tuomilehto J; Stengard J; Pekkanen J; Nissinen A; Kromhout D

Diabetes Care 1995 Aug; 18(8):1104–12

This study shows that consumption of saturated fatty acids is associated with a higher risk of glucose intolerance and diabetes. On the other hand, intake of vitamin C, vegetables, legumes, fish, and potatoes was found to have a protective effect.

"Effects of High-Carbohydrate or High-Fat Diet on Carbohydrate Metabolism and Insulin Secretion in the Normal Rat"

Ramirez R; Lopez JM; Bedoya FJ; Goberna R

Diabetes Res 1990 Dec; 15(4):179–83

This study shows that rats fed a high fat/protein diet gained more weight and developed marked glucose intolerance, compared to rats on a high-glucose diet.

"Dietary n-3 PUFA Increases the Apoptotic Response to 1,2-dimethylhydrazine, Reduces Mitosis and Suppresses the Induction of Carcinogenesis in the Rat Colon"

Latham P; Lund EK; Johnson IT

Carcinogenesis 1999 Apr; 20(4):645–50

In this study, rats fed a diet rich in fish oil had significantly lower carcinogen-induced aberrant crypt foci in their distal colon compared to rats fed a diet rich in corn oil.

"Effects of Dietary Gamma-Linolenic Acid on Blood Pressure and Adrenal Angiotensin Receptors in Hypertensive Rats"

Engler MM; Schambelan M; Engler MB; Ball DL; Goodfriend TL

Proc Soc Exp Biol Med 1998 Jul; 218(3):234–37

This study shows that dietary gamma-linolenic acid from borage oil lowers the systolic blood pressure in spontaneously hypertensive rats.

"Modulation of Eosinophil Chemotactic Activities to Leukotriene B4 by n-3 Polyunsaturated Fatty Acids"

Kikuchi S; Sakamoto T; Ishikawa C; Yazawa K; Torii S

Prostaglandins Leukot Essent Fatty Acids 1998 Mar; 58(3):243–48

This study shows that rats supplemented with docosahexaenoic acid (DHA) and eicosapentaenoic acid (EPA) exhibited a dose-dependent reduction in the accumulation of eosinophils, likely to reduce the manifestations of allergic disease.

"The Incorporation of Dietary n-3 Polyunsaturated Fatty Acids into Porcine Platelet Phospholipids and Their Effects on Platelet Thromboxane A2 Release"

Murray MJ; Zhang T

Prostaglandins Leukot Essent Fatty Acids 1997 Mar; 56(3):223–28

This study demonstrates that pigs preferred a diet enriched with fish oil or with a combination of fish oil and borage oil, showed a significantly reduced production of thromboxane A2 after platelet stimulation, compared to pigs fed a corn oil enriched diet.

"Supplementation with Flaxseed Oil Versus Sunflowerseed Oil in Healthy Young Men Consuming a Low Fat Diet: Effects on Platelet Composition and Function"

Allman MA; Pena MM; Pang D

Eur J Clin Nutr 1995 Mar; 49(3):169–78

This study shows that individuals receiving a diet supplemented with flaxseed oil showed a decrease in the response of platelet aggregation compared to individuals whose diet was supplemented with sunflower seed oil.

"Effects of Four Doses of n-3 Fatty Acids Given to Hyperlipidemic Patients for Six Months"

Harris WS; Windsor SL; Dujovne CA

J Am Coll Nutr 1991 Jun; 10(3):220–27

This study shows that supplementation with fish oil significantly lowers the triglyceride serum levels of hyperlipidemic patients.

"Effects of Fatty Acids and Eicosanoid Synthesis Inhibitors on the Growth of Two Human Prostate Cancer Cell Lines"

Rose DP; Connolly JM

Prostate 1991 May; 18(3):243–54

This study shows that the in vitro growth of the prostate cancer cell line PC3 is inhibited by 65 percent when docosahexaenoic acid and eicosapentaenoic acid, two omega-3 fatty acids present in fish oils, are added to the culture.

"Dietary Intake of Alpha-Linolenic Acid and Rick of Fatal Ischemic Heart Disease among Women"

Hu FB; Stampfer MJ; Manson JE; Rimm EB; Wolk A; Colditz GA; Hennekens CH; Willett WC

Am J Clin Nutr 1999 May; 69 (5):890–97

This study, performed on a group of 76,283 women without history of cancer or cardiovascular disease, shows that those with the highest versus the lowest intake of alpha-linolenic acid, a polyunsaturated fat, had a 45 percent reduction in the risk of fatal ischemic heart disease.

"Fat Intake and Fatty Acid Profile in Plasma Phospholipids and Adipose Tissue in Patients with Crohn's Disease, Compared with Controls"

Geerling BJ; v Houwelingen AC; Badart-Smook A; Stockbrugger RW; Brummer RJ
Am J Gastroenterol 1999 Feb; 94(2):410–17

This study shows that patients with Crohn's disease have a significantly lower percentage of total n-3 fatty acid content in the plasma phospholipids and adipose tissue compared to controls. Since fatty acids participate in the immune and inflammatory responses of Crohn's disease, these findings may be relevant to the course of the disease.

"Omega-3 Fatty Acids in Adipose Tissue and Risk of Myocardial Infarction: The EURAMIC Study"

Guallar E; Aro A; Jimenez FJ; Martin-Moreno JM; Salminen I; van't Veer P; Kardinaal AF; Gomez-Aracena J; Martin BC; Kohlmeier L; Kark JD; Mazaev VP; Ringstad J; Guillen J; Riemersma RA; Huttunen JK; Thamm M; Kok FJ
Arterioscler Thromb Vasc Biol 1999 Apr; 19(4):1111–18

This study, performed on a sample of 639 patients with occurrence of myocardial infarction and 700 controls, found that individuals with the highest versus the lowest quintile of alpha-linolenic acid intake had a 32 percent reduction in risk of myocardial infarction.

"Fish Consumption and Risk of Sudden Cardiac Death"

Albert CM; Hennekens CH; O'Donnell CJ; Ajani UA; Carey VJ; Willett WC; Ruskin JN; Manson JE
JAMA 1998 Jan 7; 279(1):23–28

This study, performed on a cohort of 20,551 U.S. male physicians, found that those consuming fish at least once per week had a 52 percent decreased risk of sudden death, compared to those with a fish intake of less than monthly.

"The Effect of Dietary Omega-3 Fatty Acids on Coronary Atherosclerosis. A Randomized, Double-Blind, Placebo-Controlled Trial"

von Schacky C; Angerer P; Kothny W; Theisen K; Mudra H
Ann Intern Med 1999 Apr 6; 130(7):554–62

This study shows that daily consumption of fish oil concentrates mitigates the course of coronary artery atherosclerosis and reduces the number of cardiovascular events in patients with documented coronary artery disease.

"Antithrombotic Effects of (n-3) Polyunsaturated Fatty Acids in Rat Models of Arterial and Venous Thrombosis"

Andriamampandry MD; Leray C; Freund M; Cazenave JP; Gachet C
Thromb Res 1999 Jan 1; 93(1):9-16

This study shows that a diet enriched with n-3 fatty acids exerts antithrombotic effects in rats which are arterial thrombosis models.

"Effect of Omega-3 Fatty Acids on the Progression of Metastases after the Surgical Excision of Human Breast Cancer Cell Solid Tumors Growing in Nude Mice"

Rose DP; Connolly JM; Coleman M

Clin Cancer Res 1996 Oct; 2(10):1751–56

This study shows that supplementation with the omega-3 fatty acids eicosapentaenoic acid or docosahexaenoic acid inhibits the development of breast tumor metastasis in the lungs of nude mice.

"Effect of Serum Fatty Acid Composition on Coronary Atherosclerosis in Japan"

Hojo N; Fukushima T; Isobe A; Gao T; Shiwaku K; Ishida K; Ohta N; Yamane Y

Int J Cardiol 1998 Sep 1; 66(1):31–38

This study shows that the serum levels of high-density-lipoprotein cholesterol and eicosapentaenoic acid in patients with coronary stenosis are significantly lower compared to those of controls and suggests that supplementation with omega-3 fatty acids may have a protective effect on coronary atherosclerosis progression.

"Effects of Dietary Fish and Weight Reduction on Ambulatory Blood Pressure in Overweight Hypertensives"

Bao DQ; Mori TA; Burke V; Puddey IB; Beilin LJ

Hypertension 1998 Oct; 32(4):710–17

This study shows that daily consumption of fish and weight loss produced a fall in blood pressure of 6.0/3.0 mmHg and 5.5/2.2 mmHg, respectively, in a sample of sixty-nine overweight, medication-treated, hypertensive patients. The combination of daily fish intake and weight loss reduced blood pressure by 13.0/9.3 mmHg, suggesting a substantial reduction in cardiovascular risk and medication requirements in these patients.

"Omega-3 Polyunsaturated Fatty Acid Levels in the Diet and in Red Blood Cell Membranes of Depressed Patients"

Edwards R; Peet M; Shay J; Horrobin D

J Affect Disord 1998 Mar; 48(2–3):149–55

This study shows that depressed patients have a significantly lower content of n-3 polyunsaturated fatty acids (PUFAs) in their red blood cells membranes compared to healthy controls. The level of PUFA depletion correlates with the severity of the depression.

"A Diet Rich in Walnuts Favourably Influences Plasma Fatty Acid Profile in Moderately Hyperlipidaemic Subjects"

Chisholm A; Mann J; Skeaff M; Frampton C; Sutherland W; Duncan A; Tiszavari S

Eur J Clin Nutr 1998 Jan; 52(1):12–16

This study shows that two types of diet, one rich in walnuts and with 38 percent of calories intake from fat, the other low-fat, with a 30 percent of total calories intake from fat, both lowered total and LDL cholesterol levels and increased the HDL cholesterol levels, changes that are likely to reduce the risk of cardiovascular disease.

"Intake of Macronutrients and Risk of Breast Cancer"

Franceschi S; Favero A; Decarli A; Negri E; La Vecchia C; Ferraroni M; Russo A; Salvini S; Amadori D; Conti E; et al

Lancet 1996 May 18; 347(9012):1351–56

This study, performed on a cohort of 2,569 women with breast cancer and 2,588 controls, shows that high intakes of polyunsaturated fatty acids and unsaturated fatty acids are associated with a 30 percent and 25 percent reduction in breast cancer risk, respectively.

"Dietary Fat Intake and Risk of Lung Cancer: A Prospective Study of 51,452 Norwegian Men and Women"

Veierod MB; Laake P; Thelle DS

Eur J Cancer Prev 1997 Dec; 6(6):540–49

This study, performed on a sample of 51,452 individuals aged sixteen to fifty-six years, shows that the ratio of lung cancer decreased by 50 percent in individuals supplementing their diet with cod liver oil.

THE BENEFITS OF FIBER

"Long-term Intake of Dietary Fiber and Decreased Risk of Coronary Heart Disease among Women"

Wolk A; Manson JE; Stampfer MJ; Colditz GA; Hu FB; Sepizer FE; Hennekens CH; Willett WC.

JAMA 1999 Jun 2; 281(21):1998–2004

This study, conducted in a cohort of 68,782 U.S. women, found that those in the highest versus the lowest quintile of dietary fiber intake had a 23 percent decreased risk of major coronary heart disease events. The risk reduction was especially associated with consumption of cereal fiber, which conferred a 37 percent risk reduction for each 5 gram per day of increased intake.

"Vegetable, Fruit, and Cereal Fiber Intake and Risk of Coronary Heart Disease among Men"

Rimm EB; Ascherio A; Giovannucci E; Spiegelman D; Stampfer MJ; Willett WC

JAMA 1996 Feb 14; 275(6):447–51

This study, conducted on a cohort of 43,757 U.S. women, found that those in the highest versus the lowest quintile of fiber intake had a 41 percent lower risk of fatal and nonfatal myocardial infarction. When fatal myocardial infarction was the only outcome considered, the risk was even lower, with a 55 percent risk reduction associated with the highest versus the lowest quintile of fiber intake.

"Wheat Bran Fiber and Development of Adenomatous Polyps: Evidence from Randomized, Controlled Clinical Trials"

Macrae F

Am J Med 1999 Jan 25; 106(1A):38S–42S

This article reviews some of the randomized controlled trials assessing the relationship between wheat bran fiber intake and colon adenomas. In one study, conducted on patients with familial polyposis, daily intake of vitamin C, vitamin E, and fiber for four years inhibited the development of rectal polyps. Another study showed a significant reduction of fecal bile acids concentrations—supposedly a risk factor for colon cancer—associated with dietary wheat bran intake. The Australian Polyp Prevention Project showed a decreased incidence of colorectal cancer associated with a combination of wheat bran supplementation and fat intake reduction.

"Mechanisms by Which Wheat Bran and Oat Bran Increase Stool Weight in Humans"

Chen HL; Haack VS; Janecky CW; Vollendorf NW; Marlett JA

Am J Clin Nutr 1998 Sep; 68(3):711–19

This study shows that the increase in stool weight associated with oat bran consumption is due mainly to an increase of fecal bacterial mass and lipids, and that the stool weight increase associated with wheat bran intake is due mainly to undigested plant fiber. The fiber provided by oat bran is 96 percent digestible and stimulates the growth of intestinal bacteria.

THE BENEFITS OF NUTRIENTS

"Effects of Selenium Supplementation for Cancer Prevention in Patients with Carcinoma of the Skin. A Randomized Controlled Trial. Nutritional Prevention of Cancer Study Group"

Clark LC; Combs GF Jr; Turnbull BW; Slate EH; Chalker DK; Chow J; Davis LS; Glover RA; Graham GF; Gross EG; Krongrad A; Lesher JL Jr; Park HK; Sanders BB Jr; Smith CL; Taylor JR.

JAMA 1996 Dec 25; 276(24):1957–63

This study, performed on a total of 1,312 patients with skin cancer, shows that daily supplementation with selenium is associated with a 50 percent reduction in total cancer mortality and a 37 percent reduction in total cancer incidence.

"Vitamin E and Vitamin C Supplement Use and Risk of All-Cause and Coronary Heart Disease Mortality in Older Persons: The Established Populations for Epidemiologic Studies of the Elderly"

Losonczy KG; Harris TB; Havlik RJ

Am J Clin Nutr 1996 Aug; 64(2):190–96

This study, performed on a sample population of 11,178 persons 67 to 105 years old, showed that supplementation with vitamin E was associated with a 34 percent reduced risk of death from all causes, a 47 percent reduced risk of death from coronary artery disease, and a 59 percent reduced risk of death from cancer. Simultaneous supplementation with vitamin E and C was associated with a 42 percent decreased risk of overall mortality and with a 53 percent decreased risk of coronary mortality.

"Reduced Risk of Colon Cancer with High Intake of Vitamin E: The Iowa Women's Health Study"

Bostick RM; Potter JD; McKenzie DR; Sellers TA; Kushi LH; Steinmetz KA; Folsom AR
Cancer Res 1993 Sep 15; 53(18):4230–37

This study shows that, in a cohort of 35,215 Iowa women aged fifty-five to sixty-nine years, those with the highest versus the lowest quintile of vitamin E intake had an overall 68 percent decreased risk of colon cancer. Multivariate analyses showed that women fifty-five to fifty-nine years old had a risk reduction of 84 percent.

"Average Intake of Anti-Oxidant (pro)Vitamins and Subsequent Cancer Mortality in the 16 Cohorts of the Seven Countries Study"

Ocke MC; Kormhout D; Menotti A; Aravanis C; Blackburn H; Buzina R; Fidanza F; Jansen A; Nedeljkovic S; Nissienen A; et al
Int J Cancer 1995 May 16; 61(4):480–44

This study shows that the average intake of vitamin C of a population of sixteen cohorts in the Seven Countries Study was associated with a 34 percent reduction in stomach cancer mortality.

"Decreased Incidence of Prostate Cancer with Selenium Supplementation: Results of a Double-Blind Cancer Prevention Trial"

Clark LC; Dalkin B; Krongrad A; Combs GF Jr; Turnbull BW; Slate EH; Witherington R; Herlong JH; Janosko E; Carpenter D; Borosso C; Falk S; Rounder J
Br J Urol 1998 May; 81(5):730–34

This study shows that, in a cohort of 974 men with a history of skin cancer, those taking daily supplements of 200 micrograms of selenium had a 63 percent reduced incidence of prostate cancer, compared to those taking placebo. The incidence decreased further in individuals with initially normal levels of prostate-specific antigen, where supplementation with selenium versus placebo was associated with a 75 percent reduction in prostate cancer incidence.

"The Linxian Trials: Mortality Rates by Vitamin-Mineral Intervention Group"

Blot WJ; Li JY; Taylor PR; Guo W; Dawsey SM; Li B
Am J Clin Nutr 1995 Dec; 62(6 Suppl):1424S–26S

This study shows that, in a sample population of 30,000 individuals in Lixian, China, daily supplementation for five years with beta-carotene, alpha-tocopherol, and selenium reduced overall mortality and cancer mortality by 9 percent and 13 percent, respectively. In another trial involving 3,318 individuals, multivitamin/mineral supplementation was associated with a 55 percent reduction in death from cerebrovascular disease in males and a 10 percent reduction in females.

"Lowered Risks of Hypertension and Cerebrovascular Disease after Vitamin/Mineral Supplementation: The Linxian Nutrition Intervention Trial"

Mark SD; Wang W; Fraumeni JF Jr; Li JY; Taylor PR; Wang GQ; Guo W; Dawsey SM; Li B; Blot WJ

Am J Epidemiol 1996 Apr 1; 143(7):658–64

This study shows that, in a cohort of 3,318 individuals from a rural region in China, daily supplementation with a multivitamin/mineral versus placebo was associated with a 57 percent decreased risk of hypertension in men and an 8 percent decrease in women.

"Double Blind, Cluster Randomised Trial of Low Dose Supplementation with Vitamin A or Beta Carotene on Mortality Related to Pregnancy in Nepal. The NNIPS-2 Study Group."

West KP Jr; Katz J; Khatry SK; LeClerq SC; Pradhan EK; Shrestha SR; Connor PB; Dali SM; Christian P; Pokhrel RP; Sommer A

BMJ 1999 Feb 27; 318(7183):570–75

This study shows that, in women of a rural area of Nepal, three and a half years of daily vitamin A and beta-carotene supplementation lowered the pregnancy-related mortality ratio by 44 percent and the maternal mortality ratio by 40 percent.

"Efficacy of Vitamin A in Reducing Preschool Child Mortality in Nepal"

West KP Jr; Pokhrel RP; Katz J; LeClerq SC; Khatry SK; Shrestha SR; Pradhan EK; Tielsch JM; Pandey MR; Sommer A

Lancet 1991 Jul 13; 338(8759):67–71

This randomized, placebo-controlled study shows that children in a rural area of Nepal aged six to seventy-two months receiving vitamin A supplementation had a 30 percent reduction in mortality, compared to children receiving placebo.

"Do Nutritional Supplements Lower the Risk of Stroke or Hypertension?"

Mark SD; Wang W; Fraumeni JF Jr; Li JY; Taylor PR; Wang GQ; Dawsey SM; Li B; Blot WJ

Epidemiology 1998 Jan; 9(1):9–15

This study, performed on a cohort of 29,584 persons in China, shows that individuals receiving selenium supplementation had a 9 percent reduction in stroke mortality, a 13 percent reduction in total cancer mortality, and a 9 percent reduction in overall mortality.

"The Effect of Oral Selenium Supplementation on Human Sperm Motility"

Scott R; MacPherson A; Yates RW; Hussain B; Dixon J

Br J Urol 1998 Jul; 82(1):76–80

This study shows that three months of selenium supplementation significantly increased sperm motility and chance of successful conception in subfertile men. Eleven percent of men in the selenium group achieved paternity versus 0 percent of men in the control group.

"Prostate Cancer and Supplementation with Alpha-Tocopherol and Beta-Carotene: Incidence and Mortality in a Controlled Trial"

Heinonen OP; Albanes D; Virtamo J; Taylor PR; Huttunen JK; Hartman AM; Haapakoski J; Malila N; Rautalahti M; Ripatti S; Maenpaa H; Teerenhovi L; Koss L; Virolainen M; Edwards BK

J Natl Cancer Inst 1998 Mar 18; 90(6):440–46

This study shows that daily supplementation with 50 mg alpha-tocopherol in male smokers reduces the incidence of prostate cancer by 32 percent and of prostate cancer mortality by 41 percent.

"Calcium Supplements for the Prevention of Colorectal Adenomas. Calcium Polyp Prevention Study Group"

Baron JA; Beach M; Mandel JS; van Stolk RU; Haile RW; Sandler RS; Rothstein R; Summers RW; Snover DC; Beck GJ; Bond JH; Greenberg ER

N Engl J Med 1999 Jan 14; 340(2):101–7

This study shows that daily supplementation with 3 g calcium carbonate reduces the risk of recurrence of colorectal adenomas by 15 percent.

"A Case-Control Study of the Relationship between Dietary Factors and Risk of Lung Cancer in Women of Shenyang, China.

Zhou B; Wang T; Sun G; Guan P; Wu JM

Oncol Rep 1999 Jan-Feb; 6(1):139–43

This study shows that intake of beta-carotene, vitamin C, and fiber is associated with a reduction in lung cancer risk of 16 percent, 25 percent, and 54 percent, respectively.

"Vitamin and Calcium Supplement Use Is Associated with Decreased Adenoma Recurrence in Patients with a Previous History of Neoplasia"

Whelan RL; Horvath KD; Gleason NR; Forde KA; Treat MD; Teitelbaum SL; Bertram A; Neugut AI

Dis Colon Rectum 1999 Feb; 42(2):212–17

This study shows that daily supplementation with multivitamins, vitamin E, and calcium reduces the risk of recurrence of colorectal adenomas by 53 percent, 38 percent, and 49 percent, respectively.

"Antioxidant Intake and Risk of Incident Age-Related Nuclear Cataracts in the Beaver Dam Eye Study"

Lyle BJ; Mares-Perlman JA; Klein BE; Klein R; Greger JL

Am J Epidemiol 1999 May 1; 149(9):801–9

This study shows that individuals with the highest versus the lowest intake of the carotenoid lutein have a 50 percent decreased risk of developing cataracts.

"The Linxian Cataract Studies. Two Nutrition Intervention Trials"

Sperduto RD; Hu TS; Milton RC; Zhao JL; Everett DF; Cheng QF; Blot WJ; Bing L; Taylor PR; Li JY; et al

Arch Ophthalmol 1993 Sep; 111(9):1246–53

This study shows that individuals sixty-five to seventy-four years of age receiving daily multivitamin/mineral supplementation versus placebo had a 36 percent reduction in prevalence of cataract. Supplementation with riboflavin/niacin versus placebo in people of the same age group was associated with a 44 percent reduction in prevalence of cataract.

"Clinical Trial Experience with Extended-Release Niacin (Niaspan): Dose-Escalation Study"

Goldberg AC

Am J Cardiol 1998 Dec 17; 82(12A):35U–38U; discussion 39U–41U

This randomized, placebo-controlled study shows that daily supplementation with 2,000 mg extended-release niacin verus placebo decreased levels of total serum cholesterol by 12 percent, of LDL cholesterol by 16.7 percent, of triglycerides by 34.5 percent, of lipoprotein(a) by 23.6 percent, and increased levels of HDL cholesterol by 25.8 percent.

"Intake of Vitamins B6 and C and the Risk of Kidney Stones in Women"

Curhan GC; Willett WC; Speizer FE; Stampfer MJ

J Am Soc Nephrol 1999 Apr; 10(4):840–45

This study, conducted on a cohort of 85,557 women with no history of kidney stones, shows that those with the highest versus the lowest intake of vitamin B6 had a 34 percent decreased risk of kidney stone formation.

BENEFITS OF A VEGETARIAN DIET

"Dietary Habits and Mortality in 11,000 Vegetarians and Health-Conscious People: Results of a 17-Year Follow-up"

Key TJ; Thorogood M; Appleby PN; Burr ML

BMJ 1996 Sep 28; 313(7060):775–79

This study found that the mortality rate of a sample of 10,771 vegetarians or health-conscious individuals, 19 percent of whom smoked, was about half that of the general population. Consumption of fresh fruit was associated with 24 percent less mortality from ischemic disease, 32 percent less mortality from cerebrovascular disease, and 21 percent less mortality from all causes.

"Mediterranean Dietary Pattern in a Randomized Trial: Prolonged Survival and Possible Reduced Cancer Rate

de Lorgeril M; Salen P; Martin JL; Monjaud I; Boucher P; Mamelle N

Arch Intern Med 1998 Jun 8; 158(11):1181–87

In this study, 605 patients with coronary artery disease were randomized to follow for four years either a Mediterranean-type diet, rich in fruit, vegetables, cereals, and omega-3 fatty acids, or a control diet close to the step 1 American Heart Association prudent diet. A 56 percent reduction of risk of total deaths and a 61 percent reduction of risk of cancer was found in the individuals following the Mediterranean-type diet.

"A Clinical Trial of the Effects of Dietary Patterns on Blood Pressure. DASH Collaborative Research Group"

Appel LJ; Moore TJ; Obarzanek E; Vollmer WM; Svetkey LP; Sacks FM; Bray GA; Vogt TM; Cutler JA; Windhauser MM; Lin PH; Karanja N
N Engl J Med 1997 Apr 17; 336(16):1117–24

This study finds that hypertensive patients receiving for eight weeks a diet low in saturated and total fat and rich in fruits, vegetables, and low-fat dairy products show a decrease in systolic and diastolic blood pressure of 11.4 and 5.5 mmHg compared to patients consuming a control diet low in fruit, vegetables, and dairy with a fat content typical of the average American diet.

"Intensive Lifestyle Changes for Reversal of Coronary Heart Disease"

Ornish D; Scherwitz LW; Billings JH; Gould KL; Merritt TA; Sparler S; Armstrong WT; Ports TA; Kirkeeide RL; Hogeboom C; Brand RJ
JAMA 1998 Dec 16; 280(23):2001–7

This study investigates the effects of a five-year program consisting of a low-fat (10 percent) vegetarian diet, smoking cessation, exercise, and stress management on coronary artery disease. The experimental group showed a 4.5 percent relative improvement in coronary artery stenosis after one year and a 7.9 percent relative improvement after five years. By contrast, the control group showed a 5.4 percent relative worsening at one year and a 27.7 percent relative worsening at five years. The experimental group experienced less than half the cardiac events than the control group.

"The 'Diet Heart' Hypothesis in Secondary Prevention of Coronary Heart Disease"

de Lorgeril M; Salen P; Monjaud I; Delaye J
European Heart Journal 1997 Jan; 18(1):13–18

This study reviews the results of two recent trials in which the increase in consumption of natural antioxidants, oligoelements, and vegetable proteins resulted in a 30 to 70 percent reduction in the recurrence rate of coronary artery disease.

"Blood Pressure and Atherogenic Lipoprotein Profiles of Fish-Diet and Vegetarian Villagers in Tanzania: The Lugalawa Study"

Pauletto P; Puato M; Caroli MG; Casiglia E; Munhambo AE; Cazzolato G; Bittolo Bon G; Angeli MT; Galli C; Pessina AC
Lancet 1996 Sep 21; 348(9030):784–88

This study shows that consumption of freshwater fish is associated with a lower incidence of hypertension; a lower concentration of plasma cholesterol, triglycerides, and lipoprotein; and a higher plasma concentration of n-3 polyunsaturated fatty acids. The frequencies of definite and borderline hypertension in a group of villagers consuming freshwater fish compared to a group with a vegetarian diet was 2.8 percent versus 16.4 percent and 9.7 percent versus 22.3 percent, respectively.

"Dietary Flavonoid Intake and Risk of Cardiovascular Disease in Postmenopausal Women"

Yochum L; Kushi LH; Meyer K; Folsom AR
Am J Epidemiol 1999 May 15; 149(10):943–49

This study finds a decreased risk of coronary heart disease associated with flavonoids intake. Consumption of broccoli is strongly associated with reduced risk of death from coronary heart disease.

"Risk Factors for Cardiovascular Disease and Diabetes in Two Groups of Hispanic Americans with Differing Dietary Habits"

Alexander H; Lockwood LP; Harris MA; Melby CL
J Am Coll Nutr 1999 Apr; 18(2):127–36

This study finds that Hispanic Seventh-Day Adventists, eating a plant-based diet, had significantly lower body mass index and waist-to-hip ratios compared to the Hispanic Catholic omnivores. The Seventh-Day Adventists also showed significantly lower levels of fasting insulin and glucose concentration, systolic blood pressure, total serum cholesterol and triglycerides, and higher levels of serum high-density lipoprotein cholesterol.

"Ethnic Variation in Cardiovascular Disease Risk Factors among Children and Young Adults: Findings from the Third National Health and Nutrition Examination Survey, 1988–1994"

Winkleby MA; Robinson TN; Sundquist J; Kraemer HC
JAMA 1999 Mar 17; 281(11):1006–13

This study analyzes the ethnic differences in the risk of cardiovascular disease and finds that black and Mexican American girls have significantly higher body mass indexes compared to white girls. The differences, evident by age six, become wider with increasing age. The intake of dietary fat parallels these findings. Blood pressure levels are also significantly higher in black compared to white girls.

"Dietary Antioxidants and Risk of Myocardial Infarction in the Elderly: The Rotterdam Study"

Klipstein-Grobusch K; Geleijnse JM; den Breeijen JH; Boeing H; Hofman A; Grobbee DE; Witteman JC
Am J Clin Nutr 1999 Feb; 69(2):261–66

This study finds that, in a sample population of 4,802 individuals, those with the highest versus the lowest tertile of dietary beta-carotene intake have a 45 percent reduction in the risk of myocardial infarction. Beta-carotene intake from supplements provides an even more marked protection.

"Cardiovascular Disease Risk Factors Are Lower in African-American Vegans Compared to Lacto-Ovo-Vegetarians"

Toohey ML; Harris MA; DeWitt W; Foster G; Schmidt WD; Melby CL

J Am Coll Nutr 1998 Oct; 17(5):425–34

This study shows that vegans, compared to lacto-ovo vegetarians, have significant lower body mass index, serum total cholesterol, LDL cholesterol, and triglycerides. The ratio of total to HDL cholesterol is significantly lower in vegans compared to lacto-ovo vegetarians.

"Whole-Grain Intake May Reduce the Risk of Ischemic Heart Disease Death in Postmenopausal Women: The Iowa Women's Health Study"

Jacobs DR Jr; Meyer KA; Kushi LH; Folsom AR

Am J Clin Nutr 1998 Aug; 68(2):248–57

This study, performed on a sample population of 34,492 postmenopausal women, finds that those with the highest quintiles of whole-grain intake have a 35 percent lower risk of death from ischemic heart disease.

"Serum Ascorbic Acid and Cardiovascular Disease Prevalence in U.S. Adults"

Simon JA; Hudes ES; Browner WS

Epidemiology 1998 May; 9(3):316-21

This study finds that, in a sample population of 6,624 individuals, those with the highest versus the lowest levels of serum ascorbic acid have a 27 percent decreased prevalence of coronary artery disease and a 26 percent decreased prevalence of stroke.

"Rapid Reduction of Serum Cholesterol and Blood Pressure by a Twelve-Day, Very Low Fat, Strictly Vegetarian Diet"

McDougall J; Litzau K; Haver E; Saunders V; Spiller GA

Journal of the American College of Nutrition 1995 Oct; 14(5):491-96

This study shows that, in a group of 500 men and women, twelve days of a vegetarian, very low-fat diet lowered the total serum cholesterol level of 11 percent, the blood pressure level of 6 percent, and caused a weight loss of 2.5 kg in men and 1 kg in women.

"Effects of Dietary Patterns on Blood Pressure: Subgroup Analysis of the Dietary Approaches to Stop Hypertension (DASH) Randomized Clinical Trial"

Svetkey LP; Simons-Morton D; Vollmer WM; Appel LJ; Conlin PR; Ryan DH; Ard J; Kennedy BM

Arch Intern Med 1999 Feb 8; 159(3):285–93

This study shows that a diet rich in fruits and vegetables, with or without low-fat dairy products, significantly lowered systolic and diastolic blood pressure in hypertensive and nonhypertensive patients.

"Changes in Cardiovascular Risk Factors and Hormones during a Comprehensive Residential Three-Month Kriya Yoga Training and Vegetarian Nutrition"

Schmidt T; Wijga A; Von Zur Muhlen A; Brabant G; Wagner TO
Acta Physiologica Scandinavica 1997; 640(Suppl):158–62

This study finds that a three-month program including a low-fat, lacto-vegetarian diet and yoga causes a significant reduction of the body mass index, total serum and LDL cholesterol, fibrinogen, and blood pressure level in participants.

"Lifestyle and the Use of Health Services"

Knutsen SF
American Journal of Clinical Nutrition 1994 May; 59(5 Suppl):1171S–1175S

This study, performed on a sample population of 27,766 Seventh-Day Adventists, finds that nonvegetarians have significantly more hospitalizations and surgeries compared to vegetarians. Use of medication was more than doubled in nonvegetarian males and increased by 70 to 115 percent in nonvegetarian females. An omnivorous diet was also associated with increased prevalence of chronic diseases and asthma.

"Protective Effect of Fruits and Vegetables on Stomach Cancer in a Cohort of Swedish Twins"

Terry P; Nyr'en O; Yuen J
Int J Cancer 1998 Mar 30; 76(1):35–37

This study shows that people consuming the lowest intake of fruit and vegetables have a 5.5 percent increased risk of developing stomach cancer compared to people with the highest intake of these food groups.

"Vegetable Consumption and Risk of Chronic Disease"

La Vecchia C; Decarli A; Pagano R
Epidemiology 1998 Mar; 9(2):208–10

This study evaluates the relationship between vegetable consumption and prevalence of chronic disease in a sample of 46,693 individuals. People consuming the highest tertile of vegetables had an over 20 percent lower risk of myocardial infarction and peptic ulcer; 11 percent lower risk of angina pectoris; 30 percent lower risk of chronic bronchitis, bronchial asthma, liver cirrhosis and kidney stones; and 16 percent lower risk of arthritis.

"Vegetarianism, Dietary Fibre and Gastro-Intestinal Disease"

Nair P; Mayberry JF
Digestive Diseases 1994 May-Jun; 12(3):177–85

This article reviews the literature demonstrating that vegetarians have longer life expectancies and lower incidence of gastrointestinal cancer, gallstones, diverticular disease, and constipation, while meat eating is associated with increased mortality from all causes.

"Food-Group Consumption and Colon Cancer in the Adelaide Case-Control Study. I. Vegetables and Fruit"

Steinmetz KA, Potter JD
Int J Cancer 1993 Mar 12; 53(5):711-19

In this study, women consuming onions and legumes had a reduction in risk of colon cancer of about 50 percent. Increased intake of raw fruit and cabbage was associated with a 24 percent and 29 percent risk reduction, respectively. In males, greater intake of these foods was associated with a risk reduction of about 25 percent.

"Vegetarian Diets and Colon Cancer: The German Experience"

Frentzel-Beyme R; Chang-Claude J
American Journal of Clinical Nutrition. 59(5 Suppl):1143S-1152S, 1994 May

This study shows that a vegetarian diet of long duration is associated with decreased total and cancer mortality.

"Prospective Study of Diet and Ovarian Cancer"

Kushi LH; Mink PJ; Folsom AR; Anderson KE; Zheng W; Lazovich D; Sellers TA. Am J Epidemiol 1999 Jan 1; 149(1):21–31

This study analyzes the association between diet and ovarian cancer in a cohort of 29,083 postmenopausal women. Women with the highest versus the lowest quartile of lactose and cholesterol intake had a 60 percent and 55 percent increased risk of cancer, respectively. Consumption of eggs was also associated with increased risk. Green, leafy vegetables were found to be protective, with a 56 percent decreased risk of cancer in women with the highest versus the lowest quartile of intake.

"A Case-Control Study of the Relationship between Dietary Factors and Risk of Lung Cancer in Women of Shenyang, China"

Zhou B; Wang T; Sun G; Guan P; Wu JM
Oncol Rep 1999 Jan-Feb; 6(1):139–43

This study shows that the intake of beta-carotene, vitamin C, and fiber reduces the risk of lung cancer in a dose-dependent manner.

"Mortality Risks of Oesophageal Cancer Associated with Hot Tea, Alcohol, Tobacco and Diet in Japan"

Kinjo Y; Cui Y; Akiba S; Watanabe S; Yamaguchi N; Sobue T; Mizuno S; Beral V
J Epidemiol 1998 Oct; 8(4):235–43

This study shows that either alcohol or smoking more than double the risk of esophageal cancer. The combined effect of alcohol and smoking is more than additive, conferring an almost fourfold increased risk. Consumption of hot tea confers a 60 percent increased risk compared with nonhot tea. The risk also doubles for low intake of green and yellow vegetables (one to three times per month versus daily).

"Malignant Epithelial Tumours in the Upper Digestive Tract: A Dietary and Socio-Medical Case-Control and Survival Study

Freng A; Daae LN; Engeland A; Norum KR; Sander J; Solvoll K; Tretli S
Eur J Clin Nutr 1998 Apr; 52(4):271-78

In this study, smoking is associated with a 29-fold increase in the risk of tumors of the upper digestive tract, and alcohol with a 6.6-fold increase. Beta-carotene and vitamin C, on the other hand, lower the risk by 80 percent and 70 percent, respectively.

"Dietary Fiber and Colorectal Cancer Risk"

Le Marchand L; Hankin JH; Wilkens LR; Kolonel LN; Englyst HN; Lyu LC Epidemiology 1997 Nov; 8(6):658–65

This study shows that the intake of fiber from vegetable sources reduces the risk of colorectal cancer by 40 percent in men and by 50 percent in women with the highest versus the lowest quartile of intake.

"Multivitamin Use, Folate, and Colon Cancer in Women in the Nurses' Health Study"

Giovannucci E; Stampfer MJ; Colditz GA; Hunter DJ; Fuchs C; Rosner BA; Speizer FE; Willett WC
Ann Intern Med 1998 Oct 1; 129(7):517–24

This study shows that in a cohort of 88,756 women, those supplementing their diet daily with 400 or more micrograms folate had 31 percent lower risk of colon cancer compared to women with folate intake of 200 or less micrograms. Women using multivitamins containing folic acid had 75 percent reduction in risk of colon cancer after fifteen years of use.

"Long-term Effects of a Change from a Mixed Diet to a Lacto-Vegetarian Diet on Human Urinary and Faecal Mutagenic Activity"

Johansson G; Holmen A; Persson L; Hogstedt B; Wassen C; Ottova L; Gustafsson JA
Mutagenesis 1998 Mar., 13(2):167–71

This study shows that a shift from an omnivorous to a lacto-vegetarian diet is associated with a decrease in mutagenic activity of urine and feces.

"Consumption of Vegetables Reduces Genetic Damage in Humans: First Results of a Human Intervention Trial with Carotenoid-Rich Foods"

Pool-Zobel BL; Bub A; Müller H; Wollowski I; Rechkemmer G
Carcinogenesis 1997 Sep; 18(9):1847–50

This study shows that consumption of tomato, carrot, or spinach protects against DNA strand breaks and oxidative base damage, and thus supports the hypothesis that their cancer-protective effects may be exerted through protection against DNA damage.

"Dietary Fiber, Glycemic Load, and Risk of Non-Insulin-Dependent Diabetes Mellitus in Women"

Salmeron J; Manson JE; Stampfer MJ; Colditz GA; Wing AL; Willett WC
JAMA 1997 Feb 12; 277(6):472–77

This study, performed on a sample population of 65,173 women, found that those in the highest versus the lowest quintile of glycemic load had a 47 percent increased risk of diabetes. Cereal fiber intake was associated with an almost 30 percent reduction in risk of diabetes in women with the highest versus the lowest intake. The combination of high glycemic load and low fiber consumption conferred a 2.5–fold increase in the risk of developing diabetes.

"An in Vivo 13C Magnetic Resonance Spectroscopic Study of the Relationship between Diet and Adipose Tissue Composition"

Thomas EL; Frost G; Barnard ML; Bryant DJ; Taylor-Robinson SD; Simbrunner J; Coutts GA; Burl M; Bloom SR; Sales KD; Bell JD
Lipids 1996 Feb; 31(2):145–51

This study shows that the adipose tissue composition of vegans, compared to omnivores and vegetarians, has a higher concentration of unsaturated fatty acids and a lower concentration of saturated fatty acids. Vegans also have significantly lower serum total cholesterol levels and low-density lipoprotein cholesterol compared to omnivores.

"Selected Vitamins and Trace Elements in Blood of Vegetarians"

Krajcovicova-Kudlackova M; Simoncic R; Babinska K; Bederova A; Brtkova A; Magalova T; Grancicova E.
Annals of Nutrition & Metabolism 1995; 39(6):334–39

This study shows that individuals consuming a vegetarian or lacto-ovo-vegetarian diet have significantly higher blood concentration of vitamin C, beta-carotene, vitamin A, and selenium compared to that of omnivores. The vegetarians also have a higher plasma molar ratio of vitamin E/total lipids, indicative of effective protection against polyunsaturated fatty acids peroxidation.

"Antioxidant Status in Long-Term Adherents to a Strict Uncooked Vegan Diet"

Rauma AL; Torronen R; Hanninen O; Verhagen H; Mykkanen H
American Journal of Clinical Nutrition 1995 Dec; 62(6):1221–27

This study shows that the blood concentration of beta-carotene, vitamin C, vitamin E, and erythrocyte superoxide dismutase activity in vegans following a raw diet is significantly higher than that of omnivores and reflects a better antioxidant status.

"Randomised Controlled Trial of Effect of Fruit and Vegetable Consumption on Plasma Concentrations of Lipids and Antioxidants"

Zino S; Skeaff M; Williams S; Mann J
BMJ 1997 Jun 21; 314(7097):1787–91

This study shows that the intake of eight servings of fruit and vegetables per day for an eight-week period results in increased plasma concentration of vitamin C, alpha-carotene, and beta-carotene, likely to result in reduced cancer incidence.

"Does a Vegetarian Diet Control Wilson's Disease?"

Brewer GJ; Yuzbasiyan-Gurkan V; Dick R; Wang Y; Johnson V

Journal of the American College of Nutrition 1993 Oct; 12(5):527–30

This study reports on two patients with Wilson's disease, almost totally noncompliant with anticopper therapy, managed by a vegetarian diet. This could be due to the reduced bioavailability of copper from a vegetarian source.

"A Review of the Clinical Effects of Phytoestrogens"

Knight DC; Eden JA

Obstetrics & Gynecology 1996 May; 87(5 Pt 2):897–904

This study reviews 861 articles on phytoestrogens and soy products. All studies agreed that phytoestrogens inhibit the growth of different types of tumor cell lines in in-vitro and in-vivo models. Experimental results have been supported by epidemiological studies that provided evidence to the hypothesis that phytoestrogens inhibit the formation and growth of tumors in humans. Phytoestrogens also have been associated with reduced cholesterol levels, thus protecting against heart disease, and have been shown to improve osteoporosis.

"Soy Protein, Isoflavones and Cardiovascular Disease Risk"

Lichtenstein AH

J Nutr 1998 Oct; 128(10):1589–92

This article reviews the information available in literature showing that the soybean isoflavone fraction reduces cholesterol levels in animals and humans and seems to improve arterial compliance.

"Socioeconomic Determinants of Health. The Contribution of Nutrition to Inequalities in Health"

James WP; Nelson M; Ralph A; Leather S

BMJ 1997 May 24; 314(7093):1545–49

This article highlights how lower socioeconomic groups have higher incidence of premature and low birthweight babies, heart disease, stroke, and certain type of cancers, and have, together with other risk factors, a diet especially based on meat, milk, fats, sugars, preservatives, and potatoes. The potential health gain that could result from changing dietary habits is enormous.

ALCOHOL: A MIXED BAG

"Alcohol and Breast Cancer in Women: A Pooled Analysis of Cohort Studies"

Smith-Warner SA; Spiegelman D; Yaun SS; van den Brandt PA; Folsom AR; Goldbohm RA; Graham S; Holmberg L; Howe GR; Marshall JR; Miller AB; Potter JD; Speizer FE; Willett WC; Wolk A; Hunter DJ

JAMA 1998 Feb 18; 279(7):535–40

This study analyzes data from six prospective studies including a total of 322,647 women to evaluate the relationship between alcohol intake and risk of breast cancer. Intake of two to five drinks per day versus nondrinking conferred a 40 percent increased risk regardless of the type of alcoholic beverage.

"A Cohort Study of Alcohol Consumption and Risk of Breast Cancer"

Friedenreich CM; Howe GR; Miller AB; Jan MG
Am J Epidemiol 1993 Mar 1; 137(5):512–20

This study shows a positive association between alcohol intake and risk of breast cancer in premenopausal women. From the lowest to the highest quartiles of alcohol intake, compared to abstinence, the risk increased by 10, 37, 50, and 86 percent, respectively. This association was not present in postmenopausal women.

"The Association between Alcohol and Breast Cancer Risk: Evidence from the Combined Analysis of Six Dietary Case-Controlled Studies"

Howe G; Rohan T; Decarli A; Iscovich J; Kaldor J; Katsouyanni K; Marubini E; Miller A; Riboli E; Toniolo P; et al
Int J Cancer 1991 Mar 12; 47(5):707–10

This article reviews data from six case-control studies conducted on a total of 1,575 breast cancer cases and 1,974 controls, and concludes that women consuming up to 40 grams per day of alcohol do not have an increased risk of breast cancer, while for alcohol intake of 40 or more grams per day there is a 70 percent increased risk of breast cancer.

"Alcohol Consumption and Breast Cancer Risk in Denmark"

Ewertz M
Cancer Causes Control 1991 July; 2(4):247–52

This study finds a significant statistical association between alcohol intake and breast cancer only in women fifty to fifty-nine years of age in the lowest quartile of fat intake; for them, consumption of 24 or more grams of alcohol per day compared to abstinence was associated with an eighteen-fold increased risk of breast cancer.

"Alcohol and Breast Cancer Risk: A Case-Control Study from Northern Italy"

Ferraroni M; Decarli A; Willett WC; Marubini E
Int J Epidemiol 1991 Dec; 20(4):859–64

This study finds an 80 percent increased risk of breast cancer in women with high alcohol intake (more than 24 grams per day) and a 50 percent increased risk associated with low levels of intake.

"Alcohol Consumption and Risk of Breast Cancer: The Framingham Study Revisited"

Zhang Y; Kreger BE; Dorgan JF; Splansky GL; Cupples LA; Ellison RC
Am J Epidemiol 1999 Jan 15; 149(2):93–101

This study, conducted on a cohort of 2,764 women, shows that light alcohol intake is associated with a 20 to 30 percent reduction in risk of breast cancer, regardless of the type of alcoholic beverage.

"Moderate Alcohol Consumption and the Risk of Endometrial Cancer"

Swanson CA; Wilbanks GD; Twiggs LB; Mortel R; Berman ML; Barrett RJ; Brinton LA
Epidemiology 1993 Nov; 4(6):530–36

This study shows that increasing levels of alcohol intake are associated with decreasing risk of endometrial cancer. Increasing tertiles of alcohol intake versus abstinence are associated with a 22, 36, and 60 percent decreased risk of endometrial cancer, respectively.

"Alcohol Consumption and Ovarian Cancer Risk"

Gwinn ML; Webster LA; Lee NC; Layde PM; Rubin GL
Am J Epidemiol 1986 May; 123(5):759–66

This study finds a 50 percent decreased risk of ovarian cancer in women drinking twenty or more alcoholic beverages per week versus nondrinkers. Overall, there is a 10 percent risk reduction associated with alcohol intake.

"Alcohol Consumption and Risk of Cancer in Humans: An Overview"

Longnecker MP
Alcohol 1995 Mar-Apr; 12(2):87–96

This article reports the epidemiological evidence that alcohol intake is associated with increased risk of cancer of the mouth, pharynx, larynx, esophagus, and liver. The association between alcohol and pancreatic cancer is weak.

"Cancer Morbidity in Alcohol Abusers"

Tonnesen H; Moller H; Andersen JR; Jensen E; Juel K
Br J Cancer 1994 Feb; 69(2):327–32

This study, performed on a cohort of 18,368 alcohol abusers, found a 60 percent increased cancer incidence in men and a 50 percent increased incidence in women, compared to the general population. This increase was due to increased incidence of cancer of the tongue, mouth, pharynx, esophagus, liver, larynx, lung and pleura, and secondary cancer. Women in this cohort had a twofold increased risk of cervical cancer but not a statistically significant increase in breast cancer. Men had a 40 percent increased risk of prostate cancer.

"Alcoholism: Independent Predictor of Survival in Patients with Head and Neck Cancer"

Deleyiannis FW; Thomas DB; Vaughan TL; Davis S
J Natl Cancer Inst 1996 Apr 17; 88(8):542–49

This study shows that in patients with head and neck cancer, alcohol abuse is associated with an over twofold increased risk of death, whereas abstinence (intake of less than a drink per week) is associated with a 39 percent decreased risk.

"Second Cancers Following Oral and Pharyngeal Cancers: Role of Tobacco and Alcohol"

Day GL; Blot WJ; Shore RE; McLaughlin JK; Austin DF; Greenberg RS; Liff JM; Preston-Martin S; Sarkar S; Schoenberg JB; et al

J Natl Cancer Inst 1994 Jan 19; 86(2):131–37

In this study, performed on a cohort of 1,090 patients with oral and pharyngeal cancer, intake of fifteen or more beers per week is associated with an almost fourfold increased risk of second primary cancers.

"Smoking and Drinking in Relation to Oral and Pharyngeal Cancer"

Blow WJ; McLaughlin JK; Winn DM; Austin DF; Greenberg RS; Preston-Martin S; Bernstein L; Schoenberg JB; Stemhagen A; Fraumeni JF Jr

Cancer Res 1988 Jun 1; 48(11):3282–87

This study estimated that approximately three-quarters of all oral and pharyngeal cancers in the United States can be attributed to alcohol consumption and tobacco smoking.

"Alcoholism and Cancer of the Larynx: A Case-Control Study in Western Washington (United States)."

Hedberg K; Vaughan TL; White E; Davis S; Thomas DB

Cancer Causes Control 1994 Jan; 5(1):3–8

In this study, conducted on a cohort of 235 laryngeal cancer cases and 547 controls, alcohol intake of forty-two or more drinks per week versus seven or less was associated with a threefold increased risk of laryngeal cancer.

"Prospective Study on Alcohol Consumption and the Risk of Cancer of the Colon and Rectum in the Netherlands"

Goldbohm RA; Van den Brandt PA; Van 't Veer P; Dorant E; Sturmans F; Hermus RJ

Cancer Causes Control 1994 Mar; 5(2):95–104

This study, conducted on a cohort of 120,852 individuals, finds no association between beer and wine intake and risk of colon cancer. Consumption of liquor was significantly associated with a decreased risk of colon cancer.

"Alcohol Intake and the Risk of Lung Cancer: Influence of Type of Alcoholic Beverage"

Prescott E; Gronbaek M; Becker U; Sorensen TI

Am J Epidemiol 1999 Mar 1; 149(5):463–70

This study, conducted on a cohort of 28,160 men and women, shows that intake of one to thirteen glasses of wine per week or more than thirteen per week was associated with a 22 percent and 56 percent decreased risk of lung cancer, respectively. The corresponding intake of beer was associated with a 9 percent and 36 percent increased risk; that of spirits with a 21 and 46 percent increased risk, respectively.

"Effect of Preoperative Abstinence on Poor Postoperative Outcome in Alcohol Misusers: Randomised Controlled Trial"

Tonnesen H; Rosenberg J; Nielsen HJ; Rasmussen V; Hauge C; Pedersen IK; Kehlet H

BMJ 1999 May 15; 318(7194):1311–16

This study finds that alcohol abusers who adopted abstinence for the month prior colorectal surgery had an over 50 percent reduction in postoperative morbidity rates compared to continuous drinkers.

"Alcohol and Pancreatic Cancer in Blacks and Whites in the United States"

Silverman DT; Brown LM; Hoover RN; Schiffman M; Lillemoe KD; Schoenberg JB; Swanson GM; Hayes RB; Greenberg RS; Benichou J; et al

Cancer Res 1995 Nov 1; 55(21):4899–905

This study does not find any association between light and moderate alcohol intake and risk of pancreatic cancer. Heavy alcohol intake (57 or more drinks per week) was associated with an over twofold increased risk in black men and with a 40 percent increased risk in white men. In black women, intake of eight to twenty drinks per week and of twenty-one or more drinks per week as associated with an 80 percent and 2.5-fold increased risk, respectively. The increase in risk was not present in white women.

Alcohol consumption and risk of pancreatic cancer.

Tavani A; Pregnolato A; Negri E; La Vecchia C

Nutr Cancer 1997; 27(2):157–61

This study finds no significant association between relatively high and frequent alcohol intake (more than eight glasses per day) and risk of pancreatic cancer.

"Alcohol Use and Prostate Cancer in U.S. Whites: No Association in a Confirmatory Study"

Lumey LH; Pittman B; Wynder EL

Prostate 1998 Sep 1; 36(4):250–55

This study finds no significant association between any level of alcohol intake and risk of prostate cancer.

"Alcohol Consumption and Mortality among Women"

Fuchs CS; Stampfer MJ; Colditz GA; Giovannucci EL; Manson JE; Kawachi I; Hunter DJ; Hankinson SE; Hennekens CH; Rosner B

N Engl J Med 1995 May 11; 332(19):1245–50

This study, performed on a cohort of 85,709 women, finds that light and moderate drinking (one to three drinks per week and three to nineteen drinks per week) is associated with a 17 and 12 percent reduction in risk of death from coronary heart disease compared to abstinence. Heavy drinking (twenty or more drinks per week) is associated with a 19 percent increased risk of death, particularly from breast cancer and cirrhosis.

"Alcohol Consumption and Mortality from All Causes, Coronary Heart Disease, and Stroke: Results from a Prospective Cohort Study of Scottish Men with 21 Years of Follow-Up"

Hart CL; Smith GD; Hole DJ; Hawthorne VM

BMJ 1999 Jun 26; 318(7200):1725–29

This study, conducted on a cohort of 5766 men, finds that alcohol intake of up to 22 units per week does not significantly affect mortality rates from all causes. Mortality risk increased in men consuming twenty-two or more units of alcohol per week with a twofold increased risk of mortality from stroke in men drinking thirty-five or more units per week.

"Lifestyle Modifications to Prevent and Control Hypertension. 3. Recommendations on Alcohol Consumption. Canadian Hypertension Society, Canadian Coalition for High Blood Pressure Prevention and Control, Laboratory Centre for Disease Control at Health Canada, Heart and Stroke Foundation of Canada"

Campbell NR; Ashley MJ; Carruthers SG; Lacourciere Y; McKay DW

CMAJ 1999 May 4; 160(9 Suppl):S13–20

This article evaluates the literature from 1966 to 1996 on the effects of alcohol consumption on blood pressure. It finds that reducing alcohol intake to two drinks per day reduces blood pressure levels in hypertensive and normotensive individuals. This level of alcohol intake was associated with the lowest overall mortality rates.

"Moderate Drinking and Cardiovascular Health"

Zakhari S; Gordis E

Proc Assoc Am Physicians 1999 Mar-Apr; 111(2):148–58

In this article moderate drinking (one to two drinks per day) is described as beneficial in reducing the risk of coronary artery disease, while avoidance of drinking is recommended for pregnant women and for individuals who are about to operate motor vehicles or heavy machinery.

"Alcohol Intake and Cardiovascular Mortality in Hypertensive Patients: Report from the Department of Health Hypertension Care Computing Project"

Palmer AJ; Fletcher AE; Bulpitt CJ; Beevers DG; Coles EC; Ledingham JG; Petrie JC; Webster J; Dollery CT

J Hypertens 1995 Sep; 13(9):957–64

This study, conducted on a cohort of 6,369 treated hypertensive individuals, shows that men drinking up to ten units of alcohol per week had the lowest overall mortality rates. Alcohol intake of more than twenty-one units per week was associated with the lowest risk of death from ischemic heart disease in men and women, and with a twofold increased risk of noncirculatory death in men.

"Alcohol and Blood Pressure: The INTERSALT Study"

Marmot MG; Elliott P; Shipley MJ; Dyer AR; Ueshima H; Beevers DG; Stamler R; Kesteloot H; Rose G; Stamler J

BMJ 1994 May 14; 308(6939):1263–67

This study shows that alcohol intake of three to four or more drinks per day, compared to nondrinking, is associated with a higher level of blood pressure in both men and women.

"Prospective Study of Moderate Alcohol Consumption and Mortality in US Male Physicians"

Camargo CA Jr; Hennekens CH; Gaziano JM; Glynn RJ; Manson JE; Stampfer MJ

Arch Intern Med 1997 Jan 13; 157(1):79–85

This study, performed on a sample population of 22,071 men, shows that alcohol intake of two to four drinks per week versus less than one per week is associated with a 28 percent reduced risk of overall mortality. Consumption of five to six drinks per week is associated with a 21 percent risk reduction; of fourteen or more drinks per week, with a 50 percent increased risk of mortality.

"Follow-up Study of Moderate Alcohol Intake and Mortality among Middle-aged Men in Shanghai, China"

Yuan JM; Ross RK; Gao YT; Henderson BE; Yu MC

BMJ 1997 Jan 4; 314(7073):18–23

This study, conducted in a sample population of 18,244 Chinese men, shows that alcohol intake up to fourteen drinks per week is associated with a 19 percent reduction in mortality from all causes, regardless of the type of alcoholic beverage. Alcohol intake up to twenty-eight drinks per week is associated with a 36 percent reduction in death from ischemic heart disease. Higher doses are significantly associated with a higher risk of death from stroke, cirrhosis, and upper aerodigestive tract tumors.

"Mortality and Light to Moderate Alcohol Consumption after Myocardial Infarction"

Muntwyler J; Hennekens CH; Buring JE; Gaziano JM

Lancet 1998 Dec 12; 352(9144):1882–85

This study, conducted in a cohort of 5,358 men with a history of myocardial infarction, shows that intake of two to four drinks per week versus abstinence is associated with a 28 percent reduction in risk of total mortality; intake of one and two or more drinks per day is associated with a 21 percent and 16 percent risk reduction, respectively.

Regular Light-to-Moderate Intake of Alcohol and the Risk of Ischemic Stroke. Is There a Beneficial Effect?

Palomaki H; Kaste M

Stroke 1993 Dec; 24(12):1828–32

This study shows that light to moderate alcohol intake (up to 150 g per week) is associated with a 46 percent reduction in risk of stroke; heavy alcohol intake (more than 300 g per week) is associated with a 4.4-fold increased risk.

"Alcohol Consumption, Serum Low Density Lipoprotein Cholesterol Concentration, and Risk of Ischaemic Heart Disease: Six Year Follow-up in the Copenhagen Male Study"

Hein HO; Suadicani P; Gyntelberg F
BMJ 1996 Mar 23; 312(7033):736–41

This study shows that the association between alcohol consumption and risk of ischemic heart disease is highly dependent on serum LDL cholesterol levels. In men with high LDL cholesterol levels, drinking up to twenty-one drinks per week or twenty-two and more drinks per week is associated with a 60 percent and 80 percent decreased risk of ischemic heart disease, respectively, compared to nondrinking. The protective effect of alcohol on the risk of ischemic heart disease is not present in men with low serum levels of LDL cholesterol.

"Insulin Sensitivity and Regular Alcohol Consumption: Large, Prospective, Cross-Sectional Population Study"

Kiechl S; Willeit J; Poewe W; Egger G; Oberhollenzer F; Muggeo M; Bonora E
BMJ 1996 Oct 26; 313(7064):1040–44

This study shows that regular light-moderate drinking decreases fasting and postglucose load plasma insulin levels and improves insulin sensitivity. These effects predict changes in risk of cardiovascular disease.

"Alcohol Consumption and Insulin Concentrations. Role of Insulin in Associations of Alcohol Intake with High-Density Lipoprotein Cholesterol and Triglycerides"

Mayer EJ; Newman B; Quesenberry CP Jr; Friedman GD; Selby JV
Circulation 1993 Nov; 88(5 Pt 1):2190–97

This study shows that light to moderate drinking is associated with decreased levels of fasting and postglucose load insulin levels, with a higher concentration of serum HDL cholesterol, and with a lower concentration of serum triglycerides. These effects may partially explain the protective effects of alcohol on the risk of cardiovascular disease.

"Alcohol Consumption and Risk of Deep Venous Thrombosis and Pulmonary Embolism in Older Persons"

Pahor M; Guralnik JM; Havlik RJ; Carbonin P; Salive ME; Ferrucci L; Corti MC; Hennekens CH
J Am Geriatr Soc 1996 Sep; 44(9):1030–37

This study, conducted on a cohort of 7,959 individuals sixty-eight or more years old, shows that, compared to nondrinkers, individuals in progressively higher tertiles of light to moderate alcohol intake had a 30, 40, and 50 percent decreased risk of deep venous thrombosis and pulmonary embolism, respectively.

"Weight, Diet, and the Risk of Symptomatic Gallstones in Middle-aged Women"

Maclure KM; Hayes KC; Coldtiz GA; Stampfer MJ; Speizer FE; Willett WC
N Engl J Med 1989 Aug 31; 321(9):563–69

This study, performed on a cohort of 88,837 women, found a sixfold increased risk of symptomatic gallstones associated with being very obese. Women who were slightly overweight had a 70 percent increased risk. High versus low energy intake doubled the risk of symptomatic gallstones, whereas alcohol intake of at least 5 grams per day versus abstinence was associated with a 40 percent risk reduction.

"Sex Differences in the Association between Alcohol Consumption and Cognitive Performance. EVA Study Group. Epidemiology of Vascular Aging"

Dufouil C; Ducimetiere P; Alperovitch A

Am J Epidemiol 1997 Sep 1; 146(5):405–12

This study shows that moderate alcohol intake improves cognitive functions in women fifty-nine to seventy-one years of age. Intake of two or more drinks per day versus nondrinking was associated with a 2.5–fold higher probability of being a high cognitive performer.

"Alcohol Consumption and Hip Fractures: The Framingham Study"

Felson DT; Kiel DP; Anderson JJ; Kannel WB

Am J Epidemiol 1988 Nov; 128(5):1102–10

This study found that men and women less than sixty-five years old had a 26 percent and 54 percent increased risk of hip fractures, respectively, associated with heavy alcohol intake (seven or more ounces per week). Past light alcohol consumption was associated with a reduced risk of fractures.

"A Prospective Study of Pancreatic Disease in Patients with Alcoholic Cirrhosis: Comparative Diagnostic Value of ERCP and EUS and Long-term Significance of Isolated Parenchymal Abnormalities"

Hastier P; Buckley MJ; Francois E; Peten EP; Dumas R; Caroli-Bosc FX; Delmont JP

Gastrointest Endosc 1999 Jun; 49(6):705–9

This study found signs of chronic pancreatitis in 19 percent of alcoholic cirrhotic patients.

"Alcohol and Mortality"

Klatsky AL; Armstrong MA; Friedman GD

Ann Intern Med 1992 Oct 15; 117(8):646–54

This study found a 60 percent increased risk of noncardiovascular mortality in heavy drinkers with intake of six or more drinks per day compared to nondrinkers. The higher risk was mainly attributable to cirrhosis, unnatural death, and tobacco-related cancers. In women, heavy drinking was associated with a 2.2–fold increased risk of overall mortality. Lighter drinkers had a 30 percent reduced risk of death from coronary artery disease, with a further reduction found in older persons.

"Prediction of Risk of Liver Disease by Alcohol Intake, Sex, and Age: A Prospective Population Study"

Becker U; Deis A; Sorensen TI; Gronbaek M; Borch-Johnsen K; Muller CF; Schnohr P; Jensen G

Hepatology 1996 May; 23(5):1025–29

This study, performed on a sample population of 13,285 individuals, shows that intake of seven to thirteen alcoholic drinks per week in women and of fourteen to twenty-seven drinks per week in men is associated with a significant higher risk of developing liver disease and cirrhosis. The risk is significantly higher in women compared to men.

"Economic Costs of Substance ABuse, 1995"

Rice DP

Proc Assoc Am Physicians 1999 Mar-Apr; 111(2):119–25

This study estimates the 1995 cost of alcohol abuse in the range of $176 billion, when healthcare expenses, lost productivity, and indirect costs are considered.

"Teratogenic Effects of Alcohol in Humans and Laboratory Animals"

Streissguth AP; Landesman-Dwyer S; Martin JC; Smith DW

Science 1980 Jul 18; 209(4454):353–61

This article reviews the teratogenic effects of alcohol intake, which range from low birthweight to fetal alcohol syndrome and mental retardation in the offspring of women with chronic alcohol intake.

"Ethanol Suppression of the Functional State of Polymorphonuclear Leukocytes Obtained from Uninfected and Simian Immunodeficiency Virus Infected Rhesus Macaques"

Stoltz DA; Zhang P; Nelson S; Bohm RP Jr; Murphey-Corb M; Bagby GJ

Alcohol Clin Exp Res 1999 May; 23(5):878–84

This study shows that polymorphonuclear leukocytes from uninfected and simian immunodeficiency virus–infected rhesus macaques, exposed in vitro to high concentration of ethanol, showed reduced phagocytic activity and expression of adhesion molecules, indicating reduced function.

"Acute Ethanol Intoxication Inhibits Neutrophil beta2-integrin Expression in Rats During Endotoxemia"

Zhang P; Bagby GJ; Xie M; Stoltz DA; Summer WR; Nelson S

Alcohol Clin Exp Res 1998 Feb; 22(1):135–41

This study shows that acute ethanol intoxication in rats is associated with decreased expression of adhesion molecules on neutrophil polymorphonuclear leukocytes, which may explain the observed defects in neutrophil recruitment into sites of infections.

"Acute Ethanol Intoxication Suppresses the Pulmonary Inflammatory Response in Rats Challenged with Intrapulmonary Endotoxin"

Zhang P; Nelson S; Summer WR; Spitzer JA

Alcohol Clin Exp Res 1997 Aug; 21(5):773–78

This study shows that acute alcohol intoxication in rats is associated with suppressed immune responses partially explained by defects in alveolar macrophage and polymorphonuclear leukocyte activities.

MOVE TO ESSENTIAL FATTY ACIDS

"Frequent Nut Consumption and Risk of Coronary Heart Disease in Women: Prospective Cohort Study"

Hu FB; Stampfer MJ; Manson JE; Rimm EB; Colditz GA; Rosner BA; Speizer FE; Hennekens CH; Willett WC

BMJ 1998 Nov 14; 317(7169):1341–45

This study, conducted on a population of 86,016 women, found that those consuming more than five ounces of nuts per week had a 39 percent decreased risk of fatal coronary heart disease and a 32 percent decreased risk of nonfatal myocardial infarction, compared to women who consumed nuts rarely (less than one ounce of nuts per month).

DANGERS OF ABDOMINAL OBESITY

"Abdominal Obesity and Its Metabolic Complications: Implications for the Risk of Ischaemic Heart Disease"

Lamarche B

Coron Artery Dis 1998; 9(8):473–81

This article reviews the epidemiological studies showing that abdominal obesity is more strongly correlated to the risk of ischemic heart disease and adult-onset diabetes than obesity per se.

"Hyperinsulinemia in Hypertension: Associations with Race, Abdominal Obesity, and Hyperlipidemia"

Spangler JG; Bell RA; Summerson JH; Konen JC

Arch Fam Med 1998 Jan-Feb; 7(1):53–56

This study shows that hypertensive patients with abdominal obesity or hyperlipidemia had a 2.7-fold increased risk of hyperinsulinemia compared to patients with hypertension alone; the combination of abdominal obesity and hyperlipidemia in hypertensive patients was associated with a fivefold increased risk of elevated serum insulin levels.

"Relationships of Abdominal Obesity and Hyperinsulinemia to Angiographically Assessed Coronary Artery Disease in Men with Known Mutations in the LDL Receptor Gene"

Gaudet D; Vohl MC; Perron P; Tremblay G; Gagné C; Lesiège D; Bergeron J; Moorjani S; Després JP.
Circulation 1998 Mar 10; 97(9):871–77

This study shows that, among patients with familial hypercholesterolemia—a condition associated with high levels of serum LDL cholesterol—those with abdominal obesity and high levels of plasma insulin had a thirteen-fold increased risk of cardiovascular disease.

"The Association of Cardiovascular Disease Risk Factors with Abdominal Obesity in Canada. Canadian Heart Health Surveys Research Group"

Reeder BA; Senthilselvan A; Després JP; Angel A; Liu L; Wang H; Rabkin SW
CMAJ 1997 Jul 1; 157 Suppl:S39–45

This study shows that, among a cohort of 16,007 individuals, those with abdominal obesity had a significantly increased risk of elevated systolic blood pressure and of high serum levels of triglycerides.

"Relationship of Glucose and Insulin Levels to the Risk of Myocardial Infarction: A Case-Control Study"

Gerstein HC; Pais P; Pogue J; Yusuf S
J Am Coll Cardiol 1999 Mar; 33(3):612–19

This study shows an increased risk of myocardial infarction associated with abdominal obesity, high serum glucose and lipids levels, hypertension, and smoking. Impaired glucose intolerance and diabetes were associated with a 4- and 5.5-fold increased risk of myocardial infarction, respectively.

"Risk Factors for Acute Myocardial Infarction in Indians: A Case-Control Study"

Pais P; Pogue J; Gerstein H; Zachariah E; Savitha D; Jayprakash S; Nayak PR; Yusuf S
Lancet 1996 Aug 10; 348(9024):358–63

This study, conducted on a cohort of 200 Indian patients with acute myocardial infarction and 200 matched controls, shows that smoking, abdominal obesity, and fasting glucose levels are strong predictors of acute myocardial infarction. Individuals with abdominal obesity had a 2.2-fold increased risk of acute myocardial infarction compared to controls. Being vegetarian was associated with a 50 percent risk reduction.

"Body Size and Colorectal-Cancer Risk"

Russo A; Franceschi S; La Vecchia C; Dal Maso L; Montella M; Conti E; Giacosa A; Falcini F; Negri E
Int J Cancer 1998 Oct 5; 78(2):161–65

This study, conducted on a sample population of 1,943 colorectal cancer cases and 4,136 controls, shows that men in the highest versus the lowest quintile of body mass index had a 70 percent increased risk of colorectal cancer. Women with abdominal obesity had a 60 percent increased risk compared to lean controls.

"Body Size and Fat Distribution as Predictors of Stroke among US Men.
Walker SP; Rimm EB; Ascherio A; Kawachi I; Stampfer MJ; Willett WC
Am J Epidemiol 1996 Dec 15; 144(12):1143–50

This study, performed on a cohort of 28,643 U.S. men, shows that those in the highest versus the lowest quintile of body mass index had a 30 percent increased risk of stroke. Being in the highest versus the lowest quintile of abdominal obesity was associated with a 2.3-fold increased risk of stroke.

"Relation of Total and Beverage-Specific Alcohol Intake to Body Mass Index and Waist-to-Hip Ratio: A Study of Self-Defense Officials in Japan
Sakurai Y; Umeda T; Shinchi K; Honjo S; Wakabayashi K; Todoroki I; Nishikawa H; Ogawa S; Katsurada M
Eur J Epidemiol 1997 Dec; 13(8):893–98

This study, performed on a sample population of 2,227 Japanese men, shows that alcohol intake is strongly associated with abdominal obesity but not with body mass index.

THE DANGERS OF CERTAIN FATS

"Estimated Effects of Reducing Dietary Saturated Fat Intake on the Incidence and Costs of Coronary Heart Disease in the United States"
Oster G; Thompson D
J Am Diet Assoc 1996 Feb; 96(2):127–31

This study estimates that a reduction in the intake of total energy from saturated fats of one to three percentage points would reduce the incidence of coronary heart disease by 32,000 to 99,700 events, with corresponding savings in medical expenses and lost earnings ranging from $4.1 to $12.7 billion over a ten-year period.

"Association of Trans Fatty Acids (Vegetable Ghee) and Clarified Butter (Indian Ghee) Intake with Higher Risk of Coronary Artery Disease in Rural and Urban Populations with Low Fat Consumption"
Singh RB; Niaz MA; Ghosh S; Beegom R; Rastogi V; Sharma JP; Dube GK
Int J Cardiol 1996 Oct 25; 56(3):289–98; discussion 299–300

This study shows that the prevalence of coronary heart disease in a sample population of 1,769 rural and 1,806 urban individuals was almost tripled in urban versus rural men and more than doubled in urban versus rural women. The prevalence of coronary heart disease was significantly associated with consumption of milk, trans fatty acids, and clarified butter in both rural and urban men and women.

"Association of Higher Saturated Fat Intake with Higher Risk of Hypertension in an Urban Population of Trivandrum in South India"

Beegom R; Singh RB

Int J Cardiol 1997 Jan 3; 58(1):63–70

This study shows that the prevalence of hypertension is significantly increased in individuals with higher saturated fat intake and body mass index, and lower consumption of fruits, vegetables, and legumes.

"Relationship between Dietary Intake and Coronary Heart Disease Mortality: Lipid Research Clinics Prevalence Follow-up Study"

Esrey KL; Joseph L; Grover SA

J Clin Epidemiol 1996 Feb; 49(2):211–16

This study shows that, in a cohort of 4,546 individuals, those thirty to fifty-nine years of age consuming a higher percentage of energy intake as saturated fats had 11 percent higher risk of dying from coronary heart disease.

"It Is More Important to Increase the Intake of Unsaturated Fats than to Decrease the Intake of Saturated Fats: Evidence from Clinical Trials Relating to Ischemic Heart Disease"

Oliver MF

Am J Clin Nutr 1997 Oct; 66(4 Suppl):980S–986S

This article reviews five secondary prevention trials in which supplementation of low-fat diets with polyunsaturated fats, particularly n-3 fatty acids, was associated with reduced mortality from coronary heart disease and from all causes.

"Association between Multiple Cardiovascular Risk Factors and Atherosclerosis in Children and Young Adults. The Bogalusa Heart Study"

Berenson GS; Srinivasan SR; Bao W; Newman WP 3rd; Tracy RE; Wattigney WA

N Engl J Med 1998 Jun 4; 338(23):1650–56

This study examines the extent of the correlation between four cardiovascular risk factors (body mass index, blood pressure, serum lipid profile, and cigarette smoking) and the presence of atherosclerosis in individuals two to thirty-nine years of age. Individuals with zero, one, two, and three or four risk factors had progressively increased percentage of aortic and coronary arteries interior surface covered with fatty streaks and collagenous fibrous plaques.

"Premenopausal Black Women Have More Risk Factors for Coronary Heart Disease than White Women"

Gerhard GT: Sexton G; Malinow MR; Wander RC; Connor SL; Pappu AS; Connor WE

Am J Cardiol 1998 Nov 1; 82(9):1040–45

This study shows that premenopausal black women have higher saturated fat and cholesterol intake; higher body mass index, blood pressure, plasma lipoprotein(a), and homocysteine levels; and a two- to three-fold increased risk of coronary heart disease compared to premenopausal white women.

"Diet and Plasma Lipids in Women. I. Macronutrients and Plasma Total and Low-Density Lipoprotein Cholesterol in Women: The Framingham Nutrition Studies"

Millen BE; Franz MM; Quatromoni PA; Gagnon DR; Sonnenberg LM; Ordovas JM; Wilson PW; Schaefer EJ; Cupples LA
J Clin Epidemiol 1996 Jun; 49(6):657–63

This study, performed on a cohort of 1,422 women, shows that plasma total and LDL cholesterol levels are directly associated with saturated fat intake.

"Association of Higher Saturated Fat Intake with Higher Risk of Hypertension in an Urban Population of Trivandrum in South India"

Beegom R; Singh RB
Int J Cardiol 1997 Jan; 58:1 63–70

This study shows that consumption of saturated fat, flesh foods, milk, yogurt, and sugar is significantly associated with the risk of hypertension.

"Dietary Fat Intake and the Risk of Coronary Heart Disease in Women"

Hu FB; Stampfer MJ; Manson JE; Rimm E; Colditz GA; Rosner BA; Hennekens CH; Willett WC
N Engl J Med 1997 Nov 20; 337(21):1491-99

This study, performed on a sample population of 80,082 women ages thirty-four to fifty-nine years, estimated that substituting 5 percent of the energy intake from saturated fat with energy from unsaturated fats would reduce the risk of coronary Heart Disease by 42 percent and that substitution of 2 percent of trans fat intake with polyunsaturated fat would lower the risk by 53 percent.

"Offspring of Normal and Diabetic Rats Fed Saturated Fat in Pregnancy Demonstrate Vascular Dysfunction"

Koukkou E; Ghosh P; Lowy C; Poston L
Circulation 1998 Dec 22–29; 98(25):2899–904

This study shows that the offspring of rats fed a diet with 30 percent of total energy intake from saturated fats during pregnancy had signs of deleterious vascular functioning as shown by blunted endothelium relaxation to acetylcholine and enhanced constrictor response to norepinephrine.

"Microalbuminuria Is Positively Associated with Usual Dietary Saturated Fat Intake and Negatively Associated with Usual Dietary Protein Intake in People with Insulin-Dependent Diabetes Mellitus"

Riley MD; Dwyer T
Am J Clin Nutr 1998 Jan; 67(1):50–57

This study shows that the prevalence of microalbuminuria, a strong predictor of renal disease and mortality in patients with diabetes, was five times higher in those with the highest versus the lowest quintile of saturated fat intake.

"Epidemiologic Analysis of Crohn Disease in Japan: Increased Dietary Intake of n-6 Polyunsaturated Fatty Acids and Animal Protein Relates to the Increased Incidence of Crohn Disease in Japan"

Shoda R; Matsueda K; Yamato S; Umeda N

Am J Clin Nutr 1996 May; 63(5):741-45

This study shows that the incidence of Crohn's disease is strongly associated with a higher consumption of dietary total fat, animal protein, milk protein, and with a higher ratio of n-6 to n-3 fatty acid intake.

"Diet and Cancer of the Prostate: A Case-Control Study in Greece"

Tzonou A; Signorello LB; Lagiou P; Wuu J; Trichopoulos D; Trichopoulou A

Int J Cancer 1999 Mar 1; 80(5):704–8

This study, performed on a sample of 320 individuals with prostate cancer and 246 controls, shows that the intake of polyunsaturated fats is positively associated with the risk of prostate cancer.

"Mediterranean Dietary Pattern in a Randomized Trial: Prolonged Survival and Possible Reduced Cancer Rate"

de Lorgeril M; Salen P; Martin JL; Monjaud I; Boucher P; Mamelle N

Arch Intern Med 1998 Jun 8; 158(11):1181–87

This study shows that patients with coronary heart disease consuming a diet rich in fruits, vegetables, cereals, and omega-3 fatty acids had a 56 percent reduction in total mortality and a 61 percent reduction in cancer incidence compared to patients following a diet close to the American Heart Association Prudent Diet.

"Essential Fatty Acids and Breast Cancer: A Case-Control Study in Uruguay"

De Stefani E; Deneo-Pellegrini H; Mendilaharsu M; Ronco A

Int J Cancer 1998 May 18; 76(4):491–94

This study, performed on 365 patients with breast cancer and 397 controls, shows that consumption of polyunsaturated fat and linoleic acid is associated with a 75 percent reduction in the risk of breast cancer. On the other hand, women in the highest versus the lowest quartile of intake of alpha-linolenic acid had an almost fourfold increase in breast cancer risk.

"Dietary Fat and Advanced Prostate Cancer"

Bairati, I; Meyer F; Fradet Y; Moore L

J Urol 1998 Apr; 159(4):1271–75

This study shows that, in a cohort of 384 individuals with prostate cancer, those with the highest intake of saturated fat had more than twice the risk of advanced prostate cancer compared to those with the lowest intake. Consumption of polyunsaturated fatty acids, linoleic acid, and vegetable fat seemed to exert a protective effect, whereas total animal fat intake was a risk factor for advanced disease.

"Dietary Fat and Lung Cancer: A Case-Control Study in Uruguay"
De Stefani E; Deneo-Pellegrini H; Mendilaharsu M; Carzoglio JC; Ronco A
Cancer Causes Control 1997 Nov; 8(6):913–21

This study shows that consumption of saturated fat increases the risk of lung adenocarcinoma more than twofold while cholesterol intake is associated with an almost threefold increase in risk of small-cell lung cancer.

"Relation between Fat Intake and Mortality: An Ecological Analysis in Belgium"
Staessen L; De Bacquer D; De Henauw S; De Backer G; Van Peteghem C
Eur J Cancer Prev 1997 Aug; 6(4):374–81

This study shows a positive association between consumption of saturated fat and mortality from all causes in men ages twenty-five to seventy-four years.

"An Ecological Study of the Correlation between Diet and Tumour Mortality Rates in Italy"
Farchi S; Saba A; Turrini A; Forlani F; Pettinelli A; D'Amicis A
Eur J Cancer Prev 1996 Apr; 5(2):113–20

This study suggests that the estimated 35 percent of cancer cases attributed to nutrition could be a conservative assessment since increasing the intake of vegetable protein by 1 gram would translate to 2.5 less cases of cancer out of 100 while an increase in intake of fiber by 1 gram would result in four less cancer cases out of 100. Increasing consumption of animal fat by 1 gram would result in 1 more cancer case out of 100.

"Iron Intake, Body Iron Stores and Colorectal Cancer Risk in Women: A Nested Case-Control Study"
Kato I; Dnistrian AM; Schwartz M; Toniolo P; Koenig K; Shore RE; Zeleniuch-Jacquotte A; Akhmedkhanov A; Riboli E
Int J Cancer 1999 Mar 1; 80(5):693–98

This study shows that individuals with high fat intake and high total iron intake have a 2.5-fold increased risk of colorectal carcinoma.

DANGERS OF A HIGH PROTEIN DIET

"The Role of Diet in the Pathogenesis and Therapy of Nephrolithiasis"
Goldfarb S
Endocrinol Metab Clin North Am 1990 Dec; 19(4):805–20

This review indicates that consumption of a high-protein diet in the Western world is possibly the most important factor in the epidemic of renal stone disease of these affluent nations.

"A Prospective Study of Dietary Calcium and Other Nutrients and the Risk of Symptomatic Kidney Stones"

Curhan GC; Willett WC; Rimm EB; Stampfer MJ
N Engl J Med 1993 Mar 25; 328(12):833–38

This study evaluates 45,619 men who had no history of kidney stones and found that a high dietary calcium intake decreases the risk of symptomatic kidney stones and that the intake of animal protein is directly associated with the risk of stone formation.

"The Influence of Diet on Urinary Risk Factors for Stones in Healthy Subjects and Idiopathic Renal Calcium Stone Formers"

Trinchieri A; Mandressi A; Luongo P; Longo G; Pisani E
Br J Urol 1991 Mar; 67(3):230–36

This study shows a significant increase in the consumption of animal and vegetable protein and purine in renal stone formers compared to controls and concludes that renal stone formers could be predisposed to stones because of their dietary habits.

"Functional Alterations in the Rat Kidney Induced Either by Diabetes or High Protein Diet"

Dunger A; Berg S; Kloting I; Schmidt S
Exp Clin Endocrinol Diabetes 1997; 105 Suppl 2:48–50

This study demonstrates that a high-protein diet causes marked alteration in kidney function and induces cellular changes in renal glomeruli comparable to those associated with diabetes mellitus. It concludes that an unbalanced high-protein diet represents a considerable risk factor for kidney damage and should absolutely be avoided in patients suffering from diseases associated with kidney alterations.

"Genetic versus Environmental Factors in Renal Stone Disease"

Jaeger P
Curr Opin Nephrol Hypertens 1996 Jul; 5(4):342–46

This review shows that renal stone formers eat more oxalate, more flesh protein, and less vegetable fibers, and have lower urine volume, than their normal counterparts.

"Renal Mass and Serum Calcitriol in Male Idiopathic Calcium Renal Stone Formers: Role of Protein Intake.

Hess B; Ackermann D; Essig M; Takkinen R; Jaeger P
J Clin Endocrinol Metab 1995 Jun; 80(6):1916–21

This study finds that overconsumption of proteins may cause an increase in renal mass and up-regulate calcitriol production in recurrent idiopathic calcium stone formers, thus causing "idiopathic" hypercalciuria.

"Prevention of Recurrent Calcium Stones: Diet versus Drugs"

Jaeger P
Miner Electrolyte Metab 1994; 20(6):410–13

This review emphasizes the role of excessive intake of meat protein, oxalate, and potentially sodium as well as insufficient intake of vegetables, fibers, calcium, and fluid as risk factors in the development of renal stones. It also highlights how, most of the time, the dietary approach to renal stone disease prevents recurrence of renal stone formation and stresses that a pharmacological approach should be reserved for refractory cases only.

"Relationship of Animal Protein-Rich Diet to Kidney Stone Formation and Calcium Metabolism"

Breslau NA; Brinkley L; Hill KD; Pak CY
J Clin Endocrinol Metab 1988 Jan; 66(1):140–46

This study shows that an animal protein diet confers an increased risk for uric acid stones formation and is a potential risk factor for the development of osteoporosis.

"Correlation between Protein and Sodium Intake and Calciuria in Calcium Lithiasis"

Jungers P; Daudon M; Hennequin C; Lacour B
Nephrologie 1993; 14(6):287–90

This study shows that hypercalciuric stone formers have a higher protein and sodium intake than normocalciurics and suggests that hypercalciuric stone formers are electively sensitive to the hypercalciuric effect of high protein intake.

"Dietary Habits of Calcium Stone Formers"

Martini LA; Heilberg IP; Cuppari L; Medeiros FA; Draibe SA; Ajzen H; Schor N
Braz J Med Biol Res 1993 Aug; 26(8):805–12

This study compares the eating habits of calcium stone formers versus healthy subjects and found that while both groups had similar consumption of nutrients during the week, the calcium stone formers had a higher consumption of animal protein during weekends.

"Acute Effects of Dietary Protein on Calcium Metabolism in Patients with Osteoporosis"

Licata AA; Bou E; Bartter FC; West F
J Gerontol 1981 Jan; 36(1):14–19

This study shows that a high-protein diet causes increased urinary calcium excretion and negative calcium balance in osteoporotic patients, and therefore potentially contributes to bone loss in this disease.

"Excess Dietary Protein Can Adversely Affect Bone"

Barzel US; Massey LK
J Nutr 1998 Jun; 128(6):1051–53

This review shows that a diet high in protein and low in fruits and vegetables generates a large amount of acid that must be excreted by the kidneys and induces bone reabsorption as compensatory mechanism to buffer the acid load. Consumption of fruits and vegetables, on the other hand, provide exogenous buffers that could halt bone reabsorption and promote bone accretion.

"Osteoporosis—A Review and Update"

Lukert BP

Arch Phys Med Rehabil 1982 Oct; 63(10):480–87

This article emphasizes prevention as the most desirable treatment for osteoporosis, and recommends consumption of adequate dietary calcium, exercise, and avoidance of excess protein and phosphorus intake.

"High Protein Diets Are Associated with Increased Bacterial Translocation in Septic Guinea Pigs"

Nelson JL; Alexander JW; Gianotti L; Chalk CL; Pyles T

Nutrition 1996 Mar; 12(3):195–99

Previous work has shown that diets low in protein (5 percent of total calories) improve survival in septic animals as compared to high-protein (20 percent) diets. This study shows that septic animals receiving high-protein diets have more bacterial translocation and suggests that a low-protein, enterally fed diet might improve survival in septic patients by decreasing the incidence of bacterial translocation.

"Motor, but Not Sensory, Cortical Potentials Are Amplified by High-Protein Diet"

Brock JW; Prasad C

Physiol Behav 1991 Nov; 50(5):887–93

This study shows that animals fed a high-protein diet are hyperactive and more responsive to nociceptive stimuli than those fed either a normal- or low-protein diet. The consumption of a high-protein diet results in increased excitability of the motor cortex.

"High Protein Intake Promotes the Growth of Hepatic Preneoplastic Foci in Fischer #344 Rats: Evidence That Early Remodeled Foci Retain the Potential for Future Growth"

Youngman LD; Campbell TC

J Nutr 1991 Sep; 121(9):1454–61

This study evaluates the effects of successive administration, withdrawal, and readministration of high-protein diets on the growth, regression, and regrowth of induced preneoplastic liver lesions. Switching from the high-protein diet to a low-protein diet resulted in marked regression of the growing lesions, and refeeding the high-protein diet caused significant reappearance of these lesions.

THE DANGERS OF MEAT

"Dioxins in U.S. Food and Estimated Daily Intake"

Schecter A; Startin J; Wright C; Kelly M; Papke O; Lis A; Ball M; Olson J

Chemosphere 1994 Nov-Dec; 29(9–11):2261–65

In this study, eighteen dairy, meat, and fish samples from a supermarket in upstate New

York were tested for presence of polychlorinated dioxins. The dioxin levels found in the samples greatly exceeded those estimated by the U.S. Environmental Protection Agency to cause one excess cancer per million people, and so did the reported dioxin levels in human breast milk and in the nursing infant.

"Health Risks of Heterocyclic Amines"

Felton JS; Malfatti MA; Knize MG; Salmon CP; Hopmans EC; Wu RW
Mutat Res 1997 May 12; 376(1–2):37–41

This study describes how broiling, frying, barbecuing, heat processing, and pyrolysis of meat produce carcinogenic heterocyclic amines. These potent mutagenic compounds have been shown to induce multiple tumors in animals. Cancer risk in humans varies according to different exposure to these compounds and genetic susceptibility, and could range between individuals more than a thousandfold.

MEAT AND COLON CANCER

"Attributable Risks for Colorectal Cancer in Northern Italy"

La Vecchia C; Ferraroni M; Mezzetti M; Enard L; Negri E; Franceschi S; Decarli A
Int J Cancer 1996 Mar 28; 66(1):60–64

The results of this study show that, in a sample population of 1,326 colorectal cancers and 2,024 controls, 43 percent of all colorectal cancers could be attributed to a low intake of vitamin C and beta-carotene, 17 percent to a high intake of red meat, 13 percent to a high frequency of meals per day, and 4 percent to a high intake of seasoning fats. Overall, more than two-thirds of all colorectal cancers could be attributed to these five dietary factors.

"Intake of Fat, Meat, and Fiber in Relation to Risk of Colon Cancer in Men"

Giovannucci E; Rimm EB; Stampfer MJ; Colditz GA; Ascherio A; Willett WC
Cancer Res 1994 May 1; 54(9):2390–97

This study, performed on a sample population of 47,949 U.S. males, shows that consumption of red meat was associated overall with a 70 percent increased risk of colon cancer. Men who consumed red meat five or more times per week, compared to those who ate it less than once per month, had a 3.6 times increased risk of cancer.

"Vegetable and Animal Products as Determinants of Colon Cancer Risk in Dutch Men and Women"

Kampman, E; Verhoeven D; Sloots L; Van 't Veer P
Cancer Causes Control 1995 May; 6(3):225–34

This study, performed on a sample population of 232 colon cancer cases and 259 controls, shows that consumption of red meat is associated with a 2.4 times increased risk of colon cancer in women and with a threefold increased risk in women with low intake of fruits and vegetables. Highest versus lowest quartile of vegetables and fruits intake, on the other hand, was associated with a 60 percent reduction in colon cancer risk in men and women.

"Food Groups and Colorectal Cancer Risk"

Levi F; Pasche C; La Vecchia C; Lucchini F; Franceschi S

Br J Cancer 1999 Mar; 79(7–8):1283–87

This study shows that intake of red meat, refined grain, and alcohol is associated with a 54, 32, and 28 percent increased risk of colorectal cancer, respectively. Whole grain, fruits, and raw vegetables were each associated with a 15 percent risk reduction, while garlic and cooked vegetables showed a 68 and 31 percent risk reduction for the highest versus the lowest tertile of intake.

"Rarity of Colon Cancer in Africans Is Associated with Low Animal Product Consumption, Not Fiber"

O'Keefe SJ; Kidd M; Espitalier-Noel G; Owira P

Am J Gastroenterol 1999 May; 94(5):1373–80

This study analyzes the relationship between dietary factors and rarity of colon cancer in black South Africans, who have a prevalence of colon cancer of less than 1 in 100,000. The risk of cancer was significantly lower in black compared to whites. Blacks were consuming a diet low in animal products and high in maize-meal content, while whites had a diet rich in animal products, cheese, and wheat. Since blacks had below RDA levels of protective factors such as fiber, vitamin A, C, folic acid, and calcium, it is likely that the very low prevalence of colon cancer in this population can be attributed to lack of aggressive factors rather than presence of protective ones.

"Lipid Peroxyl Radicals from Oxidized Oils and Heme-Iron: Implication of a High-Fat Diet in Colon Carcinogenesis"

Sawa T; Akaike T; Kida K; Fukushima Y; Takagi K; Maeda H

Cancer Epidemiol Biomarkers Prev 1998 Nov; 7(11):1007–12

This study shows that oxidized refined vegetable oils generate lipid peroxyl radicals in the presence of hemoglobin, capable of inducing DNA damage in rats. Animals fed a diet rich in fat and heme-iron compounds had significantly increased colon cancer incidence compared to rats fed a diet without hemoglobin. A possible explanation of the higher incidence of colon cancer in individuals with high intake of red meat and fat is the production of DNA-cleaving peroxyl radicals.

"Dietary Risk Factors for Colon Cancer in a Low-Risk Population"

Singh PN; Fraser GE

Am J Epidemiol 1998 Oct 15; 148(8):761–74

This study shows that individuals consuming white and red meat one or more times per week, versus those with no meat intake, had a 3.3 times and 90 percent higher risk of colon cancer, respectively. Intake of legumes more than twice a week, versus less than once, was associated with a 47 percent risk reduction. Colon cancer risk was increased by more than threefold in individuals with high meat intake and body mass and low legumes consumption.

"A Prospective Study of N-acetyltransferase Genotype, Red Meat Intake, and Risk of Colorectal Cancer"

Chen J; Stampfer MJ; Hough HL; Garcia-Closas M; Willett WC; Hennekens CH; Kelsey KT; Hunter DJ

Cancer Res 1998 Aug 1; 58(15):3307–11

The NAT1 and NAT2 genes encode for enzymes responsible for the activation of carcinogenic heterocyclic amines. This study shows that among men sixty years old or older having polymorphisms in these genes, eating one or more servings of red meat per day conferred an almost sixfold increased risk of colon cancer compared to eating half or less serving per day.

"Diet, Acetylator Phenotype, and Risk of Colorectal Neoplasia"

Roberts-Thomson IC; Ryan P; Khoo KK; Hart WJ; McMichael AJ; Butler RN
Lancet 1996 May 18; 347(9012):1372–74

This study shows that polymorphisms in the genes that encode for the enzyme N-acetyltransferase, responsible for the metabolic formation of carcinogens from cooked meat and fish, increases the risk of colon cancer from meat intake by 90 percent.

"Risk Factors for Colorectal Cancer in a Prospective Study among U.S. White Men"

Hsing AW; McLaughlin JK; Chow WH; Schuman LM; Co Chien HT; Gridley G; Bjelke E; Wacholder S; Blot WJ
Int J Cancer 1998 Aug 12; 77(4):549–53

This study, performed on a cohort of 17,633 white males, show that smoking thirty or more cigarettes per day was associated with a 2.3 times increased risk of colon cancer, drinking more than fourteen beers per month with a 90 percent increase, and eating red meat more than twice a day with an 80 percent increased risk.

"Eating Patterns and Risk of Colon Cancer"

Slattery ML; Boucher KM; Caan BJ; Potter JD; Ma KN
Am J Epidemiol 1998 Jul 1; 148(1):4–16

This study shows that the Western diet, compared to the "prudent," "high fat/sugar dairy," "substituters," or "drinkers" diet, is associated with a twofold increase in risk of colon cancer.

"Diet Diversity, Diet Composition, and Risk of Colon Cancer (United States)"

Slattery ML; Berry TD; Potter J; Caan B
Cancer Causes Control 1997 Nov; 8 (6):872–82

This study, performed on a sample population of 1,993 colon cancer cases and 2,410 controls, shows that men with a high intake of meat, fish, poultry, and eggs had a 70 percent increased risk of distal colon cancer. Women with the highest intake of fruits, vegetables, and whole grains had a 30 percent reduction in colon cancer risk.

"A Sigmoidoscopy-Based Case-Control Study of Polyps: Macronutrients, Fiber and Meat Consumption"

Haile RW; Witte JS; Longnecker MP; Probst-Hensch N; Chen MJ; Harper J; Frankl HD; Lee ER

Int J Cancer 1997 Nov 14; 73(4):497–502

This study finds a positive association between total calories intake, animal fat, saturated fat, and red meat and risk of colon adenomas, and an inverse association with vegetable proteins, carbohydrates, and fiber.

"Smoking, Alcohol Use, Dietary Factors and Risk of Small Intestinal Adenocarcinoma"

Wu AH; Yu MC; Mack TM

Int J Cancer 1997 Mar 4; 70(5):512–17

This study found a threefold increased risk of adenocarcinoma of the small bowel in heavy drinkers (80 or more grams of ethanol per day) compared to moderate or nondrinkers. Intake of fried bacon and ham, barbecued or smoked meat and smoked fish six or more times per week versus less than two times was associated with a 4.5–fold increased risk of small intestinal adenocarcinoma in men. Individuals in the medium and high tertile of sugar intake had a 2.5- and 3.8-fold increased risk, respectively.

"Risk Factors for Colorectal Cancer in Subjects with Family History of the Disease"

Fernandez E; La Vecchia C; D'Avanzo B; Negri E; Franceschi S

Br J Cancer 1997; 75(9):1381–84

This study, performed on a sample population of 1,584 colorectal cancer cases and 2,879 controls, found a 4.6- and 5.2-fold increased risk of "familial" colorectal cancer in individuals with a history of diabetes and cholelithiasis, respectively. Individuals with the highest versus the lowest intake of pasta, pastries, red meat, cheese, and butter had, respectively, a 2.5-, 2.4-, 2.9-, 3.5-, and 1.9-fold increased risk. Consumption of tomatoes, lettuce, peppers, and poultry were associated with a 60 to 70 percent decreased risk.

"Dietary Factors and Risk of Colon Cancer: A Prospective Study of 50,535 Young Norwegian Men and Women"

Gaard M; Tretli S; Loken EB

Eur J Cancer Prev 1996 Dec; 5(6):445–54

This study finds that women who ate sausages five or more times a month had a 3.5-fold increased risk of colon cancer compared to women who ate it less than once per month.

"Relationship of Food Groups and Water Intake to Colon Cancer Risk"

Shannon J; White E; Shattuck AL; Potter JD

Cancer Epidemiol Biomarkers Prev 1996 Jul; 5(7):495–502

This study, performed on cohort of 424 individuals with colon cancer and 414 controls, shows that total meat intake increases the risk of distal colon cancer in men by 2.2 times.

Women with the highest versus the lowest quartile of fruits and vegetables intake had a 52 percent reduction in risk. Cereals and water intake was also associated with a reduced risk in both sexes.

"Does Increased Endogenous Formation of N-nitroso Compounds in the Human Colon Explain the Association between Red Meat and Colon Cancer?"

Bingham SA; Pignatelli B; Pollock JR; Ellul A; Malaveille C; Gross G; Runswick S; Cummings JH; O'Neill IK

Carcinogenesis 1996 Mar; 17(3):515–23

This study shows that red meat intake produces a 3–fold increase in the formation of endogenous N-nitroso compounds in the colon. Since these alkyating agents cause a type of DNA damage that is also found in the mutated K-ras gene in colon cancer, it is possible that red meat intake could increase colon cancer incidence through formation of these carcinogenic compounds.

"Risk Factors for Colon Neoplasia—Epidemiology and Biology"

Potter JD

Eur J Cancer 1995 Jul-Aug; 31A(7–8):1033–38

This review shows that epidemiological studies have consistently reported a reduced risk of colon cancer incidence associated with plant-food intake and exercise, and an increased risk associated with elevated meat and alcohol intake.

"Physical Activity, Obesity, and Risk for Colon Cancer and Adenoma in Men"

Giovannucci E; Ascherio A; Rimm EB; Colditz GA; Stampfer MJ; Willett WC

Ann Intern Med 1995 Mar 1; 122(5):327–34

This study shows that individuals in the highest versus the lowest quintile of physical activity had a 47% reduction in colon cancer risk. A high versus low waist to hip ratio, an indicator of abdominal adiposity, was associated with a 3.4-fold increased risk.

"Alcohol, Low-Methionine—Low-Folate Diets, and Risk of Colon Cancer in Men"

Giovannucci E; Rimm EB; Ascherio A; Stampfer MJ; Colditz GA; Willett WC

J Natl Cancer Inst 1995 Feb 15; 87(4):265–73

This study, performed in a cohort of 47.931 U.S. males, shows that intake of 2 versus < or = 0.25 drinks per day, more than doubles the risk of colon cancer. The combination of high alcohol and low methionine and folate intakes was associated with a 3.3-fold increased risk of cancer of the total colon, and with a 7.4-fold increased risk of cancer of the distal colon.

"Dietary Factors and Risk of Colon Cancer"

Giovannucci E; Willett WC

Ann Med 1994 Dec; 26(6):443–52

This review presents the consistent and strong evidence collected from epidemiological studies that sedentary lifestyle, excess energy intake compared to requirements and meat consumption increase the risk of colon cancer. On the other hand, consumption of fruits and vegetables and avoidance of refined sugar appeared to exert protective effects.

Meat and Urinary Tract Cancer

"Risk Factors for Renal-Cell Cancer in Shanghai, China"

McLaughlin JK; Gao YT; Gao RN; Zheng W; Ji BT; Blot WJ; Fraumeni JF Jr
Int J Cancer 1992 Oct 21; 54(4):562–65

This study found an over 2-fold increased risk of renal-cell cancer associated with cigarette smoking; an elevated risk was also observed for increasing categories of body weight and meat consumption, while reduced risks were seen for increasing categories of fruit and vegetable intake.

"Diet and Risk of Renal Cell Cancer: A Population-Based Case-Control Study"

Lindblad P, Wolk A, Bergstrom R, Adami HO
Cancer Epidemiol Biomarkers Prev 1997 Apr; 6(4):215–23

This study found a 60% increased risk of renal cell cancer associated with frequent intake of fried and sauteed meat. Non smokers in the highest versus the lowest quartile of fruit intake had a 50 to 60 percent reduction in risk of renal cancer.

"International Renal Cell Cancer Study. VII. Role of Diet"

Wolk A; Gridley G; Niwa S; Lindblad P; McCredie M; Mellemgaard A; Mandel JS; Wahrendorf J; McLaughlin JK; Adami HO
Department of Cancer Epidemiology, University Hospital, Uppsala, Sweden

This study, performed on a sample population of 1,185 renal cell cancer cases and 1,526 controls, shows that those with the highest versus the lowest quartile of total energy intake had a 70 percent increased risk of renal cell cancer. Intake of fried meat was also associated with increased risk, while fruits and vegetables were protective.

"Protein Intake and Risk of Renal Cell Cancer"

Chow WH; Gridley G; McLaughlin JK; Mandel JS; Wacholder S; Blot WJ; Niwa S; Fraumeni JF Jr
J Natl Cancer Inst 1994 Aug 3; 86(15):1131–39

This study, performed on a cohort of 690 renal cell cancer patients and 707 controls, showed significantly increased cancer risk with increasing intake of red meat, high-protein foods, grains, breads and potatoes.

"Risk Factors for Lower Urinary Tract Cancer: The Role of Total Fluid Consumption, Nitrites and Nitrosamines, and Selected Foods"

Wilkens LR; Kadir MM; Kolonel LN; Nomura AM; Hankin JH
Cancer Epidemiol Biomarkers Prev 1996 Mar; 5(3):161–66

This study, performed on a cohort of 261 individuals with lower urinary tract cancer, shows that those in the highest versus the lowest tertile of nitrites and nitrosamines intake, had a two- and threefold increased risk of cancer, respectively. Processed meat intake was also significantly associated with increased risk.

"Bladder Cancer in a Low Risk Population: Results from the Adventist Health Study"

Mills PK; Beeson WL; Phillips RL; Fraser GE
Am J Epidemiol 1991 Feb 1; 133(3):230–39

This study, conducted in a cohort of 34,198 Seventh-Day Adventists, showed that high consumption of meat, poultry and fish was associated with a 2.6-fold increased bladder cancer risk.

"Nutrition and Bladder Cancer"

La Vecchia C; Negri E
Cancer Causes Control 1996 Jan; 7(1):95–100

This study reviews the results of seven ecological studies, six of which found a 30 to 50 percent reduction in risk of bladder cancer associated with the highest versus the lowest intake of fruits and vegetables. Three case-control studies found a 40 to 70 percent increased risk associated with the highest versus the lowest intake of total fat.

Meat and Lung Cancer

"Fatty Foods and the Risk of Lung Cancer: A Case-Control Study from Uruguay"

De Stefani E; Fontham ET; Chen V; Correa P; Deneo-Pellegrini H; Ronco A; Mendilaharsu M
Int J Cancer 1997 May 29; 71(5):760–66

This study, performed in a sample population of 377 lung cancer cases and 377 controls, showed that intake of fried foods was associated with a 54 percent increased risk of lung cancer, while dairy products and desserts were associated with an over 2.5-fold increased risk. In particular, milk products intake was associated with an over 4-fold increase in the risk of lung adenocarcinoma.

"Meat Consumption and Risk of Lung Cancer; A Case-Control Study from Uruguay"

Deneo-Pellegrini H; De Stefani E; Ronco A; Mendilaharsu M; Carzoglio JC
Lung Cancer 1996 Jun; 14(2–3):195–205

Results from this study show that red meat, beef, and fried meat are significantly associated with an increased risk of lung cancer, particularly squamous cell lung cancer.

"Estimating the Effect of Dietary Fat on the Risk of Lung Cancer in Nonsmoking Women"

Alavanja MC; Brownson RC; Benichou J
Lung Cancer 1996 Mar; 14 Suppl 1:S63–74

This study identified saturated fat consumption as the leading cause of lung cancer in non-smokers and former smokers. It was estimated that reducing the saturated fat intake levels in nonsmokers in the upper half of saturated fat intake to the levels of the ones in the lower half, would prevent 23 percent of lung cancers in this population. A further reduction in risk could be achieved by reducing the levels of saturated fat intake to the 20th percentile of consumption.

"A Case-Control Study of Diet and Lung Cancer in Kerala, South India"

Sankaranarayanan R; Varghese C; Duffy SW; Padmakumary G; Day NE; Nair MK
Int J Cancer 1994 Sep 1; 58(5):644–49

This study, performed on a cohort of 281 lung-cancer cases and selected controls, found a 68 percent reduction in risk of lung cancer associated with the highest versus the lowest quartile of fruits and vegetables intake. A predisposing effect was found with meat and dairy products intake.

"Fried, Well-Done Red Meat and Risk of Lung Cancer in Women"

Sinha R; Kulldorff M; Curtin J; Brown CC; Alavanja MC; Swanson CA
Cancer Causes Control 1998 Dec; 9(6):621–30

This study found a 50, 60, and 80 percent increase in lung cancer risk associated with fried meat, total meat, and red meat intake, respectively.

Meat and Lymphoid Cancers, Sarcomas, and Childhood Cancers

"Diet and Risk of Lymphoid Neoplasms and Soft Tissue Sarcomas"

Tavani A; Pregnolato A; Negri E; Franceschi S; Serraino D; Carbone A; La Vecchia C
Nutr Cancer 1997; 27(3):256–60

This study shows that individuals with the highest versus the lowest tertile of liver intake had a 60 and 80 percent higher risk of non-Hodgkin's lymphomas and Hodgkin's lymphomas, respectively, and a twofold increased risk of myelomas. The highest versus the lowest tertile of ham intake was associated with a 70 percent increased risk of Hodgkin's lymphomas.

"Diet and Risk of non-Hodgkin Lymphoma in Older Women"

Chiu BC; Cerhan JR; Folsom AR; Sellers TA; Kushi LH; Wallace RB; Zheng W; Potter JD
JAMA 1996 May 1; 275(17):1315–21

This study, performed on a sample population of 35,156 Iowa women, shows that those with the highest versus the lowest tertile of red meat intake had twice the risk of non-Hodgkin's lymphoma. Consumption of hamburger, in particular, was associated with a 2.3-fold increased risk. Greater intake of fruits reduced the risk by 36 percent.

"Cured and Broiled Meat Consumption in Relation to Childhood Cancer: Denver, Colorado"

Sarasua S; Savitz DA

Cancer Causes Control 1994 Mar; 5(2):141–48

In this study, performed on a cohort of 234 childhood cancer cases and 206 controls, consumption of hot dogs more than once per week by the mother was associated with a 2.3-fold increased risk of childhood brain tumors. In children, consumption of hamburgers and hot dogs more than once per week was associated with a twofold increased risk of acute lymphocytic leukemia and brain tumors. Combination of meat intake and no vitamins produced a two- to sevenfold increase in risk.

"Processed Meats and Risk of Childhood Leukemia (California, USA)"

Peters JM; Preston-Martin S; London SJ; Bowman JD; Buckley JD; Thomas DC

Cancer Causes Control 1994 Mar; 5(2):195–202

This study found that children eating twelve or more hot dogs per month have a 9.5-fold increased risk of childhood leukemia. The risk was eleven times higher for children whose fathers were in the highest category of hot-dog intake.

"Maternal Diet during Pregnancy and Risk of Brain Tumors in Children"

Bunin GR

Int J Cancer Suppl 1998; 11:23–25

This article reports several studies in which a significant association between maternal intake of cured meat and childhood brain tumors is reported.

"Maternal Consumption of Cured Meats and Vitamins in Relation to Pediatric Brain Tumors"

Preston-Martin S; Pogoda JM; Mueller BA; Holly EA; Lijinsky W; Davis RL

Cancer Epidemiol Biomarkers Prev 1996 Aug; 5(8):599–605

This study, performed on a cohort of 540 mothers of children with brain tumors and 801 controls, found that mother consumption of processed meat two or more times per day versus no intake doubled the risk of childhood brain tumors. Daily intake of vitamins throughout pregnancy was associated with a 46 percent reduction in risk.

"Dietary Carcinogens and the Risk for Glioma and Meningioma in Germany"

Boeing H; Schlehofer B; Blettner M; Wahrendorf J

Int J Cancer 1993 Feb 20; 53(4):561–65

This study found a significant association between processed meat intake and risk of glioma. In particular, a higher risk was found for ham, processed pork meat, and fried bacon.

Meat and Upper Aerodigestive Tract Cancer

"Food Groups and Risk of Oral and Pharyngeal Cancer"

Levi F; Pasche C; La Vecchia C; Lucchini F; Franceschi S; Monnier P

Int J Cancer 1998 Aug 31; 77(5):705–9

This study found an over 2–fold increase in risk of oral and pharyngeal cancer associated with frequent intake of red meat and eggs. Intake of pork and processed meat was associated with a 3.2-fold increased risk. The highest versus the lowest tertile of raw vegetables, fruits, and cooked vegetables intake was associated with a 70, 80, and 90 percent decreased risk, respectively.

"Dietary Factors and the Risk of Squamous Cell Esophageal Cancer Among Black and White Men in the United States"

Brown LM; Swanson CA; Gridley G; Swanson GM; Silverman DT; Greenberg RS; Hayes RB; Schoenberg JB; Pottern LM; Schwartz AG; Liff JM; Hoover R; Fraumeni JF Jr

Cancer Causes Control 1998 Oct; 9(5):467–74

This study found a 2.7-fold higher risk of squamous cell esophageal cancer associated with high versus low intake of red meat in blacks and a 1.5-fold higher risk in whites. High versus low intake of raw fruits and vegetables was associated with a 70 percent risk reduction in both blacks and whites. Supplementation with vitamins, especially vitamin C, conferred a 60 percent risk reduction.

"Case-Control Study on the Role of Heterocyclic Amines in the Etiology of Upper Aerodigestive Cancers in Uruguay"

De Stefani E; Ronco A; Mendilaharsu M; Deneo-Pellegrini H

Nutr Cancer 1998; 32(1):43–48

This study found a 2.8-fold increased risk of cancer of the oral cavity, pharynx, larynx, and esophagus associated with red meat intake.

"Salted Meat Consumption and the Risk of Laryngeal Cancer"

De Stefani E; Oreggia F; Rivero S; Ronco A; Fierro L

Eur J Epidemiol 1995; Apr; 11(2):177–80

In this study salted meat intake was significantly associated with increased risk of laryngeal cancer. Consumption of beef conferred a twofold increased risk.

"Diet and Squamous-Cell Cancer of the Oesophagus: A French Multicentre Case-Control Study"

Launoy G; Milan C; Day NE; Pienkowski MP; Gignoux M; Faivre J

Int J Cancer 1998 Mar 30; 76(1):7–12

This study found a strong association between butter intake and low consumption of fresh fish, fruits and vegetables, and risk of esophageal cancer. It also suggests that over one-third of the esophageal cancers in northwest France could be due to excess butter intake.

Meat and Pancreatic Cancer

"Diet, Alcohol, Coffee and Pancreatic Cancer: Final Results from an Italian Study"

Soler M; Chatenoud L; La Vecchia C; Franceschi S; Negri E

Eur J Cancer Prev 1998 Dec; 7(6):455–60

This study, performed on a sample population of 362 pancreatic cancer patients and 1,552 controls, found that meat and liver intake was associated with a 43 percent increased risk of pancreatic cancer and ham and sausages with a 64 percent increased risk. Thirty-six percent of the pancreatic cancers could be attributed to the combination of these foods items. Consumption of fresh fruit, fish, and olive oil was associated with about a 40 percent risk reduction.

"Nutrition and Pancreatic Cancer"

Howe GR; Burch JD

Cancer Causes Control 1996 Jan; 7(1):69–82

This article reports the epidemiological evidence gathered from several studies that meat, carbohydrates, and cholesterol intake is positively associated with pancreatic cancer. Consumption of fruits and vegetables, on the other hand, has consistently been associated with a risk reduction.

"Attributable Risks for Pancreatic Cancer in Northern Italy"

Fernandez E; La Vecchia C; Decarli A

Cancer Epidemiol Biomarkers Prev 1996 Jan; 5(1):23–27

This study, performed on a cohort of 362 pancreatic cancer cases and 1,408 controls, estimated that 14 percent of pancreatic cancers were attributable to smoking, 14 percent to high consumption of meat, and 12 percent to low fruit intake. Overall, these three risk factors could explain 23 percent of the pancreatic cancers in this sample population.

"Food Habits and Pancreatic Cancer: A Case-Control Study of the Francophone Community in Montreal, Canada"

Ghadirian P; Baillargeon J; Simard A; Perret C

Cancer Epidemiol Biomarkers Prev 1995 Dec; 4(8):895–99

This study found a 4-fold increased risk of pancreatic cancer associated with high consumption of salt, smoked meat, and fried food and a 2.8-fold increased risk associated with refined sugar.

"A Cohort Study of Smoking, Alcohol Consumption, and Dietary Factors for Pancreatic Cancer (United States)"

Zheng W; McLaughlin JK; Gridley G; Bjelke E; Schuman LM; Silverman DT; Wacholder, S; Co-Chien HT; Blot WJ; Fraumeni JF Jr

Cancer Causes Control 1993 Sep; 4(5):477–82

This study, performed on cohort of 17,633 U.S. men, found a fourfold increase in pancreatic cancer risk among smokers of twenty-five or more cigarettes per day compared to non-smokers and a threefold higher risk in men in the highest versus the lowest quartile of meat intake.

Meat and Prostate Cancer

"Dietary Factor and Risks for Prostate Cancer among Blacks and Whites in the United States"

Hayes RB; Ziegler RG; Gridley G; Swanson C; Greenberg RS; Swanson GM; Schoenberg JB; Silverman DT; Brown LM; Pottern LM; Liff J; Schwartz AG; Fraumeni JF Jr; Hoover RN
Cancer Epidemiol Biomarkers Prev 1999 Jan; 8(1):25–34

This study, performed on a cohort of 932 men with prostate cancer and 1,201 controls, shows that, among American blacks, those with the highest versus the lowest quartile of animal fat intake had a twofold increased risk of prostate cancer. The risk of advanced prostate cancer was three to four times higher in blacks and whites in the highest quartile of animal fat intake.

"What Causes Prostate Cancer? A Brief Summary of the Epidemiology"

Chan JM; Stampfer MJ; Giovannucci EL
Semin Cancer Biol 1998 Aug; 8(4):263–73

In this article, consumption of meat, fat, and dairy products was associated with a higher risk of prostate cancer; selenium, vitamin E, fruits, and tomatoes conferred protection.

"Dietary Fat Intake and Risk of Prostate Cancer: A Prospective Study of 25,708 Norwegian Men"

Veierod MB; Laake P; Thelle DS
Int J Cancer 1997 Nov 27; 73(5):634–38

This study, performed on a cohort of 25,708 men sixteen to fifty-five years old, found an increased risk of prostate cancer associated with high body mass index and hamburger/meatballs intake.

"An Ecological Study of Trends in Cancer Incidence and Dietary Changes in Hong Kong"

Koo LC; Mang OW; Ho JH
Nutr Cancer 1997; 28(3):289–301

This article presents the results from six government surveys showing that high meat intake significantly increases the risk of colon, rectal, prostate, and breast cancer.

"A Case-Control Study of Cancer of the Prostate in Somerset and East Devon"

Ewings P; Bowie C
Br J Cancer 1996 Aug; 74(4):661–66

The results of this study show an increasing risk of prostate cancer associated with increasing levels of meat intake.

"Prospective Study of Plasma Fatty Acids and Risk of Prostate Cancer"

Gann PH; Hennekens CH; Sacks FM; Grodstein F; Giovannucci EL; Stampfer MJ

J Natl Cancer Inst 1994 Feb 16; 86(4):281–86

This study shows that intake of alpha-linolenic acid, an indicator of red meat and butter intake, is associated with a 2- to 3.5-fold increased risk of prostate cancer. Eating meat five or more times per week versus less than once per week conferred a 2.5-fold increased risk of prostate cancer.

Meat and Stomach Cancer

"Dietary Factors and the Risk of Gastric Cancer in Mexico City"

Ward MH; Lopez-Carrillo L

Am J Epidemiol 1999 May 15; 149(10):925–32

This study shows a threefold increased risk of gastric cancer associated with a high intake of fresh or processed meat. Dairy products and fish consumption conferred an over twofold greater risk.

"Risk of Adenocarcinoma of the Stomach and Esophagus with Meat Cooking Method and Doneness Preference"

Ward MH; Sinha R; Heineman EF; Rothman N; Markin R; Weisenburger DD; Correa P; Zahm SH

Int J Cancer 1997 Mar 28; 71(1):14–19

This study shows an increased risk of stomach and esophageal cancer associated with high intake of red meat, especially barbecued and grilled. Medium and well-done meat versus rare/medium rare was associated with a 2.4- and 3.3-fold increased risk, respectively.

Meat and Gynecologic Cancer

"Dietary Factors and Breast Cancer Risk in Vaud, Switzerland"

Levi F; La Vecchia C; Gulie C; Negri E

Nutr Cancer 1993; 19(3):327–35

This study shows a 2-fold increased risk of breast cancer associated with consumption of meat. Cheese intake was associated with a 2.7-fold increased risk. On the other hand, women in the highest versus the lowest tertile of total green vegetable intake had a 40 to 60 percent reduction in breast cancer risk.

"Meat Intake, Heterocyclic Amines, and Risk of Breast Cancer: A Case-Control Study in Uruguay"

De Stefani E; Ronco A; Mendilaharsu M; Guidobono M; Deneo-Pellegrini H
Cancer Epidemiol Biomarkers Prev 1997 Aug; 6(8):573–81

This case-control study found a strong association between the intake of red meat and heterocyclic amine (chemicals formed during the cooking process) and the risk of breast cancer. Individuals in the highest quartile of heterocyclic amine intake had a 3.3-fold increased risk of cancer.

"A Comparison of Food Habit and Food Frequency Data as Predictors of Breast Cancer in the NHANES I/NHEFS Cohort"

Byrne C; Ursin G; Ziegler RG
J Nutr 1996 Nov; 126(11):2757–64

This study assesses the relationship between eating habits and breast cancer incidence in a cohort of 6,156 women aged thirty-two to eighty-six years. Intake of salad dressings other than low fat, eating poultry with the skin, and eating beef other than lean were associated with a 30 percent, 70 percent, and 2.2-fold increased risk of breast cancer, respectively.

"Meat, Fat and Risk of Breast Cancer: A Case-Control Study from Uruguay"

Ronco A; De Stefani E; Mendilaharsu M; Deneo-Pellegrini H
Int J Cancer 1996 Jan 26; 65(3):328–31

This study finds that women in the highest versus the lowest quartile of meat intake had an over fourfold increased risk of breast cancer.

"Nutritional, Socioeconomic, and Reproductive Factors in Relation to Female Breast Cancer Mortality: Findings from a Cross-National Study"

Herbert JR; Rosen A
Cancer Detect Prev 1996; 20(3):234–44

In this study, intake of animal products was the strongest predictor of breast cancer mortality. Consumption of fish and cereals was shown to exert protective effects.

"Dietary Fat and the Risk of Breast Cancer: A Prospective Study of 25,892 Norwegian Women"

Gaard M; Tretli S; Loken EB
Int J Cancer 1995 Sep 27; 63(1):13–17

This study, performed on a sample population of 25,892 Norwegian women, shows that those eating meat more than five times per week had a two- to fourfold increased risk of breast cancer compared to those eating meat two or less times per week. Drinking 0.75 liters of milk versus 0.15 or less was associated with an almost threefold increased risk.

"Diet and the Risk of Breast Cancer in Spain"

Landa MC; Frago N; Tres A

Eur J Cancer Prev 1994 Jul; 3(4):313–20

This study, performed on a cohort of 100 women with breast cancer and 100 controls, finds a 3.2-fold increased risk of breast cancer in women in the highest versus the lowest tertile of processed meat intake and a 3.8 times higher risk in women in the lowest tertile of fruit intake.

"Consumption of Meat, Animal Products, Protein, and Fat and Risk of Breast Cancer: A Prospective Cohort Study in New York"

Toniolo P; Riboli E; Shore RE; Pasternack BS

Epidemiology 1994 Jul; 5(4):391–97

This study finds that, among a cohort of 14,291 New York City women, those in the upper versus the lower quintile of meat intake had a 90 percent increased risk of breast cancer.

"The Effect of Dietary Exposures on Recurrence and Mortality in Early Stage Breast Cancer"

JR, Hurley TG; Ma Y

Breast Cancer Res Treat 1998 Sep; 51(1):17–28

This study shows an over 60 percent increased risk of breast cancer recurrence and mortality in women with high intake of butter, margarine, and lard. The risk almost doubled with each increase in daily serving of red meat, liver, and bacon.

"Well-Done Meat Intake and the Risk of Breast Cancer"

Zheng W; Gustafson DR; Sinha R; Cerhan JR; Moore D; Hong CP; Anderson KE; Kushi LH; Sellers TA; Folsom AR

J Natl Cancer Inst 1998 Nov 18; 90(22):1724–29

This study finds an increased risk of breast cancer associated with increasing doneness level of meat consumed. Very well done versus rare or medium done hamburger and bacon were associated with a 54 and 64 percent increased risk of breast cancer respectively; very well done beef steak was associated with a 50 percent increased risk.

"Mammary Gland Carcinogenicity of 2-amino-1-methyl-6-phenylimidazo [4,5-b]Pyridine in Sprague-Dawley Rats on High- and Low-Fat Diets"

Snyderwine EG; Thorgeirsson UP; Venugopal M; Roberts-Thomson SJ

Nutr Cancer 1998; 31(3):160–67

This study shows that 45 percent and 24 percent of the rats fed a high- and low-fat diet, respectively, developed mammary tumors when treated with a carcinogenic heterocyclic amine derived from cooked meat, thus suggesting that a high-fat diet increases the tumorigenicity of heterocyclic carcinogenic amine.

"Intake of Fried Meat and Risk of Cancer: A Follow-up Study in Finland"

Knekt P; Steineck G; Jarvinen R; Hakulinen T; Aromaa A

Int J Cancer 1994 Dec 15; 59(6):756–60

In this study, performed on a cohort of 9,990 Finnish men and women, women in the highest versus the lowest tertile of fried meat intake had an 80 percent increased risk of endometrial, ovarian, and breast cancer.

"A Population-Based Case-Control Study of Dietary Factors and Endometrial Cancer in Shanghai, People's Republic of China"

Shu XO; Zheng W; Potischman N; Brinton LA; Hatch MC; Gao YT; Fraumeni JF Jr

Am J Epidemiol 1993 Jan 15; 137(2):155–65

This study shows a 3.5-fold increased risk of developing endometrial cancer associated with animal fat consumption; consumption of animal protein conferred a 3-fold increased risk of endometrial cancer. The association between fat and protein and risk of endometrial cancer was restricted to foods of animal origin in the diet.

"Dietary Intake of Energy and Animal Foods and Endometrial Cancer Incidence. The Iowa Women's Health Study"

Zheng W; Kushi LH; Potter JD; Sellers TA; Doyle TJ; Bostick RM; Folsom AR

Am J Epidemiol 1995 Aug 15; 142(4):388–94

This study, performed on a cohort of 23,000 postmenopausal Iowa women, finds a 50 percent increased risk of endometrial cancer in those in the highest versus the lowest intake of processed meat and fish.

"Diet, Body Size, Physical Activity, and the Risk of Endometrial Cancer"

Goodman MT; Hankin JH; Wilkens LR; Lyu LC; McDuffie K; Liu LQ; Kolonel LN

Cancer Res 1997 Nov 15; 57(22):5077–85

This case-control study shows that women in the highest quartile of body mass index had a fourfold increased risk of endometrial cancer compared to women in the lowest quartile. High intake of fat was associated with a 60 percent increased risk whereas consumption of fruits and vegetables conferred protection.

"Dietary Factors and Epithelial Ovarian Cancer"

Shu XO, Gao YT, Yuan JM, Ziegler RG, Brinton LA

Br J Cancer 1989 Jan; 59(1):92–96

This study found an 80 percent increased risk of ovarian cancer associated with the highest versus the lowest quartile of animal fat intake. Consumption of vegetable fat was not related to the risk of ovarian cancer.

"Selected Food Intake and Risk of Vulvar Cancer"

Parazzini F; Moroni S; Negri E; La Vecchia C; Dal Pino D; Cavalleri E

Cancer 1995 Dec 1; 76(11):2291–96

This study finds an inverse association between vegetable intake and risk of vulvar cancer. On the other hand, increasing levels of body mass index were associated with increasing risk, with women in the highest quartile of body mass having a threefold increased risk of vulvar cancer.

Meat and Heart Disease

"The Medical Costs Attributable to Meat Consumption"

Barnard ND; Nicholson A; Howard JL

Prev Med 1995 Nov; 24(6):646–55

This study analyzes the prevalence of diseases in omnivorous compared to vegetarians, as reported from published controlled trials. The computed 1992 healthcare costs attributable to meat intake were in the range of $28.6 to $61.4 billion, this amount deriving from an estimated cost of $2.8 to $8.5 billion for hypertension, $9.5 billion for heart disease, $16.5 billion for cancer, $14.0 to $17.1 billion for diabetes, $0.2 to $2.4 billion for gallbladder disease, $1.9 billion for obesity-related musculoskeletal disorders, and $0.25 to $5.5 billion for foodborne illness.

"Risk of Death from Cancer and Ischaemic Heart Disease in Meat and Non-Meat Eaters"

Thorogood M; Mann J; Appleby P; McPherson K

BMJ 1994 Jun 25; 308(6945):1667–70

This study estimates the mortality ratio for ischemic heart disease and cancer in a cohort of 6,115 vegetarians and 5,015 omnivores. Vegetarians had 28 percent less deaths from ischemic heart disease and 39 percent less deaths from cancer, compared to omnivores.

"A Multi-State Survey of Consumer Food-Handling and Food-Consumption Practices"

Altekruse SF; Yang S; Timbo BB; Angulo FJ

Food and Drug Administration, Center for Food Safety and Applied Nutrition, Washington, DC, USA

In this study, 19,356 individuals from eight states were interviewed to assess the correctness of food-handling practices. Nineteen percent of respondents failed to wash hands and cutting boards properly after contact with raw meat. Changes in these practices would reduce the likelihood of foodborne infections, estimated to cause 6.5 to 33 million illnesses a year.

THE DANGERS OF MILK

"Adolescent Milk, Dairy Product and Fruit Consumption and Testicular Cancer"

Davies TW; Palmer CR; Ruja E; Lipscombe JM

Br J Cancer 1996 Aug; 74(4):657–60

This study finds that milk consumption during adolescence was significantly higher in men with testicular cancer compared to healthy controls. Each extra quarter pint of milk consumed by cases versus controls increased the risk of testicular cancer by 39 percent.

"Dietary Factors and Lung Cancer among Men in West Sweden"

Axelsson G; Liljeqvist T; Anderson L; Bergman B; Rylander R
Int J Epidemiol 1996 Feb; 25(1):32–39

This study shows that individuals consuming high quantities of milk have a 73 percent increase in risk of lung cancer. On the other hand, people with the highest intake of vegetables had 63 percent less risk of lung cancer.

"Dietary Factors and Risk of Lung Cancer in Never-Smokers"

Nyberg F; Agrenius V; Svartengren K; Svensson C; Pershagen G
Int J Cancer 1998 Nov 9; 78(4):430–36

This study finds that cultured milk products are associated with a twofold increased risk of lung cancer in both genders, while milk intake is positively associated with lung cancer in men.

"Lung Cancer, Smoking and Diet among Swedish Men"

Rylander R; Axelsson G; Andersson L; Liljequist T; Bergman B
Lung Cancer 1996 Mar; 14 Suppl:S75–83

This study shows that milk intake is associated with increased risk of lung cancer in both smokers and non-smokers, while vegetable intake is inversely associated with it.

"Review of the Evidence for an Association between Infant Feeding and Childhood Cancer"

Davis MK
Int J Cancer 1998; Suppl:29–33

This article reviews the results of nine published case-control studies and finds an increased risk of Hodgkin's disease in children never breast-fed or breast-fed for short term compared to children breast-fed for six or more months.

"Diet and Risk of Lymphoid Neoplasms and Soft Tissue Sarcomas"

Tavani A; Pregnolato A; Negri E; Franceschi S; Serraino D; Carbone A; La Vecchia C
Nutr Cancer 1997; 27(3):256–60

This study shows that individuals with the highest versus the lowest tertile of milk intake had an 80 percent higher risk of non-Hodgkin's lymphomas and a 90 percent increased risk of sarcomas. Intake of ham was associated with a 70 percent increased risk of Hodgkin's lymphomas and intake of butter with a 2.8-fold increased risk of myelomas. Consumption of green vegetable and whole grains gave a 60 percent reduction in risk of myelomas and non-Hodgkin's lymphomas, respectively.

"Dietary Risk Factors for Renal Cell Carcinoma in Denmark"

Mellemgaard A; McLaughlin JK; Overvad K; Olsen JH

Eur J Cancer 1996 Apr; 32A(4):673–82

This study shows that women in the highest quartile of total energy intake, fat intake, and carbohydrates intake had a threefold increased risk of renal cell cancer compared to women in the lowest quartile. Women drinking more than one glass of milk per day compared to those who never drank it had a 3.7 times increased risk, while the risk in women using thickly spread versus thinly spread butter was eleven times higher. For men, the association between renal cell cancer and total energy intake and fat intake was weaker but still present, with a 70 percent and 90 percent increased risk associated with the highest quartile of total energy and fat intake, respectively.

"Fermented Milk Products Are Associated to Ulcer Disease. Results from a Cross-Sectional Population Study"

Elmståhl S; Svensson U; Berglund G

Eur J Clin Nutr 1998 Sep; 52(9):668–74

This study shows that a high intake of milk, meat, bread, and total fat is associated with an increased risk of peptic ulcer, whereas fermented milk products and vegetable are associated with decreased risk.

"Milk and Other Dietary Influences on Coronary Heart Disease"

Grant WB

Altern Med Rev 1998 Aug; 3(4):281–94

Results from this study, which used a statistical approach involving thirty-two countries, show that the highest statistical association between dietary factors and ischemic heart disease was found for milk in men aged thirty-five years or more and in women aged sixty-five years or more, and for sugar in women thirty-five to sixty-four years of age.

"Intolerance of Cow's Milk and Chronic Constipation in Children"

Iacono G; Cavataio F; Montalto G; Florena A; Tumminello M; Soresi M; Notarbartolo A; Carroccio A

N Engl J Med 1998 Oct 15; 339(16):1100–4

This study shows that 68 percent of children suffering from chronic constipation and severe perianal lesions who undertook a two-week period of cow's milk withdrawal and soy milk replacement responded with resolution of the constipation and of the lesions.

"Five-Year Follow-up of High-Risk Infants with Family History of Allergy Who Were Exclusively Breast-Fed or Fed Partial Whey Hydrolysate, Soy, and Conventional Cow's Milk Formulas

Chandra RK

J Pediatr Gastroenterol Nutr 1997 Apr; 24(4):380–88

This study shows that infants who were breast-fed or who received a whey hydrolysate formula had a 58 and 68 percent lower incidence of eczema and asthma, respectively, compared to children fed with a conventional cow's milk formula.

"Persistent Cow's Milk Protein Intolerance in Infants: The Changing Faces of the Same Disease"

Iacono G; Cavataio F; Montalto G; Soresi M; Notarbartolo A; Carroccio A

Clin Exp Allergy 1998 Jul; 28(7):817–23

This study shows that children with persistent cow's milk protein intolerance had increased frequency of constipation, wheezing, multiple food intolerance, and allergic disease such as asthma, rhinitis, and eczema.

"Cell-Mediated Immune Response to Beta Casein in Recent-Onset Insulin-Dependent Diabetes: Implications for Disease Pathogenesis"

Cavallo MG; Fava D; Monetini L; Barone F; Pozzilli P

Lancet 1996 Oct 5; 348(9032):926–28

In this study, 51 percent of patients with insulin-dependent diabetes showed proliferation of a specific clone of T lymphocytes in response to beta-casein, a protein present in cow's milk. Such a response was seen in only 2.7 percent of healthy individuals. These results suggest that early exposure to cow's milk generates clones of T lymphocytes that may cross-react with an antigen present on the surface of pancreatic beta cells.

"Breastfeeding and Incidence of Non-Insulin-Dependent Diabetes Mellitus in Pima Indians"

Pettitt DJ; Forman MR; Hanson RL; Knowler WC; Bennett PH

Lancet 1997 Jul 19; 350(9072):166–68

This study shows that, in a population with high prevalence of subsequent non-insulin-dependent diabetes mellitus, exclusive breast-feeding in the first two months of life versus exclusive bottle-feeding reduces the risk of diabetes by 59 percent. These results suggest that the increasing prevalence of non-insulin-dependent diabetes in certain populations may be due to an increase in bottle-feeding practice.

"Cow's Milk Consumption, Disease-Associated Autoantibodies and Type 1 Diabetes Mellitus: A Follow-up Study in Siblings of Diabetic Children. Childhood Diabetes in Finland Study Group"

Virtanen SM; Hyppönen E; Läärä E; Vähäsalo P; Kulmala P; Savola K; Räsänen L; Aro A; Knip M; Akerblom HK

Diabet Med 1998 Sep; 15(9):730–38

This study shows that drinking three or more glasses of milk per day is associated with an approximately fourfold increased risk of developing autoantibodies associated with insulin-dependent diabetes mellitus.

"Relation between Antibodies to Islet Cell Antigens, Other Autoantigens and Cow's Milk Proteins in Diabetic Children and Unaffected Siblings at the Clinical Manifestation of IDDM. The Childhood Diabetes in Finland Study Group"

Vähäsalo P; Petäys T; Knip M; Miettinen A; Saukkonen T; Karjalainen J; Savilahti E; Akerblom HK

Autoimmunity 1996; 23(3):165–74

This study shows increased levels of antibodies against cow's milk proteins in siblings of diabetic children who were positive for islet cell antibodies, a marker of pancreatic beta-cells destruction.

"IDDM and Milk Consumption. A Case-Control Study in São Paulo, Brazil"

Gimeno SG; de Souza JM

Diabetes Care 1997 Aug; 20(8):1256–60

This study shows that a shorter time of exclusive breast-feeding and intake of cow's milk products before age eight days are associated with a higher risk of developing insulin-dependent diabetes mellitus.

"Rodent Malaria in Rats Exacerbated by Milk Protein, Attenuated by Low-Protein Vegetable Diet"

van Doorne CW; Eling WM; Luyken R

Trop Med Int Health 1998 Jul; 3(7):596–600

This study shows that rats with induced malaria and fed a diet enriched with milk protein showed increased weight gain, parasitemia, paralysis, and mortality compared to rats fed a milk protein-free diet.

"Investigation of Multidrug-Resistant Salmonella Serotype Typhimurium DT104 Infections Linked to Raw-Milk Cheese in Washington State"

Villar RG; Macek MD; Simons S; Hayes PS; Godoft MJ; Lewis JH; Rowan LL; Hursh D; Patnode M; Mead PS

JAMA 1999 May 19; 281(19):1811–16

This study investigates the reason of the fivefold increase in salmonellosis reported in a Hispanic population living in Washington State. In four months, fifty-four confirmed cases of salmonellosis were reported. Nine percent of patients, whose median age was four years, were hospitalized. Seventy-seven percent of patients had eaten unpasteurized milk products that revealed contamination by a multidrug-resistant strain of Salmonella typhimurium.

"A Prolonged Outbreak of Escherichia coli O157:H7 Infections Caused by Commercially Distributed Raw Milk"

Keene WE; Hedberg K; Herriott DE; Hancock DD; McKay RW; Barrett TJ; Fleming DW

J Infect Dis 1997 Sep; 176(3):815–18

This article reports an outbreak caused by ingestion of raw milk contaminated by Escherichia coli O157:H7 in Oregon. The infections continued from December 1992 until June 1994, and their pattern of occurrence was intermittent and unpredictable.

"A Milk-Borne Campylobacter Outbreak Following an Educational Farm Visit"

Evans MR; Roberts RJ; Ribeiro CD; Gardner D; Kembrey D

Epidemiol Infect 1996 Dec; 117(3):457–62

This article reports on an outbreak of gastrointestinal infections involving 53 percent of children and 23 percent of adults on an educational farm visit. The source of the infection was found in the contamination of milk by *Campylobacter jejuni.*

"The Epidemiology of Raw Milk-Associated Foodborne Disease Outbreaks Reported in the United States, 1973 through 1992"

Headrick ML; Korangy S; Bean NH; Angulo FJ; Altekruse SF; Potter ME; Klontz KC
Am J Public Health 1998 Aug; 88(8):1219–21

This article describes forty-six raw milk-associated outbreaks reported to the Centers for Disease Control and Prevention from 1973 through 1992.

"General Outbreaks of Infectious Intestinal Disease Associated with Milk and Dairy Products in England and Wales: 1992 to 1996"

Djuretic T; Wall PG; Nichols G
Commun Dis Rep CDR Rev 1997 Mar 7; 7(3):R41–45

This article reports twenty outbreaks of food-poisoning associated with intake of milk and milk products reported to the PHLS Communicable Disease Surveillance Centre in England and Wales between 1992 and 1996, which caused a total of 600 illnesses and at least 45 hospital admissions.

"An Outbreak of Gastroenteritis and Fever Due to Listeria Monocytogenes in Milk"

Dalton CB; Austin CC; Sobel J; Hayes PS; Bibb WF; Graves LM; Swaminathan B; Proctor ME; Griffin PM
N Engl J Med 1997 Jan 9; 336(2):100–5

This study describes the identified source of an outbreak of gastroenteritis and fever due to contamination of chocolate milk with Listeria monocytogenes. Forty-five people became ill and four were hospitalized.

"Human Exposure to Mycobacterium paratuberculosis via Pasteurised Milk: A Modelling Approach"

Nauta MJ; van der Giessen JW
Vet Rec 1998 Sep 12; 143(11):293–96

This articles explains how people consuming pasteurized milk may be exposed to infection with *Mycobacterium paratuberculosis,* which is commonly shed in the milk of infected cattle. According to the suggested association between this bacterium and Crohn's disease, they may be at increased risk for this disease.

"Mycobacterium paratuberculosis: A Potential Food-Borne Pathogen?"

Collins MT
J Dairy Sci 1997 Dec; 80(12):3445–48

This article describes how cattle infection with *Mycobacterium paratuberculosis* is a relatively common event and leads to shedding of the bacterium in the feces and milk where the organism, due to its thermal resistance, may be able to survive pasteurization.

DANGERS OF PESTICIDES

"The Export of Pesticides: Shipments from U.S. Ports, 1995–1996"

Smith C., Root D

Int J Occup Environ Health 1999 Apr-Jun; 5(2):141–50

This study reports that in 1995–1996, the United States exported to developing countries forty-eight million pounds (24,000 tons) of extremely toxic pesticides and twenty-one million pounds (fourteen tons per day) of pesticides that were domestically banned or never registered.

"The History of DBCP from a Judicial Perspective"

Siegel CS; Siegel DS

Int J Occup Environ Health 1999 Apr-Jun; 5(2):127–35

This study discusses the lawsuit against U.S. manufacturers and corporate users of 1,2-di-bromo-3-chloropropane (DBCP), filed by more than 26,000 workers who were damaged by exposure to this chemical.

"The Toxicology of 1,2-dibromo-3-chloropropane (DBCP): A Brief Review"

Teitelbaum DT

Int J Occup Environ Health 1999 Apr-Jun; 5(2):122–26

This article reviews the toxicity profile of 1,2-dibromo-3-chloropropane (DBCP), a widely used nematocide. Toxicity includes male infertility; adverse effects on the female reproductive system; depressed respiratory, hepatic, and renal function; depressed central nervous system activity; skin and ocular irritation; and, presumably, carcinogenicity.

"Azoospermia and Oligospermia among a Large Cohort of DBCP Applicators in 12 Countries"

Slutsky M; Levin JL; Levy BS

Int J Occup Environ Health 1999 Apr-Jun; 5(2):116–22

This article shows that, among a cohort of 26,400 workers on banana and pineapple plantations from twelve developing countries, 64.3 percent of all men and 90.1 percent of those from Philippines who were exposed for a median of three years to 1,2-dibromo-3-chloropropane (DBCP) developed azo- or oligospermia. Of these men, 28.5 percent had no children.

"Sterilization of Workers from Pesticide Exposure: The Causes and Consequences of DBCP-Induced Damage in Costa Rica and Beyond"

Thrupp LA

Int J Health Serv 1991; 21(4):731–57

This article discusses the lawsuit presented by approximately 1,500 banana plantation workers in Costa Rica who became sterile after exposure to the nematicide DBCP. The manufacturers concealed the experimental evidence of toxicity to the reproductive system and continued to utilize the chemical in developing countries.

"Pentachlorophenol Exposure in Women with Gynecological and Endocrine Dysfunction"

Gerhard I; Frick A; Monga B; Runnebaum B

Environ Res 1999 May; 80(4):383–88

This study, performed on a cohort of 171 women with gynecological problems, found a significant association between exposure to the pesticide pentachlorophenol (PCP), detected in sixty-five women, and presence of mild ovarian and adrenal insufficiency, suggesting a role for this chemical in fertility problems.

"Pentachlorophenol Concentrations in Human Cerebrospinal Fluid"

Jorens PG; Janssens JJ; van Tichelen WI; van Paesschen W; de Deyn PP; Schepens PJ

Neurotoxicology 1991 Spring; 12(1):1–7

This study reports the finding of substantial concentrations of pentachlorophenol (PCP), a pesticide widely used in wood preservation, in the cerebrospinal fluid of sixteen patients with neurological symptoms.

"Association between Renal Function Tests and Pentachlorophenol Exposure"

Begley J; Reichert EL; Rashad MN; Klemmer HW

Clin Toxicol 1977; 11(1):97–106

In this study, analysis of urine and blood samples from eighteen workers at a wood treatment plant exposed to pentachlorophenol (PCP) revealed that serum concentrations of PCP were positively associated with reduced kidney function.

"Non-Occupational Exposure to Pentachlorophenol: Clinical Findings and Plasma-PCP-Concentrations in Three Families"

Sangster B; Wegman RC; Hofstee AW

Hum Toxicol 1982 Mar; 1(2):123–33

This study finds high levels of pentachlorophenol (PCP) in the blood of the members of three families who were exposed to large amounts of this pesticide in their household. Three people showed signs of local toxicity manifested by burning painful sensation, erythema, dryness, and scaling.

"Pentachlorophenol, An Assessment of the Occupational Hazard"

Williams PL

Am Ind Hyg Assoc J 1982 Nov; 43(11):799–810

This study presents the fetotoxic and teratogenic properties of pentachlorophenol (PCP). By uncoupling mitochondrial oxidative phosphorylation, PCP can induce local or systemic toxicity. In addition, chemical contaminants of PCP in commercial preparations can cause chloracne and chronic liver damage.

"Aplastic Anemia and Red Cell Aplasia Due to Pentachlorophenol"

Roberts HJ

South Med J 1983 Jan; 76(1):45–48

This study reports the occurrence of aplastic anemia and pure red cell aplasia in four and two patients, respectively, exposed to pentachlorophenol (PCP). In two patients the blood disorder evolved in Hodgkin's lymphoma and acute leukemia.

"Human Pentachlorophenol Poisoning"

Jorens PG; Schepens PJ

Hum Exp Toxicol 1993 Nov; 12(6):479–95

This study describes the toxicological profile of pentachlorophenol (PCP), one of the most frequently used fungicides and pesticides. Signs of chronic intoxication include: dermatological toxicity, fever, hematopoietic disorders, respiratory and central and peripheral nervous system depression, renal dysfunction, and gastrointestinal toxicity. Exposure to PCP has been linked to higher risk of nasal carcinoma and soft tissue sarcoma, which may be due to the contaminants present in PCP preparations.

"Pentachlorophenol-Associated Aplastic Anemia, Red Cell Aplasia, Leukemia and Other Blood Disorders"

Roberts HJ

J Fla Med Assoc 1990 Feb; 77(2):86–90

This article discusses the potential mutagenic and carcinogenic effects of the pesticide pentachlorophenol (PCP). Exposure to products containing PCP has been associated, after several decades of latency, with the development of hematologic disorders such as aplastic anemia, pure red cell aplasia, leukemia, and lymphoma.

"Pentachlorophenol Carcinogenicity: Extrapolation of Risk from Mice to Humans"

Reigner BG; Bois FY; Tozer TN

Hum Exp Toxicol 1993 May; 12(3):215–25

This article discusses the potential public health hazard caused by the widespread use of pentachlorophenol (PCP). PCP has been shown to induce tumors in mice. When extrapolating the toxicity data from mice to humans, the authors found that the average daily exposure to PCP in humans is several times higher than the estimated safe levels, indicating that the extra risk of cancer for lifetime exposure is 20 to 140 times higher than the acceptable extra risk.

"Selected Incidents of Illnesses and Injuries Related to Exposure to Pesticides Reported by Physicians in California in 1986"

Maddy KT; Edmiston S

Vet Hum Toxicol 1988 Jun; 30(3):246–54

This article presents data on severe pesticide-related cases—defined as those involving death, hospitalization for more than twenty-four hours, or cases where five or more people at once became ill after exposure to pesticides—reported to local agencies in California in 1986. There were 67 reported incidents involving 583 people. Of these, 38 percent occurred after indoors pesticide exposure.

"Pesticides and Childhood Cancers"

Daniels JL; Olshan AF; Savitz DA

Environ Health Perspect 1997 Oct; 105(10):1068–77

This article presents evidence, gathered from epidemiologic studies, of a strong association between pesticide exposure and childhood leukemia, brain cancer, Wilms' tumor, Ewing's sarcoma, and germ-cell tumors.

"Pesticides and Non-Hodgkin's Lymphoma"

Zahm SH; Blair A

Cancer Res 1992 Oct 1; 52(19 Suppl):5485S–5488S

This article reviews results from published studies, showing a significant association between pesticide exposure and non-Hodgkin's lymphoma. In particular, a two- to eightfold increased risk of non-Hodgkin's lymphoma was associated with exposure to 2,4–dichlorophenoxyacetic acid. An increased risk also was shown to be associated with the use of triazine herbicides, organophosphate insecticides, fungicides, and fumigants. It is suggested that pesticide use could have contributed to the 50 percent increase in non-Hodgkin's lymphoma incidence observed in the past fifteen years.

"Mortality Due to Cancers of the Brain and Lymphatic Tissues and Leukemia as a Function of Agriculture Pesticide Use in Quebec (1976–1985)"

Godon D; LaJoie P; Thouez JP

Can J Public Health 1991 May-Jun; 82(3):174–80

This study details a significantly increased mortality from cancers of the brain, the lymphatic tissues, and leukemias in areas exposed to high levels of pesticides. In particular, living in areas of high exposure was associated with a 90 percent increased risk of cancers of the lymphatic tissues.

"Pesticides and Childhood Cancer"

Zahm SH; Ward MH

Environ Health Perspect 1998 Jun; 106 Suppl 3:893–908

This article reviews the results from published studies that link pesticide exposure to increased risk of childhood cancers, in particular leukemia, neuroblastoma, Wilms' tumor, soft-tissue sarcoma, Ewing's sarcoma, non-Hodgkin's lymphoma, and cancers of the brain, colorectum, and testes. The reported risks were of greater magnitude compared to those found in adults, suggesting a greater susceptibility of children to these carcinogens.

"Correlation Analysis of Pesticide Use Data and Cancer Incidence Rates in California Counties"

Mills PK

Arch Environ Health 1998 Nov-Dec; 53(6):410–13

This study evaluates the relationship between pesticide exposure and cancer incidence using data from the California Cancer Registry and the California Department of Pesticide Regulation. A significant association was found between exposure to atrazine and increased incidence of leukemia, brain cancer, and testicular cancer in Hispanic males. In this population there was also a significant association between exposure to captan and 2,4-dichlorophenoxyacetic acid and increased risk of leukemia. Exposure to atrazine and captan also was significantly associated with increased risk of prostate cancer in black males. These segments of the population are often employed as farm workers and are potentially exposed to high doses of pesticides. It is noteworthy that these results were extrapolated without allowing any latency time between presumed pesticide exposure and cancer diagnosis.

"Household Pesticides and Risk of Pediatric Brain Tumors"

Pogoda JM; Preston-Martin S

Environ Health Perspect 1997 Nov; 105(11):1214–20

This study found an over ten times increased risk of childhood brain tumors associated with mother's use of sprays or foggers used for flea/tick control. Harvesting food right after pesticide treatment and using pesticides without following the manufacturer's recommendations was associated with a 3.6-fold increased risk of childhood cancer.

"A Case-Control Study of Non-Hodgkin Lymphoma and Exposure to Pesticides"

Hardell L; Eriksson M

Cancer 1999 Mar 15; 85(6):1353–60

This study, conducted on a cohort of 404 patients with non-Hodgkin's lymphoma and 741 controls, found a 60 percent increased risk of disease associated with herbicides exposure and a 3.7-fold higher risk associated with fungicide exposure.

"Pesticides and Other Agricultural Risk Factors for Non-Hodgkin's Lymphoma among Men in Iowa and Minnesota"

Cantor KP; Blair A; Everett G; Gibson R; Burmeister LF; Brown LM; Schuman L; Dick FR

Cancer Res 1992 May 1; 52(9):2447–55

This study, performed on a cohort of 622 individuals with non-Hodgkin's lymphoma and 1,245 controls, found an over 50 percent increased risk of disease in individuals handling several pesticide groups.

"Childhood Leukaemia and Exposure to Pesticides: Results of a Case-Control Study in Northern Germany"

Meinert R; Kaatsch P; Kaletsch U; Krummenauer F; Miesner A; Michaelis J

Eur J Cancer 1996 Oct; 32A(11):1943–48

This study shows that pesticides use in household gardens is associated with a 2.5-fold increased risk of childhood leukemia.

"Cancer in Offspring of Parents Engaged in Agricultural Activities in Norway: Incidence and Risk Factors in the Farm Environment"

Kristensen P; Andersen A; Irgens LM; Bye AS; Sundheim L
Int J Cancer 1996 Jan 3; 65(1):39–50

This study finds a threefold increased risk of brain tumors in the offspring of pig farm workers and an increased risk of osteosarcoma and Hodgkin's lymphoma in the offspring of chicken farmers. Horticulture and pesticide use was associated with higher risk Wilms' tumor, non-Hodgkin's lymphoma, retinoblastoma, and neuroblastoma.

"Mortality among Male Licensed Pesticide Users and Their Wives"

Sperati A; Rapiti E; Settimi L; Quercia A; Terenzoni B; Forastiere F
Am J Ind Med 1999 Jul; 36(1):142–46

This study, conducted on a cohort of 2,978 male farmers and 2,586 of their wives, finds a 2.3 times higher risk of non-Hodgkin's lymphoma in women and a 1.4- and 2.4-fold increased risk of leukemia in men and women, respectively, compared to the general population.

"Occupational, Environmental, and Life-style Factors Associated with the Risk of Hematolymphopoietic Malignancies in Women"

Miligi L; Seniori Costanini A; Crosignani P; Fontana A; Masala G; Nanni O; Ramazzotti V; Rodella S; Stagnaro E; Tumino R; Vigano C; Vindigni C; Vineis P
Am J Ind Med 1999 Jul; 36(1):60–69

This study, conducted on a cohort of 1183 women with hematolymphopoietic disorders and 828 controls, finds an increased risk of Hodgkin's and non-Hodgkin's lymphoma, leukemia, and multiple myeloma in women working as hairdressers and textile workers.

"Environmental Risk Factors and Parkinson's Disease: A Case-Control Study in Taiwan"

Liou HH; Tsai MC; Chen CJ; Jeng JS; Chang YC; Chen SY; Chen RC
Neurology 1997 Jun; 48(6):1583–88

This study, performed on a cohort of 120 patients with Parkinson's disease and 240 controls, shows that previous use of herbicides/pesticides and paraquat is associated to a significant increased risk of disease.

"Parkinson's Disease and Exposure to Agricultural Work and Pesticide Chemicals"

Semchuk KM; Love EJ; Lee RG
Neurology 1992 Jul; 42(7):1328–35

This study, performed on a cohort of 130 patients with Parkinson's disease and 260 controls, found a significant increased risk of Parkinson's associated with previous exposure to herbicides. The risk increased with increasing levels of exposure.

"Incidence of Cancers of the Brain, the Lymphatic Tissues, and of Leukemia and the Use of Pesticides among Quebec's Rural Farm Population, 1982–1983"

Godon D; Thouez JP; Lajoie P; Nadeau D
Geogr Med 1989; 19:213–32

This study found a 2.2-fold increased risk of leukemia in men living in a rural area with high pesticide exposure, compared to the urban general male population. In addition, a 2-fold increased risk was observed among rural men drinking water from wells compared to those who drank water from the river.

"Acute Pesticide Morbidity and Mortality: California"

Mehler LN; O'Malley MA; Krieger RI
Rev Environ Contam Toxicol 1992; 129:51–66

This article presents data from the California Pesticide Illness Surveillance Program showing that the number of reported illnesses possibly, probably, or definitely related to pesticides exposure has ranged from 970 in 1989 to 1,372 in 1988. Exposure to antimicrobials accounted for an additional 746 to 813 cases annually. Cases of nonoccupational death included suicide, accidental ingestion, and entry into fumigated structures. Occupational deaths were described as rarer and differed in nature.

"Brain Cancer Mortality among French Farmers: The Vineyard Pesticide Hypothesis"

Viel JF; Challier B; Pitard A; Pobel D
Arch Environ Health 1998 Jan-Feb; 53(1):65–70

This study finds a 25 percent increased risk of death from brain cancer in workers exposed to vineyard pesticides compared to the overall population.

"Family Pesticide Use and Childhood Brain Cancer"

Davis JR; Brownson RC; Garcia R; Bentz BJ; Turner A
Arch Environ Contam Toxicol 1993 Jan; 24(1):87–92

This study finds a significant association between the use of pesticides for household pest control and of herbicides for garden weed control and increased risk of brain cancer in children.

"Mutagenic and Carcinogenic Effects of Pesticides"

Saleh MA
J Environ Sci Health [B] 1980; 15(6):907–27

This study discusses some of the effects of commonly used pesticides. Halogenated hydrocarbons have been shown to have carcinogenic properties and to cause sterility. Mutagenic and carcinogenic activity has been reported for several organophosphorus insecticides and for tetrachlorodibenzodioxin (TCDD) and maleic hydrazide present in herbicides.

"Summary of Illnesses and Injuries Reported in California by Physicians in 1986 as Potentially Related to Pesticides"

Edmiston S; Maddy KT

Vet Hum Toxicol 1987 Oct; 29(5):391–97

This study reports data from the California Department of Food and Agriculture, documenting, in the year 1986, 2,099 reports of pesticide-related illnesses, 51 percent of which were confirmed as occupational and 7 percent of which were nonoccupational.

"High Incidence of Lung Cancer in Persons with Chronic Professional Exposure to Pesticides in Agriculture"

Barthel E

Z Erkr Atmungsorgane 1976 Sep; 146(3):266–74

This study finds a twenty-fold increased incidence of lung cancer in a cohort of 316 workers with history of long-term use of pesticides, compared to the general population.

"Pesticide Use in the U.S. and Policy Implications: A Focus on Herbicides"

Short P, Colborn T

Toxicol Ind Health 1999 Jan-Mar; 15(1–2):240–75

This article reports that, in 1995, a total of 556 million pounds of herbicide active ingredients were applied in the United States. Sixty percent of the herbicides have been shown to negatively affect the endocrine and reproductive systems in animals, and at least seventeen types of inert ingredients, which account for 90 percent or more of the pesticide product, have been shown to potentially disrupt the endocrine system.

"A Case-Control Study of Self-Reported Exposures to Pesticides and Pancreas Cancer in Southeastern Michigan"

Fryzek JP; Garabrant DH; Harlow SD; Severson RK; Gillespie BW; Schenk M; Schottenfeld D

Int J Cancer 1997 Jul 3; 72(1):62–67

This study, performed on a cohort of 66 prostate cancer patients and 131 controls, shows a significant increased risk of prostate cancer associated with ethylan exposure.

"Exposures of Children to Organophosphate Pesticides and Their Potential Adverse Health Effects"

Eskenazi B; Bradman A; Castorina R

Environ Health Perspect 1999 Jun; 107(Suppl 3):409–19

This article discusses the higher risk of children exposed to environmental contaminants and reports data showing that pesticide exposure may adversely affect the neurobiochemistry of developing animals, resulting in impaired performance, movement, and balance. It also discusses experimental evidence for a role of pesticides in the etiology of respiratory disorders in children.

"Worldwide Trends in DDT Levels in Human Breast Milk"

Smith, D

Int J Epidemiol 1999 Apr; 28(2):179–88

This study shows that reported DDT levels in human breast milk vary around the world but are still higher, in some areas, than the World Health Organization's recommended limit set for infants.

"Mortality in a Cohort of Licensed Pesticide Applicators in Florida"

Fleming LE; Bean JA; Rudolph M; Hamilton K

Occup Environ Med 1999 Jan; 56(1):14–21

This study finds a 2.4-fold increase in prostate cancer mortality in a cohort of 33,658 licensed pesticide applicators, compared to the general population.

"Cancer Incidence in a Cohort of Licensed Pesticide Applicators in Florida"

Fleming LE; Bean JA; Rudolph M; Hamilton K

J Occup Environ Med 1999 Apr; 41(4):279–88

This study finds a 90 percent increased incidence of prostate cancer and a 2.5-fold increased incidence of testicular cancer in a cohort of licensed pesticide applicators in Florida, compared to the general population. Among women, a 3.7-fold increased incidence of cervical cancer was observed.

"Organochlorine Exposure and Risk of Breast Cancer"

Hoyer AP; Grandjean P; Jorgensen T; Brock JW; Hartvig HB

Lancet 1998 Dec 5; 352(9143):1816–20

This study, performed on a sample population of 240 women with breast cancer and 477 controls, finds a twofold increased dose-dependent risk of breast cancer associated with serum levels of dieldrin, an organochlorine compound, suggesting a role for xeno-oestrogens in the pathogenesis of breast cancer.

"Organochlorine Exposure and Breast Cancer Risk in Colombian Women"

Olaya-Contreras P; Rodriguez-Villamil J; Posso-Valencia HJ; Cortez JE

Cad Saude Publica 1998; 14 Suppl 3:125–32

This study finds a 95 percent increased risk of breast cancer in women in the highest versus the lowest tertile of serum dichlorodiphenyl-dichloroethene (DDE) concentration.

"Organochlorine Compounds (DDE and PCB) in Plasma and Breast Cyst Fluid of Women with Benign Breast Disease"

Blackwood A; Wolff M; Rundle A; Estabrook A; Schnabel F; Mooney LA; Rivera M; Channing KM; Perera FP

Cancer Epidemiol Biomarkers Prev 1998 Jul; 7(7):579–83

This study demonstrates the presence, in a cohort of twenty-four women with multiple breast cysts, or organochlorines compounds in the cyst fluid. DDE and PCB were detected in the cystic fluid of twenty-two and nineteen women, respectively. Concentration of DDE in the cyst fluid was significantly correlated to that in the plasma.

"Relative Abundance of Organochlorine Pesticides and Polychlorinated Biphenyls in Adipose Tissue and Serum of Women in Long Island, New York."

Stellman SD; Djordjevic MV; Muscat JE; Gong L; Bernstein D; Citron ML; White A; Kemeny M; Busch E; Nafziger AN

Cancer Epidemiol Biomarkers Prev 1998 Jun; 7(6):489–96

This study, conducted on a sample population of 293 women living in an area of high incidence of breast cancer, evaluates the serum and adipose concentration of some organochlorine pesticides (OCPs) and PCBs that have been linked to an increased risk of breast cancer. Adipose and serum levels of these compounds were detected in 100 percent of the samples.

"Chlororganic Pesticides and Polychlorinated Biphenyls in Breast Tissue of Women with Benign and Malignant Breast Disease"

Guttes S; Failing K; Neumann K; Kleinstein J; Georgii S; Brunn H

Arch Environ Contam Toxicol 1998 Jul; 35(1):140–47

This study finds a higher concentration of chlororganic hydrocarbons in the breast tissue samples of forty-five women diagnosed with breast cancer, compared to women with benign breast disease. Experimental evidence has demonstrated a carcinogenic, immunotoxic, and estrogenic activity associated with these compounds.

"Environmental Organochlorine Exposure and Postmenopausal Breast Cancer Risk"

Moysich KB; Ambrosone CB; Vena JE; Shields PG; Mendola P; Kostyniak P; Greizerstein H; Graham S; Marshall JR; Schisterman EF; Freudenheim JL

Cancer Epidemiol Biomarkers Prev 1998 Mar; 7(3):181–88

This study shows a higher risk of breast cancer in postmenopausal women exposed to organochlorine compounds.

"Triazine Herbicide Exposure and Breast Cancer Incidence: An Ecologic Study of Kentucky Counties"

Kettles MK; Browning SR; Prince TS; Horstman SW

Environ Health Perspect 1997 Nov; 105(11):1222–27

This study shows a significantly increased risk of breast cancer in women in the medium and higher tertile of triazine exposure, compared to women in the lower tertile.

"Increased Concentrations Octachlorodibenzo-p-Dioxin in Cases with Breast Cancer—Results from a Case-Control Study"

Hardell L; Lindstrom G; Liljegren G; Dahl P; Magnuson A

Eur J Cancer Prev 1996 Oct; 5(5):351–57

This study finds a higher concentration of the organochlorine octachlorinated dibenzo-p-dioxin in the breast tissue samples of twenty-two cancer patients, compared to the levels detected in the tissues of women with benign breast disease.

"Respiratory Symptoms, Skin Disorders and Serum IgE Levels in Farm Workers"

Bener A; Lestringant GG; Beshwari MM; Pasha MA

Allerg Immunol (Paris) 1999 Feb; 31(2):52–56

This study reports a very high prevalence of dermatological and respiratory symptoms in workers exposed to high concentrations of pesticides, compared to controls. Cough, dyspnea, bronchitis, sinusitis, asthma, pneumonia, and respiratory insufficiency were some of the most frequently reported respiratory symptoms; pruritus and contact dermatitis were the most frequently reported skin disorders.

"Prevalence of Wheeze and Asthma and Relation to Atopy in Urban and Rural Ethiopia"

Yemaneberhan H; Bekele Z; Venn A; Lewis S; Parry E; Britton J

Lancet 1997 Jul 12; 350(9071):85–90

This study estimates that the prevalence of asthma in Ethiopia is 0.31 percent in rural areas and 3.6 percent in urban areas. In the urban population, the presence of atopy is a strong risk factor for asthma. These two conditions are positively associated with housing style, bedding materials, and use of malathion insecticide.

"Fatality Associated with Inhalation of a Pyrethrin Shampoo"

Wax PM; Hoffman RS

J Toxicol Clin Toxicol 1994; 32(4):457–60

This article reports a case of death due to sudden, irreversible bronchospasm, associated with inhalational exposure to a pyrethrin insecticide.

"Asthmatic Reactions to a Commonly Used Aerosol Insect Killer"

Newton JG; Breslin AB

Med J Aust 1983 Apr 16; 1(8):378–80

This article assesses the reaction to a widely used household insecticide in seven patients with asthma and a history of insecticide sensitivity. Chest tightness occurred in all seven subjects, and objective signs of airway obstruction occurred in three.

"Worldwide Variation in Prevalence of Symptoms of Asthma, Allergic Rhinoconjunctivitis, and Atopic Eczema: ISAAC. The International Study of Asthma and Allergies in Childhood (ISAAC) Steering Committee.

Lancet 1998 Apr 25; 351(9111):1225–32

This study, conducted on a cohort of 463,801 children ages thirteen to fourteen years in 155 centers throughout the world, found a twenty- to sixty-fold difference in prevalence of asthma, allergic rhinoconjunctivitis, and atopic eczema between different centers. The highest prevalence of asthma was reported in the United Kingdom, Australia, New Zealand, and Republic of Ireland.

"Morbidity among Farm Workers in a Desert Country in Relation to Long-Term Exposure to Pesticides"

Gomes J; Lloyd O; Revitt MD; Basha M

Scand J Work Environ Health 1998 Jun; 24(3):213–19

This study finds that, among a group of 226 farm workers with history of long-term exposure to low levels of pesticides, the prevalence of blurred vision, dizziness, headache, muscular pain, and weakness was 63, 55, 64, 61, and 77 percent, respectively. These numbers are much higher than those reported among new farm workers or referents. In addition, objective measures of depleted erythrocyte acetylcholinesterase activity indicated a higher risk of pesticide toxicity in this population.

"Prevalence of Dermatoses and Skin Sensitisation Associated with Use of Pesticides in Fruit Farmers of Southern Taiwan"

Guo YL; Wang BJ; Lee CC; Wang JD

Occup Environ Med 1996 Jun; 53(6):427–31

This study, conducted on a cohort of 122 fruit farmers in Taiwan, finds that 25, 30, and 70 percent of this population presented with skin fungal infections, dermatitis, and pigmentation and thickening of the hands, respectively.

"Delayed Health Effects of Pesticides: Review of Current Epidemiological Knowledge"

Baldi I; Mohammed-Brahim B; Brochard P; Dartigues JF; Salamon R

Rev Epidemiol Sante Publique 1998 Mar; 46(2):134–42

This article reviews the epidemiological studies analyzing the possible long-term effects of pesticide exposure. These effects include cancer, neurological toxicity, and disturbances of the reproductive and endocrine systems.

"Paternal Exposure to Pesticides and Congenital Malformations"

Garcia AM; Benavides FG; Fletcher T; Orts E

Scand J Work Environ Health 1998 Dec; 24(6):473–80

This study shows that paternal occupational exposure to pyridil derivatives is associated with a 2.7-fold increased risk of congenital malformation in the offspring. Exposure to inorganic compounds, aliphatic hydrocarbons, and glufosinate also was shown to be associated with an increased risk of congenital malformation.

"Maternal Pesticide Exposure from Multiple Sources and Selected Congenital Anomalies"

Shaw GM; Wasserman CR; O'Malley CD; Nelson V; Jackson RJ

Epidemiology 1999 Jan; 10(1):60–66

This study finds a 60 percent increased risk of orofacial cleft in the offspring of men who have been occupationally exposed to pesticides. Pesticide use for gardening was associated with a 50 percent increased risk of congenital malformation, including neural tube defects, limb anomalies, and conotruncal defects. Living within 0.25 miles of an agricultural crop or having the household professionally sprayed with pesticides was associated with a 50 and 60 percent increased risk of neural tube defects, respectively.

"Parental Agricultural Work and Selected Congenital Malformations"
Garcia AM; Fletcher T; Benavides FG; Orts E
Am J Epidemiol 1999 Jan 1; 149(1):64–74

This study, conducted on a cohort of 261 infants with congenital malformations and 261 controls, shows that mother's involvement in agricultural work during the month prior to conception or in the first trimester of pregnancy was associated with a threefold increased risk of congenital malformations in the offspring.

"Cryptorchidism and Hypospadias in Sons of Gardeners and Farmers"
Weidner IS; Moller H; Jensen TK; Shakkebaek NE
Environ Health Perspect 1998 Dec; 106(12):793–96

This study, conducted on a cohort of 7,522 cases of cryptorchidism and hypospadias and 23,273 controls, found a 70 percent increased risk of cryptorchidism in the offspring of women involved in gardening activity.

"Organochlorine Pesticides and PCBs in Human Milk Collected from Mothers Nursing Hospitalized Children"
Krauthacker B; Reiner E; Votava-Raic A; Tjesic-Drinkovic D; Batinic D
Chemosphere 1998 Jul; 37(1):27–32

This study finds increased levels of organochlorine pesticides in the milk of mothers nursing neonates with neurological deficits or with inappropriate arousal responses, compared to mothers of children who were hospitalized for different conditions and who served as controls.

"Maternal Residential Proximity to Hazardous Waste Sites and Risk for Selected Congenital Malformations"
Croen LA; Shaw GM; Sanbonmatsu L; Selvin S; Buffler PA
Epidemiology 1997 Jul; 8(4):347–54

This study finds that the offspring of women who were living within a mile of a National Priority List hazardous waste site had a twofold increased risk of neural tube defects and heart defects. Living within 0.25 miles from the site was associated with an over fourfold increased risk of congenital heart defects.

"Exposure to Pesticides and Cryptorchidism: Geographical Evidence of a Possible Association"

Garcia-Rodriguez J; Garcia-Martin M; Nogueras-Ocana M; de Dios Luna-del-Castillo J; Espigares Garcia M; Olea N; Lardelli-Claret P

Environ Health Perspect 1996 Oct; 104(10):1090–95

This study finds higher rates of cryptorchidism in districts located close to intense farming areas. The higher the use of pesticides, the stronger the association with cryptorchidism.

"Reproductive Effects of Paternal Exposure to Chlorophenate Wood Preservatives in the Sawmill Industry"

Dimich-Ward H; Hertzman C; Teschke K; Hershler R; Marion SA; Ostry A; Kelly S

Scand J Work Environ Health 1996 Aug; 22(4):267–73

This study finds higher rates of congenital cataracts, anencephaly, spina bifida, and anomalies of the reproductive system in the offspring of men exposed to chlorophenate wood preservatives.

"Agricultural Work during Pregnancy and Selected Structural Malformations in Finland"

Nurminen T; Rantala K; Kurppa K; Holmberg PC

Epidemiology 1995 Jan; 6(1):23–30

This study finds a 40 percent increased risk of congenital malformations and an 80 percent increased risk of orofacial cleft in the offspring of mothers performing agricultural work during the first trimester of pregnancy.

"Environmental Trichlorfon and Cluster of Congenital Abnormalities"

Czeizel AE; Elek C; Gundy S; Metneki J; Nemes E; Reis A; Sperling K; Timar L; Tusnady G; Viragh Z

Lancet 1993 Feb 27; 341(8844):539–42

This study presents a cluster of congenital malformations that occurred in one Hungarian village. Of fifteen live births, eleven were affected by birth defects. The presumed teratogenic compound was identified in a chemical, trichlorfon, used in high concentrations in a local fish farm. All the mothers of Down syndrome babies and several pregnant women reported having eaten contaminated fish.

"Assessment of the U.S. Environmental Protection Agency Methods for Identification of Hazards to Developing Organisms, Part II: The Developmental Toxicity Testing Guideline"

Claudio L; Bearer CF; Wallinga D

Am J Ind Med 1998 Jun; 35(6):554–63

This study reviews the protocols used by the U.S. Environmental Protection Agency as guidelines for environmental toxins use and assesses their adequacy in preventing health hazards to infants and children. The protocols, compiled on the basis of scientific information provided by chemical and pesticide manufacturers were found to contain limitations that could interfere with their ability to protect infants and children from environmental toxins.

"Exposure to Children to Pollutants in House Dust and Indoor Air"

Roberts JW; Dickey P

Rev Environ Contam Toxicol 1995; 143:59–78

In this study, dust collected from carpets of seventeen houses and ten used sofas was shown to possess mutagenic activity and to contain high concentrations of potentially carcinogenic PAHs, lead, PCBs, and mite and cat allergens. Control of home exposure to these compounds could be an effective way to present and contain the epidemic of allergic diseases occurring in the United States.

ON ASPARTAME

"Increasing Brain Tumor Rates: Is There a Link to Aspartame?"

Olney JW; Farber NB, Spitznagel E; Robins LN

J Neuropathol Exp Neurol 1996 Nov; 55(11):1115–23

This study presents the evidence suggesting a potential role of aspartame in the rising incidence of brain tumors in the United States: One study reported a very high incidence of brain tumors in rats fed an aspartame-rich diet, while no tumors were found in control rats; the aspartame molecule was shown in vitro to have mutagenic properties, and there was a temporal association between the introduction of aspartame in the U.S. market and the later increase in brain tumor incidence.

THE DANGERS OF SUGAR

"Effects of Sweetness and Energy in Drinks on Food Intake Following Exercise"

King NA; Appleton K; Rogers PJ; Blundell JE

Physiol Behav 1999 Apr; 66(2):375–79

In this study, participants were given, after performing a challenging exercise, three different drinks: water, a low-energy drink artificially sweetened, or a high-energy drink sweetened with sucrose. In the test meal that followed, those who drank the artificially sweetened low-energy drink had significantly higher energy intake compared to those who drank water or the sucrose drink, and those who drank water had the lowest energy intake.

"Food Groups and Risk of Colorectal Cancer in Italy"

Franceschi S; Favero A; La Vecchia C; Negri E; Conti E; Montella M; Giacosa A; Nanni O; Decarli A

J Cancer 1997 Jul 3; 72(1):56–61

This study, performed on a sample population of 1,953 colorectal cancer cases and 4,154 controls, found that those in the highest versus the lowest quintile of refined sugar intake had a 40 percent increased risk of colorectal cancer. High intake of bread and cereal dishes was associated with a 70 percent increased risk, while consumption of fish, fruits and vegetables conferred a 30 to 40 percent decreased risk.

"Dietary Sugar and Colon Cancer"

Slattery ML; Benson J; Berry TD; Duncan D; Edwards SL; Caan BJ; Potter JD
Cancer Epidemiol Biomarkers Prev 1997 Sep; 6(9):677–85

This study, performed on a cohort of 1,993 colon cancer cases, and 2,410 controls, shows that those with the highest versus the lowest quintile of sucrose intake had a sixty percent increased risk of colon cancer. A sedentary lifestyle also increased the risk: Men and women who had a combination of high sugar intake and lack of exercise had a 3.5- and 2-fold increased risk of colon cancer, respectively, compared to individuals with an active lifestyle and low sugar intake. In individuals with sedentary lifestyle, high sucrose intake, low fiber intake, and large body mass index, the risk increased by 4.6 times.

"Dietary Sugar and Lung Cancer: A Case-Control Study in Uruguay"

De Stefani E; Deneo-Pellegrini H; Mendilaharsu M; Ronco A; Carzoglio JC
Nutr Cancer 1998; 31(2):132–37

This study, performed on a cohort of 463 lung cancer cases and 465 controls, shows a 55 percent increased risk of lung cancer in people in the highest versus the lowest category of sucrose intake. Lung cancer risk was twenty-eight times higher in individuals with a combination of high cigarettes, high total fat, and high sucrose intake.

"Smoking, Alcohol Use, Dietary Factors and Risk of Small Intestinal Adenocarcinoma"

Wu AH; Yu MC; Mack TM
Int J Cancer 1997 Mar 4; 70(5):512–17

This study, performed on a cohort of 36 patients with adenocarcinoma of the small intestine and 998 controls, finds that persons in the medium and high tertile of sucrose intake had a 2.5- and 3.8-fold increased risk of cancer of the small intestine compared to those in the lowest tertile of sucrose intake. Heavy drinking, compared to moderate or low drinking, was associated with a 3-fold increased risk.

"Diet and Risk of Breast Cancer: Major Findings from an Italian Case-Control Study"

Favero A; Parpinel M; Franceschi S
Biomed Pharmacother 1998; 52(3):109–15

This article reports the results of a large case-control study performed on a cohort of 2,569 women with breast cancer and 2,588 controls, where intake of sugar, bread, cereals, and pork meat was associated with increased risk of breast cancer.

"Adverse Effects on Risk of Ischaemic Heart Disease of Adding Sugar to Hot Beverages in Hypertensives Using Diuretics. A Six-Year Follow-up in the Copenhagen Male Study"

Suadicani P; Hein HO; Gyntelberg F

Blood Press 1996 Mar; 5(2):91–97

Results of this study show that, among hypertensive patients on diuretic therapy, those with a high sugar intake have a threefold increased risk of ischemic heart disease compared to those with a low sugar intake.

"Diet, Physical Activity, and Gallstones—A Population-Based, Case-Control Study in Southern Italy"

Misciagna G; Centonze S; Leoci C; Guerra V; Cisternino AM; Ceo R; Trevisan M

Am J Clin Nutr 1999 Jan; 69(1):120–26

This study finds a significant association between body mass index, consumption of refined sugar and animal fats, and increased risk of gallstones.

"Relationship between Changes in Dietary Sucrose and High Density Lipoprotein Cholesterol: The CARDIA study. Coronary Artery Risk Development in Young Adults"

Archer SL; Liu K; Dyer AR; Ruth KJ; Jacobs DR Jr; Van Horn L; Hilner JE; Savage PJ

Ann Epidemiol 1998 Oct; 8(7):433–38

This study finds a consistent inverse association between sucrose intake and serum levels of high density lipoprotein cholesterol (HDL-C).

"Milk and Other Dietary Influences on Coronary Heart Disease"

Grant WB

Altern Med Rev 1998 Aug; 3(4):281–94

This study uses a multicountry statistical approach to assess the relationship between intake of certain categories of foods and risk of mortality from ischemic heart disease. It found that milk in men of thirty-five or more years of age and sugar in women sixty-five years or older were the most strongly correlated to ischemic heart disease mortality.

DIET AND ARTHRITIS

"Controlled Trial of Fasting and One-Year Vegetarian Diet in Rheumatoid Arthritis"

Kjeldsen-Dragh J; Haugen M; Borchgrevink CF; Laerum E; Eek M; Mowinkel P; Hovi K; Førre O

Lancet 1991 Oct 12; 338(8772):899–902

This randomized, controlled study assesses the effect of fasting followed by one year of a vegetarian diet in rheumatoid arthritis patients. This regimen produced a significant improvement in the number of tender joints, number of swollen joints, pain score, duration of morning stiffness, grip strength, erythrocyte sedimentation rate, C-reactive protein, white blood cell count, and a health assessment questionnaire score. In the control group, only pain score improved significantly. The benefits in the diet group were still present after one year.

"Diet and Disease Symptoms in Rheumatic Diseases—Results of a Questionnaire-Based Survey"

Haugen M; Kjeldsen-Kragh J; Nordv ag BY; Førre O
Clin Rheumatol 1991 Dec; 10(4):401–7

In this study, one-third of patients with rheumatoid arthritis, ankylosing spondylitis, and psoriatic anthropathy reported worsening of symptoms after intake of certain foods, while 43 percent of patients with juvenile rheumatoid arthritis and 42 percent of patients with primary fibromyalgia stated the same. Less pain and stiffness were reported by 46 percent of the patients who tried certain diets in the attempt to alleviate disease symptoms, and 36 percent reported reduced joint swelling.

"Uncooked, Lactobacilli-Rich, Vegan Food and Rheumatoid Arthritis"

Nenonen MT; Helve TA; Rauma AL; Hänninen OO
Br J Rheumatol 1998 Mar; 37(3):274–81

This study shows that consumption of an uncooked vegan diet, rich in lactobacilli and chlorophyll, decreases the subjective symptoms of rheumatoid arthritis, while returning to an omnivorous diet produces worsening of the symptoms.

"Is Diet Important to Rheumatoid Arthritis?"

Buchanan HM; Preston SJ; Brooks PM; Buchanan WW
Br J Rheumatol 1991 Apr; 30(2):125–34

This article shows that milk, milk products, corn, and cereals are implicated in food allergy and cause aggravation of symptoms in rheumatoid arthritis patients. It also suggests that patients with rheumatoid arthritis might have a "leaky" intestinal mucosa that allows food allergens to be absorbed more easily.

"Faecal Microbial Flora and Disease Activity in Rheumatoid Arthritis during a Vegan Diet"

Peltonen R; Nenonen M; Helve T; Hänninen O; Toivanen P; Eerola E
Br J Rheumatol 1997 Jan; 36(1):64–68

In this study forty-three rheumatoid arthritis patients were randomized into two groups: A test group received living food, a form of uncooked vegan diet rich in lactobacilli, and the control group continued their ordinary omnivorous diets. Patients on a vegan diet showed changes in the fecal microbial flora that were associated with improvement in rheumatoid arthritis activity.

"Food Intolerance in Rheumatoid Arthritis: A Double-Blind, Controlled Trial of the Clinical Effects of Elimination of Milk Allergens and Azo Dyes"

van de Laar MA; van der Korst JK
Ann Rheum Dis 1992 Mar; 51(3):298–302

In this study ninety-four patients were randomly assigned to a twelve-week allergen-free or allergen-restricted (containing only lactoproteins and yellow dyes) diet. Nine patients (three in the allergen-restricted group, six in the allergen-free group) showed favorable responses, followed by marked disease exacerbation during rechallenge.

"Nutritional Status of Danish Patients with Rheumatoid Arthritis and Effects of a Diet Adjusted in Energy Intake, Fish Content and Antioxidants"

Hansen G; Nielsen L; Kluger E; Thysen MH; Emmertsen H; Stengård-Pedersen K;
Lund EC; Unger B
Ugeskr Laeger 1998 My 18; 160(21):3074–78

This prospective, single-blinded study shows that rheumatoid arthritis patients who increased the consumption of fish and antioxidants for six months demonstrated a significant improvement in the duration of morning stiffness, the number of swollen joints, pain status, and reduced the cost of medicine.

"Diet and Rheumatoid Arthritis in Women: A Possible Protective Effect of Fish Consumption"

Shapiro JA; Koepsell TD; Voigt LF; Dugowson CE; Kestin M; Nelson JL
Epidemiology 1996 May; 7(3):256–63

This study shows that women consuming two or more servings of broiled or baked fish per week have a 43 percent decreased risk of rheumatoid arthritis compared to women who have a fish intake of less than once per week. The association with fish was even stronger when the analysis was restricted to cases positive for rheumatoid factor.

"A Fish Oil Diet Reduces the Severity of Collagen-Induced Arthritis after Onset of the Disease"

Leslie CA; Conte JM; Hayes KC; Cathcart ES
Clin Exp Immunol 1988 Aug; 73(2):328–32

This study shows that mice with collagen-induced arthritis had much less severe arthritis when a fish oil diet was fed instead of a corn oil diet.

"The Effects of Dietary Supplementation with n-3 Polyunsaturated Fatty Acids in Patients with Rheumatoid Arthritis: A Randomized, Double-Blind Trial"

Nielsen GL; Faarvang KL; Thomsen BS; Teglbjaerg KL; Jensen LT; Hansen TM; Lervang HH;
Schmidt EB; Dyerberg J; Ernst E
Eur J Clin Invest 1992 Oct; 22(10):387–91

This randomized, placebo-controlled, double-blind study shows that twelve weeks of dietary supplementation with n-3 polyunsaturated fatty acids in patients with rheumatoid arthritis produces significant improvement of morning stiffness and joint tenderness with no side effects.

"Suppression of Monosodium Urate Crystal-Induced Acute Inflammation by Diets Enriched with Gamma-Linolenic acid and Eicosapentaenoic Acid"

Tate GA; Mandell BF; Karmali RA; Laposata M; Baker DG; Schumacher HR Jr; Zurier RB
Arthritis Rheum 1988 Dec; 31(12):1543–51

This study shows that a combined diet of fish oil and plant seed oil (EPA-enriched and GLA-enriched) reduces both the cellular and fluid phases of acute inflammation induced in rats by monosodium urate crystals.

"Fish-Oil Fatty Acid Supplementation in Active Rheumatoid Arthritis. A Double-Blinded, Controlled, Crossover Study"

Kremer JM; Jubiz W; Michalek A; Rynes RI; Bartholomew LE; Bigaouette J; Timchalk M; Beeler D; Lininger L
Ann Intern Med 1987 Apr; 106(4):497–503

This nonrandomized, double-blinded, placebo-controlled, crossover trial shows that fish oil ingestion results in subjective alleviation of active rheumatoid arthritis and reduction of neutrophil leukotriene B4 production.

"Changes in Laboratory Variables in Rheumatoid Arthritis Patients during a Trial of Fasting and One-Year Vegetarian Diet"

Kjeldsen-Kragh J; Mellbye OJ; Haugen M; Mollnes TE; Hammer HB; Sioud M; Forre O
Scandinavian Journal of Rheumatology 1995; 24(2):85–93

This study shows that arthritis patients who underwent a fast followed by a month of vegetarian diet had a significant reduction in inflammatory activity, as measured by a decrease in platelet and leukocyte count, calprotectin, total IgG, IgM rheumatoid factor, C3-activation products, and the complement components C3 and C4.

"Nutrient Intake and Obesity in a Multidisciplinary Assessment of Osteoarthritis"

White-O'Connor B; Sobal J
Clin Ther 1986; 9 Suppl B:30–42

This study finds that 79 percent of a group of seventy-seven osteoarthritis patients were obese and that pain from this disease was positively related to obesity. Dietary intake of vitamin D, folacin, vitamin B6, zinc, and pantothenic acid in this group of patients was 80 percent below the recommended dietary allowance.

"Inadequate Calcium, Folic Acid, Vitamin E, Zinc, and Selenium Intake in Rheumatoid Arthritis Patients: Results of a Dietary Survey"

Stone J; Doube A; Dudson D; Wallace J
Semin Arthritis Rheum 1997 Dec; 27(3):180–85

This study determines the adequacy of calcium, folic acid, vitamin E, zinc, and selenium intake in patients with rheumatoid arthritis. The percentage of patients who achieved the recommended daily intake was 23 percent for calcium, 46 percent for folic acid, 29 percent for vitamin E, 10 percent for zinc, and only 6 percent for selenium. Patients on methotrexate had a significantly reduced intake of folic acid as a percentage of RDI compared with those on other therapies.

DIET AND BREAST CANCER

"Dietary Carotenoids and Vitamins A, C, and E and Risk of Breast Cancer"

Zhang S; Hunter DJ; Forman MR; Rosner BA; Speizer FE; Colditz GA; Manson JE; Hankinson SE; Willett WC
J Natl Cancer Inst 1999 Mar 17; 91(6):547–56

This study, performed on a cohort of 83,234 women, finds a strong inverse association for increasing intake of alpha-carotene, beta-carotene, lutein/zeaxanthin, vitamin C, and vitamin A and risk of breast cancer. Premenopausal women with a family history of breast cancer and eating five or more servings of fruits and vegetables per day had a 71 percent reduction in breast cancer risk compared to women consuming less than two servings per day. For women without history of familial breast cancer, the risk decreased by 23 percent.

"Beta-Carotene Intake and Risk of Postmenopausal Breast Cancer"

Jumaan AO; Holmberg L; Zack M; Mokdad AH; Ohlander EM; Wolk A; Byers T
Epidemiology 1999 Jan; 10(1):49–53

This study, conducted on a sample of 273 women with breast cancer and 371 controls, shows that increasing doses of reported beta-carotene intake are associated with decreased breast cancer risk.

"Diet and Breast Cancer Risk. Results from a Population-Based, Case-Control Study in Sweden"

Holmberg L; Ohlander EM; Byers T; Zack M; Wolk A; Bergstrom R; Bergkvist L; Thurfjell E; Bruce A; Adami HO
Arch Intern Med 1994 Aug 22; 154(16):1805–11

This study shows that women with the highest versus the lowest quartile of beta-carotene intake had a 40 percent reduction in risk of developing breast cancer. Consumption of the highest versus the lowest quartile of alcohol, on the other hand, was associated with a 60 percent increased risk.

"Dietary Factors and Risk of Breast Cancer: Combined Analysis of 12 Case-Control Studies"

Howe GR; Hirohata T; Hislop TG; Iscovich JM; Yuan JM; Katsouyanni K; Lubin F; Marubini E; Modan B; Rohan T, et al

J Natl Cancer Inst 1990 Apr 4; 82(7):561–69

This study evaluates the results of twelve case-control studies and finds a consistent association between saturated fat intake and risk of breast cancer. Postmenopausal women with the highest versus the lowest intake of saturated fat had a 46 percent increased risk of breast cancer. On the other hand, highest versus lowest vitamin C intake was associated with a 31 percent risk reduction. Implementing these two dietary factors was estimated to prevent 24 percent of breast cancer in postmenopausal women and 16 percent in premenopausal women.

"Dietary effects on Breast-Cancer Risk in Singapore"

Lee HP; Gourley L; Duffy SW; Esteve J; Lee J; Day NE

Lancet 1991 May 18; 337(8751):1197–200

This study shows that red meat intake is a significant predisposing factor for breast cancer, while beta-carotene intake and soya protein are significant protective factors.

"Premenopausal Breast Cancer Risk and Intake of Vegetables, Fruits, and Related Nutrients"

Freudenheim JL; Marshall JR; Vena JE; Laughlin R; Brasure JR; Swanson MK; Nemoto T; Graham S

J Natl Cancer Inst 1996 Mar 20; 88(6):340–48

This case-control study finds that intake of several foods and supplements is associated with reduced risk of breast cancer in a group of premenopausal women of forty or more years of age. Specifically, the reduction in risk of breast cancer in women with the highest versus the lowest quartile of intake was on the order of 47 percent for vitamin C, 45 percent for alpha-tocopheral, 50 percent for folic acid, 33 percent for alpha-carotene, 54 percent for beta-carotene, 53 percent for lutein and zeaxanthin, and 52 percent for fiber from fruits and vegetables.

"Tofu and Risk of Breast Cancer in Asian-Americans"

Wu AH; Ziegler RG; Horn-Ross PL; Nomura AM; West DW; Kolonel LN; Rosenthal JF; Hoover RN; Pike MC

Cancer Epidemiol Biomarkers Prev 1996 Nov; 5(11):901–6

This study shows that, in pre- and postmenopausal Asian American women, the risk of breast cancer decreased by 15 percent for every additional serving of tofu per week.

"Dietary Factors and the Risk of Endometrial Cancer: A Case-Control Study in Greece"

Tzonou A; Lipworth L; Kalandidi A; Trichopoulou A; Gamatsi I; Hsieh CC; Notara V; Trichopoulos D

Br J Cancer 1996 May; 73(10):1284–90

This study shows that intake of monounsaturated fat, mostly from olive oil, and calcium are both significantly associated with a decreased risk of endometrial cancer.

"Dietary Fat, Olive Oil Intake and Breast Cancer Risk"

Martin-Moreno JM; Willett WC; Gorgojo L; Banegas JR; Rodriguez-Artalejo F; Fernandez-Rodriguez JC; Maisonneuve P; Boyle P

Int J Cancer 1994 Sep 15; 58(6):774–80

This study shows that, in a cohort of 762 pre- and postmenopausal women and 988 controls, consumption of the highest versus the lowest quartile of olive oil is associated with a 34 percent reduction in risk of breast cancer.

Index